Oxford Textbook of
Correctional Psychiatry

Oxford Textbook of
Correctional Psychiatry

Edited by

Robert L. Trestman, Ph.D., M.D.
Professor of Medicine, Psychiatry, and Nursing
University of Connecticut Health Center

Kenneth L. Appelbaum, M.D.
Clinical Professor of Psychiatry
University of Massachusetts Medical School

Jeffrey L. Metzner, M.D.
Clinical Professor of Psychiatry
University of Colorado School of Medicine

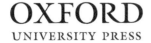

OXFORD
UNIVERSITY PRESS

OXFORD

UNIVERSITY PRESS

Oxford University Press is a department of the University of
Oxford. It furthers the University's objective of excellence in research,
scholarship, and education by publishing worldwide.

Oxford   New York
Auckland   Cape Town   Dar es Salaam   Hong Kong   Karachi
Kuala Lumpur   Madrid   Melbourne   Mexico City   Nairobi
New Delhi   Shanghai   Taipei   Toronto

With offices in
Argentina   Austria   Brazil   Chile   Czech Republic   France   Greece
Guatemala   Hungary   Italy   Japan   Poland   Portugal   Singapore
South Korea   Switzerland   Thailand   Turkey   Ukraine   Vietnam

Oxford is a registered trademark of Oxford University Press
in the UK and certain other countries.

Published in the United States of America by
Oxford University Press
198 Madison Avenue, New York, NY 10016

Library of Congress Cataloging-in-Publication Data
Oxford textbook of correctional psychiatry / edited by Robert L. Trestman,
Kenneth L. Appelbaum, Jeffrey L. Metzner.
     p. ; cm.
Textbook of correctional psychiatry
Includes bibliographical references.
ISBN 978–0–19–936057–4 (alk. paper)
I. Trestman, Robert L., editor.   II. Appelbaum, Kenneth L., editor.   III. Metzner, Jeffrey L.,
editor.   IV. Title: Textbook of correctional psychiatry.
[DNLM: 1. Forensic Psychiatry—methods.   2. Mental Health Services.   3. Prisoners—
psychology.   4. Prisons.   W 740]
RC451.4.P68
365'.6672—dc23
2014022223

9 8 7 6 5 4 3 2 1
Printed in the United States of America
on acid-free paper

We dedicate this book to our wives, Bonnie, Cary, and Linda, and to our children. They have tried to keep our lives grounded and balanced. They have supported us in our professional careers even when our work pulled us away from family time. They have not hesitated to show us that despite our accomplishments there are many things we do not know and about which they continue to teach us. Best of all, they give us their unqualified love while accepting ours in return.

Contents

Foreword

I have worked at the intersection of mental health and criminal justice policy and practice, and in active collegial engagement with forensic psychiatrists, for more than four decades. Over these years, I have watched correctional psychiatry move to the very center of the profession's interests and commitments. It is not difficult to understand why.

"Mass incarceration" has become one of the most disturbing and challenging social problems we face in the United States. The huge scale of this problem has become increasingly salient not only to correctional psychiatrists but to every informed and ethically engaged citizen. Our nation's penal population is the largest in the world and accounts for a quarter of the prisoners in all of the world's prisons, even though we account for only five percent of the world's population (NRC, 2014). This distinct form of "American exceptionalism" does not go back to the Founding or even to Second World War. It is distinctly connected to crime policy during the last third of the Twentieth Century.

The rate of incarceration in this country has more than quadrupled over the past four decades. The daily census of state and federal prisons rose from about 200,000 in 1973 to 1.5 million at its peak in 2009. Another 700,000 inmates are held daily in local jails. This brings the incarcerated population in the United States on any given day to about 2.3 million (Walmsley, 2013). About 700,000 prisoners are released from state and federal prisons each year. Even these startling figures don't reveal the full scope of mass incarceration and its impact on the lives of the incarcerated individuals and their families and communities: Every year, about 12 million individual are booked into (and released from) local jails. About 4.8 million persons are on probation or parole (Maruschack and Parks, 2012). Altogether, more than seven million individuals are under correctional supervision. How did this happen?

Crime policy took a strongly punitive turn at all levels of criminal justice administration beginning in the late 1970s. It has been marked by an increase in arrests, especially for drug crimes, higher rates of incarceration per arrest, and increasing severity of sentences for crimes involving violence as well as drugs. Mandatory prison terms for these crimes increased markedly in the 1980s, and during the 1990s, more than half the states, as well as Congress, enacted "three strikes" laws (or even "two strikes" laws) mandating terms of 25 years or longer for offenders covered by these laws. Most states also abolished, or significantly limited,

opportunity for discretionary release (indeterminate sentences) in favor of so-called "truth in sentencing" laws that required prisoners to serve at last 85% of the actual sentence. Ameliorative principles and procedures, including any overt attempt at rehabilitation, were erased from the prevailing ideology of criminal punishment.

The turn toward mass incarceration has had huge costs, of course, and these costs (like the costs of street crime itself) fall unevenly on marginalized individuals and poor communities. The association between incarceration rates and race is inescapable. The number and proportion of prisoners with behavioral health disorders and comorbid medical afflictions, including infectious disease, are very high, although estimates vary widely (Prins, 2014). According to a recent survey by researchers from the Bureau of Justice Statistics, more than half of all inmates in jails and prisons have a current, treatable "mental health problem" (James and Glaze, 2006). Other surveys consistently show that at least 15% of inmates have a serious mental metal illness (Steadman, et al, 2009). Although the causal connection between deinstitutionalization of mental health services and the increase of the number of mentally ill inmates in prisons remains in dispute, there is little doubt that a significant proportion of mentally ill inmates in local jails are arrested and held in custody there due to gaps in mental health services that could have prevented or ameliorated the acute crises that landed them in jail. Moreover, confinement and the stresses of prison life tend to make the inmate's clinical situation worse, especially for individuals with serious mental illness. In short, one of the most pronounced effects of mass incarceration has been to substantially increase the demands on prison health systems and on community services of all kinds after prisoners are released. These pressures and needs are especially high for mental health services.

All of these factors have placed psychiatrists on the front lines of the society's effort to cope with the humanitarian challenges of mass incarceration. The needs are huge and the capacity of correctional agencies to respond to them is typically severely constrained. Quality of care varies widely across the country as does the financial structure of care. Although there are several accrediting bodies, only about 500 of 3000 facilities have been accredited. (NRC, 2014) The challenge is both individual and collective. At the individual level, correctional psychiatrists must respond to the demands of conscience. The larger the population under care, the larger the challenge. Clinical skill is only the minimum prerequisite for the job. The psychiatrist needs the ability to cope with scarcity and to manage resources in an ethically reasonable way. The psychiatrist also needs to learn how to use his or her voice effectively in advocating for change within the organization responsible for health care delivery as well as within the correctional agency. He or she may often encounter an authoritarian culture where the caring is not the overriding value. At the collective level, psychiatry and allied professions must stand up for the needs and rights of the patients and for the psychiatrists who bear the responsibility for serving those needs. These ethical imperatives are not unlike those that confronted psychiatrists in large mental hospitals under siege in the 1970s.

Are correctional psychiatrists (and other correctional health care providers) standing alone in facing these challenges? Fortunately, psychiatrists and their professional comrades do have some allies. One is the federal courts, where the threat of a lawsuit aiming to remediate inadequate medical and mental health care can still provide an incentive for negotiation when the conditions fall below minimally acceptable standards, notwithstanding the limitations imposed by Congress in the Prison Litigation Reform Act (1996). The California litigation leading to and following the Supreme Court's decision in Brown v. Plata, 131 S. Ct. 1910 (2011), demonstrates that, if necessary, the federal courts will order states to reduce the number of prisoners in order to assure adequate health care. A second influence is the authority of professional organizations. Revival of the rehabilitative aspiration of correctional services and a commitment to humanitarian ideals is evident in recent statements and standards issued by or under the auspices of the American Correctional Association (2003), the American Bar Association (2010), and the American Psychiatric Association (2014). A third force is the investment of several major philanthropic foundations in consolidating knowledge about causes and consequences of the growth of incarceration in the United States and in pointing the way forward. One important contribution to this discussion is a recently released report by the National Research Council, *The Growth of Incarceration in the United States*. (NRC, 2014)

A fourth emerging influence is political, as a backlash against over-incarceration takes hold, calling attention to the high costs of current policies and the potential financial benefits of reducing reliance on incarceration, providing rehabilitative services during confinement, and assuring a seamless transition in healthcare services (and other rehabilitative services) upon release and reentry into the community. Successful implementation of the Affordable Care Act could play an important role (NRC, 2014), as can prisoner reentry programs supported under the Second Chance Act and the Justice Reinvestment Act. (See Pew Center on the States, 2012; Council of State Governments Justice Center, 2013).

These are hopeful signs that the number of incarcerated individuals with serious mental illness will decline over the next few decades. For now and the foreseeable future, however, publication of *The Oxford Textbook of Correctional Psychiatry* responds to an urgent need for authoritative guidance by psychiatrists and professional staff in facilities and communities across the country and by a growing number of psychiatrists and other mental health professionals in forensic fellowships. It will serve equally well as a reference book and as a reader for concentrated study. It is hard to imagine that practitioners will encounter a clinical, ethical or organizational challenge relating to the patient, the treatment or the setting not addressed in this volume. In addition, it creates a solid foundation improving practice that goes beyond existing guidelines and resources. My personal hope and expectation is that the psychiatrists who choose to serve patients in correctional settings will become the next generation of advocates for humanitarian values in corrections, leaders of the profession, and allies of proponents of criminal justice reform. This volume will help point the way.

Richard J. Bonnie
Harrison Foundation Professor of Law and Medicine
Professor of Psychiatry and Neurobehavioral Sciences
Professor of Public Policy
Director of the Institute of Law, Psychiatry and Public Policy
University of Virginia

References

American Bar Association, 2010. *Standards for Treatment of Prisoners.*

American Correctional Association, 2003. *Standards for Adult Correctional Institutions.*

American Psychiatric Association, 2014. *Psychiatric Services in Jails and Prisons.*

Council of State Governments Justice Center, 2013. *Reentry Matters; Strategies and Successes of Second Chance Act Grantees Across the United States.*

James, DJ and Glaze, LE, 2006. *Mental Health Problems of Prison and Jail Inmates,* U.S. Bureau of Justice Statistics.

Maruschack, JM and Parks, E, 2012. *Probation and Parole in the United States, 2011.* U.S. Bureau of Justice Statistics

National Research Council, 2014. *The Growth of Incarceration in the United States.*

Steadman, HJ, Osher, FC, Robbins, PC, et al, 2009. Prevalence of Serious Mental Illness Among Jail Inmates. *Psychiatric Services* 60:761-765.

Pew Center on the States, 2012. *Time Served: The High Cost and Lower Return of Long Prison Terms.*

Prins, SJ, 2014. Prevalence of Mental Illnesses in U.S. State Prisons: A Systematic Review. *Psychiatric Services,* 65:862-872.

U.S. Department of Justice, Bureau of Justice Assistance, 2013. *Justice and Mental Health Collaboration Program*

Walmsley, R. 2013. *World Prison Population List.* International Center for Prison Studies.

Acknowledgments

A work such as this is always a complex collaboration. We thank all the contributors for their efforts to present the best available information and guidance to the reader. We specifically thank Stacey K. Rich for her organizational skills, support, and phenomenal attention to detail; it made this project far more manageable than it might otherwise have been. We also thank Christopher Reid, our editor at Oxford University Press. His problem solving and encouragement made this project possible.

We undertook this project to develop a resource for correctional psychiatrists. We hope that they and our colleagues from other mental health and medical disciplines will find this textbook useful. Correctional health care providers have not always received the recognition they deserve. Many persevere under challenging conditions with limited resources. They have followed many of the patients we serve into unfortunate circumstances of detention. If they did not do this, our profession would be woefully remiss by abandoning so many people in need of competent care. We offer them our encouragement and respect, and we look forward to the day when they receive more universal recognition and needed resources.

In addition to our colleagues from health care, we acknowledge our partners who work in custody positions. We are no longer seen as guests in their house. We are an integral and undeniable part of the correctional family. Not all families, however, have harmonious relationships. With that in mind, we thank those on the custody side of the house who appreciate our contributions. We hope they, too, may find useful information for their work in this textbook. We, in turn, could not provide effective services without their support, collaboration, and professionalism. They did not ask to become the locus of care for ever-growing numbers of people with serious mental disorders.

While this textbook provides a resource for our colleagues, it has the underlying and fundamental goal of enhancing care for the population we serve. Far too many of our fellow citizens have found themselves imprisoned for reasons sometimes rooted in our collective failure to provide them with meaningful access to basic necessities, including mental health care. We find it tragic that many of them have had to wait for incarceration to receive services that no one should lack in our society. We want to acknowledge them for their patience with us and for often offering us their appreciation, which increases the meaning of the work that we do.

Contributors

Frederick L. Altice, MD, MA
Section of Infectious Diseases, AIDS Program
Yale School of Medicine and School of Public Health

Joel T. Andrade, PhD
Massachusetts Partnership for Correctional Healthcare

Kenneth L. Appelbaum, MD
Center for Health Policy and Research, Commonwealth
  Medicine
University of Massachusetts Medical School

Bruce A. Arrigo, PhD
Department of Criminal Justice & Criminology
University of North Carolina at Charlotte

Dean Aufderheide, PhD, MPA
Florida Department of Corrections

Virginia Barber-Rioja, PhD
Department of Psychiatry
New York University Medical Center

Carl C. Bell, MD
Retired—Department of Psychiatry
College of Medicine
University of Illinois at Chicago

Robert H. Berger, MD
Correctional Managed Health Care
University of Connecticut Health Center

Ingrid A. Binswanger, MD, MPH, MS
Department of Medicine
University of Colorado School of Medicine

Brad Bogue, MA
Justice System Assessment and Training, Inc.
Boulder, Colorado

Richard J. Bonnie, LLB
Institute of Law, Psychiatry and Public Policy
University of Virginia School of Law

Arthur Brewer, MD
Department of Family Medicine
University Correctional Health Care
Rutgers University—Robert Wood Johnson Medical School

Johann Brink, MB, ChB
Department Psychiatry
University of British Columbia

Brittany Brizendine, PsyD, MBA
California Department of Corrections and Rehabilitation

Melody C. Brown, BA

Craig G. Burns, MD
Connecticut Department of Correction

Kathryn A. Burns, MD, MPH
Ohio Department of Rehabilitation and Correction and
Department of Psychiatry and Behavioral Health
Ohio State University

Philip J. Candilis, MD
St. Elizabeth's Hospital
Department of Behavioral Health

Shama Chaiken, PhD
California Department of Corrections and Rehabilitation

M. Paul Chaplin, PhD
Correctional Managed Health Care
University of Connecticut Health Center

Kristin G. Cloyes, PhD, RN
College of Nursing
University of Utah

James F. DeGroot, PhD
Georgia Department of Corrections

Pamela M. Diamond, PhD
Division of Health Promotion and Behavioral Sciences
School of Public Health
University of Texas Health Science Center at Houston

Charles Dike, MD
Department of Psychiatry
Yale School of Medicine

Henry A. Dlugacz, MSW, JD
Department of Psychiatry and Behavioral Sciences
New York Medical College

Doris A. Dumond, MA
Consultants for Improved Human Services

Robert W. Dumond, MA
Department of Psychology
Southern New Hampshire University

Joel Dvoskin, PhD
Department of Psychiatry
University of Arizona College of Medicine

Bernice S. Elger, MD, PhD
Institute of Biomedical Ethics
Universities of Geneva and Basel

Brian Falls, MD
Division of Psychiatry and the Law
Department of Psychiatry and Behavioral Science
University of California, Davis

Jamie Fellner, JD
United States Program
Human Rights Watch

Warren J. Ferguson, MD
Department of Family Medicine and Community Health
University of Massachusetts Medical School

Bruce C. Gage, MD
Washington State Department of Corrections and
Department of Psychiatry and Behavioral Sciences
University of Washington School of Medicine

Gerard G. Gagné, Jr., MD
Correctional Managed Health Care
University of Connecticut Health Center

Erik J. Garcia, MD
Department of Family Medicine and Community Health
University of Massachusetts Medical School

Graham D. Glancy, MB, ChB
Department of Psychiatry
University of Toronto, Windsor

Ezra E. H. Griffith, MD
Department of Psychiatry
Yale School of Medicine

Albert J. Grudzinskas, Jr., JD
Department of Psychiatry
University of Massachusetts Medical School

Patrece Hairston, PsyD
Department of Psychiatry
University of Colorado School of Medicine

Annette L. Hanson, MD
Department of Psychiatry
University of Maryland School of Medicine

Brian J. Holoyda, MD, MPH
Department of Psychiatry & Behavioral Sciences
University of California, Davis

Kerry C. Hughes, MD

Eric D. Huttenbach, MD, JD
Department of Psychiatry
University of Massachusetts Medical School

André M. Ivanoff, PhD
School of Social Work
Columbia University

Mohamedu F. Jones, LLM
Partner, Pannone Lopes Devereaux & West LLC

Jayesh Kamath, MD, PhD
Department of Psychiatry
University of Connecticut Health Center

Kevin Kapila, MD
Fenway Health
Harvard Medical School

Reena Kapoor, MD
Department of Psychiatry
Yale School of Medicine

Randi Kaufman, PsyD
Department of Psychiatry
Harvard Medical School

Emily A. Keram, MD
Department of Psychiatry
University of California, San Francisco

James L. Knoll, IV, MD
Department of Psychiatry
SUNY Upstate Medical University

Catherine M. Knox, MN, RN

Li-Wen Lee, MD
Department of Psychiatry
Columbia University College of Physicians and Surgeons

Catherine F. Lewis, MD
Department of Psychiatry
University of Connecticut Health Center

Ingrid Li, MD
Department of Psychiatry
Rutgers University—Robert Wood Johnson Medical School

Rebecca Lubelczyk, MD
Department of Family Medicine and Community Health
University of Massachusetts Medical School

H. Martin Malin, PhD
The Institute for Advanced Study of Human Sexuality

Michael P. Maloney, PhD
Department of Psychiatry and the Biobehavioral Sciences
The David Geffen School of Medicine
University of California

Barbara E. McDermott, PhD
Department of Psychiatry and Behavioral Sciences
University of California

Jeffrey L. Metzner, MD
Department of Psychiatry
University of Colorado School of Medicine

Jaimie P. Meyer, MD, MSc
Section of Infectious Diseases, AIDS Program
Yale School of Medicine

Kevin R. Murphy, PhD
Department of Psychiatry
University of Massachusetts Medical School

Michael A. Norko, MD, MAR
Department of Psychiatry
Yale School of Medicine

Maureen L. O'Keefe, MA
Colorado Department of Corrections

Jason D. Ourada, MD
Suffolk County House of Correction

Ira K. Packer, PhD
Department of Psychiatry
University of Massachusetts Medical School

Raymond F. Patterson, MD
Department of Psychiatry
Howard University

Joseph V. Penn, MD
Department of Psychiatry
Correctional Managed Care
University of Texas Medical Branch

Mary Perrien, PhD

Tasha R. Phillips, PsyD
Department of Psychiatry
University of Massachusetts Medical School

Debra A. Pinals, MD
Department of Psychiatry
University of Massachusetts Medical School

Rusty Reeves, MD
Department of Psychiatry
University Correctional Health Care
Rutgers University—Robert Wood
    Johnson Medical School

Josiah D. Rich, MD, MPH
Departments of Medicine and Epidemiology
The Warren Alpert Medical School
Brown University

Stacey K. Rich, AS
Correctional Managed Health Care
University of Connecticut Health Center

Erik J. Roskes, MD
Department of Psychiatry
University of Maryland School of Medicine

Merrill Rotter, MD
Department of Psychiatry
Albert Einstein College of Medicine

Fabian M. Saleh, MD
Department of Psychiatry
Harvard Medical School

Henry Schmidt, III, PhD
Behavioral Affiliates, Inc.

Charles L. Scott, MD
Department of Psychiatry & Behavioral Sciences
University of California, Davis

Ajay Shah, MD
Department of Psychiatry
University of Connecticut Health Center

Anthony C. Tamburello, MD
University Correctional Health Care
Department of Psychiatry
Rutgers University—Robert Wood Johnson Medical School

Faye S. Taxman, PhD
Department of Criminology, Law and Society
Center for Advancing Correctional Excellence
George Mason University

Stuart D. M. Thomas, PhD
Faculty of Social Sciences
University of Wollongong

Lindsay D. G. Thomson, MB, ChB, MPhil, MD
Division of Psychiatry
The University of Edinburgh

Todd Tomita, MD
Department Psychiatry
University of British Columbia

Stefan R. Treffers, MA
Department of Criminology
University of Windsor

Robert L. Trestman, PhD, MD
Correctional Managed Health Care
University of Connecticut Health Center

S. Lorén Trull, JD
Department of Interdisciplinary Studies,
    Public Policy Program
University of North Carolina at Charlotte

Donna Vanderpool, MBA, JD
Professional Risk Management Services, Inc.

Sundeep Virdi, JD, MD
Department of Psychiatry
University of Connecticut Health Center

Robyn J. Wahl, PharmD, MBA
Correctional Managed Health Care
University of Connecticut Health Center

Sarah E. Wakeman, MD
Department of Medicine
Harvard Medical School

Nancy Wolff, PhD
Center for Behavioral Health Services &
    Criminal Justice Research
Rutgers, The State University of New Jersey

Sohrab Zahedi, MD
Correctional Managed Health Care
University of Connecticut Health Center

Introduction

Correctional psychiatry has evolved with great speed over the past two decades. The number of incarcerated mentally ill and addicted individuals has more than quadrupled to levels that frequently exceed those in community systems of care. The challenges and opportunities of correctional psychiatry are substantial, indeed profound. Most sources acknowledge that correctional systems are now the de facto mental health systems of care. Complex, comorbid disorders are now common presentations in correctional settings. Typically 12% to 16% of the incarcerated population has a serious mental illness; 75% to 80% have comorbid substance use disorders. Psychotic disorders, personality disorders, posttraumatic stress disorders, traumatic brain injury, and intellectual disability are highly prevalent and challenging to manage. The costs of psychopharmacological treatment represent a substantial proportion of correctional health care costs in the context of limited resources and single-payer capitated systems of care. An entire, and distinctly challenging, continuum of care exists in jails and prisons, each level presenting unique demands of collaboration with other disciplines, including custody. Further, knowledge of effective interventions with mentally ill or addicted patients while incarcerated contributes to successful community re-entry.

The field of correctional psychiatry has reached the point where a formal textbook is in order. *The Oxford Textbook of Correctional Psychiatry* is designed for use either as part of an organized course or for self-directed study. Chapters contain a literature review with supportive references and typically focus on areas of clarity and areas still lacking an evidence basis; a critical examination of best practices; a discussion of implementation in the correctional context; and appropriate case examples. We have worked to bring together contributions of leaders in the field—clinicians who deliver care, administrators and monitors who shape the systems of care, researchers and ethicists who help guide care improvement, educators who mentor new correctional psychiatrists and clinicians of other disciplines, and lawyers who participate in formative litigation.

Section I: Section I, *Context and Perspective*, provides relevant background. The first chapter reviews the evolution of the US imprisonment system and the system's development in relation to correctional psychiatry. The chapter examines the history of American prisons, including their shifting purposes, standards, and practices and their limited regard for prisoners with mental illness. The chapter goes on to explain how rehabilitation theory has intersected with the diagnosis and treatment of inmates with psychiatric disorders. The chapter concludes by discussing the current status of imprisonment in the United States, which includes systematic mass incarceration that adversely and unequally affects people of color. The next chapter summarizes the historical context of correctional versus community mental health; factors resulting in the increasing management of people with mental illness in correctional settings; and similarities and differences between mental health care in correctional versus community settings. Next, formative case law and litigation are discussed, with a review of the legal and constitutional background for correctional mental health care in the United States and the critical ways courts influence policy and care delivery. The next chapter focuses on human rights, with a review of the challenges and controversies that exist in correctional mental health care in North America and internationally and an overview of the key internationally recognized human rights that should inform the work of correctional mental health professionals. The final chapter in this section shares the insights of 10 individuals currently or recently incarcerated in the Colorado prison system. The transcribed autobiographical interviews present core elements and themes in their own words. We believe they speak eloquently of human struggle, coping, failure, regret, and hope.

Section II: Section II, *Organization, Structure, and Function of Correctional Institutions*, begins with a chapter on jails and prisons. Distinctions between prisons (post-sentence facilities) and jails (housing detainees awaiting trial) in service delivery and treatment challenges in the long-term management of prisoners with serious mental illness are discussed. The next chapter focuses on a pragmatic discussion of what it is like for psychiatrists to work inside the walls of a jail or prison. The psychiatrist must come to terms with the realities of the correctional setting to feel secure, satisfied with the work, and clinically effective. The subsequent chapter deals with many, often unique, ethical concerns that jails and prisons present to the psychiatrist. Obligations to the law, professional standards, the community, and public health require a complex appreciation of competing values. This chapter discusses the critical concerns, including informed consent and coercion, dual agency, appropriate access to care, and managing professional boundaries and standards. As with any health care setting, communication is a critical component of effective care delivery, and the next chapter explicitly discusses the inherent cultural differences among interdisciplinary staff, the special challenges to effective communication faced by correctional psychiatrists, and the importance of that communication given the central role that psychiatrists play in the overall mission of jail and prison health care. The final chapter in this section deals with the cost and financing of correctional mental health care. The funding of correctional health care is a complex enterprise, driven by constitutionally mandated care obligations on the one hand and resource constraints on the other. This chapter includes a discussion of global capitation, per-inmate costs, at-risk contracting, liability concerns, performance indicators, and other contractual relationships.

Section III: Section III addresses correctional *Patient Management Processes*. The first chapter focuses on a core component of psychiatric care in any setting—screening and assessment. In jails and prisons, the process, structure, content, and timing of screenings and assessments are vital parts of the health care system. This chapter reviews the initial mental health screening of persons entering prisons and jails, with a special emphasis on suicide risk screening and follow-up clinical assessments when intake screening suggests a need for treatment or suicide prevention efforts. Learning to conduct an interview is fundamental to psychiatric training and treatment. Consequently, the next chapter addresses the challenges, requirements, importance, and complexity of clinical interviews in jails and prisons, with particular attention given to how the correctional population and setting can influence the interview process. Managing correctional populations is the topic of the following chapter. Jails and prisons share population management challenges with hotels—what beds are available to meet the explicit requirements for which individuals? The management of large facilities and systems must incorporate ways to recognize many safety and clinical demands in real time. Levels of security risk; medical, mental health, and addiction treatment needs; and sex offender status, among others, must all be taken into account in placement decisions. The chapter discusses these pragmatic issues, particularly in the context of psychiatric management, and details issues concerning disciplinary infractions and restricted housing. It should surprise no one that misbehavior occurs within jails and prisons. A formal disciplinary process generally handles such misbehavior. Because inmates with mental illness may be more prone to rule infractions due to their illness, they are more likely to receive discipline and be segregated unless specific rules limit such sanctions. The next chapter reviews segregation practices, the data on the potential effect of segregated housing on mental illness, and the role of psychiatry in the disciplinary process. The last chapter in this section focuses on community re-entry. Approximately 97% of inmates return to the community. This simple reality makes it in society's enlightened self-interest to be concerned with the readiness of these former inmates to live a productive life. This chapter presents the current understanding of transition support needs and practices to optimize successful community reentry for those with mental illness.

Section IV: Section IV tackles *Common Management Issues*. The first chapter deals with a common management challenge—sleep. Inmates often seek health care for sleep problems, but studies on insomnia in correctional institutions are scarce. Correctional health professionals need appropriate education regarding insomnia evaluation and management. This chapter outlines treatment guidelines that apply in community settings, presents an overview of the clinical and ethical issues of insomnia management in correctional institutions, and provides evidence-based recommendations. The following chapter attempts to educate the correctional clinician on the common presentations of intoxication and withdrawal syndromes. Drugs and/or alcohol were being used at the time of the offense by more than half of all detainees, necessitating screening at intake for both intoxication and risk of withdrawal from substances. The similarities and distinctions of such syndromes with mental illnesses are discussed. Standardized medical management approaches to ensure patient safety during supervised withdrawal are also presented. Incarceration is intrinsically stressful, and the next chapter addresses the presentation, assessment, and management of adjustment disorders, which frequently arise in jail or prison.

Incarceration presents an opportunity to reexamine medications and diagnoses of people with mental illness. The next two chapters address these issues. Community medications may have been prescribed while ongoing illicit drug use confounded the diagnostic picture. Collaboration between clinician and patient may have been poor, and treatment adherence may have been marginal. This chapter discusses the issues and pragmatic management opportunities that can lead to improved patient care and enhanced functioning. Diagnostic review and revision are addressed in the chapter that follows. Psychiatric hospitals have great constraints on the time available for observation and accurate diagnosis; the correctional setting, as an unintended consequence of mass incarceration, affords an extended opportunity to achieve improved diagnostic accuracy, as this chapter reflects.

The next chapter describes how individuals with mental illness may be diverted from the correctional system to programs and other alternatives. It reviews the major models used to divert those with serious mental illness from incarceration, paying attention to legal and clinical issues that arise. Brief overviews of drug and mental health courts, jail diversion programs, and alternatives to incarceration for defendants with mental illness are presented. As in community settings, a continuum of care exists for inmates with mental illness, which the following chapter describes. Levels of care typically found in prisons and many jails include outpatient care, emergency services, day treatment, supported residential housing, infirmary care, and inpatient psychiatric hospitalization. The chapter reviews how to successfully adapt each level to meet the mental health needs of inmates. Recognizing when someone is not being truthful is challenging, but detection of malingering in corrections helps ensure judicious use of limited resources and brings diagnostic accuracy to assessments. The next chapter explains the use of structured tests of malingering and other clinical skills to make treatment decisions in jails and prisons. The final chapter in this section concerns intoxication and drug abuse in correctional settings. Knowledge about substance use in correctional facilities fosters competent clinical intervention and enhances management at all levels. Psychiatrists working in jails and prisons have the difficult task of maintaining therapeutic alliances with patients who have co-occurring and often active substance use disorders. The clinical challenges in jails and prisons differ, and the substances found in facilities vary geographically. Correctional psychiatrists make important contributions by providing direct assessment and treatment to inmates and by offering educational, clinical, and policy consultations to other staff.

Section V: Section V includes topics regarding *Emergencies* in correctional settings. Although psychiatric emergencies are common, sometimes they present in unusual ways in penal settings.

The first chapter focuses on crisis assessment and management. Crisis calls occur commonly in correctional settings, with psychiatrists often involved in triage and management. The pragmatics of evaluating and managing common events that lead to mental health crisis calls and the range of concerns, typical practices and procedures used in correctional settings, and best interventions receive attention in this chapter. The use of restraints and emergency medication is the topic of the subsequent chapter, including legal precedents that guide their use and best practices to minimize their routine application in jails and prisons. Acute hospitalization, which is often required in psychiatric care, is the focus of the final chapter in this section. The relationship between acute psychiatric care in jails and prisons on the one hand and forensic or community hospitals on the other varies by jurisdiction. This chapter discusses models that link psychiatric care across institutional boundaries.

Section VI: Section VI contains *General Pharmacology Issues.* The first chapter addresses formulary management. Because pharmaceutical expenditures represent a substantial percentage of a health care organization's budget, medication use is closely scrutinized. Clinicians must consider the appropriateness, effectiveness, and safety of medications prescribed to incarcerated patients. Evidence-based best practices that inform the development of, and adherence to, disease management guidelines and a preferred, restricted medication formulary enhance the quality, safety, and effectiveness of care. This chapter also details the process and procedures used to develop, implement, and monitor prescription practice change by establishing an effective pharmacy and therapeutics committee. The use of hypnotic agents and controlled substances is the topic of the next chapter. Sleep medications are among the most frequently prescribed medications in the community. Many other class II controlled substances such as benzodiazepines and opiate medications have become a major public health concern through overuse and abuse. The chapter evaluates best practices in this arena of prescription practice. The following chapter targets medication administration and management. For many inmates with mental illness, incarceration offers an opportunity to receive treatment that was not accessible in the community; in one study only one third of those diagnosed with schizophrenia or bipolar disorder were receiving medication at the time of arrest compared to two thirds during incarceration. There are many steps, people, and processes involved in getting medication to the patient within a correctional facility. This chapter reviews the structural, procedural, and clinical concerns of medication administration and management in jails and prisons. The last chapter deals with prescription medication abuse in jails and prisons. Community abuse of prescription medication is typically limited to overuse or inappropriate sharing of medication. In jails and prisons, the demand characteristics are dramatically altered, creating an elaborate laboratory for medication alteration, diversion, and abuse. This chapter presents data on specific classes of abused medication, methods of abuse, and approaches to minimize abuse or diversion of prescribed medications.

Section VII: Section VII reviews *Disorders and Syndromes,* starting with a chapter on diagnostic prevalence and comorbidity. One longstanding issue is the perceived increase in the prevalence of mental disorders found in correctional settings compared to the community. This chapter outlines the best available data on the correctional prevalence of common mental disorders and considers the key assumptions and methodological challenges involved in ascertaining these rates. The next chapter focuses on psychotic disorders and their complex and diverse presentation in jails and prisons. In addition to the schizophrenia spectrum disorders, many disorders of unclear etiology occur or are secondary to the neurotoxic effects of substance abuse. This chapter discusses the evidence basis for appropriate treatment of the psychotic disorders and opportunities for psychotherapy and psychopharmacology in correctional settings. Mood disorders are the topic of the following chapter, as depression and bipolar disorder represent a substantial percentage of all psychiatric care in community and correctional settings. The review includes core management, best practices, and evidence-based therapeutic approaches to the treatment of major depressive disorders and bipolar disorders in jails and prisons.

The next chapter turns to anxiety disorders, including posttraumatic stress disorder. Unrecognized anxiety disorders can result in disruptive behavior that may appear to be volitional. They can also lead to overuse of general medical health services that are already facing substantial demands. Appropriate, available, consistent, and well-integrated assessment, diagnosis, and treatment can be used to successfully manage anxiety disorders that present in correctional settings. Personality disorders, the topic of the following chapter, are highly prevalent and problematic in jails and prisons. Four personality disorders of particular clinical relevance to correctional psychiatry exist: borderline personality disorder, antisocial personality disorder, narcissistic personality disorder, and paranoid personality disorder. The review of each disorder contains a description, management concerns and challenges, data on correctional prevalence, appropriate psychotherapy, and potential psychopharmacological interventions. Attention-deficit disorders are being recognized and treated more frequently in the community; the next chapter addresses differential diagnosis and management challenges in a population with epidemic substance abuse and presents an evidence-based treatment model. The penultimate chapter examines general medical disorders with psychiatric implications, including medical conditions that can mimic or exacerbate the presenting symptoms of delirium, mood disorders, and psychosis. This section concludes with a review of the psychiatric aspects of chronic pain management in correctional settings. It provides information on what to elicit in a chronic pain interview, the methods used to assess chronic pain, and the assessment factors that are appropriate for integration into a management plan. The methods used to manage chronic pain, including close coordination with a treatment team, cognitive-behavioral interventions, and pharmacological management, are presented. Tracking treatment outcomes from a psychiatric perspective in the correctional setting is then discussed.

Section VIII: Section VIII is dedicated to the *Psychotherapeutic Options* that are available or appropriate for jails and prisons. First, the applicability of the recovery model in corrections is discussed. President Bush's New Freedom Commission on Mental Health spoke to important yet challenged aspects of mental health care systems, recognizing that "care must focus on increasing consumers' ability to successfully cope with life's challenges, on facilitating recovery, and on building resilience, [and] not just on managing symptoms." Prisons and jails, however, are built around confinement and the general principles of sentencing that include retribution, deterrence, incapacitation, and rehabilitation. This chapter presents feasible and potentially helpful considerations related to recovery-oriented services within correctional environments and some of the tensions between recovery and responsibility when working with an offender population. The next chapter brings our attention to individual psychotherapy with a discussion of practical and fundamental aspects of individual psychotherapy with inmate patients, followed by an overview of evidence-based paradigms for psychotherapy in corrections. Therapeutic style, strategies to minimize the risks of therapeutic nihilism, the context of the treatment setting, and the limits of confidentiality are reviewed. While much of the evidence base supports cognitive-behavioral approaches (e.g., motivational interviewing and mindfulness), the enduring importance of maintaining competence in psychodynamically informed therapy and recognition of countertransference in correctional settings are discussed. The final chapter reviews group psychotherapy, which has become a standard practice in community settings, prisons, and, to a lesser degree, jails. Although simple process groups still play a limited role in some settings, the field of group therapy has evolved substantially, with some significant work adapting evidence-based therapies for use in correctional settings or designing them de novo. This chapter presents evidence-based best practices that are currently in use and discusses appropriate patient selection, required therapist training, sustainability, and outcomes.

Section IX: Section IX centers on *Suicide Risk Management*. Prevalence, demographics, trends, screening and assessment, recognition of key risk factors, and safe and appropriate suicide risk management in jails are presented. Factors that increase suicide risk in prisons are often distinct from factors in other correctional settings. Restrictive housing, facility transfers, loss of community social supports, chronic management, and other considerations all play potential roles. Proactive recognition of these concerns and active management are critical to risk reduction. This chapter discusses such factors in the context of changing prison dynamics and trends. Following a completed suicide, formal protocols assist staff in understanding the precipitating event and in intervening to address staff feelings; these protocols are also used in quality improvement initiatives (e.g., root cause analysis). Best practice approaches to postmortem review and staff intervention/support have been developed and used in many facilities. Reducing the frequency of suicide attempts requires a staff culture that is committed to continued learning and improving of knowledge and skills.

Section X: Section X focuses on *Addictions Treatment*. According to recent US data, approximately half of the individuals incarcerated in state and federal prisons meet criteria for drug abuse or dependence. Tobacco and alcohol use are also more common in correctional populations than in the general, noninstitutionalized population. Thus, criminal justice populations have a significant need for evidence-based treatment of addiction and for interventions to reduce the medical complications of drug use. The first chapter reviews the basics of treatment programming. Although programs to address substance use disorders among correctional populations exist, many individuals fail to receive adequate care and continue to experience complications of those disorders. This chapter describes the evolution of addiction programming within correctional settings from the late 1700s to the present. Current levels of care and specialized modalities for individuals involved in the criminal justice system, such as cognitive-behavioral interventions, drug courts, therapeutic

communities, pharmacologically supported therapy, and harm reduction approaches, are presented. The next chapter deals with dually diagnosed individuals. Nearly half of female inmates and one third of male inmates with substance use disorders have a diagnosable mental illness. Treatment for this population needs to address the syndemic of criminal lifestyle, mental illness, and substance abuse to effectively reduce recidivism and symptoms. This chapter includes a discussion of the factors that are unknown or unclear in the literature and also discusses best practices and implementation of treatment for dual-diagnosis patients. Effective implementation of treatment requires support from the correctional system. The chapter concludes with a research agenda for the future of dual-diagnosis treatment in corrections.

The following chapter reviews pharmacotherapy for substance use disorders in correctional facilities. Drug addiction treatment is increasingly complex. Only 5% of prisons and 34% of jails offer detoxification services, and only 1% of jails offer methadone for opioid withdrawal. Even fewer facilities offer medication-assisted therapy (MAT) for alcohol or substance use disorders, despite the tremendous evidence base supporting this therapy. There is a growing role for MAT in jails and, to a lesser degree, in prisons for the treatment of alcohol and opiate dependence. This chapter presents the current state of evidence-based practice in correctional MAT models. This section concludes with a chapter on successful support of the transition back to the community for incarcerated patients with substance use disorders. Re-incarceration of former prisoners is commonly associated with relapse to drug and alcohol use because of ineffective treatment of substance use disorders after release. This chapter discusses best practice and evidence-based models in use by jails and prisons to support successful community re-entry.

Section XI: Section XI focuses on the generic and unique correctional characteristics of *Aggression, Self-Injury, and Misconduct*. The first chapter reviews aggression and the importance of correctional psychiatrists' recognizing opportunities for appropriate assessment and intervention. Studies reflect significant risks of violence for correctional officers and inmates. This chapter reviews the factors that contribute to assaultive behavior in correctional settings; pragmatic issues and opportunities for assessment, diagnosis, and treatment of those behaviors, both impulsive and predatory, are also presented. One of the greatest management challenges in correctional settings is self-injurious behavior, the topic of the next chapter. Often, the motivations, demographics, and characteristics are distinct from self-injury in the community. Effective management in correctional settings almost always requires partnership and cooperation between health care and custody staff. This chapter reviews context and nosology, epidemiology, and best practices for assessment, diagnosis, and intervention in jails and prisons. The following chapter articulates specific management approaches for difficult or disruptive behaviors through the use of behavior management plans. Treatment is viewed as a series of interventions designed to reduce the frequency, intensity, and/or severity of a behavior. This chapter describes concepts related to behavior management and the creation of behavior management plans.

Section XII: Section XII addresses *Distinct Populations* of patients. The first chapter focuses on gender-specific treatment. The US correctional system was confronted with an increase in female inmates in part because of the War on Drugs from the mid-1980s to the mid-1990s. During this period, the number of women incarcerated rose 888%. This chapter describes the current knowledge base on incarcerated women, including their patterns of offending and arrests versus those of men, their sociodemographics, their psychopathology, and, finally, how best to treat them and implement this treatment within jails and prisons. Next, we turn to the treatment of incarcerated individuals with developmental disabilities. Although the research is inconsistent, most studies suggest that offenders with developmental delays commit less serious offenses yet serve more time in prison than other offenders. This chapter outlines the progress in identification and habilitation of individuals with developmental disabilities in the criminal justice system. Definitions, legal issues, and prevalence rates are discussed, as well as the vulnerabilities individuals with developmental delays present to the correctional system. The chapter concludes with guidance on screening, management, and habilitation. The subsequent chapter deals with individuals who have had traumatic brain injuries (TBIs). Recent studies have confirmed a 50% to 60% prevalence of TBIs among prisoners, with most experiencing multiple injuries beginning in their mid-teens. This chapter reviews the prevalence of TBIs in correctional settings, its impact on co-occurring mental illness and substance use, and opportunities to recognize, intervene, and treat these patients.

Incarcerated veterans are the topic of the next chapter. The demographics, criminogenic risk factors, and life experiences of incarcerated veterans, both combat and noncombat, differ substantially from nonveteran offenders. The pervasive trauma and posttraumatic stress disorders in this population can be profound. There is a critical need to create and implement evidence-based programs to treat the emotional, behavioral, and neurological needs of mentally ill and traumatized veterans. Society also struggles with the ambivalence of wanting to simultaneously punish and rescue them. This chapter delineates the challenges and interventions involved in working with incarcerated veterans. Lesbian, gay, bisexual, and transsexual (LGBT) issues are reviewed in the following chapter. The unique needs of incarcerated LGBT individuals with mental illness are often invisible, and they are generally misunderstood and underserved. This chapter seeks to add to the clinical knowledge of practitioners working with this population, to clarify legal precedent, and to establish best practices. As described in the next chapter, juveniles are incarcerated in both juvenile systems and adult correctional systems, depending on jurisdiction, age, and criminal charges. Suicide risk, developmental disabilities such as fetal alcohol spectrum disorder, and trauma histories have particular importance in this age group. The complexity of the mental, emotional, and behavioral disorders of youth in corrections leads to several best practice approaches for screening, assessment, and treatment. This chapter reviews the history of juvenile incarceration and best or evidence-based practices in the management and treatment of incarcerated juvenile offenders. From the young, we turn our attention to the old in the following chapter on geriatric patients. Screening for impairment and developing effective interventions and treatment for the incarcerated elderly have become substantial challenges. The number of inmates aged 60 and older in prisons in the United Kingdom increased by 120% between 2002 and 2013; similar growth trends are reported in the United States, Sweden, Japan, Australia, and Canada. This growth is complicated because chronological age

does not necessarily match "health age" or health status in prison. As a result, many prison systems have adjusted their definition of "elderly" down to age 55 (and some as low as age 40) to reflect the relatively poor health status of aging men and women in their institutions. This chapter reviews the current status and prevalence of the incarcerated elderly and presents best practice models for their care.

Gangs are a fact of life in jails and prisons, as reviewed in the next chapter. The extent and impact of gang activity on a facility depend on size and geographic location. Psychiatrists need an awareness of the dynamics of gang leadership, membership, and involvement, as these factors affect a gang member's ability to participate in and interest in collaborative treatment. This chapter presents these issues and best practices for intervention. Sex offenders are incarcerated in substantial numbers for nonviolent and violent crimes, with or without diagnoses of paraphilias. The next chapter provides information on this population. The treatment of sex offenders is arguably one of the most challenging undertakings for psychiatrists. This chapter reviews the nosology, assessment, diagnosis, and best and evidence-based practices for the care of convicted sex offenders in correctional settings. This section concludes with a discussion of the need for psychiatrists to have cultural competence in care provision within correctional settings. Disparities exist in the rate of incarceration of minorities in the United States, with substantial elevations occurring in black, Latino, and Native American populations. Cultural competence is an essential aspect of providing mental health care. This chapter reviews the evolution of cultural competence skills and current best practices in jails and prisons to optimize effective treatment outcomes.

Section XIII: Section XIII includes a range of *Special Topics* and begins with a chapter on forensic issues faced by correctional psychiatrists. This chapter reviews competency restoration, court collaboration, litigation-related concerns, and other relevant areas. The next chapter shifts to a discussion of psychological testing, which offers substantial value and a helpful adjunct to standard clinical assessments in correctional situations. Tests provide additional sources of data for use in comprehensive assessments but do not substitute for clinical evaluations. This chapter presents some of the history of psychological testing and contexts for when it is done, can be done, and should not be done on the basis of best practice and evidence-based practice. The evolution of correctional health care standards and accreditation parallels community developments. This next chapter presents a brief historical narrative of the events that resulted in the development and adoption of national jail, prison, and juvenile correctional health care standards; a cogent review of jail and prison standards with particular relevance to psychiatry and mental health; and a discussion of accreditation programs.

Hunger strikes are the next special topic chapter. The management of hunger strikes in correctional settings presents the psychiatrist with unique clinical and ethical challenges. The potential for such complex tensions between medical decision making and medical ethics rarely exists in other practice locations. This chapter provides correctional psychiatrists with the historical, clinical, legal, and ethical background for working with hunger strikers. The following chapter deals with the growing recognition of and commitment to eliminate sexual assaults in jails and prisons. Sexual abuse in detention has been called "the most serious and devastating of non-lethal offenses which occur in corrections" because of its profound impact on survivors, and, ultimately, society. This chapter explores sexual violence in US detention centers in the twenty-first century; examines current knowledge about sexual victimization in America's jails, prisons, and juvenile facilities; discusses the successes and promising practices facilitated by the Prison Rape Elimination Act of 2003; considers the challenges that continue to exist; and makes recommendations to address the problem. Correctional facilities and systems in the United States sometimes fail to provide constitutionally adequate care. The next chapter addresses the monitoring of systems and the significant role for quality assurance and improvement. This chapter summarizes the monitoring process in a class-action lawsuit settlement agreement using a single prison mental health system as an illustrative example. Emphasis is also placed on the importance of developing a quality improvement process that should ultimately eliminate the need for an external monitor.

Correctional settings present opportunities for psychiatrists to assume leadership roles, as reviewed in the next chapter. The increase in the number of detainees and inmates who require mental health services, the need for dedicated and qualified leadership of complex systems of care, and the importance of education and training in correctional mental health practices have created many administrative and clinical opportunities for psychiatrists. The following chapter shifts attention to the role of clinical trainees in jails and prisons, which offer important and worthy training sites for medical students, general psychiatry residents, child and adolescent psychiatry residents, and forensic psychiatry fellows. The opportunities to match current psychiatric training requirements with these facilities abound. Caring for individuals with mental illness where they live increasingly means providing that care in jails and prisons.

The next chapter expands the context to include international perspectives and practice differences. Across the developed world, services for those in prison with mental disorders have been established but are seldom equivalent to those found in the community. Prisoners frequently grew up in socioeconomically deprived settings and experience high rates of mental disorder. They have often been victimized. Prisons are our new asylums. In the United States, three times as many mentally ill people are in prison than in psychiatric hospitals. It is essential that whatever our geographic location, we learn from other jurisdictions and systems. This chapter examines correctional psychiatry in an international context and explores similarities and differences in our practices and the cultural, political, and economic background to these practices. Research and program evaluation opportunities are addressed in the following chapter. Research in mental health issues in prisoner populations essentially stopped in the mid-1970s. This chapter reviews the definition of research, how it informs policy and practice, the history of prisoner research, the evolution of federal regulations in the United States to protect prisoners as human subjects, and the impact of regulation. This is followed by recommendations for building the correctional mental health research evidence base.

The final chapter envisions the future of correctional psychiatry. No one can predict with certainty what the future holds. We feel safe, however, in saying that changes, incremental and perhaps revolutionary, will occur. We identify opportunities to expand the evidence base of correctional psychiatry, the need to refine practice guidelines, and the role that psychiatry might play in influencing the use of incarceration. As part of our review, we describe what we believe the future may hold for our subspecialty. We hope that this textbook contributes to a picture of where things stand and a vision of where we need to go.

SECTION I

Context and perspective

CHAPTER 1

History of imprisonment

Bruce A. Arrigo and S. Lorén Trull

Introduction

In the United States, the use of criminal confinement as a form of punishment commenced during the colonial era (Rothman, 2002; Scull, 2006). Since then, criminal confinement has continued to evolve, with fluctuating commitments to punishment's transitory purpose and the variable penal philosophies that justify it. This chapter focuses on the evolution of the US imprisonment system and examines the relevance of the system's development in relation to correctional psychiatry. The first section of the chapter reviews the history of American prisons, including their shifting purposes, standards, and practices. The second portion highlights the persistent lack of regard for prisoners with mental illness throughout the history of American penology, and it explains how rehabilitation theory has intersected with the diagnosis and treatment of persons experiencing psychiatric disorders while criminally confined. The chapter concludes by discussing the current status of imprisonment in the United States, noting the impact that the War on Drugs campaign has had on minority communities.

History of american prisons and punishment

The prisons of the colonial era were based on religion, English tradition, and practical wisdom (Meskell, 1999). With relatively small populations to police, the criminal justice system administered swift and public punishments that were intended to humiliate, enslave, or even torture (Pfohl, 2009). Moreover, given the strong sense of kinship that shaped colonial hamlets, punishment existed to deter transgression and to discipline waywardness (Foucault, 1979). Deterrence philosophy was fueled through Calvinist religious doctrine and dogma (Barnes, 1968). For Calvinists, it was wasteful and futile to rely on and invest in a reformist-based penal system because humans were innately sinful, wicked, and evil. Operating from within this no-nonsense and religiously driven framework, the colonies drew from English criminal codes to define specific capital offenses, ranging from murder to blasphemy (Barnes, 1968). For noncapital offenses, retribution increased in severity as recidivism continued, and punishment could eventually result in banishment (Cullen & Gilbert, 1982). This English-based, Calvinist-inspired system of punishment persisted until the late 1700s when reform movements emerged as a response to rapid population growth and the call for a more humane "corrections" system (Barnes, 1968; Rothman, 2002). Utilitarians such as Jeremy Bentham and John Stuart Mill began criticizing the English system of punishment and imprisonment.

They argued that people were not innately cruel or sinful but rather that they were capable of weighing the costs and benefits of committing a crime and making a decision on how best to behave based on this reasoned calculus (Barnes, 1968).

During the post-Revolutionary era, the Italian criminologist Cesare Beccaria emerged as the most significant theorist to influence the American system of corrections (Hirsch, 1982). A notable objection to the English penal system was his disdain for the practice of meting out severe punishment that exceeded the harshness of the crime (Meskell, 1999). Beccaria posited that the source for crime was the criminal code itself and not the individual (Gillin, 1926). Specifically, he maintained that to overcome the arbitrary and draconian criminal codes found in countries such as England, governments should enact legislation that strictly defines punishments, appropriately limits the power of judges, clearly and publicly codifies laws, comprehensively creates punishments that instill fear in and thus deter potential offenders from engaging in criminal behavior, and purposely develops punishments that were the least harsh and the least necessary to achieve the goal of deterrence (Gillin, 1926). By the late 1700s, America's acceptance of Beccaria's recommendations led to the revision of its criminal codes and the introduction of a reformist-based system of punishment (Cullen & Gilbert, 1982).

The early US prisons were harsh, often housing men and women together. They lacked discipline, humane treatment, and sanitary living conditions (Rothman, 2002; Scull, 2006). In 1786, following the acceptance of arguments put forward by the Classical school of criminology (i.e., the integration of utilitarianism's reasoned calculus and Beccaria's fear of punishment philosophy), Benjamin Rush, along with the Society for Assisting Distressed Prisoners (SADP), drafted a new criminal code in the United States (Barnes, 1968). One of the most notable correctional facilities to emerge following this codification was the Walnut Street Jail in Philadelphia (Roth, 2006). The origins of its system of punishment and imprisonment can be traced to a law passed by the Pennsylvania legislature on April 5, 1790, based on an SADP draft report that called for solitary confinement combined with the administration of hard labor (Barnes, 1968). The law specifically substituted hard labor as punishment, called for the segregation of prisoners by gender and type of crime, and also permitted solitary confinement for the most serious of offenders (Barnes, 1968). Prisoners in the Walnut Street Jail were required to read the Bible and participate in religious instructions, and they were not allowed to drink alcohol. This model of criminal confinement encouraged introspection and the elimination of bad habits, and it purged the "moral contamination" of other inmates through the use of segregated or isolative confinement (Roth, 2006).

The penal culture changed along with the law undergirding the American penal system. Jails were no longer run for profit, as they had been under the colonial system; the organization of imprisonment was standardized; and they were less vulnerable to extortion by the keepers of the kept (McGowen, 1995). While the Walnut Street Jail limited solitary confinement to the most egregious of offenders, the facility lacked a full-fledged model of prisoner isolative segregation that did not include hard labor (De Beaumont, De Tocqueville, & Lieber, 1833). Moreover, while the Walnut Street Jail experienced some success, as evidenced by declining crime rates, it lacked proper prison-based controls, suitable plans for expansion, and sufficient financial support. The facility deteriorated in the 1820s and was officially shut down in 1835 (Lewis, 1965).

A new wave of reformers began to take part in shaping the burgeoning US system of imprisonment and punishment. The origin of crime shifted sharply to a new view of criminality rooted in the ills of a failed social order (Gillin, 1926). From this perspective, the purpose of confinement was to advance the well-being of the individual offender; that is, the aim of criminal confinement was to ensure the safety and to further the good of society as a whole while disciplining (i.e., normalizing) the transgressor (Foucault, 1979). In 1816, a New York prison was constructed in Auburn modeled after this philosophy (De Beaumont et al., 1833).

The attempt at solitary confinement without hard labor was unsuccessful at the Auburn Prison. As a penal practice, some questioned whether isolative segregation ultimately led to insanity (Barnes, 1968). Eventually, this criticism eliminated isolative segregation as a broadly applied penal practice. The Auburn Prison then implemented the congregate system of correctional management (Meskell, 1999). Under the congregate system, prisoners were allowed to work together during the day. However, at night, they were required to sleep in different cells and were prohibited from speaking, effectively preventing communication with other inmates (Lewis, 1965). The Auburn system used intense observation of prisoners to monitor inmate behavior, and it relied on consistent discipline throughout the prison to manage and correct inmates.

The Eastern Penitentiary at Cherry Hill in Pennsylvania was constructed in 1821, and it departed from the example set at the Auburn facility (Barnes, 1968). Eastern Penitentiary implemented a system of imprisonment that focused on the reform of prisoners as soon as they began serving their sentences. Convicts were placed in solitary confinement, not allowed to work, and expected to reflect on their criminal wrongdoings. Eventually, inmates were given permission to work, had access to the Bible, and were taught to read during their incarceration if they entered the prison illiterate (De Beaumont et al., 1833). These reforms were driven by Quaker religious convictions and based on a philosophy of both moral reform and social rehabilitation (Dumm, 1987). Known as the Philadelphia model, this approach to penal practice required less intense supervision of convicts than did the Auburn model. Both of these structures, or models, of correctional management shaped the American prison system through much of the nineteenth century. However, the approach developed at the Auburn Prison was more widely adopted throughout the United States and came to dominate nineteenth-century practices (US Department of Justice, 1939). This was due, in large part, to the health repercussions of isolative segregation without labor (as experienced at

Eastern Penitentiary) and the financial savings that followed from the imprisonment model at Auburn (i.e., the per-inmate costs were nearly half those of Eastern Penitentiary).

In the late 1800s through the mid-1900s, a series of international mobilization events and national reform efforts emerged to improve the treatment of convicts. In 1885, an international prison conference led to radical changes in penal philosophy and practice. During this period, the focus on scientific approaches to the confinement and rehabilitation of prisoners propelled efforts to reduce reliance on incarceration, to pursue alternative sanctions for less severe crimes, and to introduce new strategies such as probation (Ferracuti, 1989). Two more international conferences were held—one in Amsterdam in 1901, the other in London in 1925. These conferences shifted the focus to the criminal offender's psychopathology (Palermo, 2013). This clinically oriented understanding of delinquent and criminal behavior resulted in better inmate treatment and improved patient outcomes. Moreover, these gains fostered the development of alternative measures of detention and ushered in a new focus on the social reintegration of prisoners (Ferracuti, 1989).

This rehabilitative turn in correctional philosophy led to improvements in prison conditions. Notwithstanding the mostly nominal gains that followed, many deficiencies remained in US correctional institutions up until the 1960s. Indeed, the penal system had reached a point where inmates were afforded a decent diet, had access to reading materials, benefitted from several forms of recreation, and were able to buy certain personal items. However, prisoners served longer sentences, were under constant surveillance, and still lacked access to much-needed health and mental health services and community recovery programming (Palermo & White, 1998).

As the twentieth century progressed, urban centers became more densely populated, and crime rates as well as jail populations increased. These realities contributed to overcrowded prisons, substandard living conditions, and a heightened threat of inmate violence (Morris, 1995). Once again, the increased prison population led to strict supervision, reduced access to rehabilitative services, and a decline in living conditions. American prisons became undisciplined and dangerous, a breeding ground for the recruitment of gang members, for the sale and purchase of drugs, and for the development of a pariah prison economy (e.g., sexual violence; Wortley, 2003). In an effort to improve the deteriorating conditions, judicial intervention surged from the 1960s to the 1980s (Dilulio, 1990). A coalesced concern for civil liberties, prisoners' rights, and scholarly research documenting the physical and psychological impact of incarceration in the absence of social and psychological supports led to progressive, constitutionally supported reforms within the American penal system (Appelbaum, 1994).

Beginning in the late twentieth century, researchers noted that a significant decline in criminality had occurred across the United States. However, unprecedented prison population growth coupled with rapid correctional facility expansion continued unabated (Mauer, 2011). In 2014, by most accounts, the number of criminally confined individuals in jails and/or prisons exceeds 2.7 million. This figure does not account for the collateral harm that extends to the family members of those incarcerated (Chesney-Lind & Mauer, 2003; Clear & Frost, 2013). Moreover, the total number of persons with serious mental illness in prisons and jails is larger than the total number of psychiatric hospital patients (Lamb & Weinberger, 1998), making the delivery of effective correctional psychiatric services and social programming both fiscally unsustainable and clinically untenable. These institutional dynamics persist today, especially when noting that at least 40% of persons with severe mental illnesses are at some point in their lives housed in jails and/or prisons (Torrey, Kennard, Lamb, & Pavle, 2010). Moreover, the conditions of imprisonment in the twenty-first century remain problematic (e.g., overcrowded and underfunded), with an emphasis on retributive penal practices. Examples include reliance on "supermax" secure housing units to mass incarcerate, deployment of long-term disciplinary and administrative solitary confinement, and dependence on digitized security and surveillance systems to officially monitor inmates (Arrigo, Bersot, & Sellers, 2011).

Mental illness and the american correctional system

Just as correctional institutions have evolved over time by way of their shifting purposes, standards, and practices, so too has the type of treatment inmates receive. Throughout the nineteenth and early twentieth centuries, the purpose of imprisonment in the United States was to rehabilitate (McGee, 1969). Indeed, the very name *penitentiary*—a popular descriptor used during this period—indicated that prisons were more than just a place to house transgressors (Cullen & Gendreau, 2000). Religious values principally motivated this commitment to the rehabilitative ideal until it was professionalized in the twentieth century in the form of individual treatment (Palermo, 2013). The professionalization of correctional treatment changed the way recovery and reform were defined and the conditions under which both occur.

Throughout the latter portion of the twentieth century to the present, individualized rehabilitation has dominated prison psychiatry. An important part of this philosophy is determining which antisocial characteristics an inmate possesses and/or which critical thinking errors an inmate exhibits that cause criminal conduct (Andrews & Bonta, 2010). This assessment and diagnostic approach to offender treatment became a starting point for predicting and controlling criminal predispositions, thoughts, and behaviors. The aim was to better address the offender's clinical needs and to better protect the community's security (Cullen & Gendreau, 2000).

Diagnosis requires clinicians to examine individual behavior, symptoms, and mental capacity in ways that label or classify offenders (Shipley & Arrigo, 2001). Critics of this approach have suggested that "almost any offender in a correctional setting is hypothetically entitled to a diagnosis of antisocial personality disorder (ASPD)" (Toch, 1998, p. 149). Moreover, by focusing on criminal behavior, clinical symptoms, and mental capacity, other researchers have warned that an "overdiagnosis of psychopathy in criminal populations" is likely to follow (Hart & Hare, 1997, p. 23). As predicted, the prevalence rates for ASPD and psychopathy are alarmingly high. According to most estimates, nearly 50% to 80% of offenders are diagnosed with ASPD, and 15% to 30% are diagnosed with psychopathy (e.g., Gacono, 2000). The justification for relying on the diagnosis of psychopathy is that accurate identification is "for the offender's own good and for the good of those with

whom the psychopath interacts" (Shipley & Arrigo, 2001, p. 409). Conversely, some mental health practitioners question whether investing in this sort of deficit-oriented language and logic furthers the collective goal of structurally transforming correctional treatment by humanizing offender rehabilitation (Polizzi, Braswell, & Draper, 2014).

Arguably, clinical risk assessment, diagnosis, and treatment have become more sophisticated given advances in psychopharmacological medicine, actuarial rigor in social science methodologies, and precision in diagnostic techniques and analytics. Regrettably, the fate of prisoners classified as mentally ill has not similarly progressed. Incarceration is difficult on one's mental health because of the "overcrowding, violence, lack of privacy, lack of meaningful activities, isolation from family and friends, uncertainty about life after prison, and inadequate health services" (Fellner, 2006, p. 391). Numerous studies report the rise in the number of mentally ill persons in the prison system (Torrey et al., 2010). Moreover, the swelling number of inmates with psychiatric disorders found in correctional settings today has converted jails and prisons into ill-equipped de facto institutions that warehouse the mentally ill, much like in the nineteenth century. Indeed, while American prison systems are beginning to implement some novel accommodations for persons with psychiatric disorders (e.g., specialized rehabilitation units, diversion through mental health court), those with mental illness are often subjected to the same punitive treatment of isolative confinement that was popular during the nineteenth century (Fellner, 2006). Prison segregation only amplifies the lack of adequate care available for those who need or could benefit from mental health treatment, and it exacerbates the detrimental impact such custodial care has on prisoners who experience or are otherwise susceptible to psychiatric symptoms and/or illness (Haney, 2006).

The US prison system has always struggled to determine clinical correctives and rehabilitative treatments to assist mentally ill offenders. Current correctional policies that target inmates with psychiatric disorders balance the ideals of individual liberty against the demands of institutional safety and the need for public welfare (Arrigo et al., 2011). Mindful of the inadequate delivery of psychiatric services found in many American prisons, several international covenants and a number of human rights activists have called for an overhaul of policies that affect persons with a mental disability (Perlin, 2011). In fact, the United Nations Standard Minimum Rules for the Treatment of Prisoners recognizes that some prisoners with serious mental illness should not be subjected to imprisonment at all (Fellner, 2006; Haney, 2006). While much of the focus is on improving conditions within correctional institutions, researchers contend that the "most effective way to ensure that the rights of mentally ill offenders are protected is to try to keep them out of prison in the first place" (Fellner, 2006, p. 411). This would require an increase in community-based programming and court-ordered mental health services, a consideration of the offender's mental status in judicial policies such as mandatory minimum sentencing, and a restructuring of the pretrial process in which psychiatrically disordered offenders would be identified (e.g., Appelbaum, 1994). Thus, while the diagnosis of mental illness has become more sophisticated over time, the treatment of the mentally ill within the prison system has not nearly similarly progressed.

The current era of mass incarceration

Beginning in the 1980s a transition in judicial and penal policy emerged that would have an unprecedented impact on the US imprisonment system. The "law-and-order" philosophy began to resurface, especially during the presidential campaign of Richard Nixon (Beckett, 1997). This tough-on-crime agenda gained momentum during the 1970s and peaked in 1982 when President Ronald Reagan announced his infamous War on Drugs campaign (Alexander, 2010). This initiative was accompanied by a sizeable increase in antidrug initiatives and the emergence of crack cocaine markets in inner-city communities. It set the stage for the current and disproportionate rates of incarceration for black and brown men in the United States. This shift also marked a significant change in public opinion. By 1989, 64% of Americans believed that the sale and distribution of illicit drugs was the most important societal issue confronting the country (Beckett, 1997). By the early 1990s, with mounting support from the public and with surges in county, state, and federal law enforcement budgets, a system of racialized justice began to populate American cities and towns (Alexander, 2010). By 1991, nearly a fourth of young African American males were under some form of incarceration or social control administered by the correctional industry. Between 1985 and 2000, convictions for drug offenses accounted for about two thirds of the rise in federally housed prisoners (Mauer, 2006). To date, the most telling consequence of the War on Drugs initiative is that more than 31 million people have been arrested and convicted for these criminal offenses, leading to systematic mass incarceration that adversely and unequally affects people of color (Alexander, 2010; Mauer & King, 2007).

The number of African Americans incarcerated under the guise of the War on Drugs campaign is alarming. By 2000, seven states reported that African Americans accounted for 80% to 90% of all criminally confined drug offenders (Human Rights Watch, 2000). Nationwide, between 1983 and 2000, the number of African Americans incarcerated for drug crimes increased by a factor of 26; for Latino offenders during the same period the number increased by a factor of 22 (Travis, 2002). These figures stand in stark contrast to the rate of incarceration for white offenders, who witnessed only an 8% increase compared to their minority counterparts. This finding is particularly troubling given that the majority of illegal drug users and dealers in the United States are white (Mauer, King, & Young, 2004).

By 2013, both national and state governments began to recognize the fiscal and social impact of the 40-year overincarceration trend (Clear & Frost, 2013). Since 1980, the federal prison population has increased every year. In 2009, Americans were in prison at the rate of 760 per 100,000 citizens; this is 5 times the rate in Britain, 8 times the rate in Germany, and 12 times the rate in Japan (Global Public Square, 2013). The reality of US imprisonment is that the country incarcerates the largest number of people worldwide at a rate that is four times that of the planet's average (Hartney, 2006). While the sheer number of convicts represents a considerable social control and institutional management problem—particularly as it disproportionately affects low-income minority males—a fiscal problem also undeniably exists. The United States spends nearly $42 billion annually on the prison-industrial complex. Despite this exorbitant spending, the system is still regularly sued by individuals for failure to meet minimum standards of health and safety (Hartney, 2006).

Summary

Confronted with the reality of racialized justice and an imprisonment culture that struggles to cultivate, much less implement, sorely needed rehabilitative prescriptions, correctional psychiatry now increasingly directs its clinical attention to the challenges of treating the psychopathology of Internet harassers, cyber stalkers, and virtual sexual predators (Gunn, 2000). Coupled with these novel and mostly untested directions is the application of cognitive neuroscience to forensic and correctional settings (Garland, 2011; Gazzaniga, 2009). For example, restoring the death row inmate's competence for purposes of state-sanctioned execution raises serious questions about the legal limits of individual privacy rights, the "soft" science of functional magnetic resonance imaging technology, and medicine's responsibilities to professionally navigate the clinical ethics of both (e.g., Arrigo, 2007). Thorny directions and complex developments such as these await the attention of correctional psychiatry as it responds to the legal, fiscal, and social constraints of penal policy and the future of American imprisonment.

References

Alexander, M. (2010). *The new Jim Crow: Mass incarceration in the age of colorblindness*. New York: New Press.

Andrews, D. A., & Bonta, J. (2010). *The psychology of criminal conduct* (5th ed.). Cincinnati, OH: Anderson Publishing.

Appelbaum, P. S. (1994). *Almost a revolution: Mental health law and the limits of change*. New York: Oxford University Press.

Arrigo, B. A. (2007). Punishment, freedom, and the culture of control: The case of brain imaging and the law. *American Journal of Law and Medicine, 33*(3), 457–482.

Arrigo, B. A., Bersot, H., & Sellers, B. G. (2011). *The ethics of total confinement: A critique of madness, citizenship and social justice*. New York: Oxford University Press.

Barnes, H. E. (1968). *The evolution of penology in Pennsylvania: A study in American social history*. Montclair, NJ: Patterson Smith.

Beckett, K. (1997). *Making crime pay: Law and order in contemporary American politics*. New York: Oxford University Press.

Chesney-Lind, M., & Mauer, M. (2003). *Invisible punishment: The collateral consequences of mass incarceration*. New York: New Press.

Clear, T. R., & Frost, N. A. (2013). *The punishment imperative, the rise and failure of mass incarceration in America*. New York: NYU Press.

Cullen, F. T., & Gendreau, P. (2000). Assessing correctional rehabilitation: Policy, practice and prospects, United States. *Criminal Justice, 3*, 109–175.

Cullen, F. T., & Gilbert, K. E. (1982). *Reaffirming rehabilitation*. Cincinnati, OH: Anderson Publishing.

De Beaumont, G. A. D., De Tocqueville, C. A., & Lieber, F. (1833). *On the penitentiary system in the United States and its application in France*. Translated from the French, with an introduction, notes and additions by F. Lieber. Philadelphia: Carey, Lea & Blanchard.

Dilulio, J. J. (1990). *Courts, corrections, and the constitution*. New York: Oxford University Press.

Dumm, T. L. (1987). *Democracy and punishment*. Madison: University of Wisconsin Press.

Fellner, J. (2006). A corrections quandary: Mental illness and prison rules. *Harvard Civil Rights-Civil Liberties Law Review, 41*, 391–412.

Ferracuti, F. (1989). *Carcere e trattamento [prisons and treatment], Trattato di Criminologia, Medicina Criminologica e Psichiatria Forense [Treatise on Criminology, Criminological Medicine and Forensic Psychiatry]* (vol. 11). Milan: Giuffre.

Foucault, M. (1979). *Discipline and punish: The birth of the prison* (A. Sheridan, Trans.). New York: Vintage.

Gacono, C. (2000). *The clinical and forensic assessment of psychopathy: A practitioner's guide.* New York: Routledge.

Garland, B. (2011). *Neuroscience and the law: Brain, mind, and the scales of justice.* New York: Dana Press.

Gazzaniga, M. S. (2009). *The ethical brain.* New York: Dana Press.

Gillin, J. L. (1926). *Criminology and penology.* London: Jonathan Cape.

Global Public Square (2013). U.S. wakes up to prison nightmare. Retrieved from http://globalpublicsquare.blogs.cnn.com/2013/08/17/u-s-wakes-up-to-its-prison-nightmare/.

Gunn, J. (2000). Future directions for treatment in forensic psychiatry. *British Journal of Psychiatry, 176,* 332–338.

Haney, C. (2006). *Reforming prisons: Psychological limits to the pains of imprisonment.* Washington, DC: APA Books.

Hart, S. D., & Hare, J. D. (1997). Psychopathy: Assessment and association with criminal conduct. In D. M. Stoff, J. Breiling, & J. D. Maser (Eds.), *Handbook of antisocial behavior* (pp. 22–35). New York: John Wiley.

Hartney, C. (2006). U.S. rates of incarceration: A global perspective (FOCUS). Retrieved from http://www.issuelab.org/permalink/resource/2634.

Hirsch, A. J. (1982). *From pillory to penitentiary: The rise of criminal incarceration in early Massachusetts.* Ann Arbor: Michigan Law Review Association.

Human Rights Watch (2000). Punishment and prejudice: racial disparities in the war on drugs. *HRW Reports, 12,* 2.

Lamb, H. R., & Weinberger, L. E. (1998). Persons with severe mental illness in jails and prisons: A review. *Psychiatric Services, 49,* 483–492.

Lewis, W. D. (1965). *From Newgate to Dannemora: The rise of the penitentiary in New York, 1796–1848.* Ithaca, NY: Cornell University Press.

Mauer, M. (2006). *Race to incarcerate* (rev. ed.). New York: New Press.

Mauer, M. (2011). Sentencing reform: Amid mass incarcerations-guarded optimism. *Criminal Justice, 26,* 27–36.

Mauer, M., & King, R. S. (2007). *A 25-year quagmire the war on drugs and its impact on American society.* Washington, DC: Sentencing Project.

Mauer, M., King, R. S., & Young, M. C. (2004). *The meaning of "life": Long prison sentences in context.* Washington, DC: Sentencing Project.

McGee, R. A. (1969). What's past is prologue. *Annals of the American Academy of Political and Social Science, 381,* 1–10.

McGowen, R. (1995). Well-ordered prison: England, 1780–1865. In N. Morries & D. Rothman (Eds.), *Oxford history of the prison: The practice of punishment in Western society* (pp. 79–109). New York: Oxford.

Meskell, M. W. (1999). An American resolution: The history of prisons in the United States from 1777 to 1877. *Stanford Law Review, 51,* 839–865.

Morris, N. (1995). The contemporary prison. In N. Morries & D. Rothman (Eds.), *Oxford history of the prison: The practice of punishment in Western society* (pp. 227–259). New York: Oxford.

Palermo, G. B. (2013). Evolution of punishment and incarceration. In N. Konrad, B. Vollm, & D. N. Weisstub (Eds.), *Ethical issues in prison psychiatry.* New York: Springer.

Palermo, G. B., & White, M. A. (1998). *Letters from prison: A cry for justice.* Springfield, IL: Charles C. Thomas.

Perlin, M. L. (2011). *International human rights and mental disability law: When the silenced are heard.* New York: Oxford University Press.

Pfohl, S. J. (2009). *Images of deviance and social control: A sociological history.* Grove, IL: Waveland Press.

Polizzi, D., Braswell, M., & Draper, M. (2014). *Transforming corrections: Humanistic approaches to corrections and offender treatment* (2nd ed.). Durham, NC: Academic Press.

Roth, M. P. (2006). *Prisons and prison systems.* Westport, CT: Greenwood Press.

Rothman, D. J. (2002). *Conscience and convenience: The asylum and its alternatives in progressive America.* New York: Aldine Transaction.

Scull, A. (2006). *The insanity of place/the place of insanity: Essays on the history of psychiatry.* New York: Routledge.

Shipley, S., & Arrigo, B. A. (2001). The confusion over psychopathy (II): Implications for forensic (correctional) practice. *International Journal of Offender Therapy and Comparative Criminology, 45,* 407–420.

Toch, H. (1998). Psychopathy or antisocial personality disorder in forensic settings. In T. Millon, E. Simonsen, M. Birket-Smith, & R. D. Davis (Eds.), *Psychopathy: Antisocial, criminal and violent behavior* (pp. 144–158). New York: Guilford.

Torrey, E. F., Kennard, A. D., Lamb, H. R., & Pavle, J. (2010). *More mentally ill persons are in jails and prisons than hospitals: A survey of the states.* Arlington, VA: Treatment Advocacy Center.

Travis, J. (2002). *But they all come back: Facing the challenges of prisoner reentry.* Washington, DC: Urban Institute Press.

US Department of Justice (1939). *The Attorney General's survey of release procedures digest of federal and state laws on release procedures.* Washington, DC: US Government Printing Office.

Wortley, R. (2003). *Situational prison control: Crime prevention in correctional institutions.* New York: Cambridge University Press.

CHAPTER 2

Mental illness management in corrections

Charles L. Scott and Brian Falls

Introduction

An increasing number of individuals with mental illness are now treated in correctional environments instead of community settings. In the incarcerated population, prevalence estimates of serious mental illness (SMI) range from 9% to 20% (Beck & Maruschak, 2000; Diamond, Wang, Holzer, Thomas, & Cruser, 2001; Regier, Farmer, Rae, Locke, Keith, Judd, & Goodwin, 1990; Steadman, Osher, Robbins, Case, & Samuels, 2009) compared to 6% in the community (Kessler, Chiu, Demler, & Walters, 2005). More astonishingly, in 2005, more than three times as many persons with serious mental illness in the United States were located in jails and prisons than in hospitals (Torrey, Kennard, Eslinger, Lamb, & Pavle, 2010). It was not always like this. How did US correctional systems become *de facto* mental health institutions for so many? Scholars point to a number of reasons for the increasing prevalence of mental illness among incarcerated individuals, including deinstitutionalization, limited community resources, prominent court decisions and legislative rulings, and the "revolving door" phenomenon (Talbott, 2004; Yohanna, 2013). This chapter summarizes the historical context of correctional versus community mental health; factors that result in the increasing management of people with mental illness in correctional settings; and similarities and differences between the provision of mental health care in correctional versus community settings.

Historical context of correctional versus community mental health care

Mental illness has existed in the United States since the nation began (de Young, 2010; Eldridge, 1996). Individuals with mental illness who lived during colonial times often relied on families or friends to care for them. If their relatives or friends could not or would not care for them, they typically became homeless or incarcerated. Until the mid-eighteenth century, this segment of the "insane," as they were called, ended up in the same institutions as criminals—houses of correction and workhouses—even if they had not committed a crime (de Young, 2010).

The establishment of Philadelphia's Pennsylvania Hospital in 1751 marked the start of a new era, one in which the disposition of these two populations differed. Shortly after this general hospital—the nation's first—opened, it accepted patients with mental illness (de Young, 2010; Graham, 2008), almost assuredly diverting some from correctional settings.

Despite a dedicated environment for the treatment of mental illness in the new hospital, patients initially encountered conditions similar to those previously experienced by people with psychiatric problems in correctional settings. For example, they were locked in the "damp and unwholesome" cellar of the hospital (Graham, 2008) and, not uncommonly, chained (de Young, 2010). However, a noteworthy distinction existed between the purposes of confinement in houses of correction and those of the new hospital: instead of simply enclosing individuals, the hospital attempted to treat their mental illnesses.

By 1773, Virginia had constructed the "Public Hospital for Persons of Insane and Disordered Minds," the country's first building devoted solely to treating individuals with mental illness. The hospital's first patient was transferred from the local jail (Zwelling, 1985), perhaps a progressive recognition that people with mental illness deserve treatment instead of punishment. By today's standards, the available treatments were undoubtedly inadequate. However, the shift represented, if nothing more, a developing contrast in the physical location between those with mental illness and those convicted of a crime.

In the following years, the number of individuals institutionalized for mental illness grew, and states accordingly built more asylums. Most of these institutions emphasized a more humane psychological approach to the custody and care of individuals with psychiatric disease, which was in accordance with French physician Philippe Pinel's "moral treatment" (de Young, 2010).

Over time, provision of care diverged from this more humane approach. As the number of patients at facilities swelled, asylum populations outgrew their funding, effectively decreasing staff-to-patient ratios (de Young, 2010). As they became progressively less equipped to manage their ever-growing populations, the quality of care provided by understaffed hospital units deteriorated (Wright, 1997). After World War II (de Young, 2010; Torrey, Fuller, Geller, Jacobs, & Ragosta, 2012), the general public began to increasingly view psychiatric hospitals as cruel (de Young, 2010; Talbott, 2004), "run-down archaic establishments that simply housed the mentally ill" (Testa & West, 2010).

Factors resulting in increased management of persons with mental illness in correctional settings

Deinstitutionalization and limited community resources

Increasing public attention to the inhumane conditions of these facilities, along with several other sociocultural and economic factors, led to a "shift in the locus of care" from public psychiatric hospitals to the community (Koyanagi, 2007). At its peak in 1955, there were 560,000 individuals living in state hospitals across the United States (Borus, 1981; Koyanagi, 2007; Talbott, 2004). By 2010, the state hospital census was less than 9% of its 1955 total (Torrey et al., 2012). This movement of individuals from public hospitals into the community came to be known as "deinstitutionalization" (Borus, 1981; Lamb & Bachrach, 2001; Talbott, 2004).

As stated previously, several factors led to this phenomenon. After World War II, the public's attention was increasingly drawn to the poor living conditions in state psychiatric hospitals (Scull, 1981). The late 1940s and early 1950s saw the introduction of far more effective treatments, such as lithium and chlorpromazine, that allowed physicians to safely release some patients into the community (de Young, 2010). In the 1960s, a subset of attorneys advocated for the "liberation" of patients from psychiatric hospitals (Geller, 2000; Scull, 1981).

The 1960s also saw the development of programs (Supplemental Security Income [SSI], Social Security Disability Insurance, Medicaid, and Medicare) that used federal dollars to provide financial assistance for people with mental illness in the community (Koyanagi, 2007). By and large, state hospital patients were not eligible for SSI or Medicaid (Gronfein, 1985). States discharged these patients, thereby shifting the financial burden from state-funded hospitals to these federally funded programs (Gronfein, 1985; Koyanagi, 2007; Searight & Handal, 1988).

Although the intent was to support independent living in the community, deinstitutionalization, in reality, resulted in homelessness and movement into various *de facto* psychiatric institutions for many patients (Koyanagi, 2007; Lamb & Weinberger, 1998; Searight & Handal, 1988; Szasz, 2007). Such institutions included correctional settings (Lamb & Weinberger, 2005; Talbott, 2004). Although scholars disagree whether a causal relationship exists (Osher & Han, 2002; Prins, 2011), many believe deinstitutionalization is the primary contributor to the growth of inmates with psychiatric disorders in jails and prisons (Lamb & Weinberger, 2005; Talbott, 2004). A retrospective study in the 1980s determined that successful "deinstitutionalization appears to depend on the availability of appropriate programs for care in the community" (Braun, Kochansky, Shapiro, Greenberg, Gudeman, Johnson, & Shore, 1981). However, as state hospital populations transitioned back into communities, states did not provide sufficient treatment to the ever-growing nonhospitalized population (Cameron, 1989; Koyanagi, 2007).

The US Community Mental Health Act of 1963 provided federal grants to establish community mental health programs in anticipation of the discharge of state hospital patients (Koyanagi, 2007; Slovenko, 2003). Although it theoretically was a reasonable idea, the program was underfunded (Koyanagi, 2007). President Reagan's Omnibus Budget Reconciliation Act of 1981 overturned the previous administration's Mental Health Systems Act and discontinued the federal government's direct provision of services to people with mental illness (Bazelon Center for Mental Health Law, 2011; Cameron, 1989). Federal mental health spending declined by nearly a third from 1980 to 1982 (Marmor & Gill, 1989). By 1985, the federal government funded only about 11% of community mental health agency budgets (Eichman, Griffin, Lyons, Larson, & Finkel, 1992). Since the passage of the 1973 Health Maintenance Organization Act, the growth of managed care organizations has decreased inpatient lengths of stay (Parsons, 2006). Between 2009 and 2012, states cut $4.35 billion in public mental health funding, the largest reduction since deinstitutionalization (Glover, Miller, & Sadowski, 2012).

Prominent court decisions and legislative policy

In the 1960s and 1970s, courts increased the threshold for civil commitment, enhancing the right to autonomy and increasing the difficulty of hospitalizing individuals (Perlin, 2007). As a result, involuntary hospitalizations decreased in frequency and duration (Peters, Miller, Schmidt, & Meeter, 1987). Some persons with mental illness who no longer met civil commitment criteria remained unaided in the community, some unwilling or unable to pursue outpatient treatment. This lack of access to care in the community increased the likelihood of criminal behavior by untreated persons with mental illness. Unsurprisingly, there was an associated growth in correctional populations. California exemplified this pattern; the number of people with psychiatric illness in one county jail doubled within a year of passing a new civil commitment statute, the Lanterman–Petris–Short Act (Abramson, 1972).

Meanwhile, legislators passed statutes promoting harsher sentencing. Led by Texas in 1974, most states have now enacted "three-strikes" laws (Tonry, 2013), while the federal government approved lengthy determinate sentences for drug offenders. Passage of drug-related laws throughout the years has led to an inflation in drug-related incarcerations (Austin, Clark, Hardyman, & Henry, 2000; Lurigio, 2000; Spencer, 1995). US statutes that criminalize drug use and distribution date back a century to the 1914 passage of the Harrison Act. The Anti-Drug Abuse Act of 1986 mandated a 5- to 40-year sentence, without parole, for first-time offenders convicted of possession with intent to distribute certain quantities of heroin, cocaine, phencyclidine, lysergic acid diethylamide (LSD), or marijuana (Spencer, 1995). The 1994 Violent Crime Control and Law Enforcement Act expanded the use of mandatory minimums for drug and drug-related offenses (Spencer, 1995). The number and duration of drug-related incarcerations have grown with these laws (Austin et al., 2000; Lurigio, 2000; Spencer, 1995) to the point where more than four of five inmates now have a history of drug use (Karberg & James, 2005; Karberg & Mumola, 2006). As the number of incarcerated drug users has risen, so too has the percentage of inmates with psychiatric and substance use diagnoses (Lurigio, 2000).

"Revolving door" incarcerations

The "revolving door" metaphor was initially used to describe frequent rehospitalizations and decreased durations of hospitalizations of homeless individuals with mental illness (Talbott, 1974). However, it has been readapted to reflect the frequent reincarceration of persons with mental illness (Baillargeon, Binswanger, Penn, Williams, & Murray, 2009). One Texas study examined nearly 80,000 inmates from 2000 to 2006, finding that those with a serious mental illness (major depression, bipolar disorders, schizophrenia, and other psychotic disorders) were approximately twice as likely to be reincarcerated as their peers without these diagnoses (Baillargeon et al., 2009). These data are even more impressive when one considers that inmates with mental illness have fewer chances to commit new crimes that may result in reincarceration because they typically receive longer sentences and spend more time incarcerated than in the community. For example, prison inmates with mental illness are incarcerated on average for 12 months longer than other offenders (Ditton, 1999).

Correctional and community care linkages

Correctional and community environments have important similarities and distinctions about the provision of mental health care. These two settings, however, are not isolated islands. In fact, persons with mental illness who face possible arrest may travel over interlinking bridges between correctional and community settings. Figure 2.1 outlines some potential entry and exit points between correctional and community care faced by persons with mental illness upon arrest; it does not include all potential or likely combinations.

How and why an individual with mental illness enters a correctional setting instead of community treatment depends on factors that include criminal history, mental health history, local jurisdictional attitudes and approaches, police training, and, not infrequently, chance.

Vignette: Dual diagnosis and treatment non-adherence

Joe is a 28-year-old male with bipolar disorder and alcohol and methamphetamine use. He lives with his mother and has been treated in the community with a mood stabilizer, which he frequently refuses to take. One evening, after snorting methamphetamine, he became paranoid that his mother was working with the FBI to have him killed. He confronted her; she told him he needed to take his medicine and then tried to call his doctor. He pushed her while grabbing for the phone, and she fell to the floor and bruised her arm. She called 911. When the police arrived, they noticed small bruises and a small cut on the mother's arm. She acknowledged that Joe pushed her, which resulted in the injuries. Joe's mother begged the police to take Joe to the local emergency room because he "needs immediate treatment." She stated that she did not want to press charges, her injuries were an accident, and Joe had no intent to harm her.

At this point, the police play a critical role in how Joe's life will unfold. If they use their discretion and take Joe to the local emergency room instead of jail, Joe may be completely diverted from the criminal justice system. In contrast, if the police decide that Joe should be criminally charged for his actions, they will likely take him to the local jail or detention facility. Depending on Joe's local jurisdiction and available resources, he might be diverted to a mental health court or community treatment, or kept in the jail awaiting charges, where he might not have access to inpatient

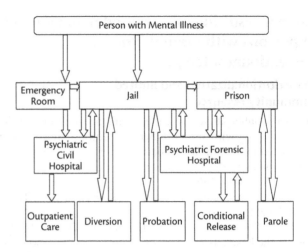

Fig. 2.1 Entry and exit points between correctional and community care.

psychiatric care. Due to Joe's mental illness, his attorney could question Joe's competency to stand trial. If Joe is found incompetent, he may be transferred to a state hospital in some jurisdictions, again crossing the threshold between corrections and community. If Joe is found to be nonrestorable, he might be released to the community for treatment or committed for a longer period depending on whether he meets statutory criteria for continued commitment. If restored to competency, Joe would reenter the correctional system, where he could accept a plea bargain (if one is offered) or proceed to trial. Because Joe has a major mental illness, his attorney could raise the issue of his mental state and criminal responsibility if allowed by state statute.

If found not criminally responsible for his assault on his mother, Joe will likely return to a state hospital for continued commitment until he is determined safe for release. If found guilty, Joe may serve time in jail or prison. Some states would allow Joe to be involuntarily committed to a state hospital at the end of his prison term as a mentally disordered offender (MDO) if his mental disorder played a substantial role in his crime and he continued to have symptoms that pose a risk of danger to others. If Joe does not qualify as an MDO and is released from prison, he may have strict parole requirements to continue mental health treatment and refrain from substance use. If Joe violates his conditions of parole, he could be returned to prison. In some states, if Joe had committed a qualifying sexual offense, he could be evaluated to determine if he meets criteria for indefinite commitment as a sexually violent predator.

As this vignette illustrates, incarcerated individuals may shuttle between correctional and community treatment systems, like a vehicle on a complicated highway with numerous on and off ramps and frequent detours. Despite this confusing maze of possibilities, there are several similarities and differences between the provision of correctional and community mental health care. These similarities and differences are summarized below.

Similarities and differences between correctional and community mental health care
Standards of care
Both community and correctional mental health providers are expected to follow general standards of care. In addressing

whether the standards should differ for incarcerated individuals, the American Psychiatric Association (2000, p. 6) stated

> The fundamental policy goal for correctional mental health care is to provide the same level of mental health services to each patient in the criminal justice process that should be available in the community. This policy goal is deliberately higher than the "community standard" that is called for in various legal contexts.

Tort law governs the legal resolution of complaints about medical treatment and applies in both correctional and community settings. Negligent torts occur when a clinician's behavior unintentionally causes an unreasonable risk of harm to another. The four elements required to establish medical negligence are commonly known as the "four Ds": Dereliction of Duty that Directly results in Damages.

Correctional mental health care differs in the availability of additional legal mechanisms that inmates may use to address concerns about their care. For example, inmates may sue, claiming that the care provided, or not provided, violates their constitutional rights. In *Estelle v. Gamble* (1976), the US Supreme Court attempted to define the constitutional standard of care for prison inmates. J.W. Gamble was a prison inmate who claimed that his constitutional rights were violated because, in part, an X-ray was not ordered to evaluate his complaint of back pain. The Court in *Gamble* noted that although a failure to obtain an X-ray or use additional diagnostic techniques may represent negligence, the presence of medical malpractice alone does not represent a constitutional violation: "Medical malpractice does not become a constitutional violation merely because the victim is a prisoner" (*Estelle v. Gamble*, 1976). The Court noted that a violation of an inmate's constitutional rights is established if prison personnel demonstrate "deliberate indifference" to a prisoner's "serious illness or injury." In the subsequent case of *Farmer v. Brennan* (1994) the Court defined "deliberate indifference" as follows:

> A prison official may be held liable under the Eighth Amendment for acting with "deliberate indifference" to inmate health or safety only if he knows that inmates face a substantial risk of danger of serious harm and disregards that risk by failing to take reasonable measures.

Provision of mental health care

There are many similarities between correctional and community mental health care services. Both systems typically provide appropriate medications, emergency care, hospitalization, medication management, and follow-up care. However, key differences often exist in correctional systems, including restricted formularies due to concerns of medication abuse or cost, alternative involuntary medication procedures, restricted access by visitors, and the inability of mental health providers to control the treatment environment. In particular, decisions on the placement of inmates with mental illness may involve important custody considerations such as security level and potential for harm from other inmates (e.g., rival gang members or known enemies). Additional treatment considerations in custodial environments include increased limitations on confidentiality and "dual-role" issues when correctional providers need to reveal information for inmate discipline or placement evaluations.

Discharge and follow-up care

Correctional settings are increasingly expected to arrange follow-up care for released inmates. Several cases that examine this expectation suggest the following guidelines (*Brad H v. City of New York*, 2000; *Lugo v. Senkowski*, 2000; *Wakefield v. Thompson*, 1999):

♦ Provide psychiatric medications sufficient for an inmate to reasonably access a treating provider in the community;

♦ Coordinate discharge planning and reentry into the community when feasible; and

♦ Consider monitoring and further intervention necessary for treatment that is begun but not completed.

Such increasing expectations for correctional providers pose potential challenges because of key differences when compared to community settings. In particular, inmate release is generally not under the control of the correctional provider and, in some circumstances, inmates may be released with little or no notice. In addition, depending on the location of the jail or prison, the correctional provider may have a limited, if any, relationship with community treatment providers, particularly when the inmate returns to a community far from the correctional institution.

Summary

What began as a good-intentioned separation of criminals and people with mental illness in the late eighteenth century has ended in mass incarceration of individuals with psychiatric and substance use disorders. The population of incarcerated individuals with psychiatric illness continues to grow in the wake of deinstitutionalization, scant community resources, and a changing legal landscape. Many factors determine how and why individuals with mental illness are treated in correctional settings as opposed to community settings. There are numerous interlinking bridges between these two worlds. Understanding these multiple pathways is crucial for navigating the mental health care delivery systems inside and outside the walls of detention.

References

Abramson, M. F. (1972). The criminalization of mentally disordered behavior: Possible side-effect of a new mental health law. *Hospital and Community Psychiatry*, 23, 101–105.

American Psychiatric Association (2000). *Psychiatric services in jails and prisons* (2nd ed.). Washington, DC: American Psychiatric Association.

Austin, J., Clark, J., Hardyman, P., & Henry, D. A. (2000). Three strikes and you're out: The implementation and impart of strike laws. Retrieved from https://www.ncjrs.gov/pdffiles1/nij/grants/181297.pdf

Baillargeon, J., Binswanger, I. A., Penn, J. V., Williams, B. A., & Murray, O. J. (2009). Psychiatric disorders and repeat incarcerations: The revolving prison door. *American Journal of Psychiatry*, 166(1), 103–109.

Bazelon Center for Mental Health Law (2011). Funding for mental health services and programs. Retrieved from http://www.bazelon.org/LinkClick.aspx?fileticket=GzmAbAweikQ%3D&tabid=436

Beck, A. J., & Maruschak, L. M. (2000). Mental health treatment in state prisons, 2000. Retrieved from http://www.bjs.gov/content/pub/pdf/mhtsp00.pdf

Borus, J. F. (1981). Sounding board. Deinstitutionalization of the chronically mentally ill. *New England Journal of Medicine*, 305, 339–342.

Brad H v. City of New York, 712 N.Y.S.2d 336 (Sup. Ct. 2000); 716 N.Y.S.2d 852 (N.Y. App. Div. 2000).

Braun, P., Kochansky, G., Shapiro, R., Greenberg, S., Gudeman, J. E., Johnson, S., & Shore, M. F. (1981). Overview: Deinstitutionalization of psychiatric patients, a critical review of outcome studies. *American Journal of Psychiatry, 138*(6), 736–749.

Cameron, J. M. (1989). A national community mental health program: Policy initiation and progress. In: D. Rochefort (Ed.), *Handbook on mental health policy in the United States* (pp. 121–142). New York: Greenwood Press.

de Young, M. (2010). *Madness: An American history of mental illness and its treatment.* Jefferson, NC: McFarland & Company.

Diamond, P. M., Wang, E. W., Holzer, C. E., Thomas, C., & Cruser, D. A. (2001). The prevalence of mental illness in prison. *Administration and Policy in Mental Health and Mental Health Services Research, 29*(1), 21–40.

Ditton, P. M. (1999). *Mental health and treatment of inmates and probationers.* Washington, DC: Bureau of Justice Statistics. Retrieved from http://www.bjs.gov/content/pub/pdf/mhtip.pdf

Eichman, M. A., Griffin, B. P., Lyons, J. S., Larson, D. B., & Finkel, S. (1992). An estimation of the impact of OBRA-87 on nursing home care in the United States. *Hospital & Community Psychiatry, 43*(8), 781–789.

Eldridge, L. D. (1996). Crazy brained: Mental illness in colonial America. *Bulletin of the History of Medicine, 70*(3), 361–386.

Estelle v. Gamble, 429 U.S. 97 (1976).

Farmer v. Brennan, 555 U.S. 825 (1994).

Geller, J. (2000). The last half-century of psychiatric services as reflected in *Psychiatric Services. Psychiatric Services, 51*(1), 41–67.

Glover, R. W., Miller, J. E., & Sadowski, S. R. (2012). Proceedings on the state budget crisis and the behavioral health treatment gap: The impact on public substance abuse and mental health treatment systems. National Association of State Mental Health Program Directors. Retrieved from http://www.nasmhpd.org/docs/Summary-Congressional%20Briefing_March%2022_Website.pdf

Graham, K. A. (2008). *A history of the Pennsylvania Hospital.* Charleston, SC: The History Press.

Gronfein, W. (1985). Psychotropic drugs and the origins of deinstitutionalization. *Social Problems, 32*(5), 437–454.

Karberg, K. C., & James, D. J. (2005). Substance dependence, abuse, and treatment of jail inmates, 2002, Bureau of Justice Statistics, NCJ 209588. Retrieved from http://www.bjs.gov/content/pub/pdf/sdatji02.pdf

Karberg, K. C., & Mumola, C. J. (2006). Drug use and dependence, state and federal prisoners, 2004. Bureau of Justice Statistics, NCJ 213530. Retrieved from http://www.bjs.gov/content/pub/pdf/dudsfp04.pdf

Kessler, R. C., Chiu, W. T., Demler, O., & Walters, E. E. (2005). Prevalence, severity, and comorbidity of twelve-month DSM-IV disorders in the National Comorbidity Survey Replication (NCS-R). *Archives of General Psychiatry, 62*(6), 617–627.

Koyanagi, C. (2007). Learning from history: Deinstitutionalization of people with mental illness as precursor to long-term care reform. The Kaiser Commission on Medicaid and the Uninsured. Retrieved from http://www.nami.org/Template.cfm?Section=About_the_Issue&Template=/ContentManagement/ContentDisplay.cfm&ContentID=137545

Lamb, H. R., & Bachrach, L. L. (2001). Some perspectives on deinstitutionalization. *Psychiatric Services, 52*(8), 1039–1045.

Lamb, H. R., & Weinberger, L. E. (1998). Persons with severe mental illness in jails and prisons: A review. *Psychiatric Services, 49*, 483–492.

Lamb, H. R., & Weinberger, L. E. (2005). The shift of psychiatric inpatient care from hospitals to jails and prisons. *Journal of the American Academy of Psychiatry and the Law, 33*(4), 529–534.

Lugo v. Senkowski, 114 F. Supp.2s 111 (N.D. N.Y. September 25, 2001).

Lurigio, A. J. (2000). Drug treatment availability and effectiveness: Studies of the general and criminal justice populations. *Criminal Justice and Behavior, 27*(4), 495–528.

Marmor, T. R., & Gill, K. C. (1989). The political and economic context of mental health care in the United States. *Journal of Health Politics, Policy and Law, 14*(3), 459–475.

Osher, F. C., & Han, Y. L. (2002). Jails as housing for persons with serious mental illness. *American Jails Magazine, 16*(1), 36–41.

Parsons, T. (2006). Length of stay: Managed care agenda or a measure of clinical efficiency? *Psychiatry, 3*(6), 46–52.

Perlin, M. L. (2007). *Mental disability law: Civil and criminal* (2nd ed.). LexisNexis.

Peters, R., Miller, K.S., Schmidt, W., & Meeter, D. (1987). The effects of statutory change on the civil commitment of the mentally ill. *Journal Law and Human Behavior, 11*(2), 73–99.

Prins, S. J. (2011). Does transinstitutionalization explain the overrepresentation of people with serious mental illnesses in the criminal justice system? *Community Mental Health Journal, 47*(6), 716–722.

Regier, D. A., Farmer, M. E., Rae, D. S., Locke, B. Z., Keith, S. J., Judd, L. L., & Goodwin, F. K. (1990). Comorbidity of mental disorders with alcohol and other drug abuse: results from the Epidemiologic Catchment Area (ECA) study. *Journal of the American Medical Association, 264,* 2511–2518.

Scull, A. (1981). Deinstitutionalization and the rights of the deviant. *Journal of Social Issues, 37*(3), 6–20.

Searight, H. R., & Handal, P. J. (1988). The paradox of psychiatric deinstitutionalization: Historical perspective and policy implications. *Journal of Health and Human Resources Administration, 11*(2), 249–266.

Slovenko, R. (2003). The transinstitutionalization of the mentally ill. *Ohio North University Law Review, 29*(3), 641–660.

Spencer, M. P. (1995). Sentencing drug offenders: The incarceration addiction. *Villanova Law Review, 40*(2), 335–381.

Steadman, H. J., Osher, F. C., Robbins, P. C., Case, B., & Samuels, S. (2009). Prevalence of serious mental illness among jail inmates. *Psychiatric Services, 60*(6), 761–765.

Szasz, T. (2007). *Coercion as cure: a critical history of psychiatry.* New Brunswick, NJ: Transaction.

Talbott, J. A. (1974). Stopping the revolving door: A study of readmissions to a state hospital. *Psychiatric Quarterly, 48,* 159–168.

Talbott, J. A. (2004). Deinstitutionalization: Avoiding the disasters of the past (1979 reprint). *Psychiatric Services, 55*(10), 1112–1115.

Testa, M., & West, S. G. (2010). Civil commitment in the United States. *Psychiatry, 7*(10), 30–40.

Tonry, M. (2013). *Oxford handbook of crime and criminal justice.* New York: Oxford University Press.

Torrey, E. F., Fuller, D.A., Geller, J., Jacobs, C., & Ragosta, K. (2012). *No room at the inn: Trends and consequences of closing public psychiatric hospitals.* Arlington, VA: Treatment Advocacy Center. Retrieved from http://tacreports.org/storage/documents/no_room_at_the_inn-2012.pdf

Torrey, E. F., Kennard, A. D., Eslinger, D., Lamb, R., & Pavle, J. (2010). *More mentally ill persons are in jails and prisons than hospitals: A survey of the states.* Treatment Advocacy Center and National Sheriffs' Association, May.

Wakefield v. Thompson, 177 F.3d 1160 (9th Cir. 1999).

Wright, D. (1997). Getting out of the asylum: Understanding the confinement of the insane in the nineteenth century. *Social History of Medicine, 10*(1), 137–155.

Yohanna, D. (2013). Deinstitutionalization of people with mental illness: Causes and consequences. *American Medical Association Journal of Ethics, 15*(10), 886–891.

Zwelling, S. S. (1985). *Quest for a cure: The Public Hospital in Williamsburg, Virginia, 1773-1885.* Williamsburg, VA: Colonial Williamsburg Foundation.

CHAPTER 3

Formative case law and litigation

Mohamedu F. Jones

Introduction

While it is difficult to measure the accuracy of prevalence rates of the incarcerated mentally ill, virtually every relevant study has concluded that a significant number of prisoners have serious mental illnesses (Sarteschi, 2013; see Chapter 32). Metzner and Fellner (2010) reported that the presence of comprehensive correctional mental health treatment programs and services is often due to successful class action litigation. This chapter reviews the legal and constitutional background for correctional mental health care in the United States and addresses many of the critical ways these courts affect policy and care delivery on a daily basis.

Background and precedent

Several court decisions have shaped modern correctional mental health care delivery. Under the Eighth Amendment, officials are obligated to provide convicted prisoners with adequate medical care (*Estelle v. Gamble*, 1976), which extends to mental health treatment (*Bowring v. Godwin*, 1977). Pretrial detainees also have a right to adequate physical and mental health care under the due process clause of the Fourteenth Amendment (*Bell v. Wolfish*, 1979). To prevail on a claim of constitutionally inadequate care, inmates must show that officials acted with deliberate indifference. There are two components to proving deliberate indifference: the objective element (deprivation was sufficiently serious) and the subjective element (officials acted with a sufficiently culpable state of mind; *Farmer v. Brennan*, 1994; *Wilson v. Seiter*, 1991). In practice, given the similar high threshold of proof required to sustain a claim and the goal of adequate health care, the distinction of constitutional basis upon which the right rests between convicted prisoner and pretrial detainee makes little difference.

In 1996, acting under impressions that 42 USC § 1983 was being abused by frivolous prisoners' lawsuits and clogging up federal courts, and at the urging of several state and local law enforcement and correctional officials, Congress enacted the Prison Litigation Reform Act (PLRA) to regulate prisoners' litigation that involves federal constitutional rights and outcomes. Boston and Manville (2010) described the PLRA as making "litigation by prisoners more difficult, more expensive and less likely to succeed." Provisions of the PLRA that support their conclusion include the requirement for administrative exhaustion prior to filing a complaint and the payment of filing fees. Under the exhaustion requirement, an inmate has to first file a grievance within the correctional system.

If the response is unsatisfactory, the inmate is then required to appeal through to the highest level of the correctional administrative review process and receive a final response before a complaint may be filed and accepted in a federal court.

Limitations were also placed on courts, including restrictions on prospective relief judgments and use of special masters. In cases where prisoners prevailed by proving constitutional violations and a court ordered a remedy, the PLRA grants prison officials the right to file a motion to terminate the remedial order at any point after two years. Once a motion to terminate is filed, the court has a maximum of 90 days to rule on the motion; otherwise, the remedial order is automatically stayed and is no longer in effect. In ruling on a motion to terminate, a court must find "current and ongoing" constitutional violations in order to maintain jurisdiction in the matter and enforce its remedial orders. In some instances, this has resulted in an entirely new trial.

The US Supreme Court addressed involuntary transfers of inmates to psychiatric hospitals for acute care in *Vitek v. Jones* (1980). That decision determined that an inmate may not be involuntarily transferred to a mental hospital without the following: adequate notice that such a transfer is being considered; a written statement of why the transfer is proposed; and an adversarial hearing before an independent decision maker, with appointed counsel if the inmate cannot afford one. State law and regulation may impose more stringent requirements (see Chapter 27). In *Washington v. Harper* (1990) the US Supreme Court held that a convicted prisoner may be involuntarily medicated on a non-emergency basis if prison authorities can show that the medication is medically appropriate for treating a serious mental illness that has made the prisoner a danger to self or to others. As with transfer to psychiatric hospitals, the standard for the use of involuntary medications is often more stringent based on state law and/or regulations (see Chapter 26).

Evolving legal issues

Since the US Supreme Court proclaimed that inmates have a constitutional right to adequate health care, much has been written about the controlling decisions, their implications and applications by courts, and their implementation in correctional systems. There are, however, discrete issues related to mental health care in corrections that patients and providers in prisons and jails contend with daily that may not yet be resolved as matters of constitutional law. In many cases, intermediate appellate courts have not reviewed lower court decisions regarding these issues; these, in turn, have not reached the US Supreme Court. Decisions made by courts with limited jurisdiction or limited precedential value include the exclusion of the seriously mentally ill from segregation, an obligation to fulfill discharge services or other forms of discharge planning, and the absence of health care quality improvement as evidence of deliberate indifference. Other areas, such as mental health input in the disciplinary process, clearly influence mental health conditions in institutions but may not necessarily rise to the level of constitutionally required care. In specific instances, notably the nature of structured and unstructured programming in segregation, experienced correctional mental health experts have recommended specified minimum measures necessary for appropriate clinical care. Such measures may not be required by law but support delivery of quality mental health care. A legal overview of these issues is provided in the following sections.

Mental health input in the disciplinary process

The US Supreme Court has held that following a disciplinary infraction, inmates who violate the rules are not entitled to the full body of constitutional protections in prison disciplinary proceedings available in criminal prosecutions. Minimally, they must be afforded a hearing, timely notice of the offense, and an opportunity to call witnesses and present documentary evidence. Under certain circumstances in the disciplinary proceedings, a counsel substitute or staff assistance may be required to ensure due process protections for inmates.

Mentally ill inmates are frequently involved in the disciplinary process because of rule infractions. Mental illness may contribute to the violation; some inmates were psychotic at the time of their rule violation. Experts have not identified mental health input in the disciplinary process as a specific requirement of a constitutionally adequate prison mental health care system. However, the National Commission on Correctional Health Care (2008a, 2008b), for example, does include mental health input in the disciplinary process as a correctional mental health care compliance indicator. Apparently no court decision has found seriously mentally ill inmates to have a constitutional right to mental health evaluations as part of a prison's disciplinary process. Although it does not appear to be constitutionally required, multiple correctional systems provide for mental health input in their disciplinary process.

Theoretically, a mental health clinician could be called as a witness, and a mental health evaluation related to an infraction, where completed, could conceivably fit the role of documentary evidence in a disciplinary process under *Wolff v. McDonnell* (1974). Dvoskin, Petrila, and Stark-Riemer (1995) noted, however, that *Powell v. Coughlin* (1991) held that inmates have no right to formal mental health evaluations before undergoing disciplinary hearings. More recently, the court in *Matz v. Vandenbook* (2013) questioned whether there was any legal ground that would support a federal court prohibiting prison officials from punishing "prisoners for behavior they cannot control."

Successful lawsuits have resulted in court-ordered or -approved inclusion of mental health input in the disciplinary process in California, New Jersey, and New York. In *D.M. v. Terhune* (1999), the New Jersey Department of Corrections was required to implement disciplinary regulations to mandate mental health input in the process and to consider whether to refer the inmate to a mental health program instead of imposing disciplinary sanctions.

In New York, a court ruling initially required mental health input in the prison disciplinary process. Subsequently, the state amended its regulations to incorporate the court-ordered procedures that require mental health input in the disciplinary process and consideration by the hearing officer of the mental illness of the inmate when determining whether to dismiss, find guilty, or reduce the penalty imposed.

The court in *Coleman v. Wilson* (1995) subsequently approved a comprehensive mental health policy and procedure program that included provision of clinical input in the disciplinary process and permitted the hearing officer discretion to consider mental health conditions in mitigation of punishment.

While it may not be a constitutional right, correctional mental health experts find mental health input in prison disciplinary proceedings to be relevant to overall mental health care in institutions and recommend that it form a part of the process. They emphasize, however, that mental health input should not cross a forensic boundary and directly address responsibility for the action. They argue that doing so could create circumstances where the mental health staff become the ultimate decision makers of culpability.

Mental health care in "segregated" units

In issuing its ruling for prisoners, the court in *Indiana Protection and Advocacy Services Commission v. Commissioner, Indiana Department of Correction* (2012) acknowledged that inmates in segregation commit a disproportionately higher percentage of suicides than those in the general population. There is growing recognition and consensus around the risks associated with placing seriously mentally ill inmates in segregated housing. A position statement by the American Psychiatric Association (2012) includes the following:

> Prolonged segregation of adult inmates with serious mental illness, with rare exceptions, should be avoided due to the potential for harm to such inmates. If an inmate with serious mental illness is placed in segregation, out-of-cell structured therapeutic activities (i.e. mental health/psychiatric treatment) in appropriate programming space and adequate unstructured out-of-cell time should be permitted. Correctional mental health authorities should work closely with administrative custody staff to maximize access to clinically indicated programming and recreation for these individuals.

A substantial body of law has evolved on this point. *Toussaint v. Yockey* (1984) indicated it is constitutional to put inmates in segregation for long periods, even indefinitely. *Madrid v. Gomez* (1995) held that it is constitutional to place an incarcerated person in disciplinary or security segregation for legitimate penological reasons. The courts in *Ruiz v. Johnson* (1999) and in *Madrid* held that it is unlawful to subject inmates in segregation to systematic psychological deprivations, extreme social isolation, and reduced environmental stimulation. The *Madrid* court excluded inmates from the secured housing units (SHUs) at Pelican Bay State Prison in California who were at a "particularly high risk for suffering very serious or severe injury to their mental health, including overt paranoia, psychotic breaks with reality, or massive exacerbations of existing mental illness as a result of the conditions in the SHU. Such inmates consist of the already mentally ill, as well as persons with borderline personality disorders, brain damage or mental retardation, impulse-ridden personalities, or a history of prior psychiatric problems or chronic depression." In a "super-max" case, *Jones 'El v. Berge* (2001), the court ruled it is unconstitutional to house mentally ill inmates in segregation for extended periods where their illness may be exacerbated by the "depravity" of their confinement.

Appropriate care must be provided when mentally ill inmates are placed in segregation. In *Madrid*, the court found that there was a need for "substantial psychiatric services" in the SHU at Pelican Bay. In a number of systems encountered by this writer, policy mandated the minimum clinical and psychiatric contact that had to occur within designated timeframes. In addition, updated treatment plans, including psychotropic medication therapy, had to be completed at specified time intervals.

In assessing whether adequate care is provided in a locked unit, the court in *Indiana Protection and Advocacy Services Commission v. Commissioner, Indiana Department of Corrections* (2012) pointed out that appropriate mental health treatment in administrative segregation is different from mere mental health monitoring. In this writer's experience, ongoing multiple cell-front clinical contacts performed in a perfunctory manner by mental health clinical staff in segregation units, particularly for policy-mandated minimal periodic clinical services, are inadequate irrespective of the reasons. Inmates in segregation may sometimes refuse to come out of the cell for reasons directly related to their mental illness, or clinicians may feel compelled to interview patients at the cell-front because of high caseloads. Inmates may also be seen cell-front for custody reasons, such as security lockdowns or insufficient escort officers. None of these reasons justifies the continued use of the cell-front as the default location for clinical interventions by mental health clinicians in a locked unit.

Metzner and Dvoskin (2006) identified screening as a required standard of appropriate care to exclude the severely mentally ill from segregation (where such exclusion is required or permitted) and divert them to special mental health programs, where available. Screenings and timely evaluations are necessary to recognize mental health problems and monitor for any deterioration of mental status because of the conditions. In *Morgan v. Rowland* (2006), the district court observed favorably that inmates in segregation were screened and evaluated within 24 hours of placement.

Segregated inmates require frequent and ongoing monitoring, which the *Morgan* court recognized to include rounding of each inmate in segregation. Treatment plans must be individualized and preferably developed by a multidisciplinary treatment team. In *Troy v. State of Colorado* (2013), the district court endorsed the need for a multidisciplinary treatment team to include a psychiatrist, while pointing out it could not order it. This writer has jointly observed treatment teams with correctional mental health experts in segregation. Our observation focused on the composition and involvement of members of the treatment team, including whether or not the assigned primary clinician, psychiatrist, and correctional staff were present and interactive in the multidisciplinary team meeting.

During these observations, we looked for the presence of the patient in the treatment team meeting and whether the patient had an opportunity to participate meaningfully. We noted the availability and use of medical, mental health, and custody records during the meeting. Other areas we measured while observing treatment teams included the presentation by the primary treating clinician; references to and discussions regarding prescribed psychotropic medications, if any; and the individualization and relevance of the treatment plan to diagnosis and treatment goals. We also looked at therapeutic group assignments if indicated and their clinical relationships to treatment goals. As observers, we were attentive to whether the treatment team considered a change in the level of care where appropriate, including the need for admission to inpatient care if clinically indicated.

Correctional mental health care experts also emphasize that adequate treatment in segregated units must include sufficient hours of structured out-of-cell therapeutic and unstructured or recreation activities. Metzner and Dvoskin (2006) recommend structured out-of-cell therapeutic activities for at least 10–15 hours per week in addition to at least 10 hours of unstructured or recreation activities. The Society of Correctional Physicians (2013) endorses the exclusion of the seriously mentally ill from prolonged segregation. When placed in segregation, the society recommends adequate out-of-cell structured therapeutic activities and adequate time for outdoor exercise in appropriately designed areas.

Other core standards of appropriate care in locked units are suicide prevention protocols such as periodic documented welfare checks that are staggered and not predictable. Welfare checks are observations of affirmative indicators of a "living body." These checks may last for a designated initial period or throughout a stay in segregation.

Discharge planning

The majority of states provide some form of mental health care discharge planning. In a survey of 43 states, La Vigne, Davies, Palmer, and Halberstadt (2008) found that most states provided discharge medications, with a significantly smaller number of states also making referrals and/or appointments for postrelease health care services. The US Supreme Court, however, has not found a constitutional duty to provide health care after a person is released from incarceration. Specifically, the Supreme Court in *DeShaney v. Winnebago City Department of Social Services* (1989) pointedly declared that any constitutional obligation to provide services to persons in custody is limited to the period during which they are in custody.

The Ninth Circuit Court of Appeals in *Wakefield v. Thompson* (1999) is seemingly the sole federal appellate court to hold that corrections officials have an affirmative duty to provide a form of discharge service. That discharge service is the provision of medications at the time of release, albeit for a very limited duration. The court reasoned that the inmate's practical ability to secure medication is not immediately restored upon release from prison.

Following *Wakefield*, *Prasad v. County of Sutter* (2013) held that ignoring medical discharge instructions amounts to deliberate indifference to serious medical needs. *Lugo v. Senkowski* (2000) held that the state has a duty to provide medical services for an outgoing prisoner who is receiving continuing treatment at the time of release and needs ongoing treatment immediately following that release.

The factual circumstances of *Wakefield* and cases that followed it specifically dealt with medical procedures and medications. However, the *Wakefield* line of cases would appear to extend the continuum of care to require compliance with any mental health needs prescribed by health care providers in the form of "discharge instructions." This principle of extending a constitutional obligation beyond prison walls, at least for a period of "transition," has not been adopted in any other circuit, and only a limited number of district courts have applied it. Recently, in *Inesti v. Hogan* (2013), a US District Court in New York held that the legal obligation for the safety and well-being of an incarcerated person generally ends on release from custody.

In *Brad H v. City of New York* (2000), perhaps the most extensive and far-ranging discharge planning court decision on record to date, the city consented to providing mentally ill inmates with treatment and supportive services following their release. In addition to psychiatric treatment, which includes outpatient treatment and medications, the city agreed to assist with housing and, in cases of indigence, with the means to obtain services. *Brad H* is distinguishable from non–New York state cases because the principles of institutional mental health care and discharge planning undergirding the settlement agreement in the case were based on New York state statutory and case law.

Despite its limited precedential legal value, *Brad H* may offer a useful blueprint to systems seeking to expand postrelease services to incarcerated persons. It may also serve as a valuable aid in negotiations as a framework for effective settlement of post-discharge planning litigation. Prison officials may also be able to use *Brad H* to formulate policies for the regulation of effective discharge services as clinically indicated for their patients. Mental health staff could potentially use *Brad H* as a practical guide for articulating discharge instructions permissible under institutional policies.

Quality improvement in mental health care

Measuring the quality of care in mental health involves assessments of whether the services provided consistently achieve the desired outcomes in the mental health program. Hermann, Leff, and Logodmos (2002) concluded that fundamental principles of effective quality care models involve monitoring and evaluating processes and outcomes in order to compare current practice with evidence-based treatment guidelines and outcomes with accepted benchmarks. An effective quality improvement system must also have the capacity to identify opportunities for improvement and to develop and implement desired changes.

Several federal district courts have articulated that quality improvement played an essential role in providing adequate health care in correctional systems. *Grubbs v. Bradley* (1993), *Madrid* (1995), and *Coleman* (1995) identified quality improvement systems as part of the remedy to findings of constitutionally inadequate correctional health care by a court. *Coleman* and *Madrid* held specifically that a correctional system cannot provide adequate mental health care without quality improvement. In *Madrid*, the court found the absence of a functional quality improvement system to be a systemic deficiency and to constitute deliberate indifference. *Grubbs* held that "an appropriate quality assurance plan" was "indispensable" to remedy systemic deficiencies in correctional systems. The court described the Tennessee Department of Corrections' "resistance" to establish a quality assurance system as "inexplicable." In addition, the *Grubbs* (1993) court pointedly observed that requiring the establishment of a quality improvement system was "not unduly intrusive." In both *Grubbs* and *Coleman*, the court required the development of system-wide quality improvement programs as part of the remedial action plan.

Laube v. Campbell (2004) emphasized that quality improvement systems implemented in correctional settings must be consistent with nationally accepted standards. *Hadix v. Johnson* (2002) and *Laube* recognized continuous quality improvement (CQI) as an effective model for quality improvement in correctional systems. The *Hadix* court approvingly observed that CQI is widely used in large organizations. Also, the court distinguished CQI from traditional quality assurance, which relies on peer reviews and case audits to evaluate individual performance related to fixed outcome measures in order to discover and eliminate ineffective individual clinical practices. In contrast, the court characterized CQI as one of the most effective long-term strategies for enhancing quality "by analyzing and adjusting major systems in a never-ending quest for improvement." The *Hadix* court specifically recognized that effective CQI is dependent on management information systems that systematically gather and analyze information.

Laube described an appropriate correctional CQI system as one with capacities to quantify performance indicators, analyze them for "opportunities for improvement," and expeditiously implement remedies. The indicators would then be reassessed to measure the results of interventions as part of an ongoing process of assessing corrective action plans, with the objective of preventing future adverse outcomes.

This writer has participated in the development of an information management–based CQI system from initial discussions, design, and beta testing through piloting and expected roll-out. The benefits of an effective quality improvement system include assisting in the provision of adequate patient care and supervision, as well as the potential to inoculate a system against litigation.

Summary

Many of the developments in US correctional laws and standards discussed here have been formulated by lower courts and/or advanced by correctional mental health experts. To date, appellate review has been scant, leaving open final resolution of multiple issues. Nevertheless, case law and litigation are driving innovation in standards of care and enhancing the quality of correctional mental health. These reforms are gaining acceptance as preferred and expected standards of correctional mental health care in jails and prisons and may reflect the present-day "evolving standard of decency," in turn becoming touchstones of constitutionally adequate care across systems.

References

American Psychiatric Association (2012). Position statement on segregation of prisoners with mental illness. Retrieved from http://www.psych.org/File%20Library/Learn/Archives/ps2012_PrisonerSegregation.pdf

Bell v. Wolfish, 441 U.S. 520 (1979).

Boston, J., & Manville, D. (2010). *Prisoners' self-help litigation manual*. New York: Oxford University Press.

Bowring v. Godwin, 551 F.2d 44 (4th Cir. 1977).

Brad H v. City of New York, 185 Misc 2d 420 (Sup. Ct. N.Y. County 2000).

Coleman v. Wilson, 912 F. Supp. 1282, 1308 (E. D. Cal. 1995).

D.M. v. Terhune, 67 F. Supp. 2d 401 (D.N.J. 1999).

DeShaney v. Winnebago Cty. Dep't of Soc. Servs., 489 U.S. 189 (1989).

Dvoskin, J. A., Petrila, J., & Stark-Riemer, S. (1995). Powell v. Coughlin and the application of the professional judgment rule to prison mental health. *Mental and Physical Disability Law Reporter, 19*(1), 108–114.

Estelle v. Gamble, 429 U.S. 97 (1976).

Farmer v. Brennan, 511 U.S. 825 (1994).

Grubbs v. Bradley, 821 F.Supp 496 (M.D. Tenn. 1993).

Hadix v. Johnson, 2002 LEXIS 21283 213, 300 (S. D. Mich. 2002).

Hermann, R. C., Leff, S. H., & Logodmos, G. (2002). *Selecting process measures for quality improvement in mental healthcare.* Rockville, MD: Center for Mental Health Services.

Indiana Prot. & Advocacy Servs. Comm'n v. Comm'r, Ind. Dep't of Corr., 2012 U.S. Dist. LEXIS 182974 (S.D. Ind. Dec. 31, 2012).

Inesti v. Hogan, 2013 U.S. Dist. LEXIS 29549 (S.D.N.Y. Mar. 5, 2013)

Jones 'El v. Berge, 164 F. Supp. 2d 1096 (W. D. Wis. 2001), aff'd 374 F. 3d 541 (7th Cir. 2004).

La Vigne, N., Davies, E., Palmer, T., & Halberstadt, R. (2008). *Release planning for successful reentry: A guide for corrections, service providers, and community groups.* Washington, DC: Urban Institute Justice Policy Center. Retrieved from http://www.urban.org/UploadedPDF/411767_successful_reentry.pdf

Laube v. Campbell, 333 F. Supp. 2d 1234, 1263 (M.D. Ala. 2004).

Lugo v. Senkowski, 114 F. Supp.2s 111 (N.D. N.Y. September 25, 2001).

Madrid v. Gomez, 889 F. Supp. 1146 (N. D. Cal. 1995); rev'd in part on other grounds 190 F.3d 990 (9th Cir. 1999).

Matz v. Vandenbrook, 2013 U.S. Dist. LEXIS 116930 (W.D. Wis. Aug. 19, 2013).

Metzner, J. L., & Dvoskin, J. (2006). An overview of correctional psychiatry. *Psychiatric Clinics of North America, 29*(3), 761–772.

Metzner, J. L., & Fellner, J. (2010). Solitary confinement and mental illness in U.S. prisons: A challenge for medical ethics. *Journal of the American Academy of Psychiatry and the Law, 38*(1), 104–108.

Morgan v. Rowland, 2006 U.S. Dist. LEXIS 11081 (D. Conn. Mar. 17, 2006).

National Commission on Correctional Health Care (2008a). *Standards for health services in jails.* Chicago: National Commission on Correctional Health Care.

National Commission on Correctional Health Care (2008b). *Standards for health services in prisons.* Chicago: National Commission on Correctional Health Care.

Powell v. Coughlin. 953 F2d 744 (2d Cir. 1991).

Prasad v. County of Sutter, 2013 U.S. Dist. LEXIS 100085 (E.D. Cal. July 17, 2013).

Prison Litigation Reform Act of 1995 (PLRA), 18 U. S. C. § 3626.

Ruiz v. Johnson, 37 F. Supp. 2d 855 (S. D. Tex. 1999), rev'd on other grounds, 243 F.3d 941 (5th Cir. 2001), adhered to on remand, 154 F. Supp. 2d 975 (2001).

Sarteschi, C. M. (2013) Mentally ill offenders involved with the U.S. criminal justice system: A synthesis. Retrieved from http://sgo.sagepub.com/content/3/3/2158244013497029

Society of Correctional Physicians (2013). Restricted housing of mentally ill inmates: Position statement. Retrieved from http://societyofcorrectionalphysicians.org/resources/position-statements/restricted-housing-of-mentally-ill-inmates.

Toussaint v. Yockey, 722 F. 2d 1490 (9th Cir. 1984).

Troy v. State of Colorado, Civil Action No. 10-cv-01005-RBJ-KMT (Col. August 24, 2012). Available at http://solitarywatch.com/wp-content/uploads/2012/08/troy-anderson-v-colorado-doc.pdf.

Vitek v. Jones, 445 U.S. 480 (1980).

Wakefield v. Thompson, 177 F.3d 1160 (9th Cir. 1999).

Washington v. Harper, 494 U.S. 210 (1990).

Wilson v. Seiter, 501 U.S. 294 (1991).

Wolff v. McDonnell, 418 U.S. 539 (1974).

CHAPTER 4

Human rights

Jamie Fellner

Introduction

The participation of health professionals in the interrogation and torture of prisoners at Guantanamo has led to renewed attention in the United States to the ethical and human rights responsibilities of those who practice medicine (Institute on Medicine as a Profession, 2013; Physicians for Human Rights, University of Cape Town, 2003). This chapter provides an overview of the key internationally recognized human rights that should inform the work of correctional mental health professionals. Unfortunately, US correctional health care and correctional staffs often ignore human rights.

Human rights reflect a humanistic vision predicated on the foundation of human dignity, which complements the ethical principles of beneficence and nonmaleficence. The human rights framework supports correctional mental health staff in their efforts to protect patients from harm and provide them the treatment they need.

The human rights framework

Human rights were first articulated in modern times by the Universal Declaration of Human Rights (UDHR), the international community's 1948 affirmation of the inherent dignity and the equal and inalienable fundamental rights of all persons (United Nations [UN], 1948). Subsequent international and regional treaties codified human rights and established compliance and oversight mechanisms. Special attention has been given to the treatment of people who are involuntarily confined in correctional facilities, because they are particularly vulnerable to violations of their rights. Numerous international statements of principles and guidelines deal specifically with prisoners, conditions of detention, and correctional staff, as well as authoritative international interpretations of human rights in the prison context by treaty bodies, UN-appointed special rapporteurs, and academic experts (Coyle, 2002).

Several interrelated human rights are particularly relevant to the work of correctional health professionals: human dignity, the right to rehabilitation, the right to life, the right to mental health treatment, the right to freedom from torture or other cruel treatment or punishment, and the right to be free of discrimination based on disability. These rights are affirmed in some treaties to which the United States is a party, including the International Covenant on Civil and Political Rights (ICCPR; UN, 1966a) and the Convention Against Torture and Other Cruel, Inhuman, or Degrading Treatment or Punishment (CAT; UN, 1984). As a party, the United States is bound to comply with their provisions, and this

obligation extends not just to federal agencies but to state agencies and employees as well. The United States has signed, although not yet ratified, other relevant treaties: the International Covenant on Economic, Social, and Cultural Rights (ICESCR; UN, 1966b) and the Convention on the Rights of Persons with Disabilities (UN, 2006). As a signatory, the United States is obliged to refrain from action that would undermine the treaties' purpose.

Dignity

The UDHR begins by affirming human dignity, "[R]ecognition of the inherent dignity of all members of the human family is the foundation of freedom, justice and peace in the world" (UN, 1948). People do not forfeit their dignity simply because they are incarcerated. The ICCPR states that persons deprived of their liberty "shall be treated with humanity and with respect for the inherent dignity of the human person" (UN, 1966). This is not an optional directive, nor is it one officials can violate on budgetary or staffing grounds (UN Human Rights Committee, 1992). Prisoners retain all their human rights while in prison, with restrictions on those rights permitted only to the extent required by the fact of incarceration itself. Protecting the dignity of prisoners means that any measures that restrict their rights and freedoms within prison should be imposed only when necessary, to the extent necessary, and only for so long as is necessary.

Rehabilitation

Recognizing the inherent dignity of every human being means recognizing his or her potential for change, growth, redemption, and rehabilitation. Human rights treaties mandate a positive goal for corrections, something beyond mere punishment through deprivation of liberty. As stated in the UN-approved Standard Minimum Rules (SMR) for the Treatment of Prisoners (UN, 1977), "the purpose and justification of a sentence of imprisonment . . . is ultimately to protect society against crime. This end can only be achieved if the period of imprisonment is used to ensure, so far as possible, that upon his return to society the offender is not only willing but able to lead a law-abiding and self-supporting life . . . [The treatment of prisoners] shall be such as will encourage their self-respect and develop their sense of responsibility."

Mental health professionals play a crucial role in rehabilitation for the substantial proportion of prisoners with, or at risk of developing, mental illnesses and disorders. As summarized by the SMR, "The medical services of the institution shall seek to detect and treat any physical or mental illnesses or defects which may hamper a prisoner's rehabilitation. All necessary medical, surgical and psychiatric services shall be provided to that end" (UN, 1977).

The right to life

Prisoners have a right to life that may be violated by a preventable suicide (UN, 1966). When prison staff know a prisoner is suffering from a disorder that may make him particularly vulnerable to taking his life, respect for right to life means they must do everything that could reasonably be expected, including preventive operational measures, to prevent the suicide. In a French case, for example, the European Court of Human Rights reviewed the treatment of a French prisoner who had hanged himself. The inmate, who had a psychotic disorder, had previously attempted suicide and the prison authorities placed him in solitary confinement for a prolonged period (45 days)—a type of confinement whose very conditions of isolation aggravate the risk of suicide. Because they did not monitor him, authorities were unaware that the inmate was not taking his antipsychotic medication. The court concluded the officials had violated the inmate's right to life by not treating him in a clinically appropriate manner (*Renolde v. France*, 2008).

The right to health

The right to health, which embraces both physical as well as mental health and well-being, is affirmed in the UDHR and codified in the ICESCR. Governments must take specific steps to protect and promote health both by instituting measures and providing facilities, goods, and services to meet health needs and by protecting people from unhealthy or dangerous conditions.

Prisoners are entitled to care that meets the standards that prevail in the community (UN Committee on Economic, Social, and Cultural Rights, 2000). European prison rules that reflect human rights norms require prison authorities to "safeguard the health of all prisoners in their care" and further provide that "medical services in prison shall seek to detect and treat physical or mental illnesses or defects from which prisoners may suffer" and that "all necessary medical, surgical and psychiatric services including those available in the community shall be provided to the prisoner for that purpose" (Council of Europe Committee of Ministers, 2006).

Prison authorities may violate a prisoner's right to health when his medical condition deteriorates because they did not act promptly and diligently to identify an illness and initiate appropriate therapy (Abramsky & Fellner, 2003; European Committee for the Prevention of Torture and Inhuman or Degrading Treatment or Punishment, 2011; *Vasyukov v. Russia*, 2011). Insufficient medical care may also contravene the right to health when prisoners are kept in facilities that do not have the staffing and resources to provide proper specialized treatment for an illness (Abramsky & Fellner, 2003; *Taddei v. France*, 2010).

The right to be free of abuse

Prisoners should not be subjected to torture or other cruel, inhuman, or degrading treatment or punishment. The prohibition on cruelty is contained in Article 7 of the ICCPR and fleshed out in the CAT (UN, 1966a, 1984). Article 10 of the CAT specifically requires parties to the treaty to "ensure that education and information regarding the prohibition against torture are fully included in the training of . . . medical personnel . . . who may be involved in the custody, interrogation or treatment of any individual subjected to any form of arrest, detention or imprisonment" and that "the prohibition be included in the rules or instructions issued in regard to the duties and function of any such person" (UN, 1984).

Torture and other cruel, inhuman, or degrading treatment are not subject to precise delineation but exist on a continuum of acts by public officials (or others acting at their direction or instigation) that inflict pain or suffering, be it physical or mental. The prohibition against torture and other mistreatment should be interpreted to provide the widest possible protection against physical or mental abuse. To qualify as torture, severe suffering must be intentionally inflicted for a specific purpose such as punishment. Cruel, inhuman, or degrading treatment, however, can exist in the absence of a specific purpose and inflicts less severe pain.

With regard to prisoners, an act by prison staff that causes acute physical or mental suffering beyond that inherent in incarceration may be impermissible whatever the ostensible justification. The prohibited mistreatment of prisoners is not limited to the infliction of pain through horrific methods (e.g., electric shocks to the genitals) or even more ordinary abuses such as beatings and rape.

Even authorized prison practices and programs may inflict so much suffering that they cross the threshold of mistreatment and become tantamount to torture or cruel, inhuman, or degrading treatment or punishment. The prolonged use of restraints, the placement of prisoners with serious mental illness in solitary confinement, and the use of pepper spray and other forms of force to remove prisoners from their cells can all constitute prohibited conduct, even if staff say it was undertaken to promote safety and security. Control and restraint measures should only be used as a last resort when they are necessary and are the least restrictive option to protect the life or well-being of the inmate, other inmates, or staff. These measures also should be imposed for the shortest time possible to achieve the purpose.

Insufficient, inappropriate, or untimely mental health treatment can also constitute cruel, inhuman, or degrading treatment. Such treatment can be deliberate or the result of negligence, oversight, or ignorance. As the European Committee for the Prevention of Torture (2011) has noted, inadequate health care can "lead rapidly to situations falling within the scope of the term 'inhuman and degrading treatment.'" The touchstone is the suffering endured by the prisoner and whether staff conduct caused or aggravated that suffering. For example, if prisoners' mental health deteriorates and they endure serious suffering due to insufficient clinical staff to treat them, their right to be free of cruel or inhuman treatment may have been violated, regardless of the reason for the staff shortage.

Solitary confinement: a special case

Special attention must be paid to whether solitary confinement (i.e., a locked-down housing unit, which usually includes prisoners being locked in their cell 23 hours per day) is used in ways that violate human rights, especially the right to be free of cruel, inhuman, or degrading treatment. Round-the-clock in-cell confinement, with its lack of meaningful social contact and stimulation as well as the inherent unstructured time and idleness, can be psychologically harmful to any prisoner. The nature and severity of the harm depend on the individual, the duration of the confinement, and the particular conditions (e.g., access to natural light, books, or radio). Potential adverse psychological effects are summarized in Chapter 14.

Adverse effects of solitary confinement are especially significant for persons with serious mental illness. All too frequently, prisoners with mental illness decompensate in isolation, requiring crisis care or psychiatric hospitalization. Many simply will not get better as long as they are in such restrictive housing. Suicides occur disproportionately more often in segregation units than elsewhere in prison (Abramsky & Fellner, 2003; Metzner & Fellner, 2010).

Mental health professionals are often unable to mitigate fully the harm associated with isolation. Mental health services in segregation units are typically limited to psychotropic medication, a health care clinician periodically stopping at the cell front to ask how the prisoner is doing (i.e., mental health rounds, often derisively called "walk-bys"), and occasional meetings in private with a clinician. Individual or group therapy and structured educational, recreational, or life-skill-enhancing activities are usually not available because of insufficient resources and rules that require prisoners to remain in their cells (Metzner & Dvoskin, 2006). Depending on the specific conditions, the justification for them, their duration, and the vulnerabilities and needs of individual prisoners, solitary confinement can entail violation of the rights to dignity, rehabilitation, life, and medical treatment and the right to be free of cruelty (Metzner & Fellner, 2010; UN Committee Against Torture, 2006; UN General Assembly, 2011).

International treaty bodies and human rights experts, including the UN Human Rights Committee (1992, 2006), the UN Committee Against Torture (2006), the UN Special Rapporteur on Torture (UN General Assembly, 2011), and the European Committee for the Prevention of Torture (2011) have concluded that solitary confinement may amount to torture or other cruel, inhuman, or degrading treatment or punishment. Acknowledging the damaging consequences on mental health from prolonged isolation, they have insisted that if and when solitary confinement must be imposed, it should be for as short a period as possible.

International and national medical organizations have affirmed the ethical obligation of physicians to refrain from countenancing, condoning, participating in, or facilitating torture or other forms of cruel, inhuman, or degrading treatment (American Medical Association, 1978; World Medical Association, 1997; World Psychiatric Association, 1996). In 2007, the National Commission on Correctional Health Care issued a position statement that correctional health care professionals "should not condone or participate in cruel, inhumane or degrading treatment of inmates." Recognizing the harm that can come from solitary confinement, the American Psychiatric Association (2012) recently adopted the following position statement:

> Prolonged segregation of adult inmates with serious mental illness, with rare exceptions, should be avoided due to the potential for harm to such inmates. If an inmate with serious mental illness is placed in segregation, out-of-cell structured therapeutic activities (i.e., mental health/psychiatric treatment) in appropriate programming space and adequate unstructured out-of-cell time should be permitted. Correctional mental health authorities should work closely with administrative custody staff to maximize access to clinically indicated programming and recreation for these individuals.

The Society of Correctional Physicians (2013) also recently issued a similar position statement.

Nondiscrimination based on disability

Many of the provisions of the newest international human rights convention, the Convention on the Rights of Persons with Disabilities, have unique relevance for prisoners with mental disabilities (UN, 2006). This convention affirms that all persons with any type of disability must enjoy all human rights and fundamental freedoms. Under Article 14(2) of the convention, "if persons with disabilities are deprived of their liberty through any process, they are, on an equal basis with others, entitled to guarantees in accordance with international human rights law and shall be treated in compliance with the objectives and principles of the present Convention, including by provision of reasonable accommodation" (UN, 2006). The Special Rapporteur on Torture has pointed out that the lack of reasonable accommodation in detention facilities may increase the risk of exposure to neglect, violence, abuse, torture, and ill treatment (UN General Assembly, 2011). In addition, Article 15 of the convention affirms the right to be free of torture or cruel, inhuman, or degrading treatment or punishment; Article 16 prohibits violence, abuse, and exploitation of persons with disabilities; and Article 17 recognizes the right of every person with disabilities to respect for his or her physical and mental integrity.

The human rights of prisoners with mental illness in practice

US prisons are often highly regimented and overcrowded facilities that are fraught with the potential for violence and exploitation, lack privacy, offer only limited opportunities for meaningful education, work, or other productive activities, and permit limited contact with families and community. Prison is especially difficult for those with mental disorders and psychosocial disabilities that impair their thinking, emotional responses, and ability to cope with the unique stresses of incarceration. They are more likely to violate prison rules and to be victimized by others (Abramsky & Fellner, 2003).

Although correctional facilities may be *de facto* mental health facilities because of the high proportion of prisoners with mental illness, correctional administrators often fail to prioritize comprehensive and effective mental health services; this is usually due to inadequate funding for needed resources. Correctional psychiatrists frequently confront unreasonably large caseloads, physically unpleasant facilities, and insufficient numbers of qualified mental health staff able to provide an appropriate range of mental health interventions, as well as institutional cultures often unsympathetic to mental health services. In addition to shortages of mental health staff, correctional systems frequently lack sufficient acute care and inpatient psychiatric care resources as well as intermediate care units for inmates who need them.

Mentally ill prisoners in the United States typically remain in prison or in correctional health facilities operated according to prison rules, with treatment almost always subordinated to custody and security concerns. Prison policies and practices often make it impossible to provide appropriate mental health care and permit practices that may directly threaten prisoners' mental health, above and beyond the toxic prison environment. The overuse and misuse of prolonged solitary confinement and limitations on mental health treatment for individuals held under such conditions, in particular, present a human rights problem in almost every prison system.

There are countless individual and prison-wide examples of practices and conditions that violate the human rights of prisoners with mental illness. Five recent cases provide compelling examples:

◆ Following years of litigation, a state court found South Carolina's correctional mental health system to be severely understaffed and so riddled with flaws and deficiencies that "inmates have died ... for lack of basic mental health care, and hundreds more remain substantially at risk for serious physical injury, mental decompensation, and profound, permanent mental illness." The court also found that mentally ill inmates were disproportionately subject to the use of force and solitary confinement, often used in lieu of treatment (*T.R., P.R., K.W., et al. v. South Carolina Department of Corrections*, 2014).

◆ According to the Department of Justice, prisoners with serious mental illness at a Pennsylvania prison are often subjected to a toxic combination of conditions that include prolonged isolation, harsh housing conditions, punitive behavior modification plans, and excessive use of force. These conditions, intended to control the behavior of these prisoners, often exacerbate their mental illnesses. A prisoner with serious mental illness is placed in isolation with inadequate mental health care, causing him to decompensate and behave negatively; staff respond by subjecting the prisoner to harsher living conditions, denying him stimuli and/or using excessive force against him; the prisoner's mental health continues to deteriorate, and he begins to engage in self-injurious conduct (e.g., banging his head hard and repeatedly against a concrete wall, ingesting objects, or hurling himself against the metal furnishings of his room) or attempts to kill himself. Staff eventually respond by placing him in a unit where treatment is provided. However, as soon as the prisoner begins to stabilize, he is returned to isolation, and his mental health again spirals downward (Perez & Hickton, 2013).

◆ According to the complaint in a recent lawsuit, a Mississippi prison warehouses mentally ill prisoners under dangerous and filthy conditions with a paucity of mental health professionals and scant mental treatment. Seriously ill prisoners are isolated weeks and even years behind solid steel doors in cells that often lack working toilets or lights. Inmates scream, babble, and throw excrement. They self-mutilate—swallowing shards of glass and razors, tearing their flesh with sharp objects—and attempt suicide, sometimes successfully. Custodial staff rely on excessive force to control mentally ill prisoners; they beat them and fire Mace, pepper spray, and other chemical agents into their cells, even when they pose no threat (*Dockery v. Epps*, 2013).

◆ Edward Smith (not his real name), a mentally ill prisoner, was held in solitary confinement in a California prison. He stopped taking his medication and began hearing voices. He would not eat, smeared his cell and himself with feces, and refused to leave his cell to shower or exercise. His prison psychiatrist concluded that he had lost touch with reality and that emergency medication was needed. Since Smith would not voluntarily leave his cell to get medication, he was subject under prison rules—as the psychiatrist knew—to a forced cell extraction. As shown on a video, correctional officers sprayed the naked and screaming Smith five times in 15 minutes with pepper spray. When the chemicals subdued him sufficiently, a team of specially suited officers tackled him, put restraints on him, and strapped him to a gurney. He was kept in five-point restraints for 72 hours. A couple of months later, he was removed to a prison psychiatric hospital, where his condition improved (St. John, 2013).

◆ T.S. was a 21-year-old prisoner in Michigan with a documented history of bipolar disorder and depression. Because he kept disobeying custodial orders, he was placed in administrative segregation. After he repeatedly flooded his cell, correctional officers placed him in four-point restraint, securing his arms and legs to his bed. He became "floridly psychotic," screaming and delusional. A social worker referred T.S. to a prison psychiatric hospital. However, because of a series of mishaps and communication lapses, the transfer never occurred. During the period T.S. was restrained, he did not receive medical or psychiatric treatment. No mental health staff tried to get him released from the restraints. No custody, psychological, or nursing staff took any action to summon emergency care while his mental and physical condition deteriorated. T.S. died four days after he was placed in restraints (*Hadix v. Caruso*, 2006).

Enforcement of human rights

Few prison officials realize that their responsibilities include ensuring protection of and respect for the human rights of prisoners based on international treaties. Unfortunately, there are no direct enforcement mechanisms for internationally recognized human rights. In the United States, lawsuits cannot be predicated on these treaties, and US courts will not enforce them. Treaty bodies and authorities review US treaty compliance (with the help of submissions from nongovernmental organizations) and make recommendations, but they have no power to compel the United States to comply with those recommendations.

Officials remain responsible for fulfilling their human right obligations, even if they cannot be held legally liable for failing to do so. Internal mechanisms of accountability that incorporate human rights standards will signal that officials take violations of ethical and human rights obligations seriously and will also support health professionals to resist pressures to engage in or be complicit with practices and policies that violate inmates' rights.

Summary

As Physicians for Human Rights (2003) has stated, "for health professionals, a human rights framework provides a steady moral compass, a blueprint of a just and humane social order that at its core articulates the principles of the dignity and equality of every human being." Pursuing respect for the rights of prisoners, correctional psychiatrists can not only improve their treatment and hence their prospects for well-being but can, more generally, help humanize prison conditions.

Human rights provide a universally acknowledged set of precepts that can be used during internal and external advocacy. For example, mental health professionals who seek to remove patients from segregation or to change segregation policies can point to their ethical obligation to not only attend to the mental health needs of their patients but to protect them from inhuman treatment. Indeed, in addition to providing whatever services they can to isolated patients, mental health practitioners should advocate within the prison system for a change in segregation policies (Metzner & Fellner, 2010). Mental health professionals should not—consistent with their human rights and ethical obligations—acquiesce silently to conditions of confinement that harm prisoners and violate human rights. They are obligated not only to treat inmates with mental illness based upon clinical autonomy (i.e., clinical decisions are based on healthcare needs and delivered in an ethical manner) and with compassion but to strive to change policies and practices that abuse inmates and violate their rights, even those that involve custodial decisions (e.g., segregation, use of force, restraints). Whether individually or through their professional organizations, mental health practitioners can also provide information and analysis to the public, elected officials, and UN treaty bodies regarding the reality of mental health services in prisons and how they meet, or fail to meet, human rights norms.

In short, for practitioners who want improved policies and practices, human rights offer a powerful rationale and vision for a different kind of correctional mental health services. The more correctional mental health practitioners embrace and advocate for human rights, the greater the likelihood prisoners' rights will be respected. Prisoners will benefit—and so will mental health professionals—as prisons become a place where they can work without compromising their professional standards and ethical responsibilities.

References

Abramsky, S., & Fellner, J. (2003). *Ill-equipped: US prisons and offenders with mental illness.* New York: Human Rights Watch.

American Medical Association (1978). Health and ethics policies of the AMA House of Delegates: H-65.997 Human Rights. Retrieved from http://www.ama-assn.org/ad-com/polfind/Hlth-Ethics.pdf

American Psychiatric Association (2012). Position statement on segregation of prisoners with mental illness. Retrieved from http://www.psych.org/File%20Library/Learn/Archives/ps2012_PrisonerSegregation.pdf

Council of Europe Committee of Ministers (2006). European prison rules. Retrieved from https://wcd.coe.int/ViewDoc.jsp?id=955747

Coyle, A. (2002). *A human rights approach to prison management: Handbook for prison staff.* London: International Centre for Prison Studies.

Dockery v. Epps (2013). Complaint. S.D. Miss. 31 October 2013.

European Committee for the Prevention of Torture and Inhuman or Degrading Treatment or Punishment (2011). *CPT standards.* Strasbourg: Council of Europe.

Hadix v. Caruso (2006), 461 F.Supp.2d 574 (W.D. Mich.).

Institute on Medicine as a Profession (2013). *Ethics abandoned: Medical professionalism and detainee abuse in the "War on Terror."* New York: Institute on Medicine as a Profession.

Metzner, J., & Dvoskin, J. (2006). An overview of correctional psychiatry. *Psychiatric Clinics of North America, 29,* 761–772.

Metzner, J. L., & Fellner, J. (2010). Solitary confinement and mental illness in U.S. prisons: A challenge for medical ethics. *Journal of the American Academy of Psychiatry and the Law, 38*(1), 104–108.

National Commission on Correctional Health Care (2007). Position statement: Correctional health care professionals' response to inmate abuse. Retrieved from http://www.ncchc.org/correctional-health-care-professionals%E2%80%99-response-to-inmate-abuse

Perez, T. E., & Hickton, D. J. (2013). *Investigation of the state correctional institution at Cresson and notice of expanded investigation.* Washington, DC: United States Department of Justice. Retrieved from http://www.justice.gov/crt/about/spl/documents/cresson_findings_5-31-13.pdf

Physicians for Human Rights and School of Public Health and Primary Health Care, University of Cape Town Health Sciences Faculty (2003). *Dual loyalty and human rights in health professional practice: Proposed guidelines & institutional mechanisms.* United States: PHR and University of Cape Town. Retrieved from https://s3.amazonaws.com/PHR_Reports/dualloyalties-2002-report.pdf

Renolde v. France (2008). No. 5608/05. European Court of Human Rights.

St. John, P. (2013, October 1). Tapes show mentally ill prisoners forced from cells with pepper spray. *Los Angeles Times.* Retrieved from http://articles.latimes.com/2013/oct/31/local/la-me-ff-prison-videos-20131101

Society of Correctional Physicians (2013). Position statement: Restricted housing of mentally ill inmates. Retrieved from http://societyofcorrectionalphysicians.org/resources/position-statements/restricted-housing-of-mentally-ill-inmates

Taddei v. France (2010). No. 36435/07. European Court of Human Rights.

T.R., P.R., K.W., et al. v. South Carolina Department of Corrections (2014). Case No. 2005-CP-40-02925.

United Nations (1948). Universal declaration of human rights. Retrieved from http://www.un.org/rights/50/decla.htm

United Nations (1966a). International covenant on civil and political rights. Retrieved fromhttp://www.ohchr.org/en/professionalinterest/pages/ccpr.aspx

United Nations (1966b). International covenant on economic, social and cultural rights. Retrieved from http://www.ohchr.org/EN/ProfessionalInterest/Pages/CESCR.aspx

United Nations (1977). Standard minimum rules for the treatment of prisoners. Retrieved from http://www.unodc.org/pdf/criminal_justice/UN_Standard_Minimum_Rules_for_the_Treatment_of_Prisoners.pdf

United Nations (1984). Convention against torture and other cruel, inhuman or degrading treatment or punishment. Retrieved from http://www1.umn.edu/humanrts/instree/h2catoc.htm

United Nations (2006). Convention on the rights of persons with disabilities. Retrieved from http://www.ohchr.org/EN/HRBodies/CRPD/Pages/ConventionRightsPersonsWithDisabilities.aspx

United Nations Committee Against Torture (2006). Consideration of reports submitted by states parties under article 19 of the convention, conclusions and recommendations of the Committee Against Torture, United States of America. CAT/C/USA/CO/2. Retrieved from http://www.refworld.org/docid/453776c60.html

United Nations Committee on Economic, Social and Cultural Rights (2000). General comment no. 14: The right to the highest attainable standard of health (art. 12 of the covenant). E/C.12/2000/4. Retrieved from http://www.refworld.org/docid/4538838d0.html

United Nations General Assembly (2011). Interim report of the special rapporteur of the Human Rights Council on torture and other cruel, inhuman or degrading treatment or punishment. A/66/268. Retrieved from http://solitaryconfinement.org/uploads/SpecRapTortureAug2011.pdf

United Nations Human Rights Committee (1992). CCPR general comment no. 20: article 7 (prohibition of torture, or other cruel, inhuman or degrading treatment or punishment). Retrieved from http://www.refworld.org/docid/453883fb0.html

United Nations Human Rights Committee (2006). Consideration of reports submitted by states parties under article 40 of the covenant, concluding observations of the Human Rights Committee: United States of America. CCPR/C/USA/CO/3. Retrieved from http://www.refworld.org/docid/45c30bb20.html

Vasyukov v. Russia (2011). No. 2974/05. European Court of Human Rights.

World Medical Association (1997). Declaration of Hamburg concerning support for medical doctors refusing to participate in, or to condone, the use of torture or other forms of cruel, inhuman or degrading treatment. Adopted by the 49th WMA Assembly. Retrieved from http://www.wma.net/en/30publications/10policies/c19/index.html

World Psychiatric Association (1996). Madrid declaration on ethical standards for psychiatric practice. Retrieved from http://www.wpanet.org/detail.php?section_id=5&content_id=48

CHAPTER 5

From the inside out
Offender perspectives

Brad Bogue and Robert L. Trestman

Introduction

Incarceration is a stressful and dehumanizing process. Those who become incarcerated are shaped and changed by the experience in many ways. For those who work with people who are inmates, it can be difficult to appreciate the range and intensity of their experiences. This chapter gives voice to some of those experiences. Ten individuals currently or recently incarcerated in the Colorado prison system were interviewed in an open-ended way as part of a project to obtain narrative accounts of how incarceration has affected them. The autobiographical interviews were transcribed, and core elements and themes in their own words are presented; their names and some details are changed to protect their identities.

Every incarcerated individual experiences imprisonment through the lens of personal experience. There is fear and humiliation, hope and frustration, isolation and friendship. Some people persist in illegal behavior; others turn their lives around. The opportunity and challenge of correctional psychiatry is to engage people during this vulnerable period—to understand patients as people, treat illness, reduce suffering, and help them recover their lives. We believe the 10 individuals interviewed for this chapter speak eloquently of human struggle, coping, failure, regret, and hope.

William B.—Gang membership

WB: Well, my first time was 13, juvenile, when I first got in the game. It didn't bother me because I was young. Doing time was nothing. . . . After that, I caught a murder case in '87.

INTERVIEWER: How old were you then?

WB: 18.

INTERVIEWER: Then you must have had a full amount of challenges.

WB: Yeah, you know what I'm saying I was scared, but I couldn't show it. You show your weak spot, somebody going to get you. So that's why I couldn't show nobody that I was scared.

INTERVIEWER: Did you have any friends from the street there?

WB: I had a couple guys try to put me under their wing and show me the ropes. I was learning on my own and do it my way, because you can't always do time another person's way. . . . Then people change, but the system don't think you change though. They think just because you being in here, you're not going to change. In this place I'm doing everything I can, and they giving me a hard time to get up out of here.

INTERVIEWER: They just don't want to give you any slack?

WB: No. They're doing off my old mark, my reputation, what I used to do, and I'm trying to show them a different side of that. They still think I'm that old person, and they don't want to let that go. I tell them all the time, "That ain't me no more." They don't understand it anywhere near as much as some of the people that are in the system, because they've experienced it or they've seen other people change. . . . The system is corrupt. They want to keep the jails filled. They're sending people back for nothing, for little, bitty things, when you can give them a chance to make things right. It's a revolving door.

INTERVIEWER: How is it different for people that are in a gang in prison?

WB: Well, the people that's not in a gang, they look at it like it's stupid and they don't see why would you get in a gang. See, some ain't really live that lifestyle or grew up in the neighborhood. Most gang members grew up in a neighborhood where they was kind of raised in that. I got into it when I was 12 years old.

That's what I'm trying to do is give back. I done hurt my community so much and now I'm trying to give back. Back to what you were saying when you were talking about those people getting older, I know dudes still in the gang, right now, 50 or something years old and still gangbanging. They ain't really let it go. I look at them and laugh. "When are you going to let this go? Your kids is gangbanging now and you still calling yourself shot calling." Sooner or later, you're going to have to let it go.

Miles L.—Time

INTERVIEWER: Does time wear on you harder now that you know you're getting on in age?

ML: It does to a point because you're not getting younger and you know it. And time means more now than it did in the past. In the past, I didn't care because I figured I would live forever. And now that I'm gettin' older, I do know that the end is veritably here. So it's harder to do . . . one day is like a week, is like a month, is like a year. To where in the past, one day, I really didn't care. I could afford to lose a day, or a week, or a month, or a year. . . . And there's something about time that you lose, everything that you had when you were younger, your thought pattern changes, the way that you see things change, the way that you deal with things change. As far as when you were young and now that you're old. Whether it has to do with time or just experience, I don't know. I don't know. If it's, you think one way when you're young, and another way when you're older. If it takes growin' up all those years to reach that point, or if it's something that just happens chemically. I don't know.

A long time ago I used to think that (prison) was full of (guards) that were all-knowing. They knew how prison worked. And today I see it for actually what it is, and it's just individuals that have a job to do. And they chose that field, and they've got good days and bad days. And they're not necessarily up on current events.

Whether they're happening inside or outside. So, they're just as fallible as everybody else.

I think doin' time is, the biggest aspect to that is the time itself, is what you do. Again, you can escape by putting your mind in employment, or education. If you're stuck inside of a room to where you're constantly thinking, and you constantly got 24 hours at a time to do, that's what makes county jail time harder than prison time—is the fact that you're locked up, and you have so much time on your hands.

Pat D.—Access to treatment

PD: I was incarcerated twice. As far as prison goes, I had a short time to do: just a two-year sentence. No way to get into the mental (health) program, they're all booked up. There's no help there for you.

I look at it this way. I put myself in prison. I was in a treatment program in the community. But in prison, they're not equipped to handle mental health people. They don't carry a lot of my meds. I learned you had to tell them, "I have to have that med. You have to get it for me."

This last time what really hurt me was I had been waiting for this mental health program. I finally got into it. I was so happy. What they concentrated on is what I wanted. I wanted to get something out of prison, other than just working. But, they wouldn't switch my work schedule, so there's no way I could do it. They wouldn't switch me because I was good at what I did. I spent seven months in the kitchen, which was hard, real hard. I didn't get nothing but work.

INTERVIEWER: Did you get to see an individual psychologist or therapist?

PD: There's mental people in there that need help, and they don't get it. They're there a lot longer than I'm going to be there. My heart goes out to them, because it's hard to get help in there. For me, when I have a problem, I need to talk to a therapist now. You know, I could have hurt somebody already. When I hit my peak, I know when it is.

When that one officer that I told, "I need mental health now," he laughed at me. I said man, I'm not joking, I need mental health, I'm going to freaking flip. It's very frustrating. I realize they deal with a lot of people, but when they've been around me five, six months, they know what I am. They know what I'm about.

Regina G.—Loneliness and faith

INTERVIEWER: What was the experience of doing time like?

RG: Discipline. Usual discipline. You're really structured. It's controlled. It was hard. I don't know. It was sad at times. It was happy at times. There are things that you have no control over. You can call family. Something happens. You just have to swallow it, and live through it, get through it the best way you can.

I was put in the safe hole because they had the lesbian act going on there. I disagreed with it, so they PC'd (protective custody) me. I lived in segregation because the girls all turned on me and stuff. I lived in there. I learned to like it there. I felt safe there. I programmed from there. I worked from there. I would just roll out of seg, and then go to work and do my programs. I was segregated from the other women. I enjoyed being alone in prison, for the fact that I had time to focus on my behaviors and to focus on what I was going to do, what I had done, and where I was going. I didn't mind being alone. Actually, when they asked me if I wanted to go back into population, I refused. I liked being alone.

I got used to it, and I got strong. I would go to work, and I would tell the Lord, "OK. It's me and you. It's me and you today. You are

going to work for me because I'm going to work for you." I would get through it like that, and he would help me through it a lot. But I'm surprised I made it through some of it, some of the things that I did. There's that wood lot, where they would take tree trunks and they'd put them on this big saw, and then they'd cut them in half. Then there was this big table and they'd fall on there, and you'd have to stack them just so. Heavy: I mean heavy. I don't know how I made it through that, but I did.

Actually, when I left there I missed it, because I got used to it, and I felt good. I felt healthy. I felt strong. I really didn't want to leave. I got attached to a lot of people there.

Prison, to me, it wasn't all a bad experience. To me, it saved my life. It saved my children's future. I'm clean and sober today. I'm good. I'm here. I'm happy.

Rick W.—Penitence and fitting in

RW: There was a time when I went from, for lack of a better term, a straight-laced white guy to being surrounded by mostly murderers and gangbangers. It's just a world I wasn't prepared for, but it was a world that I fit in somehow. I couldn't tell you how, but I was able to take care of myself.

In there, you're in the fishbowl. Everything is . . . you don't know who's watching you. You don't know who's observing what.

It's such a small world. If you show any kind of weakness, you're going to get preyed upon, because it's all of society's predators. I was at a maximum-security facility, and that's where all your hard-core predators are.

At the same time, the state takes everything away from you, everything: home, family, material things. They take everything, but what they can't take away from you is your integrity, your character, so if your word's good, your business is good, and you're not about to bullshit, that goes a long way in terms of the respect factor.

You are trying to learn a new world, and it was crippling, but at the same time, you can't show any of that, because as soon as you start showing that, that's when you get preyed upon. All I could do was focus forward. All I wanted to do was wake up the next morning and deal with it then.

You're living with somebody that you don't know and you don't have any choice but to live with this person. You don't know what they're in for, so you're just trying to get along. Most people that are in prison lack the ability to know how to communicate. You have a whole lot of guys together that absolutely don't know how to communicate with one another. They don't know how to communicate with anybody. Yet, in order to survive, to make this thing work, they have to be able to communicate.

They don't know how to, so it's such chaos . . . Then you have staff whom haven't got a clue. They don't have . . . I don't want to stain all staff, but the majority don't have a clue, not just how to communicate, but they don't have don't have integrity. They don't have professionalism. They don't have the necessary tools just to have the job.

INTERVIEWER: Speak a little about introspection

RW: When you realize for the first time that you have no character, not bad character, you have no character, and that's like having no credit. It's worse than bad credit. No integrity. No principles. No values. When you find that out for the first time . . . I was sick to my stomach. When I looked back on how I treated people, how I treated my wife, how I treated my family . . . and I had to go to prison to figure this out. I had to be around the absolute scum of the freaking earth to figure out what kind of a piece of shit I was.

But what it was, was Department of Corrections (DOC) ended up being this big mirror that I had to look at, because all those that were around me, I could find a piece of me in all of them of some sort. It was just so sickening. It was so incredibly . . . I just wanted to puke for days, months, years. I couldn't shower that shit off me.

But, I wasn't going to allow the judicial system, I wasn't going to allow DOC, I wasn't going to allow convicts, I wasn't going to allow anybody to beat me. The only way that I could throw it all back at them was to be successful. In some form or fashion, I was going to be successful.

Rick M.—Doing time, idle time

RM: You make the best of a bad situation or you could make it worse; I chose to make it easy on myself. I always got along with the guards and with the inmates. And say when they had Alcoholics Anonymous (AA), Narcotics Anonymous (NA), bible study, General Education Development (GED) school, I soaked up that time. So, for me a year would fly by. Now for another inmate just sitting in their cell all day, every day, time was different. I was the type of person I like to keep busy. I had a job, I went to school, groups. It was nonstop and that's how I do time.

INTERVIEWER: So pretty much you just take it, soak it all up, whatever their givin'.

RM: Correct. To do time. Now, however, other inmates they go and they work out and they go to the gym and they play handball and stuff. Me, I was the type of person where I was always in a group.

INTERVIEWER: Those are real tools. So do you have any goals now?

RM: My goal is to complete this sentence successfully and parole successfully. In all the past, I've always been sent back for hot urine analysis (UAs) (i.e., positive drug test) and stuff like that. But this time I want to succeed ya know and then I'm tryin' to transition out of bein' in the system. See me, I kinda been institutionalized. I've asked a hundred guards and inmates, "How does a guy get uninstitutionalized?"

In the last ten years, I've completed six community corrections sentences successfully and I've always stayed in the whole time. That way when I go out the door I'll be off paper (i.e., no further stipulations) and I go party. And I'd always get right back in the system. Right back. Being out of the system I need to create my own structure and volunteer my hours to somewhere. Cuz idle time for me is, "idle hands are the devil's hands." And that's where I always mess up you know.

Rob B.—A failed system

RB: Every day I fear what life's going to be like when I get out because I worry about other things like I happen to believe . . . but I'm cut off from the world still slightly here, that we're losing more and more of our liberties on the outside, that more and more of our freedoms are disappearing, and I look at the price of stuff in stores, and I know that . . . what kind of wage am I going to be making? Am I going to be able to afford to pay rent and eat?

Yeah, I live in terror. I don't feel this place is designed to make you a better person or to reintroduce you to society, and somehow I'll just have to deal with it.

INTERVIEWER: You are skeptical about what really is going on?

RB: Yes, but the interesting thing is it makes sense to them. The DOC lobbyists can say, "We need more guards. We need more money." The system is designed for failure.

I'm surrounded by artists in my prison, I mean that. We've got artists picking up garbage on the side of the road. I noticed across the street the VFW has a mural of a battleship. I'm thinking, "Why don't you have a sign-painting crew? Why don't you have a public works crew that does public murals?" There's no imagination in the prison system for the talent they have.

All of this is designed for failure, as far as I'm concerned. It's a rest and recovery center for career criminals, because the people who get along the best here go, "All I do here is smile and lie, and then my six months are up, and then I get to go back to crime." All this did was stimulate my mind to where I'm more anti-social, more eccentric, and I notice that that's one thing prison does to people.

INTERVIEWER: Are you saying that prison makes people worse?

RB: Oh yeah. It makes them more creative at defects. This isn't always the case. People who are so self-disciplined, they're never going to commit a crime again. The problem with the system is that you have nonviolent people who are not going to reoffend, and you're trying to drive them insane so that. Yeah. Well, it's like this. I think that it's like the guy who wrote *Empire of the Sun*. He was a psychiatrist. He gets out, he's 15 years old, he's been in captivity for eight years. He decides he's going to help humanity. He becomes a psychiatrist. He practices psychiatry for a decade and he goes, "What analysis seeks to do to make you normal really doesn't help as much as it would help if people were taught theater, literature, music."

That's how you would teach people to talk to their inner self, to articulate their grievances.

Jason H.—Attitude and endurance

JH: I have done, all told, seven and a half years in prison. I got into a gang at 13 and that was my entire life right there. At 13 years old, half my life I'd been in institutions and group homes; my attitude was pretty crappy back then. It was like I found my niche in life and that was my thing.

Looking back on it now, yeah, I wish I could go back in time and slap the old me around a little bit. I guess there's some things that I learned on a positive note from all the gangbanging and all the dumb shit that I did. I've got a different sense of morals than a lot of other people do. A lot of people write off gangsters and gangbangers and people in that life as having no morals. They do, for real. I learned a real high sense of honor from gangbanging.

I remember, I was in prison one day and got called to the front office and told that I was leaving the next day. That I was going to a halfway house. Like a dumb ass, back then, I had rabbit feet real bad. I got to the halfway house, and that night, I took off. I don't even know what I was thinking, but I just took off. I got two years for taking off out of the halfway house added to the 18 months.

At 18, I went to prison and still didn't give a damn. I just went in there with an attitude, like "You know what, man, fuck this shit. Fuck you." I was there 11 months, ended up catching assault on DOC guard. They didn't take me to court or give me any more time for it, but they sent me into 23-hour-a-day lock down. For me, it changed how sociable I was. When you're locked down 23 hours a day in a cell by yourself, without even trying to, you become a bit anti-social. Then I ended up doing shit. I did two and half years in of three-year term in solitary.

INTERVIEWER: Have you now changed that attitude to not go back?

JH: When you were pointing that out, I feel everything that I'm suffering with right now is an endurance trial. I just feel that I am overcoming my greatest fear, and my greatest fear is for whatever reason going back to who I once was. I'm trying to overcome that by doing positive things instead of negative things. My treasure now is my kids, and showing my kids that Dad's different.

Tim S.—The locked door and surviving

TS: When you take that bus in, your autonomy stops. That's when you became a number, and you put on the same clothes as everybody else. You became a wave in a sea of lost souls. You don't know that at the time. You don't realize. It's terrifying. The first time you go in your cell and they close those doors, and you're alone. The brick walls and open bars, and the smells, and the screaming, and the hollering, and it was absolutely just traumatic. You have no identity in prison. You were somebody that just started their prison sentence.

INTERVIEWER: You're like a piece on a board game, and you don't know what the game is.

TS: Absolutely. All you learn is to be hypervigilant towards "respect." You had a whole different set of rules. When you're 18, you're very impressionable. When we went into prison, we were told, this is the way you have to be to be a good, solid convict or you're a piece of shit. You begin to think, "This is what I need to do, and the harder I work towards being a good convict, the faster I become somebody."

You want to survive.

From that first time, I was in and out of community corrections, getting put on probation, or parole, or whatever, violating, and going back to that revolving door system of using drugs, using cocaine, getting a hot UA (i.e., positive urine toxicology), and back to prison.

At 35, I really wanted to make changes. I did a lot of segregation time, a lot of hole time (i.e., isolation), and I still think I've come up pretty well. But you can't be locked in a box and stare at the wall day after day with no human contact, except for when they feed you and when screaming down the tier without it affecting you to some degree.

All those opportunities and all the things that I forfeited, all things to think about those dark nights all night long, they're wasted unless you use it somehow. That's why I'm so set on trying to do something and using my experiences to give back. I haven't wasted that time. I have, still, to a degree, but I'm hoping I can live with it.

When you do time there is a helplessness, a loneliness, a kind of absent feeling, which leaves you feeling empty. It's not really lonely. It's empty. It's kind of an empty kind of void. The only way to fill that empty void is to try to control your inner personal environment, what's going on around you. You can't control any of that stuff.

INTERVIEWER: That makes sense. You make the connections in yourself, that you're not helpless.

TS: You're struggling with all this negativity and humiliation and just trying to search for some sort of value as a human being, some sort of belonging to this world, some sort of attachment to the life or the existence around you. When you give up, when you can't find that way to attach, when you can't find a way to save yourself is when you lose it.

INTERVIEWER: From that experience, just an incredible experience stacking 25 years in prison, what cycles could you think of that are involved in doing time?

TS: I think there are a couple. One is trying to survive each day, trying to get through the day. It's hard. You can't think about tomorrow, but yet you have to hope in tomorrow. You have to put some faith and hope that tomorrow is coming, but you can't really plan for it, because it will drive you crazy because of the amount of time you still have to do. I'll tell you one thing that's been actually a result of doing a lot of prison time. I have a fantastic memory of everything in my life, because I've had a unique opportunity to do nothing but think about things in my life, and think about them over and over and over.

The other thing, getting back to the other part of this living, you have to, just do whatever you have to do to get through the day. There's a lot of stuff you turn off until later. I can't do this. I'm just going to turn it off until I get out. You have to do it by day, but at the same time you can't just cancel everything in your life or you succumb to that thing. You have to inspire yourself somehow. You

have to hope that tomorrow is going to be better. Otherwise you die. It's such a hard, thin line to ride.

I believe in the whole full circle. That's why I'm so into trying to make change on a larger scale happen. Especially in recovery, we teach best what we most need to learn. By helping others, it keeps you where you need to be. It keeps you grounded in what you need to do for yourself. It's almost selfish helping other people, because you're taking care of yourself.

Regina M.—Emotions, routine, consequences

RM: When I first started, I think it was exciting; it was fun. I was curious what prison would be like, and it was just a real fun experience. Chip on my shoulder, thought I was invincible, 10 feet tall and bulletproof, and I didn't give a shit about anything. I knew I barely had a little tiny 10-year sentence, and I could get through that, no problem. And towards the end, it was more of a nerve-wracking, mind-fucking, lonely, yet, crowded place to be.

Towards the end of doing my 10, I was just tired of it. It wasn't fun any more. It took things that I took for granted and things you missed when you're out there, like stopping and smelling a fucking flower or stopping and getting a burger, just even going for a walk or being able to step outside when you want to.

Those are some of the small things a lot of people on a daily basis take for granted and don't even realize things that you're going to miss when it's all taken away from you.

INTERVIEWER: What do you recall about the experience of doing time? How did you make that work for you?

RM: Routine. I had my day pretty much planned out. I knew what I was going to do. I knew I had to get up for work at 3:00. I'd come back. I had everything planned out. I was so medicated, I was asleep by 5:30, 6:00. I knew I'd be out like that, so my days just flew by. They were just monotone.

INTERVIEWER: Can you recall anything about struggles you might have had with emotions or mind while you were doing time?

RM: Yeah. I lost my children because of doing time, so it was pretty fucking hard for me. Because the days that went by, I realized I would never get back. That I would never know if one of my children fell down and got hurt. You know what I mean? I was pretty mind fucked. Again, that's why I said I was pretty medicated. Numb. All you have is time to do is sit and think. Worrying. A lot of it is worrying about what's going on out there, things you have no control over. It's hard to not worry about what's going on out there, that life still goes on.

INTERVIEWER: What do you think people need to hear that would help them?

RM: Just the severity of using drugs. When you're thinking about getting high, you're not thinking about what diseases you could be catching while you're getting high. Or the different risks that you take, or how careless you get with everyday things. How dangerous things really are. You think you want to do what you want to do, but you don't realize how dangerous drugs really are. Or how out of your mind you are: you don't even care about what you're doing. Or the consequences.

Summary

We hope that the stories told in this chapter convey some sense of the diversity of experiences of incarceration and the diversity of people who become incarcerated. In psychiatry specifically and clinical care more broadly, there is growing recognition of the need for cultural competence (see Chapter 60). The growing focus on recovery in mental illness treatment (see Chapter 40) and on partnership with patients to develop shared goals and to enhance adherence to treatment is reshaping clinical practice. At the core of these initiatives is the relationship between the patient and the clinician—the therapeutic alliance. Developing appropriate therapeutic alliances with patients enhances outcomes; growing evidence suggests that the specifics of alliance measurement and outcome definition are not critical (Martin, Garske, & Davis, 2000). What does matter is how the patient experiences the relationship with the clinician; a judgmental or negative experience impairs the alliance (Nissen-Lie, Havik, Høglend, Rønnestad, & Monsen, 2014). The better we understand our patients and can empathize with them, the greater the therapeutic alliance and the greater the likelihood of positive outcomes.

References

Martin, D. J., Garske, J. P., & Davis, M. K. (2000). Relation of the therapeutic alliance with outcome and other variables: A meta-analytic review. *Journal of Consulting and Clinical Psychology,*68(3), 438.

Nissen-Lie, H. A., Havik, O. E., Høglend, P. A., Rønnestad, M. H., & Monsen, J. T. (2014). Patient and therapist perspectives on alliance development: Therapists' practice experiences as predictors.*Clinical Psychology & Psychotherapy.* DOI:10.1002/cpp.1891. Retrieved from http://onlinelibrary.wiley.com/doi/10.1002/cpp.1891/full

Organization, structure, and function of correctional institutions

section ii

Organization, structure, and function of correctional institutions

CHAPTER 6

Jails and prisons

Joel Dvoskin and Melody C. Brown

Introduction

As noted in Chapter 3, jails and prisons have a constitutional duty to provide necessary mental health services to detainees and inmates with serious medical needs (including psychiatric needs) under the Fourteenth and Eighth Amendments to the Constitution, respectively. While the constitutional standard in both settings, deliberate indifference, is the same, the manner in which these duties are carried out may be quite different. In this chapter, we describe the most important differences between jails and prisons and the implications of these differences in providing mental health services to inmates and detainees.

Historically, jails have been used to hold defendants for trial and to confine prisoners who have been sentenced for misdemeanors, typically for sentences of less than one year. In contrast, prisons are managed by state or federal governments (either directly or by contract) and used for longer-term confinement of convicted felons who are generally serving sentences of one year or longer.

Recently, these distinctions have been blurred, especially in California, where federal courts have mandated sentence reductions to the prisons operated by the California Department of Corrections and Rehabilitation, resulting in significant numbers of sentenced felons being housed in county jails for as long as 10 years. As a result, some jails, especially larger ones, will need to change their mental health service delivery systems to accommodate long-stay prisoners, and some jails will need to incorporate services that are described in this chapter as appropriate for prison mental health services.

Six states—Alaska, Connecticut, Delaware, Hawaii, Rhode Island, and Vermont (Guerino, Harrison, & Sabol, 2011)—run combined systems, where both jails and prisons are operated by the state and where sentenced felons and pretrial detainees might be housed in the same facility. Also, many correctional systems now provide for medical and/or mental health services via contract with private, for-profit corporations. Whatever the method of service delivery, the services must meet constitutional requirements.

The differences between jails and prisons can be examined across several important axes, including the nature of the people who live there, the circumstances of their presence, and the nature of the institution.

Jail detainees compared to prison inmates: similar people in different situations

In general, there are few differences between pretrial jail detainees and prison inmates, except for the length of time they have been locked up. Jail detainees are often delivered to the jail directly by police officers, in some cases after spending a few hours in a police lockup. Newly admitted prison inmates in most cases have been in jail for some length of time, where they may have received mental health treatment and are no longer under the influence of alcohol or illicit drugs.

As a result of their very recent arrests, it is no surprise that from 62% to 86% of newly admitted jail detainees are under the influence of alcohol, stimulants, or other drugs (Office of National Drug Control Policy, 2013). This creates several challenges for jail mental health providers, some of which are discussed in the chapters on detoxification (Chapter 17) and suicide prevention (Chapter 43). Detainees may be at higher risk of suicide immediately after admission due to the disinhibiting effects of substances. The risk of suicide can also be higher for detainees who are experiencing the painful process of detoxification from addictive chemicals. An additional challenge is created by the difficulty in diagnosing a person who arrives at the jail under the influence of alcohol, stimulants, or other substances. Even experienced clinicians will have difficulty distinguishing between various forms of preexisting psychotic illness, toxic psychosis, and drug-induced disorders, especially in offenders for whom previous records are not immediately available.

At least 6% (Bolton, 1976; Teplin, 1990) of newly admitted jail detainees are psychotic upon arrival at the jail. James and Glaze (2006) stated that 24% of jail inmates reported psychotic symptoms within the 12 months preceding their jail admission; however, it is difficult to know the underlying reason for these reported symptoms (e.g., serious mental illness, drug and alcohol abuse).

In contrast, due to their longer sentences, the percentage of prison inmates who have been recently admitted, with and without mental illness, is much lower. In other words, most inmates have been in prison for a while, dramatically decreasing the amount of clinical time that is spent in initial assessment and treatment planning. Further, even new admissions have typically been off the street (i.e., in jail) for some significant length of time prior to their arrival at prison. Because of the passage of time, much more difficult access to illegal drugs, and the availability of at least some mental health treatment in most jails, it is unusual to find newly admitted prison inmates who are acutely psychotic or intoxicated upon arrival. Thus, while jail detainees and prison inmates present with similar characteristics and histories, they may appear quite different because they are in a different stage or episode of their involvement with the criminal justice system.

Perhaps the most important difference between jails and prisons, from the perspective of mental health service delivery, is the disparity in turnover. The average pretrial jail detainee remains in jail for less than 72 hours (Osher, Steadman, & Barr, 2002).

As a result, jails have many times more admissions per bed than prisons. For example, when comparing the largest jail and prison populations, the Los Angeles County (California) jails admitted approximately 143,000 inmates in 2012 (Austin, Naro-Ware, Ocker, et al., 2012) compared to only 75,378 prisoners admitted to Texas state prisons (Carson & Golinelli, 2013).

Because of the rapid turnover that occurs in jails, mental health professionals spend a far greater percentage of their time doing first-time assessments and evaluations, which are much more time-consuming than for repeat visits. Because this work involves prescribing psychotropic medication, the American Psychiatric Association (2000) has recommended a significantly larger number of psychiatrists and other prescribers (e.g., advanced-practice nurse practitioners and physician's assistants) in jails (one prescriber for every 75–100 people on psychotropic medications for a serious mental illness) than prisons (one prescriber for every 150 people on psychotropic medications for a serious mental illness).

Acute versus persistent mental health problems

Because jail detainees are more likely than prison inmates to arrive in an intoxicated or psychotic state and because arrests frequently are the cause and/or effect of extreme emotional distress, mental health professionals in jails are far more likely than their prison counterparts to encounter people suffering from acute psychological distress, including suicidal depression, various forms of psychosis, extreme anxiety, and intoxication. While each of these phenomena can also occur in prison, prison mental health professionals are far more likely to be confronted with serious and persistent mental health problems. It is important to note that acuity does not necessarily refer to severity; here, acuity is used to denote a recent onset or an episode of exacerbated distress. Persistent or chronic disorders such as schizophrenia can be extremely serious, even if the person is not experiencing an acute exacerbation at the moment.

In responding to acute psychological distress, jail mental health professionals have several immediate duties. First, they must assess the person, paying special attention to suicidality or the likelihood of violence toward others. Chapter 11 examines the methods of screening new admissions. As a result of screening, a significant portion of detainees and inmates will be identified as likely needing mental health assessment and treatment. Each of these "positive screens" will, in turn, require assessment by a mental health professional to determine the need for treatment on an emergency or routine basis.

At this stage, diagnosis is much more difficult and much less important, especially in jails. As noted previously, even experienced clinicians may have difficulty distinguishing between acute exacerbations of serious mental illness, acute psychoses brought on by stress or intoxication, toxic psychosis, and malingering. As long as the detainee is kept safe, however, there is time to sort out these diagnostic challenges.

In contrast, prison mental health professionals are less likely to encounter psychiatric emergencies upon immediate entry to the institution and, in theory, will be able to review mental health treatment records from jail, the community, or previous prison admissions. In both jails and prisons, collateral information from previous treatment records is invaluable. In addition to the diagnostic challenges presented by acute distress and intoxication, clinicians are also faced with the difficulty of assessing malingering. Although the reasons for malingering in jails and prisons are different, the need to make accurate assessments is the same.

Malingering

One of the most vexing and controversial issues in correctional mental health is the assessment of malingering. While discussed in more depth in Chapter 23, it is important to note some differences between jails and prisons in regard to malingering.

Perhaps the best way for clinicians to think about malingering is as a question rather than an answer. In other words, if a detainee or inmate is purposely and inaccurately presenting as mentally ill, presumably he or she is doing this to achieve some sort of secondary gain. For pretrial detainees, it is commonly assumed that they are trying to create the false impression that they are incompetent to stand trial. In extreme cases, such as first-degree murder, such a strategy might make sense, as commitment to a forensic psychiatric hospital might be preferable to a sentence of life without parole or even death. Other defendants might hope that a finding of incompetence to stand trial would result in the long delay that would hinder prosecution. It is important to note that competency evaluations do not typically occur immediately upon the detainee's arrival at the jail and are typically not performed by jail mental health clinicians (see Chapter 61). Competency evaluators use a variety of methods to detect malingered symptoms or disabilities, including psychological testing; however, these are beyond the scope of this chapter.

On the other hand, there are many other reasons why a detainee or inmate might feign mental illness or exaggerate his or her symptoms. The most common reason is fear. Jails and prisons can be dangerous places, especially for offenders who are unable or unwilling to defend themselves physically. First-time offenders may exaggerate these dangers, based on fictional accounts of jails and prisons. In institutions with limited or inadequate access to mental health services, a person with a moderate depression or anxiety disorder might exaggerate symptoms in the belief that "gilding the lily" is the only way to get help. When malingering is suspected, it is important to try to understand the reasons why the detainee or inmate might feign or exaggerate symptoms or disabilities. It is dangerous to simply dismiss the possibility that he or she suffers from an actual mental illness.

In jails, there are two very useful strategies for responding to the possibility of malingering. Most importantly, detainees must be kept safe when presenting with symptoms of acute psychological distress, even if there is a strong suspicion that the distress is feigned or exaggerated. If the presentation is based on fear or extreme anxiety, a nonresponsive jail mental health system might inadvertently communicate to the detainee that the only way to end his or her intolerable psychological distress is through suicide. This is also important because the assessment of malingering is not an exact science, and the consequences of a false-positive determination of malingering should not be lethal. The second strategy is to seek previous mental health records from jails, prisons, hospitals, and community providers that have treated the detainee in the past. Even when records are slow to arrive, it is possible to verify psychiatric prescriptions by calling the pharmacy that filled them.

In prison, there is a different set of likely reasons that an inmate might feign or exaggerate symptoms or disabilities. The most common of these is a desire to move from one housing location to another that is considered safer or otherwise more desirable. Other reasons include seeking medication for inappropriate purposes or sale and, in rare cases, efforts to escape (e.g., during transportation to a hospital). Treatment responses in prison might include an assessment of the likely reasons for feigned or exaggerated symptoms and often skill-building treatments aimed at improving the inmate's manner of preventing or solving problems.

Special mental health housing

Unlike other aspects of correctional mental health, housing differs less as a function of jail versus prison and more as a function of the size of the institution or system. Jails and prisons require several housing options. As explained in Chapter 43, every jail or prison must provide appropriate housing for inmates who are deemed to pose a high or imminent risk of suicide. In large jails and prisons, this is often a special unit or part of another type of special housing, such as residential mental health housing, crisis housing, or medical infirmary housing. In smaller jails, suicide watch may be performed within general population housing. Wherever they exist, however, suicide watch cells must be reasonably suicide-resistant and include ease of observation and an absence of places from which an inmate can suspend a ligature.

Special mental health housing can serve several purposes. First, separating inmates with mental illness can allow for more efficient provision of psychiatric, nursing, and other treatment services. This is especially true for the provision of group therapies aimed at psychosocial rehabilitative and skill-building treatments. Second, it allows for more diligent observation of detainees and inmates who pose a risk of suicide or interpersonal violence. Third, it can prevent detainees and inmates with mental illnesses from being frightened or harmed by predators in the general population.

Equally important, people with serious mental illnesses may be psychologically vulnerable to exacerbations caused by real or perceived dangers posed by inmates in the general population. In large jails and prisons, it is often helpful to create psychologically safer housing alternatives such as residential treatment units. Again, this will vary more as a function of institution size and less as a function of jail versus prison settings.

Treatment: symptom reduction and safety versus skill building and rehabilitation

Treatment, of course, cannot consist solely of medication. As discussed in Chapters 41 and 42, correctional mental health services include individual and group therapies. The purposes of these therapies are several, including crisis prevention and response, suicide prevention, reduction of the amount of idle and unstructured time, and psychosocial skill building.

The relative importance given to each type of therapy depends, in large part, on the setting. Because of the high turnover and higher level of acuity, therapy in jails will largely be aimed at prevention of immediate harm and symptom reduction. While psychotropic medications play an important role in reducing symptoms, it is a mistake to ignore the potential value of individual and group therapies, especially in the treatment of anxiety and depression.

In contrast, prison mental health professionals can expect to treat their patients and clients for long periods of time, creating the very real possibility of meaningful skill acquisition in psychologically relevant ways. For example, group therapy can be effective in helping inmates to manage their anger, resulting in a decrease in prison misconduct (Novaco, Ramm, & Black, 2004; Stermac, 1986).

Segregation

As discussed in Chapter 14, there is some controversy about the extent and nature of psychological harm caused by long-term segregation. However, it is clear that such settings pose a risk of exacerbating or causing mental illness or preventing inmates with serious mental illness from improving. While large jails typically have segregation housing, such housing in jails is likely to be of shorter duration than in prisons. Because lengths of stay in prison are much longer than in jail, the likelihood of long-term segregation is much higher in prisons. Court orders and settlement agreements have increasingly required states to create mental health alternatives to traditional segregation (*Disability Advocates, Inc. v. New York State Office of Mental Health, et al.*, 2002; *Disability Law Center, Inc. v. Massachusetts Department of Corrections, et al.*, 2012; *Jones' El v. Berge*, 2002; *Madrid v. Gomez*, 1995).

While jails have been less often taken to task for their treatment of offenders with mental illness in segregation housing, changes in the landscape of US corrections suggest that they should make plans for mental health alternatives for detainees and inmates who remain housed in segregation for long periods of time (New York City Department of Correction, 2013).

Transition, discharge, and reentry planning

Transition planning, also known as "discharge planning" or "reentry planning" (American Association of Community Psychiatrists, 2001), has become a vexing issue for jails and prisons alike, in part because of a community mental health system that is already stressed and inadequately funded to meet existing demand. As a result, inmates who received regular mental health treatment in prison may have difficulty receiving those same services after they are released. Further, many years in prison may have caused preexisting life skills to atrophy to the point that simple tasks such as taking a bus to the clinic become extremely difficult.

Transition planning in jails poses a very different problem. Again, because of the high turnover, there is often very little time in which to plan for the discharge and transition back into the community of a detainee with serious mental illness. The sheer number of discharges is enough to overwhelm the social work staff of most jail mental health services. An additional challenge is the unpredictability of release from jail. Cases are routinely dismissed, plea-bargained for time served, or otherwise disposed of, often with little or no warning to jail mental health providers. One good way to address this challenge is to follow the old adage "discharge planning begins at admission" and attend to the basic elements of a transition plan during the initial assessment or initial treatment plan for any detainee with serious mental illness. The essential elements of such a plan include prescriptions or medications upon release, a safe place to sleep in the community, and assistance with obtaining entitlements such as Social Security disability income or Medicaid. One evolving best practice for transition planning includes "community in-reach," whereby case managers or primary clinicians from community mental health providers are able to meet with the detainee in jail prior to release (Dlugacz, 2010; Lennox, Senior, King, et al., 2012).

It is important to note that many changes will be occurring in the immediate future, with unknown effects on correctional mental health and the community resources to which detainees and inmates will be released. These changes include implementation of the Patient Protection and Affordable Care Act, Medicaid reform and expansion, and recent legislation requiring parity between mental health and other health insurance benefits. As of this writing, we know of no one who claims to fully understand the impact of these changes. For example, if Medicaid eligibility becomes easier to obtain, many more offenders might have timely access to mental health care upon release from jail or prison (assuming the community-based capacity exists).

Equally challenging, the lack of adequate social services in most US communities (LaVigne, Davies, Palmer, & Halberstadt, 2008; Steadman & Veysey, 1997) means that there are often inadequate services to which detainees and inmates can be referred. This also reflects the lack of social and familial support systems of many frequent arrestees with serious mental illness, particularly those who are homeless at the time of their arrest.

Summary

There are many similarities between prisons and jails, especially in regard to the constitutional standard for mental health services. However, the differences are important to recognize in ensuring that the unique needs of each kind of institution are met. Predominant among these differences is the very high degree of turnover in jail populations, resulting in dramatic increases in acuity of mental illness and substance misuse, significantly increased risk of suicide, and the increases in workload due to the much higher percentage of initial assessments. As a result, staffing plans for a variety of professions must take into account this higher workload if jails are to meet their obligations. In contrast, prison mental health services are more often faced with the realities of serious and persistent mental illnesses and the hopelessness that can come after years of incarceration and in the face of very long sentences. While prison mental health clinicians have more time with which to work, they also face significantly greater expectations for treatment that goes beyond crisis response and psychotropic medication.

References

American Association of Community Psychiatrists (2001). *AACP continuity of care guidelines: Best practices for managing transitions between levels of care*. Pittsburgh, PA: American Association of Community Psychiatrists.

American Psychiatric Association (2000). *Psychiatric services in jails and prisons: A task force report of the American Psychiatric Association*. Washington, DC: American Psychiatric Association.

Austin, J., Naro-Ware, W., Ocker, R., Harris, R., & Allen, R. (2012). *Evaluation of the current and future Los Angeles County jail population*. Denver, CO: The JFA Institute.

Bolton, A. (1976). *A study of the need for and availability of mental health services for mentally disordered jail inmates and juveniles in detention facilities*. Boston: Arthur Bolton Associates.

Carson, E. A., & Golinelli, D. (2013). *Prisoners in 2012* (NCJ 243920). Washington, DC: Department of Justice. Office of Justice Programs—Bureau of Justice and Statistics.

Disability Advocates, Inc. v. New York State Office of Mental Health, et al. (2002). U.S. District Court, Southern District of New York, Case 02 CV 2002 (GEL).

Disability Law Center, Inc. v. Massachusetts Department of Corrections, et al. (2012). U.S. District Court, District of Massachusetts, Case No. 07-10463 (MLW).

Dlugacz, H. A. (2010). *Reentry planning for offenders with mental disorders*. Kingston, NJ: Civic Research Institute.

Guerino, P., Harrison, P. M., & Sabol, W. J. (2011). *Prisoners in 2010* (NCJ 236096). Washington, DC: Department of Justice. Office of Justice Programs—Bureau of Justice and Statistics.

James, D. J., & Glaze, L. E. (2006). *Mental health problems of prison and jail inmates* (NCJ 213600). Washington, DC: Department of Justice. Office of Justice Programs—Bureau of Justice and Statistics.

Jones' El v. Berge (2002). U.S. District Court, Western District of Wisconsin, Case No. 00-C-421-C.

La Vigne, N., Davies, E., Palmer, T., & Halberstadt, R. (2008) *Release planning for successful reentry: A guide for corrections, service providers, and community groups*. Washington, DC: Urban Institute Justice Policy Center. Retrieved from http://www.urban.org/UploadedPDF/411767_successful_reentry.pdf

Lennox, C., Senior, J., King, C., et al. (2012). The management of released prisoners with severe and enduring mental illness. *Journal of Forensic Psychiatry and Psychology, 23*(1), 67–75.

Madrid v. Gomez (1995). 889 F. Supp. 1146.

New York City Department of Correction (2013, May). New mental health initiative will intervene and provide treatment for seriously mentally ill among jail population. News from the NYC DOC. Retrieved from: http://www.nyc.gov/html/doc/downloads/pdf/NEWS_from_Mental_Health_051313.pdf

Novaco, R. W., Ramm, M., & Black, L. (2004). Anger treatment with offenders. In C. R. Hollin (Ed.), *The essential handbook of offender assessment and treatment* (pp. 129–144). Hoboken, NJ: John Wiley & Sons Ltd.

Office of National Drug Control Policy (2013, May). *Arrestee drug abuse monitoring program II: 2012 Annual Report*. Washington, DC: Office of National Drug Control Policy.

Osher, F., Steadman, H. J., & Barr, H. (2002). *A best practice approach to community re-entry from jails for inmates with co-occurring disorders: The APIC model*. Delmar, NY: The National GAINS Center.

Steadman, H. J., & Veysey, B. M. (1997). *Providing services for jail inmates with mental disorders*. Washington, DC: Department of Justice. Office of Justice Programs—Bureau of Justice and Statistics.

Stermac, L. (1986). Anger control treatment for forensic patients. *Journal of Interpersonal Violence, 1*, 446–457.

Teplin, L. A. (1990). The prevalence of severe mental disorder among male urban jail detainees: Comparison with the Epidemiologic Catchment Area program. *American Journal of Public Health, 80*(6), 663–669.

CHAPTER 7

Working inside the walls

Bruce C. Gage

Introduction

The moment of entry into a correctional facility is iconic. The clanging doors, the steel, stone, and concrete, and the other sensory stimuli associated with crossing this threshold mark the entry into a different world from which exit, other than by death, is governed by a faceless system. It is no wonder that those who enter have "both conscious and visceral" reactions (Appelbaum, 2010).

To work inside the walls, the psychiatrist must come to terms with the realities of the correctional setting in order to be secure, satisfied with the work, and clinically effective. This chapter examines the context in which clinical work is embedded—that is, physical environment and security, correctional culture, personal safety, typical stressors, and personal liability.

It is convenient to assume a relatively sharp distinction between jails and prisons. In the United States, jails are short-term, usually local facilities that serve as pre-arraignment or pretrial lockups and incarcerate prisoners with sentences less than one year. Prisons are state and federal facilities and generally incarcerate prisoners for more than one year. Most of what follows focuses on prisons and larger jails. Small jails share some features of larger institutions but are tremendously diverse.

Physical environment and security

While correctional facilities emphasize keeping prisoners contained, keeping the unauthorized out is also an imperative. Thus, prisons are commonly imposing fortress-like structures situated in a defendable setting, usually away from population centers. They are surrounded by walls and/or fences topped with concertina wire. Guard towers are the rule; the officers are armed. Jails are typically box-like buildings with small windows in urban settings, often co-housed with a courthouse or other public facilities.

There is almost always a single point of entry for staff and visitors and separate entries for prisoners and commerce. Visitors are intensively screened. Staff are subject to some degree of screening each time they enter as well. What staff or visitors are allowed to bring into the facility is tightly regulated. Clinicians may not be permitted to bring in unauthorized books, computers, or cell phones, and even medical instruments may be prohibited, with the clinician obligated to use facility instruments. Cameras are almost always forbidden unless approved for a specific purpose. Personal keys, identification, money, credit cards, and similar belongings are typically secured at entry.

Entry is commonly through a sally port, sometimes called a trap, which is a system of two doors with a space between. Only one door opens at a time so that those going through are temporarily trapped between the doors, limiting the opportunity for unauthorized transit.

Within the facility, correctional officers must open doors that access sections of the facility. It is prudent to have a solid relationship with these officers as they can expedite or slow your progress through the facility. Regardless, travel within a facility is time-consuming.

Most are struck by the colorless austerity of the environment. The need for clear sight lines and minimization of hiding places militates against landscaping, sculptural installations, and pleasing architectural features. Furniture is institutional in nature—durable, tamper-proof, and immovable. While this austerity stems from important utilitarian considerations, there is little effort to beautify or soften the environment; women's facilities tend to be exceptions. Cleanliness and odor vary widely among facilities, with some brushed and washed like a naval vessel and others truly rank. They are usually eerily quiet places, occasionally erupting in a reverberating din or punctuated by the screams of an isolated prisoner.

Correctional officers are responsible for the security of the facility and the safety of its occupants. It is a serious mission, and mistakes can have dire consequences. In 2012 correctional officers were one of the top seven professions for nonlethal injury and illness (Bureau of Labor Statistics, 2013). It is essential to have and to demonstrate respect for security procedures. Adherence places the clinician in good stead with correctional staff and demonstrates to prisoners that you take security seriously, reducing the chance of being targeted.

An understanding of custody levels is crucial; they determine physical security measures, staffing models, patrols, access to different parts of the facility, the nature of staff escorts, prisoner privileges, permitted possessions, and even how medications are delivered. Each prisoner's custody level is determined by classification, essentially a risk assessment. There are various systems of classification, but most generate a score based on charges, detainers and warrants, sentencing status, criminal history, escape history, institutional disciplinary history, substance abuse, and demographic variables (Austin, 1998; Federal Bureau of Prisons, 2006; Hardyman, Austin, & Tulloch, 2002). The scores are then grouped; those with the highest risk are placed at the highest custody levels. Changes in classification level are primarily driven by negative prison behavior or its absence. Scores are typically updated following a serious negative event and on a regular schedule. In some systems, this process is called external classification. The process of internal classification focuses on prisoner needs, work capacity, and specific housing requirements, including medical or mental health considerations, and may incorporate formal needs assessments, personality dimensions, and prisoner history (Hardyman, Austin, Alexander, et al., 2002).

The highest-custody settings, commonly designated maximum or super maximum, often use sally ports for entry into cell tiers or pods of tiers. The tiers are composed of single-occupancy cells with remote-controlled locks operated by a secured officer. The cells have a built-in toilet, sink, bed, and sometimes desk and stool. These areas are hardened, meaning that additional precautions are taken to ensure that prisoners cannot escape or readily destroy or weaponize anything. Prisoners typically cannot see each other, and even verbal communication can be difficult. Prisoners are usually in their cells 23 hours per day. Supervision by custody staff is virtually always indirect—that is, the officers are not in the same physical space as the prisoners but observe them visually or by camera. The observation is constant in that an officer can observe a prisoner at any time. Prisoners are moved in security containment devices (SCDs), such as a metal waist chain attached to wrist and ankle cuffs, with two or more staff directly controlling the prisoner. Visitation is limited to official visits, but some prisons allow noncontact family visits. Prisoners have few or no personal items and usually are not allowed to keep their own medications, except possibly rescue medications.

At intermediate custody levels—that is, high or medium—supervision by custody staff may be direct (with officers occupying the same space as unrestrained prisoners) or indirect and is almost always constant. Cells may be individual or house small numbers of prisoners; bathrooms are shared. Access within the facility is typically through single, locked doors rather than sally ports. Escorting is variable, but SCDs are usually not required within the facility. Unescorted group movement between discrete areas occurs at specified times. Prisoners may eat in communal areas, go to activities and programs on or off the tier, and begin to hold jobs within the facility. Contact visits are common although not universal. This is normally the lowest custody level in jails.

At minimum custody levels, but still within facilities having a secure perimeter, dormitories are common. Supervision is typically direct but intermittent. Interaction between staff and prisoners is frequent. Escorting is rarely required within the facility. Prisoners may work outside of the secure perimeter while directly supervised by custody staff. Contact visits are the rule.

The lowest-custody setting is prerelease or work release. These are transitional facilities sited in the community and have no perimeter security. Living arrangements vary widely. Supervision is direct and intermittent. Prisoners go into the community to work or engage in other specified activities during the day and return to the facility in the evening. Visiting is tracked but may not be controlled.

Correctional culture

There is no monolithic correctional culture; each system and facility has its own unique culture and has evolved in some degree of isolation, emphasizing different philosophical approaches to the correctional mission and to criminal causation. The most common formulations of the correctional mission include punishment (or retribution), deterrence, incapacitation, and rehabilitation (or correction; Feinberg, 1975; Scott, 2005). The term "corrections" thus implies a particular philosophical perspective. The degree to which rehabilitation is emphasized has varied widely, and

some would argue it has never been substantially implemented (Rotman, 1995).

The correctional culture is also deeply influenced by beliefs about the origins of criminal behavior. The polarities of free will and determinism are commonly used to bookend arguments about criminal causation. Although these absolute positions are of dubious validity, they draw systems toward one pole or the other. When free-will thinking dominates, as it has in the United States for at least three decades, retributive, tough-on-crime rhetoric ascends (Andrews et al., 1990; Fellner, 2006; Mauer, 2006). When the emphasis is on the habitual nature of human behavior, including crime, there is a move toward rehabilitation. This is not merely an ivory tower debate; the philosophy of a system influences physical plant design, policy, programs, and staff attitudes.

Despite variability, there are important commonalities among most correctional settings. One practice that has substantial impact on culture is surveillance (Rhodes, 2004). Bentham (1787/1995) coined the term "Panopticon" for facilities designed to allow observation of prisoners without their knowing whether they were being observed. No prison was clearly built on Bentham's principles, but the idea persists today, especially in maximum-security settings, where officers in a booth watch video feeds from every cell and space within the unit (Rhodes, 2004). Foucault (1979) used the notion of the Panopticon to speak to the power that surveillance has in influencing conformity to the social order. Another important practice is the separation of prisoners from staff, which is best exemplified by indirect supervision.

The present trend toward direct supervision is a move away from these practices toward engagement as a means of both effective supervision and promotion of rehabilitation rather than conformity (Bogard, Hutchinson, & Persons, 2010; Hutchinson, Keller, & Reid, 2009). Even more dramatic in this regard is the rise of prison therapeutic communities (Parker, 2007).

A great deal has been written on the nature of correctional culture, mostly in high-security male prisons (e.g., Kauffman, 1988; Rhodes, 2004; Sykes, 1958). Jails and women's prisons have received relatively less attention, although more has been written in recent decades on incarcerated women (e.g., Owen, 1998; Zaitzow & Thomas, 2003). Books by prisoners have also enriched the literature (e.g., Abbott, 1981; Hassine, 2009).

That prisoners and staff have different subcultures is perhaps self-evident; what is often not appreciated is the relationship between them. Those new to the correctional environment are often surprised at the inconsistency of rule enforcement by correctional staff and the degree to which prisoners keep the peace within their own ranks and subtly cooperate with correctional staff. As Goffman (1961) writes, "the inmate, when with fellow-inmates, will support the counter-mores and conceal from them how tractably he acts when alone with the staff." It is vital to understand that there is a gulf of varying depth between the official structure of the jail or prison, as encoded in policy, and the actual culture. Put simply, the notion of total control, even in total institutions, is a myth.

Sykes (1958) argued that the seeds of these cultural accommodations arise from several features of high-security prisons, primarily because the rewards and punishments available to the staff are insufficient to substantially influence prisoner behavior. The available punishments are little different from what the prisoner already suffers and the rewards have been "stripped away." This leaves only unofficial and uneasy accommodations between staff and prisoners to maintain a degree of order and calm.

Prominent attitudes of the prisoner culture are reflected in values such as not "snitching" (sharing information about other prisoners with staff), "doing your own time" (not getting involved in others' business), respect, and avoiding an appearance of weakness. The prisoner culture is well enough established that it has its own recognized argot (O'Brien, 1995; Sykes, 1958). It is helpful to learn some of the terminology. For instance, inmates with mental illness may be referred to as "dings," "nut jobs," "whack jobs," and other unflattering terms by both custody staff and prisoners.

Women's prisons have a different culture in some regards, although a disdain for snitching and an emphasis on respect and doing your own time are similar. The most salient difference is the tendency of women to develop more intimate, family-like relationships and to place less emphasis on the solidarity of the community of prisoners (Owen, 1998; Zaitzow, 2003).

There is debate about the origins of prisoner culture (Williams & Fish, 1974). Some authors favor the perspective that the prison culture is imported from the community criminal subculture (e.g., Irwin & Cressey, 1962) rather than a response to prison conditions, as posited by Sykes and others.

Staff culture is less well explored. Given that "[t]he very nature of the prison guard's role—the exercise of authority over an involuntary clientele—means that prisoner and guards have a potentially fraught relationship" (Hepburn, 1989), it is not surprising that custody officers tend to have a more negative view of prisoners than others (Kjelsberg, Skoglund, & Rustad, 2007). Officers may speak of "breaking" offenders rather than rehabilitating them (Weinstock, 1989). Kauffman's portrait of brutality is bleak (Kauffman, 1988), but conditions have been improving.

During the 1970s and 1980s, there were a number of prison riots, demonstrating a breakdown in order at all levels (Morris, 1995). Before and during this time, corrections had gone through substantial changes, especially in the United States. Key factors included sentencing changes that led to crowding (Rotman, 1995), the influx and impact of modern gangs (Camp & Camp, 2002; Gaes, Wallace, Gilman, et al., 2002), and growing numbers of inmates with mental illness (Fellner, 2006; Lamb & Weinberger, 2005), which created worsening conditions and fragmented the prisoner culture (Hassine, 2009). The general impact of racial tension, independent of and through gangs, must also be noted (Irwin, 2005). These problems prompted many calls for reform, including that of Justice Anthony Kennedy, who in 2003 challenged the American Bar Association to "address the inadequacies—and the injustices—in our prison and correctional systems" (Kennedy, 2003). In fact, the development of standards by professional organizations and civil suits have driven substantial improvements in general conditions (Useem & Piehl, 2006), health care (*Coleman v. Wilson*, 1995; *Estelle v. Gamble*, 1976), and mental health care (Metzner, 2002).

Personal safety

Jails have had a lower murder rate than the US national average back to at least the early 1980s. While prison homicide rates were very high during the prison chaos of the early 1980s, they declined 93% from 1980 to 2000, dropping below the national average

(Mumola, 2005). Despite reductions in homicides, the rate of staff assaults in prisons stayed about the same between 1995 and 2000 (Stephan & Karberg, 2003).

Working in a correctional facility requires vigilance—being aware of who is nearby, identifying proximate hiding places and objects that might be used as weapons, and so on. Adhering to the facility's procedures is key to promoting and maintaining safety.

Clinicians are trained to be advocates for their patients, with an attendant encouragement of credulity. Some clinicians, out of a misguided notion of advocacy, come to view prisoners as unfortunate victims of the system and harbor hostile attitudes toward the custody staff while feeling a greater allegiance to the prisoners. Clinicians may put themselves at risk of being compromised, a term connoting staff interaction with a prisoner that gives the prisoner some coercive power over the staff member. Compromise usually begins with some minor favor for a prisoner and then escalates over time (Allen & Bosta, 1981).

Proper boundaries, objectivity, and healthy skepticism are essential. Clinicians should not accept gifts from prisoners other than tokens such as letters or drawings; in some settings, even this is a violation of policy. Similarly, prisoners should not be given information barred by policy. It is necessary to dress, speak, and behave professionally and to avoid excessive use of prison argot in conversation and charting except to quote. The importance of showing respect for others cannot be overemphasized, as both prisoners and custody staff are sensitive to disrespect. In this regard, note that uniformed staff prefer to be referred to as officers rather than guards, a term seen as demeaning.

Typical stressors

Probably evident from the foregoing, finding a balanced position between custody staff and prisoners can be difficult. The correctional psychiatrist may feel pressured to choose sides; some become more like jailers than clinicians. While clinicians are typically more socially allied with the custody staff, this need not include acceptance of an outlook inconsonant with clinical values. By being honest and direct with both staff and prisoners about professional obligations and limitations and by abstaining from judgment of either prisoners or staff, the correctional psychiatrist secures the greatest cooperation from both.

General sources of stress include environmental conditions, staffing problems, prison culture, and safety concerns (Appelbaum, 2010; Bell, 1989; Nurse, Woodcock, & Ormsby, 2003). Professional frustrations include the inefficiencies attendant to security functions, limited access to communications, limited privacy, and practice limitations such as formulary restrictions. All the typical concomitants of working in an underfunded health system are present, including poor facilities for seeing patients, high caseloads, fragmented informatics, marginal ancillary services, and limited access to consultation.

Violence and force, even when legitimately used by custody staff, are difficult to witness. A terrible dilemma is created when the clinician witnesses excessive force or degradation. Does the clinician intervene, either personally or through formal processes, or remain silent? Speaking out risks alienating custody staff, while failure to speak out raises ethical concerns. There is no clear answer, but the clinician has an obligation to respond to staff misbehavior when safety or patient welfare is at stake.

Many correctional clinicians become overwhelmed by the high prevalence of personality disorders and substance-related disorders (American Psychiatric Association, 2000; Fazel & Danesh, 2002; Teplin, 1994). The correctional psychiatrist needs to be adept at managing countertransference (Bell, 1989; Weinstock, 1989) and at recognizing the distortions that this population produces and also invites from staff. Here again, healthy skepticism and collateral information prevent clinical errors based on patient self-report or staff distortion. These practices also limit professional isolation and, by minimizing unneeded prescriptions, prevent development of a reputation as a dispensing machine.

A related challenge is prescribing controlled substances, especially benzodiazepines and stimulants. While it is understandable and wise to limit these agents in the correctional setting, it is important to be aware that absolute barring of these medications deprives prisoners of potentially effective treatments (Appelbaum, 2010).

It is important to be aware that the disruptive behavior of troubled prisoners is unpopular with both staff and prisoners. Staff face the danger of containing the behavior, and other prisoners face interruption of their daily activities due to short-term lockdowns. The pressure to do something (i.e., medicate or order therapeutic restraints) can be substantial. The correctional psychiatrist must be clear about the limits of using medications or restraints to control behavior.

Personal liability

There is no doubt that prisoners bring frequent civil suits, civil rights suits (Appelbaum, 2010), and complaints to licensing boards against correctional clinicians. Most are frivolous but often require some formal response. If a case becomes reportable, malpractice insurance may be denied or premiums may increase, even if the case is without merit and is ultimately dismissed.

Correctional psychiatrist need to understand their malpractice coverage. Those who work for the public sector may be indemnified by the public entity or, less commonly, by a private carrier. Those who work for private companies that provide contractual services or who work under their own contract typically must procure their own malpractice coverage, although some companies and agencies provide indemnification.

Even when malpractice coverage is provided through agency indemnification, correctional clinicians should consider carrying their own malpractice insurance. There are two primary reasons for this. First, a public agency may find it in its interest to settle a case rather than pay the costs of litigation or potentially lose a suit, leaving the clinician with an adverse finding. Second, the interests of the public agency and the clinician may diverge, in which case the clinician may actually be in an adversarial relationship with the agency.

It is important to be aware of suits for rights violations because they are not covered by malpractice insurance. Under 42 U.S.C. Section 1983, clinicians are not automatically immune from civil rights litigation even if they follow statute, policy, or custom. However, mere malpractice does not give rise to a rights violation; there must be deliberate indifference to the medical needs of prisoners (*Estelle v. Gamble*, 1976). Protection is also provided by the Prison Litigation Reform Act (PLRA), which requires that there be physical injury before money damages can be recovered

for mental injuries. There must also be actual knowledge of the risk posed (*Farmer v. Brennan*, 1994). A psychiatrist was found deliberately indifferent and to have committed malpractice when a prisoner died from dehydration after being kept in an observation room (*Gibson v. Moskowitz*, 2008). The Americans with Disabilities Act (ADA) has been found to apply to prisoners (*Pennsylvania v. Yeskey*, 1998), who can sue for money damages (*U.S. v. Georgia*, 2006).

Liability related to involuntary treatment is rare as long as the practitioner adheres to relevant laws and the agency has appropriate policies in place for involuntary treatment. The most common concerns, covered in Chapters 9 and 26, are emergency treatment and involuntary use of antipsychotics.

Privacy and confidentiality require attention as well. A federal appellate court found that meetings with mental health staff within hearing of other inmates create a possible claim for violation of privacy (*Hunnicutt v. Armstrong*, 2005). Clinicians must also know whether their agency is considered a covered entity under the Health Insurance Portability and Accountability Act of 1996 (HIPAA); many correctional systems are not. In addition, many states have important exceptions and variations related to correctional settings that often allow or mandate release of information related to public safety.

Successful malpractice suits against correctional psychiatrists are uncommon and typically involve substantial transgression on the part of the provider. In addition to the physical injury requirement, PLRA provides additional protections from civil suits by collecting filing fees and making cases easier for judges to dismiss. Another reason for rare malpractice findings is that clinical standards for correctional treatment are poorly articulated (Hoge, Greifinger, Lundquist, & Mellow, 2009).

Suicide is one area where liability claims are common. This important topic is covered in Chapter 43.

The correctional psychiatrist must be aware that a general responsibility to ensure safety extends beyond prisoner health. This was demonstrated by a case in which a transgendered prisoner was assaulted by other prisoners (*Farmer v. Brennan*, 1994). The court held that liability could be found when officials know of the risk and disregard it. This could potentially implicate an attending correctional psychiatrist.

Correctional clinicians have no obligation to report past crimes other than legally mandated reporting requirements, such as child or elder abuse. However, there is an affirmative obligation to prevent future harm that is similar to clinicians' *Tarasoff* duty (Pinta, 2010).

Summary

The reader may be wondering why a psychiatrist would want to work under such conditions. It is clearly not for everybody, but the rewards can be tremendous. Surprisingly, the quality of care in many facilities, especially prisons, is superior to care in the community. The clinical problems are unendingly fascinating, and, despite its downsides, having a setting with limited access to drugs that provides food, clothing, shelter, and medical care can allow a degree of patient improvement that may be difficult to realize in the community. Opportunities for creativity in treatment and program development are unparalleled. In many ways, correctional psychiatry is poised to lead the way in the treatment of some of the most ill and behaviorally disordered individuals of society.

References

Abbott, J. H. (1981). *In the belly of the beast.* New York: Random House.

Allen, B., & Bosta, D. (1981). *Games criminals play.* Sacramento, CA: Rae John Publishers.

American Psychiatric Association (2000). *Psychiatric services in jails and prisons* (2nd ed.). Washington, DC: American Psychiatric Association.

Andrews, D. A., Zinger, I., Hoge, R. D., Bonta, J., Gendreau, P., & Cullen, F. T. (1990). Does correctional treatment work? A clinically relevant and psychologically informed meta-analysis. *Criminology, 28,* 369–404.

Appelbaum, K. L. (2010). The mental health professional in a correctional culture. In C. Scott (Ed.), *Handbook of correctional mental health* (2nd ed., pp. 91–117). Washington, DC: American Psychiatric Press.

Austin, J. (1998). *Objective jail classification systems: A guide for jail administrators.* Washington, DC: National Institute of Corrections.

Bell, M. H. (1989). Stress as a factor for mental health professionals in a correctional setting. In R. Rosner & R. B. Harmon (Eds.), *Correctional psychiatry* (pp. 145–154). New York: Plenum Press.

Bentham, J. (1787/1995). *The Panopticon writings,* M. Bozovic (Ed.). London: Verso.

Bogard, D., Hutchinson, V. A., & Persons, V. (2010). *Direct supervision jails: The role of the administrator.* Washington, DC: National Institute of Corrections.

Bureau of Labor Statistics (2013). Nonfatal occupational injuries and illnesses requiring days away from work 2012. Retrieved from http://www.bls.gov/news.release/osh2.nr0.htm

Camp, G., & Camp, C. (2002). *The 2002 corrections yearbook.* Middletown, CT: Criminal Justice Institute.

Coleman v. Wilson (1995). 912 F. Supp. 1282.

Estelle v. Gamble (1976). 429 U.S. 97.

Farmer v. Brennan (1994). 511 U.S. 825.

Fazel, S., & Danesh, J. (2002). Serious mental disorder in 23000 prisoners: a systematic review of 62 surveys. *Lancet, 359,* 545–550.

Federal Bureau of Prisons (2006). Inmate security designation and custody classification. Retrieved from http://www.bop.gov/policy/progstat/5100_008

Feinberg, J. (1975). Punishment. In J. Feinberg & H. Gross (Eds.), *Philosophy of law* (pp. 500–508). Encino, CA: Dickenson Publishing Company, Inc.

Fellner, J. (2006). A corrections quandary: Mental illness and prison rules. *Harvard Civil Rights-Civil Liberties Law Review, 41,* 391–412.

Foucault, M. (1979). *Discipline and punish: The birth of the prison.* (A. Sheridan, Trans.). New York: Vintage.

Gaes, G., Wallace, S., Gilman, E., Klein-Saffran, J., & Suppa, S. (2002). The influence of prison gang affiliation on violence and other prison misconduct. *The Prison Journal, 82,* 359–385.

Gibson v. Moskowitz (2008). 523 F.3d 657.

Goffman, E. (1961). *Asylums: Essays on the social situation of mental patients and other inmates.* Garden City, NJ: Anchor Books.

Hardyman, P. L., Austin, J., & Tulloch, O. C. (2002). *Revalidating external prison classification systems: The experience of ten states and model for classification reform.* Washington, DC: National Institute of Corrections.

Hardyman, P. L., Austin, J., Alexander, J., Johnson, K. D., & Tulloch, O. C. (2002). *Internal prison classification systems: Case studies in their development and implementation.* Washington, DC: National Institute of Corrections.

Hassine, V. (2009). *Life without parole: Living in prison today.* New York: Oxford University Press.

Hepburn, J. R. (1989). Prison guards as agents of social control. In L. Goodstein & D. L. MacKenzie (Eds.), *The American prison: Issues in research and policy* (pp. 191–208). New York: Plenum Press.

Hoge, S. K., Greifinger, R. B., Lundquist, T., & Mellow, J. (2009). Mental health performance measures in corrections. *International Journal of Offender Therapy and Comparative Criminology, 53,* 634–647.

Hunnicutt v. Armstrong (2005). 152 Fed. Appx. 34.

Hutchinson, V. A., Keller, K., & Reid, T. (2009). *Inmate behavior management: The key to a safe and secure jail.* Washington, DC: National Institute of Corrections.

Irwin, J., & Cressey, D. R. (1962). Thieves, convicts and the inmate culture. *Social Problems, 10,* 142–155.

Irwin, J. (2005). *The warehouse prison: Disposal of the new dangerous class.* Los Angeles: Roxbury.

Kauffman, K. (1988). *Prison officers and their world.* Cambridge, MA: Harvard University Press.

Kennedy, A. M. (2003). Speech delivered by Justice Anthony M. Kennedy at the American Bar Association Annual Meeting, August 9, 2003. *Federal Sentencing Reporter, 16,* 126–128.

Kjelsberg, E., Skoglund, T. H., & Rustad, A. (2007). Attitudes towards prisoners, as reported by prison inmates, prison employees, and college students. *BMC Public Health, 7,* 71–79.

Lamb, H. R., & Weinberger, L. E. (2005). The shift of psychiatric inpatient care from hospitals to jails and prisons. *Journal of the American Academy of Psychiatry and the Law, 33*(4), 529–534.

Mauer, M. (2006). *Race to incarcerate* (rev. ed.). New York: New Press.

Metzner, J. L. (2002).Class action litigation in correctional psychiatry. *Journal of the American Academy of Psychiatry and the Law, 30,* 19–29.

Morris, N. (1995). The contemporary prison: 1965–present. In N. Morries & D. Rothman (Eds.), *Oxford history of the prison: The practice of punishment in Western society* (pp. 227–259). New York: Oxford University Press.

Mumola, C. J. (2005). *Suicide and homicide in state prisons and local jails.* Washington, DC: Department of Justice, Office of Justice Programs.

Nurse, J., Woodcock, P., & Ormsby, J. (2003). Influence of environmental factors on mental health within prisons: focus group study. *British Medical Journal, 327,* 480–484.

O'Brien, P. (1995). The prison on the continent: Europe 1865–1965. In N. Morris & D. J. Rothman (Eds.), *Oxford history of the prison: The practice of punishment in Western society.* (New York: Oxford University Press).

Owen, B. (1998). *In the mix: Struggle and survival in a women's prison.* Albany: State University of New York Press.

Parker, M. (2007). *Dynamic security: The democratic therapeutic community in prison.* London: Jessica Kingsley Publishers.

Pennsylvania v. Yeskey (1998). 524 U.S. 206.

Pinta, E. R. (2010). *Tarasoff* duties in prisons: community standards with certain twists. *Psychiatric Quarterly, 81,* 177–182.

Rhodes, L. A. (2004). *Total confinement.* Berkeley: University of California Press.

Rotman, E. (1995). The failure of reform: United States, 1865–1965. In N. Morris & D. J. Rothman (Eds.), *The Oxford history of the prison* (pp. 169–197). New York: Oxford University Press.

Scott, C. L. (2005). Overview of the criminal justice system. In C. L. Scott & J. B. Gerbasi (Eds.), *Handbook of correctional mental health* (pp. 21–24). Washington, DC: American Psychiatric Association Publishing, Inc.

Stephan, J. J., & Karberg, J. (2003). *Census of state and federal correctional facilities, 2000.* Washington, DC: Department of Justice, Office of Justice Programs.

Sykes, G. (1958). *The society of captives: A study of a maximum security prison.* Princeton, NJ: Princeton University Press.

Teplin, L. A. (1994). Psychiatric and substance abuse disorders among male urban jail detainees. *American Journal of Public Health, 84,* 290–293.

U.S. v. Georgia (2006). 546 U.S. 151.

Useem, B., & Piehl, A. M. (2006). Prison buildup and disorder. *Punishment and Society, 8,* 87–115.

Weinstock, R. (1989). Treatment of antisocial and other personality disorders in a correctional setting. In R. Rosner & R. B. Harmon (Eds.), *Correctional psychiatry* (pp. 41–59). New York: Plenum Press.

Williams, V. L., & Fish, M. (1974). *Convicts, codes, and contraband: The prison life of men and women.* Cambridge, MA: Ballinger Publishing Company.

Zaitzow, B. H., & Thomas, J. (2003). *Women in prison: Gender and social control.* Boulder, CO: Lynn Rienner Publishers, Inc.

Zaitzow, B. H. (2003). "Doing gender" in a women's prison. In B. H. Zaitzow & J. Thomas (Eds.), *Women in prison: Gender and social control* (pp. 21–38). Boulder, CO: Lynn Rienner Publishers, Inc.

CHAPTER 8

Ethics in correctional mental health

Philip J. Candilis and Eric D. Huttenbach

Can the imposition of this kind of suffering by an institution be morally justified?. . . . To propose or construct a correctional ethic would be an oxymoron, rather like presenting oneself as a married bachelor or a violent pacifist; or closer still, like constructing an ethic for slave-masters.

Derek R. Brookes (2001)

Introduction

The ethical analysis of health care in correctional settings suffers from the simplistic balance of care and security. Indeed, there are security limitations to clinical practice in corrections because of the requirements to keep staff, inmates, and the community safe; inmates occasionally misuse sick call, the infirmary, and their medicines, and may even, under rare circumstances, threaten their health care providers. Yet solutions that restrict the ethics of health care delivery do little to solve problems that are fundamental to the deprivation of liberty. In reviewing the legal, professional, and ethical standards of correctional practice, this chapter provides health care ethics as the model for solving the tensions inherent to correctional life rather than as an adjunct to the security mission of the correctional institution.

This approach resonates strongly with the work of commentators who assert that health care professionals should not be required to perform security functions in corrections (e.g., Kipnis, 2001). The work of health care professionals is protected by fundamental requirements of trust and adequate resources, while deferring in general terms to concerns of institutional security. For correctional health care professionals the problem arises in deciding how much deference must be given to security—a balance too frequently decided in favor of institutional policies that restrict health care delivery, limit formularies, curb confidentiality and time with inmates, and provide inadequate environments for treatment.

Mainstream policies that favor security over health are based on ideas of social role (Bradley, 1988) and the conflict between obligations toward an employer, a patient, and the public health of inmates in general. The logic that clinicians wear several hats and must balance competing obligations is the crux of this approach but does little to address the ethical problems of segregation, loss of heterosexual contact, and restriction of common material goods (Brookes, 2001). Recent movement in the courts, professional societies, and the empirical literature demonstrates that social role approaches are insufficient to solve the problem and invite a simplistic deference to institutional security that at times still governs correctional ethics.

We begin by rejecting Brookes' nihilistic stance that posing a correctional ethic is an oxymoron—"a dangerous nonsense" serving to legitimize and entrench oppressive values (Brookes, 2001). The impulse to confine dangerous criminals is fundamental to the social contract and serves a legitimate purpose with certain unacceptable consequences. The vulnerability of inmates in the control of a total institution does alter the ethical equation, but not sufficiently to grant them full parity with society's imperative for self-protection. Rather, modern correctional ethics identifies obligations in numerous directions—to the law, to the health professions, and to society as a whole—that call for a strengthening of health care values, attenuation of harms to inmates, and rejection of a simplistic balance of duties.

Access to care: the legal right to mental health care

Prisoners do not have the freedom to seek and obtain their own medical treatment; rather, they rely on the correctional institution to provide it for them. This reliance creates a legal duty to provide medical and psychiatric care. In fact, prisoners are the only class of American citizens who have a constitutionally protected right to receive health care. This is a phenomenon that underscores both the vulnerability of inmates and the special nature of health care itself.

The landmark US Supreme Court decision *Estelle v. Gamble* (429 U.S. 97 [1976]) emphasized that prisoners have a constitutionally protected right against cruel and unusual punishment guaranteed by the Eighth Amendment. Based on this analysis, correctional facilities have a legal duty to provide prisoners some access to health care. This level of care has become known as the "deliberate indifference" standard—perhaps not a particularly high level of care as intended by the Court, but one that may be equated at least to a level near or above recklessness. However, based on this minimal standard alone, a facility could meet the "deliberate indifference" constitutional requirement yet still be found negligent in a medical malpractice suit for not providing the profession's standard of care (*Estelle v. Gamble*, 1976, p. 106). A medical malpractice lawsuit is based on a negligence standard, which is a higher standard than that of recklessness and brings common clinical standards into correctional ethics. It underscores strongly the influence of general medical standards, even in a setting grounded only in deliberate indifference.

Subsequent cases have raised this minimal standard for some jurisdictions. Inmates have been guaranteed access to mental health care (*Bowring v. Godwin*, 1977), and some federal courts have defined additional rights. *Ruiz v. Estelle* (1980), for example, required limits on seclusion alone as treatment, the need for trained mental health providers, reasonable medical records, and safety measures. *Madrid v. Gomez* (1995) further defined the inmate's right to speedy access to quality medical care and facilities; facilities must provide a quality assurance system and demonstrate measures to prevent suicides and respond to other emergencies. In addition to this case law, correctional facilities must meet standards set by other federal regulations (e.g., US Department of Justice, National Institute of Corrections, 2001; US Department of Justice, Office of the Inspector General Audit Division, 2008), individual state tort law requirements, and the individual state's department of corrections regulatory requirements. Responsibilities to federal, state, and professional standards are evident in identifying ethical obligations.

Given the direction of more recent court decisions, an inmate's right to care could expand further. A recent well-publicized court decision ordered that an inmate with a severe form of gender identity disorder be granted gender reassignment surgery (*Kosilek v. Spencer*, 2012). This case, currently under appeal, is notable because it grants a prisoner access to a medical procedure that would almost certainly be denied by Medicare and most private medical insurance policies. While this is an unusual case at the federal district court level (and carries limited precedent-setting influence), it relies on the notion that case law defines a floor, but not a ceiling, for the required level of care. For our purposes in identifying a health care ethic for correctional institutions, the pattern reinforces the numerous obligations of law and medicine recognized by explicit legal analysis.

Organizational policy

Professional organizations that govern corrections and mental health add their views to the appropriate standard of care. Their public statements are important not simply because they offer guidance to their members but also because they represent social statements of purpose for the professions as a whole. The National Commission on Correctional Health Care (NCCHC, 2008) Standards for Health Services in Prisons, for example, note that it is essential that inmates have access to care in order to meet their serious health needs; this reflects the Supreme Court standard of *Estelle v. Gamble*. The NCCHC sets specific standards, including that all inmates have a mental health screening within 14 days of admission to identify serious mental health needs.

The American Public Health Association (2003) has also published standards for correctional facilities. Their goal is that

"mental health services, both diagnostic and therapeutic, must be made available to all incarcerated persons with acute and/or chronic psychiatric disorders including behavioral and emotional conditions, substance use disorders, and developmental disabilities." To meet these standards, a facility must have psychiatric services that are consistent with national community standards and written standards that ensure mental health screening at intake, acute care and suicide prevention programs, and appropriate staffing and mental health facilities.

The American Psychiatric Association (2000) echoes this approach: "Timely and effective access to mental health treatment is the hallmark of adequate mental health care." Furthermore, "The fundamental policy goal for correctional mental health care is to provide the same level of mental health services to each patient in the criminal justice process that should be available in the community. This policy goal is deliberately higher than the 'community standard' called for in the various legal contexts." This policy goal effectively brings psychiatric services to a level that does not simply mirror what is available in a given community but provides services that should be available in any community.

In March 2010, a decade after the American Psychiatric Association's policy statement, President Obama signed comprehensive health reform, the Patient Protection and Affordable Care Act. One of the major tenets of this effort is that mental health services and substance abuse services achieve parity of access similar to that of medical care—a significant raising of the health care bar. Assuming that the parity provision continues to be upheld by the courts, the level of health care will continue to rise at the community level and, in turn, in the correctional setting.

Classical ethics: the conflicting roles of the correctional psychiatrist

Traditionally, clinicians' loyalties remained strictly aligned with the roles they served, primarily as advocates for their patients. Yet even the Hippocratic writings called for an allegiance to the profession, its standards, and its protection (Candilis, Weinstock, & Martinez, 2007). The reliance on role theory to define professional practice was and remains common, echoed even in the American Psychiatric Association's reports on services in jails and prisons (1989, 2000). This approach reinforces the duality of clinical and forensic functions and invites attempts to separate the roles or "manage" the conflict. In the context of correctional privations, the strategy suffers serious limitations.

As complex professional roles expand to require professionals to serve clients, employers, professional organizations, and society, it is increasingly difficult to stay firmly within bounds. For clinicians in managed care settings, for example, this problem became painfully evident as practitioners struggled to treat patients while adhering to the cost-saving priorities of their institutions. Often, physicians were limited in their consent discussions with patients, forbidden from discussing their views or knowledge of their employer's strategies—a phenomenon exemplified by the presence of "gag clauses" in professional contracts.

The inadequacy of adhering to the requirements of a single role became even clearer in the forensic writings of the past decades as commentators pointed out the importance of recognizing the interactions among individuals, institutions, and society (e.g., Ciccone & Clements, 1984; Gutheil, Bursztajn, Brodsky, et al.,

1991). Systems approaches that took into account individual, professional, legal, and medical frameworks were necessary for the nuanced work of forensic psychiatry and psychology. There were far more options for case analysis when dilemmas could be addressed by drawing on the complexities of multidirectional obligations rather than ignoring them.

In the correctional setting, psychiatrists clearly have ethical obligations outside the traditional patient–doctor relationship. Correctional psychiatrists, for example, may be required to perform forensic evaluations by court order or as a required component of their work (Cervantes & Hanson, 2013). In this role, the professional has an obligation to provide independent and objective information to the court or prison. This objectivity is required even if the forensic evaluation could cause "harm" to the inmate, violating classic requirements of beneficence or the Hippocratic admonition to "do no harm." This is the challenge—indeed, the weakness—of strict role theory.

Because of the potential conflict, most health care providers in the correctional setting are prohibited from collecting forensic information (National Commission on Correctional Health Care, 2008). However, this is not an absolute ban; in smaller correctional facilities, a psychiatrist may be required by law or regulation to perform forensic assessment (Cervantes & Hanson, 2013; National Commission on Correctional Health Care, 2008). Usual practice ensures that the individual performing the forensic evaluation is not also on the treatment team, avoiding the classic dual role with conflicting duties toward patient and institution. Furthermore, rules are in place to protect against the conflict; correctional psychiatrists have a duty, for example, to inform inmates of the nature of their role and the limits of confidentiality (American Academy of Psychiatry and the Law, 2005). NCCHC standards take this further by directing that "the services of outside providers or someone on staff who is not in a therapeutic relationship with the inmate is obtained" and that if someone on staff does a court- or parole-ordered evaluation, he or she obtain "the informed consent of the inmate." If a correctional psychiatrist were to perform a forensic evaluation on a patient with a previous or current patient–doctor relationship, even classic protections of informed consent are not sufficient to protect the inmate or practitioner.

A thought-provoking example of this conflict arises in the clinical assessments conducted to determine appropriateness for segregation, as clinicians commonly assess the risk of segregation to the inmate. This tight connection of clinical and punitive functions underscores the difficulties of separating roles within correctional systems.

For forensic practitioners this exercise is reminiscent of the debate over evaluations for competence to be executed—a critical function of forensic psychiatrists and sanctioned by leading professional organizations (Candilis et al., 2007). The difference is that there are clear protections available for inmates undergoing competence-to-be-executed evaluations; evaluators are independent and divorced from the ultimate decision about punishment. This is not so in segregation clearances.

Moreover, correctional psychiatrists can have additional obligations to institutional safety and public health. The obligations to protect the health and safety of inmates and correctional staff are legitimate requirements that challenge confidentiality and consent protections. These duties, as well as the duty to protect the outside community from criminals, complicate the simple notions of dual role and the minimal protections that confidentiality warnings can provide. Consequently, we turn to a model that offers a richer resource for analyzing the duties of professionals practicing in conflicting roles.

Multidirectional or robust professionalism

The traditional approach to forensic ethics is to apply an individualized ethical code to each setting. For example, if psychiatrists provide medicine or therapy to a patient, they are bound by the traditional rules of medical ethics, such as those propounded by the American Medical Association (2014–2015). However, if psychiatrists engage in a forensic role such as that of a court expert, then a separate set of ethical guidelines apply. Here, the ethical code established by the American Psychiatric Association and the American Academy of Psychiatry and the Law (2005) holds sway. The physician attempts to negate any conflicts by remaining loyal to the code of the specific setting. The physician "wears the hat" based on the task at hand, attempting to choose one over the other (Strasburger, Gutheil, & Brodsky, 1997).

However, correctional psychiatry requires the professional to assume more than one role simultaneously. Clinical disclosures, security, and public health concerns are so much the fabric of correctional interactions that they create a conflict far more acute than in many other health care environments. It is impossible to function under strict role requirements. One cannot simply be a treater or a forensic practitioner; the correctional psychiatrist is both.

Robust professionalism is a novel paradigm that acknowledges that an individual may be assigned unique duties that appear to operate under separate ethical principles based simply on the setting (Candilis, Martinez, & Dording, 2001; Candilis et al., 2007; Martinez & Candilis, 2005). However, robust professionalism realizes that physicians, as professionals, cannot ignore fundamental ethical roots simply because they are working in a legal or correctional setting. The American Psychiatric Association (2000) recognizes this explicitly in its correctional standards by stating that "psychiatrists are always bound by the standards of professional ethics . . . the most fundamental statements of the moral and ethical foundations of professional psychiatric practice." The physician must integrate the requirements of individual and social ethics into a single, robust professionalism.

Robust, or multidirectional, professionalism acknowledges the individual foundations of the traditional doctor–patient relationship and that of forensic work but rejects the idea that there must be strictly separate sets of professional values. Splintering the ethical foundations of professionalism into one camp or another weakens the analytical power of both paradigms. Instead, robust professionalism advocates an integrated approach where individual loyalties and community standards are woven together into a strong conceptualization of what it means to be a professional.

As it is, it is unlikely that physicians can simply abandon their medical background and training. Even in a forensic role, physicians still build on the foundations of medical ethics—they are medical practitioners before they become forensic or correctional specialists. So while forensic practitioners may attempt to offer strict objectivity and loyalty to their employers, the reality is far different. David Luban (1988) has stated this forcefully: "commitments to the duties of a profession, to a career, or to major social situations . . . these can be, they frequently are, among the deepest loyalties and commitments in our lives; and it cannot be right to ask us to reconsider them, to trade them off, again and again." Loyalty to the fundamental roots of the medical profession and to the community that privileges it remains operative even under conditions of security and confinement.

Individual values matter as well. Physicians invariably maintain a loyalty to their own internal values, duties, and ideals—standards essential for maintaining professional identity and integrity (Wynia, Latham, Kao, et al., 1999). It is this consistency over time that anchors an individual or profession and helps resist the vagaries of social and situational forces. This is particularly true when these forces influence the professional to behave in ways contrary to historical values of medicine and psychiatry (Candilis et al., 2007).

Correctional psychiatry is a crucible of these conflicting personal and professional duties. There are traditional psychiatric services such as the prescribing of medication and the engagement in psychotherapy. But correctional psychiatrists are sometimes asked to offer a psychiatric assessment for mitigating factors during disciplinary proceedings. However, physicians retain loyalties to patients, judicial bodies, the correctional facility, and even society as a whole. Under strict role requirements, it has been difficult to admit these values into the narrow view of correctional practice. But a view of correctional professionalism that replaces narrow role theory with an integrated model of personal, professional, and community values may allow exactly that.

This expanded view of correctional practice recognizes the limits of strict "two-hat" thinking. Indeed, it minimizes damage to core beliefs when they conflict by drawing on values from outside the setting. If the requirements of a correctional institution appear onerous or punitive, comparison to community standards, organizational statements, or clinical training can have an important modifying influence. Developing a multidirectional perspective, rather than an insular one, allows ethical touchstones that may be unavailable otherwise. Moreover, the dynamic processes that exist among personal, professional, and community values are recognized not merely in the politics of correctional institutions and their communities but in the contributions of its practitioners. Prison suicides, assaults, escapes, and riots have far-reaching effects on staff and communities that call on political, economic, and social solutions that extend beyond the correctional setting alone. All these elements encourage familiarity with a richer, more robust ethical framework.

One piece is still missing from the development of a robust correctional ethic: the perspective of the individual inmate. Although it may seem intuitive that inmates hold predictable views of their confinement, the literature indicates otherwise. Studies spanning civil commitment, mandated outpatient treatment, jail diversion, and inmate sex offender treatment indicate that fairness, transparency, and respect are among the factors that most influence inmates' perspectives. Even though they may be legally obligated to enter specific programs, most of these patients do not appear to view the pressure as unfair or coercive, even under conditions that meet all common definitions of compulsion (Cusack, Steadman, & Herring, 2010; Hoge, Lidz, Eisenberg, et al., 1997; Munetz, Ritter, Teller, & Bonfine, 2014; Rigg, 2002).

In one survey of sex offender inmates in Canada, for example, 63% of participants indicated little or no perceived coercion in participating in their required psychiatric treatment (Rigg, 2002). This percentage is even higher than in a separate study on voluntary and involuntary civil psychiatric admissions, in which 35% of involuntary patients did not feel coerced (Hoge et al., 1997). Individuals' interests in being included in decision making, following procedure, and being treated respectfully were important determinants of their outlook and behavior (Lidz, 1997).

These findings have important implications for correctional systems that do not spend time or resources to account for the inmate's experience—the common practice of interviews at the cell door exemplifies this and hinders the practices of informed consent, confidentiality, and mitigation of coercion. Health care professionals can be particularly useful here in ensuring that discussion, assent, and understanding lead to inmates' engagement with treatment. Reinforcing the move toward common community standards can result in exactly the kind of behavioral conformity and treatment adherence jails and prisons try so assiduously to achieve.

Because the robust professional approach is one that recognizes multiple perspectives or claims on the ethical behavior of the psychiatrist, it is one that cannot minimize the status of the inmate under the control of what has been called a "total institution"—one that controls all aspects of personal behavior. In these circumstances it is not only community standards that matter. The vulnerabilities of the inmate have been recognized in the courts, organizational statements, and guidelines for correctional practice. When the individual comes up against the total institution, protections must be in place to account for that vulnerability. This must be true when inmates face the stresses of segregation, lack of mental health units, or absence of nonpharmacological options for treating psychiatric and behavioral conditions (e.g., cognitive-behavioral therapy, coping skills training, education, or vocational support). Including the perspective of the incarcerated criminal is part of the robust view of correctional ethics and supports the view that clinical values matter and that they can lead to safer institutions.

Summary

Simply balancing care and safety appears to be insufficient for psychiatrists who practice at the intersection of total institutions, their professions, and their prisoner patients. Obligations to the law, professional standards, the community, and public health require a more complex appreciation of competing values. It is not practical to parse out professional guidelines simply based on the specific task of the day. While one may hope to separate the tasks of clinical care, institutional safety, or forensic work, it is simply not possible in practice. Instead, correctional practice is based on law, guidelines, and an empirical dataset that sets up a series of identifiable requirements for daily practice.

The first concrete manifestation of this acknowledges the fundamental influence of health care values—of "being physicians first." As a matter of daily practice, this means having sufficient resources to offer mainstream treatments or appropriate alternatives when security-related limits are required. Rather than restricting formularies, for example, this may mean having access to alternative therapies or medications that treat the common anxiety, sleep, or attention-deficit/hyperactivity problems that affect inmates. It may mean more mental health units to allay the human and financial costs of suicide watches, victimization of mentally ill inmates, and assaults on staff. It almost certainly means developing diversionary alternatives to incarceration to address the vulnerability and treatment needs of mentally ill persons who run afoul of the law. It remains an extraordinary commentary on the state of mental health that the largest mental health institutions in the United States are jails and prisons (Torrey, Kennard, Eslinger, et al., 2010).

In daily practice, acknowledging health care, individual, and professional values in a robust vision of professionalism means not participating in security functions except as needed to protect inmates and staff. It means advocating for clinical values and opposing mistreatment (Metzner & Fellner, 2010). Making the limits of confidentiality clear is a time-honored element of the informed consent process and need not be diluted in the correctional system. Honoring clear boundaries between treatment and forensic evaluation is the crux of this issue; confidentiality warnings and access to counsel cannot be one-off affairs that do not account for the cognitive, educational, and mental health vulnerabilities of the patient in a correctional setting.

Developing trust, offering transparency, and delivering clear descriptions of procedural requirements are the lessons of an empirical database that supports this approach and can lead to more collaboration and less violence. Establishing a robust correctional professionalism promises exactly that.

References

American Academy of Psychiatry and the Law. Ethics guidelines for the practice of forensic psychiatry. Retrieved from http://www.aapl.org/pdf/ETHICSGDLNS.pdf (accessed December 13, 2013).

American Medical Association (2014–2015). *Code of medical ethics of the American Medical Association: current opinions with annotations.* Chicago: American Medical Association.

American Psychiatric Association (1989). *Psychiatric services in jails and prisons: report of the task force on psychiatric services in jails and prisons.* Washington, DC: American Psychiatric Association.

American Psychiatric Association (2000). *Psychiatric services in jails and prisons: a task force report of the American Psychiatric Association.* Washington, DC: American Psychiatric Association.

American Public Health Association (2003). *Standards for health services in correctional institutions.* Washington, DC: American Public Health Association.

Bowring v. Godwin (1977). 551 F.2d 44.

Bradley, F. H. (1988). *Ethical studies* (2nd ed.). Oxford: Oxford University Press.

Brookes, D. R. (2001). The possibility of a correctional ethic. In J. Kleinig & M. L. Smith (Eds.), *Discretion, community, and correctional ethics* (pp. 39–68). Lanham, MD.: Rowman & Littlefield Publishers.

Candilis, P. J., Martinez, R., & Dording, C. (2001). Principles and narrative in forensic psychiatry: toward a robust view of professional role. *Journal of the American Academy of Psychiatry and the Law, 29,* 167–173.

Candilis, P. J., Weinstock, R., & Martinez, R. (2007). *Forensic ethics and the expert witness.* New York: Springer.

Cervantes, N. C., & Hanson, A. (2013). Dual agency and ethics conflicts in correctional practice: Sources and solutions. *Journal of the American Academy of Psychiatry and the Law, 41,* 72–78.

Ciccone, J. R., & Clements, C. D. (1984). The ethical practice of forensic psychiatry: A view from the trenches. *Bulletin of the American Academy of Psychiatry and the Law, 12,* 263–277.

Cusack, K. J., Steadman, H. J., & Herring, A. H. (2010). Perceived coercion among jail diversion participants in a multisite study. *Psychiatric Services, 61,* 911–916.

Estelle v. Gamble (1976). 429 U.S. 97.

Gutheil, T. G., Bursztajn, H., Brodsky, A, et al. (1991). *Decision making in psychiatry and the law.* Baltimore: Williams & Wilkins.

Hoge, S. K., Lidz, C. W., Eisenberg, M., et al. (1997). Perceptions of coercion in the admission of voluntary and involuntary psychiatric patients. *International Journal of Law and Psychiatry, 20,* 167–181.

Kipnis, K. (2001). Health care in the corrections setting; an ethical analysis. In J. Kleinig & M. L. Smith (Eds.), *Discretion, community, and correctional ethics* (pp. 113–24). Lanham, MD: Rowman & Littlefield Publishers.

Kosilek v. Spencer (2012). 889 F. Supp. 2d 190.

Lidz, C. W. (1997). Coercion in psychiatric care: What have we learned from research? *Journal of the American Academy of Psychiatry and the Law, 26*(4), 631–637.

Luban, D. (1988). *Lawyers and justice: an ethical study* (p. 142). Princeton, NJ: Princeton University Press.

Madrid v. Gomez (1995). 889 F. Supp. 1146.

Martinez, R., & Candilis, P.J. (2005). Commentary: Toward a unified theory of personal and professional ethics. *Journal of the American Academy of Psychiatry and the Law, 33,* 382–385.

Metzner, J. L., & Fellner, J. (2010). Solitary confinement and mental illness in U.S. prisons: A challenge for medical ethics. *Journal of the American Academy of Psychiatry and the Law, 38*(1), 104–108.

Munetz, M. R., Ritter, C., Teller, J. L., & Bonfine, N. (2014). Mental health court and assisted outpatient treatment: perceived coercion, procedural justice, and program impact. *Psychiatric Services, 65*(3), 352–358. doi:10.1176/appi.ps.002642012.

National Commission on Correctional Health Care (2008). *Standards for health services in prisons.* Chicago: National Commission on Correctional Health Care.

Patient Protection and Affordable Care Act (2010) 42 U.S.C.§ 18001.

Rigg, J. (2002). Measures of perceived coercion in prison treatment settings. *International Journal of Law and Psychiatry, 25,* 473–490.

Ruiz v. Estelle (1980). 503 F. Supp. 1265.

Strasburger, L. H., Gutheil, T. G., & Brodsky, A. (1997). On wearing two hats: Role conflict in serving as both psychotherapist and expert witness. *American Journal of Psychiatry, 154,* 448–456.

Torrey, E. F., Kennard, A. D., Eslinger, D., Lamb, R., Pavle, J., & Treatment Advocacy Center (2010). More mentally ill persons are in jails and prisons than hospitals: a survey of the states. Retrieved from at:http://www.treatmentadvocacycenter.org/storage/documents/final_jails_v_hospitals_study.pdf (accessed December 13, 2013).

US Department of Justice, National Institute of Corrections. Correctional health care: guidelines for the management of an adequate delivery system. Retrieved from http://static.nicic.gov/Library/017521.pdf (accessed November 30, 2013).

US Department of Justice, Office of the Inspector General Audit Division. The Federal Bureau of Prison's efforts to manage inmate health care. Retrieved from http://www.justice.gov/oig/reports/BOP/a0808/final.pdf (accessed November 30, 2013).

Wynia, M. K., Latham, S. R., Kao, A. C., Berg, J. W., & Emanuel, L. L. (1999). Medical professionalism in society. *New England Journal of Medicine, 341,* 1612–1616.

CHAPTER 9

Communication in correctional psychiatry

Dean Aufderheide

Introduction

The art of communication is the language of leadership.

James Humes

A national leader in the corrections field once told me that of the myriad challenges he faced during his 30-year career, the most problematic were the result of poor communication. For problems and unwanted outcomes in health care settings, the origin is not dissimilar (O'Daniel & Rosenstein, 2008). In fact, the majority of sentinel events that occur from medical errors in US health care facilities result from breakdowns in communication (Grossman, 2011).

When the competing cultures and communication styles of correctional and health care professionals clash, communication efficacy is compromised and the potential for problems and unwanted outcomes is compounded. Notwithstanding the inherent cultural differences among interdisciplinary staff (Vinokur-Kaplan, 1995), effective communication in a correctional setting is especially challenging for psychiatrists. Whether transitioning from the protective structure of a residency or moving from a private practice or other mental health setting, psychiatrists working in a jail or prison will likely experience their new environment as adversarial and replete with competing interests and priorities (Pinta, 2009). Also, unlike in a health care setting, where physicians are at the top of the hierarchy, psychiatrists working in a jail or prison are farther down in the organizational hierarchy. Since individuals on the lower end of a hierarchy tend to be uncomfortable speaking up about problems or concerns (Schyve, 2009), communication impediments in correctional psychiatry diminish the collaborative interactions necessary to ensure that proper treatment is delivered appropriately. In such an environment, psychiatrists must develop communication strategies that are successful in creating effective and sustainable working relationships not only with patients but also with the facility's leadership, security staff, treatment team members, and other interdisciplinary staff.

This chapter presents ways in which psychiatrists play a critical role in mission requirements that necessitate effective communication skills with interdisciplinary staff in jails and prisons. From identifying the variables in the correctional culture that shape communication to improving interdisciplinary collaboration, this chapter explores the ways in which correctional psychiatrists can model effective communication styles and strategies that enhance professional credibility and improve treatment outcomes.

Defining communication

The two words "information" and "communication" are often used interchangeably, but they signify quite different things. Information is giving out; communication is getting through.

Sydney J. Harris

A profusion of definitions attempt to describe the different communication modalities (e.g., verbal, nonverbal) and distinguishing variables for understanding communicative phenomena (Losee, 1999). A conventional way of thinking about communication may be that its purpose is to achieve a maximum level of accuracy and efficiency in a message. However, an organization's cultural identity and knowledge base play a role in framing a message and putting it into a context. For psychiatrists working in a correctional setting, therefore, their communication not only must accurately convey meaning but also must create a shared understanding among all the staff involved in the delivery of mental health services.

The importance of communication in correctional psychiatry

Communication works for those who work at it.

John Powell

As the key to successful real estate transactions is said to be "location, location, location," the key to the successful practice of psychiatry in a correctional setting is "communication, communication, communication." Effective communication is at the heart of correctional psychiatry and involves the knowledge, motivation, and skills to interact effectively with all the interdisciplinary staff in the jail or prison environment. Communication competence, therefore, becomes the bridge between the distinct professional cultures and missions, creates shared values, and generates opportunities for interdisciplinary training. As Appelbaum, Hickey, and Packer (2001, p. 1346) note, ongoing communication is critical, whether through formal or informal interactions with staff:

> Shared values and training bear fruit when security staff and mental health staff engage in ongoing communication and cooperation, both formally and informally and at the level of both line staff and administrators. Regular but informal interactions can help both groups move beyond preconceived notions and create an atmosphere of trust

and communication. These casual interactions provide opportunities for mental health staff to become more sensitive to the concerns and perspective of security staff while they further inform officers about the nature and impact of mental disorders on inmate patients.

Whether in a patient interview, treatment team meeting, consultation with the facility's leadership, or discussion with security staff, there are opportunities for the correctional psychiatrist to communicate in a way that builds credibility, strengthens cooperation, and generates collaboration (Aufderheide & Brown, 2005). When psychiatrists model effective communication, they reinforce active participation by other members of the multidisciplinary treatment team. But when communication is constrained, distorted, fragmented, or misinterpreted, a vacuum is created. Misunderstandings multiply and inaccurate information is perceived as fact. Ultimately, the psychiatrist loses credibility with facility leadership and other interdisciplinary staff, and the treatment delivery system becomes vulnerable to destabilization. In the provision of psychiatric services in correctional settings, it is effective communication that results in good treatment outcomes, and it is poor communication that results in poor outcomes.

Communicating in the corrections culture

Think like a wise man, but communicate in the language of the people.
William Butler Yeats

Psychiatrists must be aware of the multicultural issues in the organization in which they work (Gaines, 1992; Kirmayer, Gutder, Blake, & Jarius, 2003; Sue, 1998). An organizational culture consists of implicit and explicit assumptions to address its problems and is considered a valid way for its constituents to conceptualize and deal with those problems (Triandis, 1989; Trompenaars & Turner, 1993). The basic assumption in correctional settings is the predominant supposition that the criminogenic characteristics of the inmate population present an omnipresent threat to public, staff, and inmate safety. The visible cues, including razor wire, uniformed officers, and security restraints, are constant reminders for psychiatrists that their communication style and strategy must be contextualized within the framework of the correctional culture. This culture inculcates all staff with the primacy of safety and security. As Hagberg and Heifetz (2000. p. 2) note, "The culture of an organization operates at both a conscious and subconscious level."

To be effective in their communications, psychiatrists must understand the jail or prison culture, its mission, and its chain of command. Undermining organizational assumptions, displays of professional condescension, disregarding the chain of command, or being dismissive of input from others can destroy credibility in the correctional culture (Aufderheide & Baxter, 2010). Consider the following case example of discrediting and counterproductive communication in a treatment team meeting.

Scenario: the wrong way to be right
It is Tuesday afternoon and the treatment team is ready to meet. Dr. Red, the prison psychiatrist, is already running late for the meeting and still has many patients to see before the end of the day. She generally finds treatment team meetings unhelpful and views them as an imposition on her time with patients. As usual, the other members of the treatment team are waiting for Dr. Red to arrive

and are becoming increasingly irritated. They also have patients to see, Dr. Red is often late, and they feel she tends to take over the meeting and not listen to their viewpoints. In fact, some team members have stopped offering their clinical input, preferring to adjourn the meeting as quickly as possible. Dr. Red finally arrives. The first patient for discussion is inmate Taylor, a 27-year-old man serving a life sentence. He has a history of treatment in prison for psychosis as well as multiple disciplinary reports. Dr. Moore, a relatively new psychologist at the prison, has put inmate Taylor on the list for discussion because the dorm sergeant expressed concerns about his deteriorating hygiene and behavior when he was conducting rounds this week. As Dr. Moore begins to share the concerns reported by security, Dr. Red interrupts, turns to inmate Taylor's case manager, Mr. Hanky, and reproaches him, stating, "Isn't this the inmate who was caught hoarding his medications several months ago? Aren't you aware he was probably planning to sell them?" Mr. Hanky does not always agree with Dr. Red but has learned over time that she interprets case discussion as a challenge to her professional authority during treatment team meetings. This tends to result in Dr. Red becoming more intransigent about her clinical opinion of the patient. Dr. Moore interjects that she reviewed the chart and, in fact, there appears to be a relationship between inmate Taylor's deteriorating behavior and thought processes and the discontinuation of the medication. She turns to Nurse Jiminy, who has worked at the prison for years, and asks her opinion about inmate Taylor. Nurse Jiminy feels put on the spot. She has to work directly with Dr. Red every day and wishes that Dr. Moore would leave her out of it. After all, she is a nurse, not a mental health expert like Dr. Red, many of these inmates do manipulate the system, and inmate Taylor does have a history of hoarding medication. As Nurse Jiminy is presenting pertinent information about inmate Taylor's history of disciplinary reports, Dr. Red interrupts again, exclaiming, "You must have overlooked my progress note! Here it is in the chart. When I discontinued his medication, inmate Taylor admitted that he is not really mentally ill. He is just trying to get his sentence reduced. I documented it right here. You are so naive. You have got to learn how to work with these inmates or they are just going to manipulate you. Plus, you have never even met this inmate." Dr. Moore feels her face beginning to turn red with embarrassment. She realizes that she still has a lot to learn and vows to be more prepared before she brings up a case again. While Mr. Hanky feels badly for Dr. Moore, he also surmises that Dr. Red's ego was injured when the sergeant didn't bring his concerns directly to her as the psychiatrist. Mr. Hanky is also worried about inmate Taylor and has had more success discussing cases individually with Dr. Red in her office. Rather than publicly supporting Dr. Moore, he suggests they move on to the next patient and thinks to himself, "I'll talk to Dr. Red in private about this whole thing and hopefully she will put inmate Taylor back on his medication. These treatment team meetings sure are a waste of time!"

Conversely, psychiatrists must be aware of the pressures inherent in the correctional environment to "go along to get along." Pinta (2009, p. 150) warns that "the adversarial nature of the prison environment and security needs can affect mental health care in a variety of ways. . . . Balancing security and treatment needs can create role ambiguities and ethics-related concerns for psychiatrists and other correctional mental health professionals."

Engaging in idiomatic vernacular to describe inmate behavior that is disparaging or demeaning in order to build an alliance with the security staff, for example, is professionally improper, unnecessary, and counterproductive. When this happens, a tendency to classify an inmate's maladaptive behavior as "mad or bad" can emerge and subvert the diagnostic and treatment process. As Aufderheide (2004, p. 5) points out in the assessment of self-injurious behavior in correctional settings:

> Consequently, frustrated clinicians frequently resort to classifying selfinjurious behavior into a taxonomy of intent, labeling inmate behavior as "instrumental" or "manipulative" versus "truly suicidal" or "due to mental health reasons." This dichotomous taxonomy derives from the spurious assumption that self-harm threats and behavior associated with mental illness are "mad" behaviors, while risk with instrumental intent is manipulative and should be classified as "bad" behavior. Some correctional mental health experts have identified this tendency to classify disturbed behavior as "mad or bad" as a distinguishing characteristic of the correctional environment.

Discussions with colleagues, other mental health professionals, supervisors, and security staff can help in developing a perspective to sharpen awareness of the effects of the correctional culture on communication. Talking with others, either on a formal or informal basis, can also help to guard against the "go along to get along" proclivity. As increased awareness deepens insight, the psychiatrist's communication style and strategy can be capably contextualized within the framework of the correctional culture.

Communication to improve treatment efficacy

The single biggest problem in communication is the illusion that it has taken place.

George Bernard Shaw

In much the same way that collaboration between health care professionals leads to improvement in decision making, communication increases staff awareness of the importance of each other's type of knowledge and skills, which leads to improved treatment outcomes (O'Daniel & Rosenstein, 2008). With effective communication skills, correctional psychiatrists can use their expertise for input into the decision-making process and for the development of strategies to address the complexities associated with patient care and management. But psychiatrists must be acutely sensitive that when the content of their communication is not understood, it literally "falls on deaf ears" and results in a loss of credibility, as illustrated in this case example.

Scenario: psychiatric psychobabble

After engaging in an act of self-injurious behavior, inmate Smith was placed in a suicide-resistant cell. He continued being disruptive and threatening further self-harm unless his demands were met. De-escalation attempts by nursing staff were unsuccessful, and inmate Smith was refusing to talk. After an emergency staff referral to mental health, the psychiatrist arrived at the cell and attempted to calm him down and conduct a risk assessment. As the crisis intervention continued, the warden, who had been notified of the escalating disruption, arrived on the mental health unit and asked the psychiatrist his assessment of the situation. "Well,"

the psychiatrist replied, "it appears this inmate has symptomatology suggestive of a disruptive mood dysregulation disorder and instrumental self-harm tendencies associated with narcissism and selective mutism." "Thanks, Doc," replied the warden. "Now, tell me about the inmate and what we're going to do."

This is an evident exaggeration of poor communication but underscores the importance that communication is only as effective as its intelligibility is to the recipient of the communication. When communication is not understandable, psychiatric treatment may be unsupported or opposed by other staff. Aufderheide and Baxter (2010, p. 173) warn that "a failure to communicate regarding inmates in treatment, whether due to choice or benign neglect, results in less effective treatment." Psychiatrists working in a jail or prison should use standardized communication tools that are intelligible and effective, especially in crisis intervention situations. The situation-background-assessment-recommendation technique, for example, provides a framework for effective communication among health care staff, especially in circumstances that require immediate action (Institute for Healthcare Improvement, 2002). In similar environments, where highly trained professionals must use expert judgment in rapidly changing circumstances, the adoption of such standardized communication tools is an effective strategy for enhancing collaboration and reducing risks (O'Daniel & Rosenstein, 2008).

Communication to improve interdisciplinary collaboration

If there is any great secret of success in life, it lies in the ability to put yourself in the other person's place and to see things from his point of view as well as your own.

Henry Ford

There is a plausible explanation for the relatively recent popularity of television reality programs about life in jails and prisons. Viewers seem mesmerized by the nonstop, frenzied activity and the constantly on-the-move correctional staff who are managing dangerous offenders. In these frenetic environments where security precautions are implemented promptly, intake and interviews are completed rapidly, and mental health interventions are coordinated quickly, it is readily apparent that effective communication is the *sine qua non* of adroit interdisciplinary collaboration. If decisions about care are to be consequential for offenders with serious mental health needs, correctional psychiatrists must recognize that they are part of a team, understand their role on the team, and understand that problem solving and decision making are most effective when communication underscores shared responsibility. Consider the following example of productive communication in an interdisciplinary consultation with security staff in managing a problematic inmate.

Scenario: working together works

Dr. Marks is the primary psychiatrist for a prison inpatient unit. During treatment team meetings, he often goes to great lengths to obtain input from everyone, including the security staff. He is aware that mental health staff and security staff often do not see eye to eye on how to handle inmates because of their different experiences, training, and goals. He looks for moments when he can learn from security staff as well as increase their knowledge and understanding of mental illness. One day, he receives a call about a crisis on the mental health unit. Although he is in the middle of his lunch, he knows how important it is to respond quickly and demonstrate that he is a member of the team. When he arrives a few minutes later, Nurse Charge and Lieutenant Bill explain that inmate Jay has become agitated after receiving his lunch tray. He was insisting that his food had been tampered with and, even after Sergeant Sack told him he would try to obtain a different tray, he continued banging on the door and demanding to see the Captain, whom he insisted he knew from a previous prison. He is now rapidly pacing in his cell, intermittently yelling, and banging on the door, and he has started to threaten to hurt staff.

Dr. Marks has not treated inmate Jay, who arrived over the weekend and refused to see the treatment team this morning. However, he did note a history of impulsive aggression, particularly when inmate Jay stops taking his medication. Lieutenant Bill asks Dr. Marks if he plans to write an order for emergency administration of medication, which will likely require a use of force. There are several staff at inmate Jay's door, and their presence appears to be increasing his agitation; other inmates are starting to react to the commotion as well. Aware of the prison hierarchy, Dr. Marks requests Lieutenant Bill's assistance, suggesting that he ask Sergeant Sack to select one officer to stay by inmate Jay's door to monitor his behavior, while the remaining staff begin rounds in an effort to calm the other inmates. He also suggests a quick meeting to share information and formulate a plan. Dr. Marks listens intently and asks follow-up questions as Sergeant Sack describes inmate Jay's loud, rapid speech and irrational demands, and how he even bent over backward by offering to obtain a different tray. Sergeant Sack also reports that inmate Jay has a long history of disciplinary reports, including assaults on staff. Sergeant Sack added, "We really need to show inmate Jay who runs this unit." Dr. Marks recognizes Sergeant Sack for his input and perspective and concurs that inmate Jay is certainly a dangerous patient who needs to follow the rules on the unit. He explains that inmate Jay appears to be experiencing an increase in racing, disorganized, and paranoid thoughts likely due to his medication noncompliance. He also acknowledges the value of what he has learned from Lieutenant Bill—that inmates in a highly agitated state will sometimes respond to simple commands from someone of a higher rank and/or a staff member whom they know and trust. Lieutenant Bill quickly comments that while he typically doesn't want to reinforce an inmate's demands to speak with a particular individual, all options need to be considered. A phone call to the Captain reveals that he does indeed know the inmate from a nearby prison where he previously worked. By the time he arrives, staff has done an excellent job of de-escalating the other inmates and getting them to remain on their bunks. The Captain suggests that Dr. Marks accompany him to the cell; together they are able to convince inmate Jay to cuff up so he can receive the injection of medication ordered by Dr. Marks. In a quick debriefing meeting, Dr. Marks thanks everyone, particularly Sergeant Sack and Lieutenant Bill, commenting, "Once again, talking together and working together has kept everyone safe."

This case example underscores the importance of reciprocal communication that breaks down barriers and builds a bridge of mutual respect and cooperation. Aufderheide and Baxter (2010, p. 179) emphasize the importance of reciprocal communication in building collaborative working relationships:

> Reciprocal communication is essential to the development of interdisciplinary collaboration. It is important that stereotypical labels that undermine the working relationship be addressed. For example, security officers may perceive the mental health staff as inmate advocates or dogooders. Mental health staff may see the officers as insensitive and unresponsive to the mental health needs of the inmates and lacking professionalism. Whatever the source of friction, it is imperative that the two talk. Mental health staff needs to educate the officers about what they do and the reasons for why they do what they do. Mental health staff should actively solicit the opinion and insights from officers about the problems they deal with on a daily basis.

By communicating and modeling collaboration, individuals create opportunities for improvement in an organization (Lasker & Weiss, 2003). Accordingly, psychiatrists in correctional settings can improve treatment and patient management decisions by communicating and modeling collaboration with security staff and other members of the treatment team.

Summary

Communication—the human connection—is the key to personal and career success.

Paul J. Meyer

There is no doubt that effective communication is at the heart of success for psychiatrists working in a jail or prison setting, and there is no doubt that opportunities and barriers to effective communication exist at multiple levels. It is crucial, therefore, for psychiatrists to develop communication strategies that create sustainable working relationships both with their patients and with other interdisciplinary personnel, from front-line staff to facility leadership. As Aufderheide and Baxter (2010, p. 172) note, "Communication from correctional mental health clinicians involved in treatment programs must be consistent, and presented across a variety of facility settings."

Whether with the facility's leadership, security staff, or other members of the treatment team, the goal is to communicate in ways that engender understanding and involvement in support of treatment goals. Through an understanding of how the correctional culture affects communication and by recognizing the importance of communication in interdisciplinary collaboration, correctional psychiatrists can model effective communication skills that preserve professional credibility and improve treatment outcomes.

References

Appelbaum, K. L., Hickey, J. M., & Packer, I. (2001). The role of correctional officers in multidisciplinary mental health care in prisons. *Psychiatric Services, 52*, 1343–1347.

Aufderheide, D. (2004). Assessing risk of suicide and self-injury in correctional settings. *National Psychologist, 13*, 5–6.

Aufderheide, D., & Brown, P. H. (2005). Crisis in corrections: The mentally ill in America's prisons. *Corrections Today, 2*, 30–33.

Aufderheide, D., & Baxter, J.D. (2010). Interdisciplinary collaboration in correctional practice. In T. Fagan & R. Ax (Eds.), *Correctional mental health: From theory to best practice* (pp. 169–186). Thousand Oaks, CA: Sage Publications, Inc.

Gaines, A. (1992). *Ethnopsychiatry: The cultural construction of professional and folk psychiatries.* Albany: State University of New York Press.

Grossman, D. (2011). The cost of poor communication. Retrieved from http://www.holmesreport.com/opinion-info/10645/The-Cost-Of-Poor Communications.aspx

Hagberg, J., & Heifetz, R. (2000). Corporate culture/organizational culture: Understanding and assessment. Retrieved from http://www.hegnet.com

Institute for Healthcare Improvement (2002). Guidelines for communicating with physicians using the SBAR process. Retrieved from http://www.ihi.org/IHI/Topics/PatientSafety/SafetyGeneral/Tools/SBARTechniqueforCommunicationASituationalBriefingModel.htm

Losee, R. (1999). Communication as complementary informative processes. *Journal of Information, Communication, and Library Sciences, 5*, 1–15.

Kirmayer, J. L., Gutder, J., Blake C., & Jarius, E. (2003). Cultural consultation: A model of mental health services for multicultural societies. *Canadian Journal of Psychiatry, 4*, 145–153.

Lasker, R. D., & Weiss, E. S. (2003). Broadening participation in community problem solving: A multidisciplinary model to support collaborative practice and research. *Journal of Urban Health: Bulletin of the New York Academy of Medicine, 80*, 14–60.

O'Daniel, M., & Rosenstein, A. H. (2008). Professional communication and team collaboration. In R. Hughes (Ed.), *Patient safety and quality: An evidence-based handbook for nurses* (pp. 801–814). Rockville, MD: Agency for Healthcare Research and Quality.

Pinta, E. R. (2009). Decisions to breach confidentiality: When prisoners report violations of institutional rules. *Journal of the American Academy of Psychiatry and the Law, 37*, 150–154.

Schyve, P. (2009). Communication: The bond to patient safety. In *The Joint Commission guide to improving staff communication* (2nd ed., pp. v–vii). Oakbrook Terrace, IL: Joint Commission Resources.

Sue, S. (1998). In search of cultural competence in psychotherapy and counseling. *American Psychologist, 53*(4), 440.

Triandis, H. C. (1989). The self and behavior in different cultural contexts. *Psychological Bulletin, 128*, 3–72.

Trompenaars, F., & Turner, C. H. (1993). *Riding the waves of culture.* London: McGraw-Hill.

Vinokur-Kaplan, D. (1995). Enhancing the effectiveness of interdisciplinary mental health treatment teams. *Administration and Policy in Mental Health, 22*, 521–529.

CHAPTER 10

Funding of correctional health care and its implications

Robert L. Trestman

Introduction

Correctional health care is funded through a range of mechanisms that parallel fee-for-service and managed care in the community. Like community health care, the use of health care in correctional settings is increasing. It is, however, often under more significant budgetary constraints and tighter management. This chapter includes a discussion of global capitation, per-inmate costs, at-risk contracting, and other contractual relationships.

Conceptual framework

Correctional expenditures typically account for between 2.5 percent and 2.9 percent of a state's budget. The combined state and federal expenditure on corrections in 2010 was approximately $80 billion (US Department of Justice, 2013). This translates into $29,141 per state inmate per year and slightly less for a federal inmate, $28,283. Another estimate, using a different methodology, yielded $31,286 as the total incarceration cost per year for a state prison inmate (Henrichson & Delaney, 2012). Additionally, local governments spent $28 billion on corrections in 2010, 1.6 percent of their total expenditures (Kyckelhahn, 2013).

In turn, correctional health care is also expensive: It consumes between 9 percent and 25 percent of the total correctional budget, based on a large array of location-specific characteristics (Schaenman, Davies, Jordan, & Chakraborty, 2013). The average per-inmate per-year medical cost in American prisons in 2010 was just over $6,000 (Kyckelhahn, 2012). Of that total, approximately one quarter of the medical budget was spent on mental health services. Substantial political pressures exist to contain costs, with limited advocacy in the community or legislature. This is in tension with potential judicial oversight, consent agreements or decrees, the need to address health disparities, and the desire to deliver health care consistent with community standards (Binswanger, Redmond, Steiner, & Hicks, 2011).

Funding of jail health care

In general, the county that it serves funds the jail. The only current exceptions appear to be a few small states such as Connecticut or Delaware that have integrated jails into the state prison system. Each of America's 3,283 jails (Stephan & Walsh, 2011) has a constitutionally mandated responsibility to provide health care (see Chapter 3). The system for health care delivery chosen typically varies by the size of the facility. Size is usually characterized simply as small, medium, or large, with respective bed capacities of 50 or fewer, 1,000 or fewer, and more than 1,000. Most small to medium facilities contract out care on a fee-for-service or hourly basis for nursing, mental health, and medical staff. Most connect closely with a local hospital for emergency, psychiatric, and medical care when needed. Large jails often have an internal health care system that more closely resembles a prison than a small jail, with substantial on-site staff and capacity for subacute care (see Chapter 6). The facility administrator (often the county sheriff) typically has responsibility for contract oversight and management.

Funding of prison health care

Prison health care is funded almost exclusively with state resources. As noted previously, a state department of correction typically receives between 2.5 percent and 2.9 percent of the entire state budget and dedicates between 9 percent and 25 percent of that budget to health care. The administrator, typically titled secretary or commissioner, oversees this budget and the contract structure. In some states, the governor's office or the legislative branch gives guidance or direction. The norm for prison systems is to have contract arrangements for all health care through mechanisms that are discussed in more detail later in this chapter.

Medicaid, medicare, and the patient protection and affordable care act

According to federal regulations that govern Medicaid and Medicare, the state may no longer bill Medicaid or Medicare for health care services while a person is incarcerated. The one exception to this rule has historically been overnight stays in a community hospital, other than emergency department visits and observational stays. Even with this opportunity for federal matching funds to pay (typically) 50 percent of the eligible expenses, many states have chosen not to exercise this option due to the complex billing process, which is structured on a per-inmate basis, and the need to coordinate closely with the state Medicaid authority.

With the Patient Protection and Affordable Care Act (ACA) comes the anticipated opportunity to initiate or maintain Medicaid enrollment for pretrial jail inmates (Blair, Greifinger, Stone, & Somers, 2011). This does not allow for billing but does ease access to entitlements following release because more than

60 percent of jail inmates turn over on a weekly basis (Minton, 2010). The one exception to billing remains overnight community hospital stays, with federal reimbursement initially at 100 percent of allowable charges and decreasing to 90 percent by 2020. Some states have already worked to ease reentry by linking with the state Medicaid program in order to connect people to their entitlements immediately prior to release (e.g., Trestman & Aseltine, 2014). Further, as one element of the ACA requires coverage for children up to age 26 years by a parent's health care plan, this may allow for billing and cost recovery for off-site specialty care or overnight hospitalizations of such patients (Patient Protection and Affordable Care Act, 2010; Blair et al., 2011).

Contract models

Prior to the rapid expansion of the incarcerated population in the early 1990s, most prison systems provided health care with their own employees or directly contracted for services. This changed, in most cases, with the dramatic increase in health care demands of a larger incarcerated population. States have pursued a range of approaches to meet the health care needs of their inmates. One study that included both the federal and state prison systems examined factors that distinguished high- and low-cost systems. The major findings, which accounted for 60 percent of the variability, suggested that it was not the range or number of services provided but rather the method of care delivery and the staffing mix that most affected per-capita costs (Lamb-Mechanick & Nelson, 2000). Capitated contracts and increased use of midlevel practitioners were two factors associated with decreased costs, while routine HIV screening at intake was associated with increased costs.

In-house providers versus outside providers

Most jails and prison systems contract for health care provision. Some facilities, however, still manage health care in house, with either their own employees or by directly subcontracting for specific services. This in-house approach survives as a legacy model, which may still be adequate in some settings. However, given the complexity of modern health care delivery and management, the use of outside providers and management systems has become the norm.

Outside vendor models

In by far the most common model, a jail or prison system contracts for health care services with an external partner or partners. For jails, such services often involve a local provider group. Large jails and prison systems usually go through a formal bidding process (often called a Request for Proposals or RFP) that specifies the requirements, service provisions, payment structure, oversight, and any penalties for failure to deliver services or defined staffing levels. The provider of services may be a medical school or a for-profit company that specializes in correctional health care services.

Global versus split contracting

The first decision a correctional administrator/contract manager must make is whether to contract for services as a whole or individually, carving out one or more services. Services that must be considered include acute, subacute, and chronic medical and surgical care; ambulatory though hospital-level care for mental health; dental care; nursing care; specialty care; diagnostic services; pharmacy services; medical records management; and administrative oversight/quality assurance. For example, general medical care might be contracted with one company; mental health treatment might be provided by a medical school's department of psychiatry; a pharmaceutical management firm might provide pharmacy services separately; and the correctional institution might do its own contract oversight.

There are advantages and disadvantages to each approach. The advantage to global contracting is simplicity and coordination of care delivery, administration, and oversight. One potential disadvantage is that the global care provider may have areas of weakness as well as strength. A split-service model allows for enhanced competition, selection of best-in-class providers, and the potential for optimized cost management. The negatives of such a model include the potential for duplicate administrative structures, more difficult oversight, and the potential for cost or responsibility shifting among the different vendors.

Also, services may be divided by level of care and service line. Ambulatory services may be provided by one organization within the walls of the correctional institution, while a dedicated unit at a nearby hospital may provide acute care.

Liability

According to the US Supreme Court, a government body remains responsible and, therefore, legally liable for providing inmate health care whether the care is contracted or self-run. There are multiple considerations in practice that are based on the system (federal, state, or local) and on whether the care is contracted. In the federal prison system, the Supreme Court states that sovereign immunity does not apply to contracted providers (whether individuals or corporate entities) and interprets the Constitution to implicitly authorize an action for damages (known as a Bivens action) when a prisoner is harmed as the result of deliberate indifference to his or her medical needs (*Bivens v. Six Unknown Named Agents of Fed. Bureau of Narcotics*, 1971). Contracted providers in federal prisons remain subject to liability claims brought under state law and to licensure obligations (*Correctional Services Corporation v. Malesko*, 2001; Goldman, 2013; *Minneci v. Pollard*, 2012).

In state or local correctional facilities, both the relevant government body and any involved contracted providers may be held accountable in federal court for an alleged violation of constitutional rights (with a standard of deliberate indifference). The government body is always responsible for providing inmate health care, whether or not government employees provide the care. Further, if the alleged deprivation was committed by contracted providers, the courts have determined that they were acting in lieu of a state employee and they are also held liable (e.g., *West v. Atkins, 42 U.S.C.*, 1983, 1988; Goldman, 2013). Depending on the alleged violation, suit may also be brought in state court for violation of state statutes, for negligence, and for violation of the state's constitution (see Chapter 3).

Type of funding

Consistent with the panoply of arrangements for care delivery and reimbursement in the community, correctional health care has a similar diversity of funding mechanisms. These include such compensation structures as fee-for-service, cost-based, capitation, high-cost carve-outs, hospital services, and specialty care. No model is perfect in all situations; each has specific benefits and risks. The traditional approach for health care provision is through fee-for-service arrangements. While this is still typical in small jail settings, larger jails and prison systems have generally moved away from this model to embrace some form of tighter care management system.

A cost-based model often includes divided oversight and care delivery. The correctional system negotiates a contract up front with fixed unit costs for services plus some defined percentage of compensation for administration and profit (typically 2 percent to 8 percent of care delivery costs). Once in place, correctional system employees or a separate firm oversees utilization management. This allows for control over the costs generated. The tension in this model is consistent with that of a fee-for-service model—the health care vendor may be motivated to generate more costs to create a greater profit. A burden of responsibility also rests on the correctional system to provide consistent and careful oversight.

Capitation models take two forms, in general: global risk and per-inmate capitation. As with any managed care contract, this can substantially shift the risk from the correctional system to the provider or vice versa based on the contract details. In the simplest situation, a global capitation contract guarantees a fixed amount of compensation for a defined array of service provision. This kind of contract will likely be used only in a stable, mature environment that has clear and adequate historical cost and utilization data. Here, the correctional system benefits by having a fixed, predictable budget. The contract must be structured carefully to ensure that all required care is delivered and that the care provider does not stay within budget by withholding needed services. The converse is also true, as the provider bears the risk of extraordinary costs, unless catastrophic limits are set. Such catastrophic limits typically take the form of a threshold cost per patient. An example would be contract language stating that when the annual cost of any individual patient exceeds a predetermined amount, say $40,000, the correctional system will absorb the excess cost. Another risk that the provider takes in this arrangement is the inmate population increase. The contract can address this risk by incremental modification of the compensation when the population increases by a given number, perhaps by a unit of 100 inmates, in any month. A more detailed financial arrangement involves per-inmate capitation, where the average census determines monthly or quarterly compensation.

Inpatient hospital services may be funded in many ways. While a few very large systems (e.g., Texas, California, and the Federal Bureau of Prisons) exclusively use prison-based hospitals, most systems contract with one or more hospitals for needed care. This generally saves the costs of correctional officer overtime compared to a system where inmate patients occupy scattered beds in multiple hospitals and ensures public safety by negotiating for a secure unit within a specific hospital. In contrast with medical and surgical services, some states maintain their own psychiatric inpatient level of care within defined infirmary settings with continuous nursing staff and psychiatrist coverage on site or on call during evenings and weekends.

Similar to hospital care, systems need to contract for specialty services such as oncology, rheumatology, cardiology, and radiology. They typically do this either as part of an overall contract with the care provider or as a carve-out with individual or multispecialty groups. These may be on a fee-for-service model (still quite common), by blocks of specified clinic time, or on a capitated basis.

Performance measures

Contracts typically define performance measures and specify thresholds for clinical and operational targets. Where appropriate, they might also incorporate financial targets. Each of these areas may include process and outcome measures (Asch et al., 2011). The former target such issues as whether a given percentage threshold of staff training occurred (e.g., 100 percent of clinical staff certified in cardiopulmonary resuscitation in a biennial cycle) or a defined percentage of inmates received a specific service in a timely manner (e.g., 98 percent of inmates are screened on intake within a defined timeframe). Outcome targets might include, for example, staff vacancy rates. Specifically, as staffing levels are a critical component of contracted care delivery, a monetary penalty might exist for any month where nursing staffing has a vacancy rate greater than 5 percent. These measures are becoming more the norm in contracts and often are closely linked to key quality assurance initiatives (Hoge, Greifinger, Lundquist, & Mellow, 2009).

Summary

The funding of correctional health care is a complex enterprise, driven by constitutionally mandated care obligations on the one hand and resource constraints on the other. Along with the dramatic increase in the incarcerated population during the past two decades, correctional health care has evolved as well. The costs of care are quite substantial, and the diversity of models of care delivery offers an administrative challenge, a financial challenge to the relevant jurisdiction, and a significant opportunity for cost effectiveness. Unfortunately, no comparative study of funding models has yet been done. As integrated electronic health and financial records are gradually introduced into correctional settings, opportunities for such studies, and the policy guidance provided by those results, may yield important information applicable to health care cost and outcome management in society more broadly.

References

Asch, S. M., Damberg, C. L., Hiatt, L., et al. (2011). Selecting performance indicators for prison health care. *Journal of Correctional Health Care, 17,* 138–149.

Binswanger, I. A., Redmond, N., Steiner, J. F., & Hicks, L. S. (2011). Health disparities and the criminal justice system: An agenda for further research and action. *Journal of Urban Health: Bulletin of the New York Academy of Medicine, 89*(1), 98–107.

Bivens v. Six Unknown Named Agents of Fed. Bureau of Narcotics (1971), 403 U.S. 388.

Blair, P., Greifinger, R., Stone, T.H., & Somers, S. (2011). *Increasing access to health insurance coverage for pre-trial detainees and individuals transitioning from correctional facilities under the Patient Protection and Affordable Care Act.* American Bar Association Issue Paper.

Correctional Services Corporation v. Malesko (2001), 534 U.S.C. 61.

Goldman, J. (2013). Private provider liability in eighth amendment-based damages actions. *Correct Care, 27*(2), 18–30.

Henrichson, C., & Delaney, R. (2012). *The price of prisons: What incarceration costs tax payers.* Vera Institute for Justice.

Hoge, S. K., Greifinger, R. B., Lundquist, T., & Mellow, J. (2009). Mental health performance measures in corrections. *International Journal of Offender Therapy and Comparative Criminology, 53,* 634–647.

Kyckelhahn, T. (2012). *State corrections expenditures, FY 1982–2010.* Bureau of Justice Statistics, NCJ239672.

Kyckelhahn, T. (2013). *Local government corrections expenditures, FY 2005–2011.* Bureau of Justice Statistics, NCJ243527.

Lamb-Mechanick, D., & Nelson, J. (2000). *Prison health care survey: An analysis of factors influencing per capita costs.* National Institute of Corrections, ID 015999.

Minneci v. Pollard (2012), 132 U.S.C. 617.

Minton, T. D. (2010). *Jail inmates at midyear 2009: Statistical tables.* Bureau of Justice Statistics Statistical Tables (NCJ 230122). Washington, DC: US Department of Justice.

Patient Protection and Affordable Care Act (2010). Pub. L. No. 111–148, § 2701.

Schaenman, P., Davies, E., Jordan, R., & Chakraborty, R. (2013). *Opportunities for cost savings in corrections without sacrificing service quality: Inmate health care* (p. 3). Washington, DC: The Urban Institute.

Stephan, J., & Walsh, G. (2011). *Census of jail facilities.* (December 2011, NCJ 230188). Washington, DC: Bureau of Justice Statistics.

Trestman, R. L., & Aseltine, R. (2014). *Justice-involved health information: Policy and practice advances in Connecticut.* Perspectives in Health Information Management, 2014 Winter; 11(Winter): 1e. Published online Jan 1, 2014.

US Department of Justice (2013). *Smart on crime: Reforming the criminal justice system for the 21st century* (p. 2). Washington, DC: National Association of State Budget Officers.

West v. Atkins (1983, 1988), 42 U.S.C.

SECTION III

Patient management processes

CHAPTER 11

Mental health screening and brief assessments

Michael P. Maloney, Joel Dvoskin, and Jeffrey L. Metzner

Introduction

The number of persons in the United States supervised by correctional authorities, including jails, prisons, probation, and parole, has burgeoned since the 1980s. At the end of 2009, 7,225,800 persons were under such supervision; 1,571,013 were incarcerated in jails or prisons at year-end 2012 (Carson & Golinelli, 2013). While the number of incarcerated persons is clear, the actual number of incarcerated prisoners who have a mental disorder or independent psychiatric symptoms is difficult to determine because of methodological issues (e.g., different definitions of mental illness, different thresholds of severity) and wide variation in the nature (e.g., prison, jail, police lockup), size, and mental health service delivery systems of various settings. However, despite differences in methodology, geographic area, and other issues (e.g., types of facility, when studies were conducted), virtually every relevant study has concluded that many prisoners have serious mental illnesses and that the number of mentally ill prisoners is increasing (Diamond, Wang, Holzer, Thomas, & Cruser, 2001; Prins & Draper, 2009; see Chapter 32). Because people with mental illnesses are at risk of suicide and exacerbations of their mental illnesses, correctional institutions need to identify such persons in a timely manner and provide appropriate clinical interventions.

This chapter addresses the initial mental health screening of persons entering prisons and jails, with a special emphasis on suicide risk screening and follow-up clinical assessments of prisoners (hereinafter referred to as inmates) whose receiving or intake screening results suggest a likely need for treatment or suicide prevention efforts.

Mental health screening and evaluation

Chapter 3 describes the history of the legal obligation to provide medical and mental health care to prisoners. Of particular note is *Ruiz v. Estelle* (1980), where the court established minimum requirements for mental health treatment in prisons. This included general guidelines for the treatment of inmates with mental illnesses and specifically emphasized the need for screening and evaluation to identify those needing mental health interventions (including suicide watch) and treatment.

An American Psychiatric Association task force report on psychiatric services in jails and prisons (American Psychiatric Association, 2000) describes four types of mental health screening and evaluation processes:

Receiving mental health screening consists of observation and structured inquiry into each [inmate's] mental health history and symptoms. Structured inquiry includes questions regarding suicide history, ideation, and potential; prior psychiatric hospitalizations and treatment; and current and past medications, both those prescribed and what is actually being taken . . .

Intake mental health screening is defined as a more comprehensive examination performed on each newly admitted [inmate] within 14 days of arrival at an institution. It usually includes a review of the medical screening, behavioral observation, an inquiry into any mental health history, and an assessment of suicide potential . . .

A *brief mental health assessment* is defined as a mental health examination that is appropriate to the particular, suspected level of services needed and is focused on the suspected mental illness . . . A brief mental health assessment should be completed for each individual whose screening reveals mental health problems in the procedures above . . .

A *comprehensive mental health evaluation* consists of face-to-face interview of the patient and review of all reasonably available healthcare records and collateral information. It concludes with a diagnostic formulation and, at least, an initial treatment plan . . .

Receiving screening is provided for every new inmate as soon as possible after he or she enters the facility. The mental health screen can be administered alone or as part of the receiving health screening that is typically provided by nurses. Especially in jails, many people do not remain incarcerated for long. The National Commission on Correctional Health Care (2008) recommends conducting intake health screening (which includes a mental health component) within 14 days of admission to a correctional facility. Positive results in either receiving or intake screening should result in a brief assessment by a qualified mental health professional.

Receiving screening

The NCCHC provides separate mental health standards for the care of inmates in jails as opposed to those in prisons. However, the standards regarding receiving screening are essentially identical: "Receiving screening is performed on all inmates on arrival at the intake facility to ensure that emergent and urgent health needs are met" (NCCHC, 2008).

Screening instruments and processes should generally share the following characteristics (Ford et al., 2007a):

Brevity: Large urban jails may process tens of thousands of new admissions each year. Because every new admission to a jail or prison must be screened, it is important that the screening process be brief.

Clarity: Admissions often occur at any time of the day or night, with many different people conducting admission screening. In order for any process to have validity, it must first have reliability (i.e., different evaluators should come to similar conclusions about each case). This can only be accomplished when definitions, thresholds, and criteria are clear.

Trained screeners: In order to attain consistency and reliability and because screeners usually lack advanced mental health training, it is important that every screener be explicitly trained in the screening process and supervised to ensure competence and fidelity.

Low false-negative rate: The consequences of a false-positive screen are relatively low; the person will receive a brief assessment by a mental health professional. On the other hand, false-negative findings could potentially result in an unnecessary and severe exacerbation of a mental illness or even in a preventable suicide. In other words, mental health and suicide screeners must always be trained to "err on the side of caution." It is especially important to identify those inmates who have a high risk of suicide, so that they may be kept safe pending a more complete mental health and suicide risk assessment.

Reasonable false-positive rate: An extremely high number of false-positive screens can result in many unnecessary assessments, thus wasting valuable clinical time that could otherwise be spent providing treatment.

Documentation: Every screen must be documented to enable administrators to track the process, ensure that every new admission is screened, and keep track of the percentage of positive versus negative screens. Adequate documentation of positive screens provides essential information to the mental health professionals who will perform subsequent assessments.

Receiving area mental health screening is generally conducted by either a correctional officer or by nursing staff during the booking process. Staff require training in the administration of the screening instrument. The purpose of this screening assessment is to identify inmates who need immediate evaluation by mental health staff for overt psychotic symptoms and/or potential danger to self or others.

In our experience, receiving screening and intake mental health assessments should generally have a combined positive referral rate ranging from 25 percent to 33 percent, which results in referral for further brief assessment or evaluation by a qualified mental health professional. When clinically appropriate (e.g., an inmate who is known to have a psychotic diagnosis from previous treatment at the institution), an inmate may be referred directly for a comprehensive mental health evaluation from receiving screening or intake mental health screening without receiving a brief mental health assessment. In such cases, the brief mental health screening is superfluous, as it is essentially assumed to be positive.

Intake mental health screening

Several models have been implemented in jails and prisons for providing intake mental health assessments. These can be part of an intake health care (i.e., medical) assessment performed by a nurse practitioner, physician's assistant, or physician. Also, the assessment can be completed by a qualified and licensed mental health professional (e.g., psychiatric nurse, clinical psychiatric social worker, or psychologist) independent of the intake medical assessment.

Inmates who have had a mental health evaluation because of a positive receiving screening assessment will not require the intake screening within 14 days; they have already been assessed and referred for treatment. Also, while many jails allow correctional officers to perform receiving mental health screening, the intake screens should be completed by health care professionals, usually nurses.

Brief mental health assessments and comprehensive mental health evaluations

Every positive screen must result in at least a brief mental health assessment by a qualified mental health professional, which may in turn result in a referral for a comprehensive mental health evaluation. The brief mental health assessment typically includes a brief mental status exam and inquiry into the documented reasons for a positive screen. The assessment can be very brief but, on average, should take approximately 20 to 30 minutes to complete and document. The purpose of this assessment is to determine if there is an imminent risk of suicide or an emergent need for mental health treatment or if the person is reasonably likely to need mental health treatment on a nonemergent basis during his or her incarceration.

Comprehensive mental health evaluations are also performed by qualified mental health professionals. These evaluations typically result in mental health care for the inmate and the creation of a mental health chart (often part of the inmate's health care record) and treatment plan.

There are literally hundreds of published psychological tests that are used in a broad array of social, educational, legal, and other arenas of society. However, correctional mental health personnel rarely use these instruments during the screening and brief assessment processes for many reasons, including time, cost, and relevance to correctional goals.

Mental health screening instruments

Variants of a suicide prevention screening guidelines form, developed jointly by state and county agencies in New York (Sherman & Morschauser, 1989), continue to be widely used in correctional facilities throughout the United States. The 17-question structured interview form includes 11 questions that are relevant to suicide risk factors and 5 questions specific to current behaviors that might be indicative of mental illness.

Martin and colleagues (2013) provided a succinct review of correctional screening instruments and identified 22 tools, most of which were developed for jail settings. Gebbie and colleagues (2008) also provided a comprehensive overview and analysis of multiple specific screening tools. Neither Martin nor Gebbie made specific recommendations regarding use of any of these scales.

The Brief Jail Mental Health Screen (BJMHS; Steadman, Scott, Osher, Agnesa, & Robbins, 2007) has been shown to be an effective jail mental health screening device, especially for men, who have a slightly higher false-negative rate than women. It contains no items, however, that specifically query about suicide ideation, intent, or risk. The BJMHS requires 2 to 3 minutes for administration and meets NCCHC standards for initial inmate mental health screening. The authors conclude that the BJMHS "produces a reasonable proportion for those screened (between 11% and 16%) who should be referred for more intensive assessment by medical staff." Again, this figure does not include those inmates without mental illness who are situationally suicidal and may be intoxicated. Because it does not screen for suicide risk, this instrument should be used in concert with the New York instrument or one of the suicide screening instruments described later in this chapter.

The Correctional Mental Health Screen (CMHS; Ford et al., 2007b) uses separate questionnaires for men (CMHS-M) and women (CMHS-F). The CMHS scales, like the BJMHS, take only a few minutes to administer. Martin and colleagues (2013) summarize data for the BJMHS and the CMHS, both male and female. While the data are complicated, the CMHS scales appear to have slightly higher sensitivity and specificity (sensitivity refers to the percent of true positives identified, while specificity refers to the proportion of true negatives correctly identified). Positive scores on either scale should be considered as an entry point for further triage/evaluation. A person who answers "yes" to a screening question is usually interviewed/assessed for further clinical intervention/treatment.

The Los Angeles County Sheriff's jail system provides an illustration of an initial screening for self-harm/suicide risk and for general mental health. This is accomplished through the administration of a screening instrument referred to as the "15 Questions" (Fig. 11.1). Trained custody or nursing staff ask these questions and enter the answers into the electronic medical record. All inmates answering positive to any mental health question are subsequently individually assessed (i.e., brief assessment) by a qualified mental health professional. Approximately 25 percent to 30 percent of new bookings answer positive to one or more of the 15 Questions, and approximately 50 percent of those are subsequently admitted to mental health housing following a mental health assessment or evaluation.

The 15 Questions serve as an initial screening for both general mental health problems and suicide risk. A licensed mental health clinician then does an individual clinical interview and mental health assessment for inmates with a positive screening assessment. This brief assessment results in a decision to send the detainee to specialized mental health housing or to general population housing. Those detainees admitted to mental health housing are further evaluated with a comprehensive evaluation by an assigned clinician. Most clients in mental health housing are referred for a further assessment by a psychiatrist for possible psychotropic treatment. The process of assessment is ongoing throughout the inmate's stay in mental health treatment housing.

Many factors must be considered in developing an effective mental health screening process for a correctional facility, including at least the following:

- The number of new bookings;
- The architectural layout of the jail or prison (e.g., adequate room for mental health to screen);
- Staffing and training issues; and
- Demographics of the inmate population (including the rate and severity of mental illness, history of previous arrests, availability of informational databases).

Most correctional mental health screening instruments are self-report instruments (i.e., the inmate is asked for information with little or no independent verification). In a program analysis (Maloney, Reitz, & Ward, 2001) conducted in the Los Angeles County jail system, some 16,000 new booking screens were reviewed. To the screening question, "Have you ever tried to hurt or kill yourself?" 3.5 percent responded yes. For an additional question that asked if the inmate was currently thinking about killing himself, only 0.65 percent responded yes. However, in a sample of 1,000 newly booked inmates during this same period who were personally interviewed during booking, 5.03 percent of the men and 7.50 percent of the women acknowledged that they were currently suicidal and 14.46 percent of the men and 17.86 percent of the women reported previous suicide attempts. These results underscore the need for ongoing program evaluation that involves the overall effectiveness of the screening/assessment system. One of this chapter's authors (M.M.) conducted an unpublished additional evaluation of the 15 Questions in 2008 with a sample of 60,000 newly booked inmates. He analyzed data on the efficacy of each question and also incorporated the use of two independent sources that do not require personal interviews. Follow-up performance evaluation indicated an improved and very low false-negative rate. One important lesson from the program evaluation was the need to augment jail screens by using additional observational data (e.g., bizarre or atypical behavior) and collateral sources of information (e.g., reports from arresting officers, available electronic databases, previous institutional mental health records). In selecting or developing a screening measure for a correctional facility or program, the screening systems or

NO.	QUESTION
1	Do you have a history of medical problems?
2	Do you have any medical problems now?
3	Do you have any current open cuts, sores, boils, wounds or skin problems?
4	Are you currently taking medications?
5	Have you ever taken any psychiatric medication?
6	Have ever been mentally ill?
7	Do you have any mental health problems?
8	Have you ever been in a psychiatric hospital?
9	Have you ever received Mental Health Services in jail?
10	Have you ever received mental health treatment from a psychiatrist, psychologist, or other mental health worker?
11	Do you hear voices that no one else can hear?
12	Have you ever been in a "Special Education" class considered developmentally disabled, or a client in a Regional Center?
13	Have you ever tried to kill yourself?
14	Are you thinking about hurting yourself now?
15	Does the inmate exhibit any bizarre or unusual behavior?

Fig. 11.1 Medical mental health screening questions.

tools must be designed to obtain data relevant to mental health diagnosis or history and to obtain information on the risk that an inmate will experience serious mental health problems during his or her incarceration. There is a need for ongoing quality improvement studies to ensure that changes in population characteristics or other variables are appropriately incorporated into screening methods.

Suicide risk assessments

The National Center on Institutions and Alternatives (Hayes, 2010) conducted a study commissioned by the US Justice Department's National Institute of Corrections. A significant decrease in the suicide rate was found in the nation's county jails over the past 20 years. Data from the mid-1980s indicated a jail suicide rate of 107 per 100,000 inmates compared to recent data documenting a decrease to 38 suicides per 100,000 jail inmates. This dramatic decrease in the suicide rate in detention facilities during the past 20 years is likely due to the introduction of required suicide prevention programming in correctional facilities (Hayes, 2010).

Chapter 43 provides a detailed review of suicide prevention in jails and prisons. A key component of a suicide prevention program, in addition to receiving mental health screening as previously summarized, is the development and implementation of a structured suicide risk assessment tool. Licensed mental health professionals who have the appropriate training and experience to do suicide risk evaluations should conduct these risk assessments.

Identifying inmates with a high risk of suicide is quite different from identifying risk in the nonincarcerated population. Higher suicide rates in incarcerated populations are the result of numerous factors unique to this population, including the reason for arrest, court issues, intoxication at the point of admission, the physical and social environment, and impaired family and personal relationships. These factors are in addition to general risk factors related to suicide, such as depression, personal loss, and economic distress. Assessment of suicide risk presents a critical initial demand of correctional institutions. While there is no universally accepted tool for assessing suicide risk in jails and prisons, there is essentially no disagreement that universal screening and follow-up assessment of positive screens are basic to any program of suicide prevention in these facilities.

Correctional suicide risk measures

The literature on suicide risk assessment is extensive. The Department of Veterans Affairs Evidence-Based Synthesis Program (Haney et al., 2012) conducted a wide review of self-harm and suicide risk assessment tools, citing more than 100 references. They concluded that data are insufficient to recommend implementation of any specific risk assessment tool. Brown (2002), who reviewed 30 suicide risk assessment tools, reached a similar conclusion. This was especially so in the context of correctional facilities due to significant programmatic differences among such facilities.

Hayes (2010) reported that

> intake screening and on-going assessment of all inmates is critical to a correctional facility's suicide prevention efforts. It should not be viewed as a single event, but as an on-going process because inmates

can become suicidal at any point during their confinement, including the initial admission into the facility, after adjudication when the inmate is returned to the facility from court; following receipt of bad news or after suffering any type of humiliation or rejection; confinement in isolation or segregation; and following a prolonged a stay in the facility.

In addition, although there is no single set of risk factors that mental health and medical communities agree can be used to predict suicide, there is little disagreement about the value of screening and assessment in preventing suicide. Research consistently shows that approximately two thirds of all suicide victims communicate their intent some time before death (Hayes, 2010) and that any individual with a history of one or more suicide attempts is at a much greater risk for suicide than those who have never made an attempt (Moscicki, 2001).

Suicide screening in correctional settings is not optional; however, the manner in which it is conducted is subject to variation. While no screening tool has universal application, structured suicide risk instruments often assess the following four sets of factors: static factors (e.g., history of prior attempts, past placement on suicide precautions), slowly changing factors (e.g., life or long sentence, a significant loss, physical illness), dynamic factors (e.g., recent suicide attempt, mood disturbance, psychotic illness), and protective factors (e.g., supportive family, religious beliefs, future oriented). Regardless of the structured instrument/form used, training of mental health professionals in the use of such forms for suicide risk assessment purposes is crucial.

Inmates who screen positive or who make suicidal threats or gestures should receive a comprehensive suicide risk assessment before being returned to the general population. While there is no specific instrument or format for such assessments, the following topics should always be covered during a comprehensive suicide risk assessment:

◆ History of suicidal or self-harming behaviors

◆ Current mood

◆ Current cognitions about suicide

◆ General risk factors

◆ Idiosyncratic risk factors

◆ Protective factors

◆ Changes since the inmate reported suicidal intention

◆ Stated intentions regarding suicide or self-harm

◆ Social and familial disconnectedness

◆ Presence or absence of futuristic thinking

Summary

The process of screening and assessment is basic to psychiatric care in any setting and provides the guidelines for ongoing intervention and treatment. This process is especially important in correctional settings, which deal with clients who are in transition or under significant stress, many of whom have numerous risk factors for psychological problems or suicide. Screening is critical for quickly and efficiently identifying persons who may be at high risk for self-harm and those who have significant mental health problems. Effective screening allows for efficient allocation of resources and timely attention to those requiring rapid or emergent intervention.

While all correctional programs (especially jails and prisons) are required to screen each inmate at the time of intake, there is no widely accepted method of screening. Each facility or program is unique in size, location, inmate flow patterns, local population demographics, staffing patterns, facility characteristics, availability of emergency resources, and other factors. Screening and assessment methods must be tailored to the given program or facility and require ongoing quality improvement. It is expected that these methods and programs are dynamic and that modification is an ongoing process.

References

American Foundation for Suicide Prevention (2009). *Risk factors for suicide*. New York: American Foundation for Suicide Prevention.

American Psychiatric Association (2000). *Psychiatric services in jails and prisons: a task force report of the American Psychiatric Association*. Washington, DC: American Psychiatric Association.

Brown, G. K. (2002). *A review of suicide measures for intervention research with adults and older adults*. Unpublished manuscript. NIMH contract 263-MH914950. Washington, DC: National Institute of Mental Health.

Carson, E. A., & Golinelli, D. (2013). *Prisoners in 2012—advance counts*. Washington, DC: Department of Justice, Office of Justice Programs, Bureau of Justice and Statistics.

Diamond, P. M., Wang, E. W., Holzer, C. E., Thomas, C., & Cruser, D. A. (2001). The prevalence of mental illness in prison. *Administration and Policy in Mental Health and Mental Health Services Research, 29*(1), 21–40.

Ford, J., Trestman, R. L., Osher, F., Scott, J. E., Steadman, H. J., & Robbins, P. C. (2007a). *Mental health screens for corrections*. Washington, DC: National Institute of Justice.

Ford, J. D., Trestman, R. L., Wiesbrock, V. H., & Zhang, W. (2007b). Validation of a brief screening instrument for identifying psychiatric disorders among newly incarcerated adults. *Psychiatric Services, 60*, 842–846.

Gebbie, K. M., Larkin, R. M., Klein, S. J., Wright, L., Satriano, J., Culkin, J. J., & Devore, B. S. (2008). Improving access to mental health services for New York state prison inmates. *Journal of Correctional Health Care, 14*, 122–135.

Haney, E. M., O'Neil, M. E., Carson, S., et al. (2012). *Suicide risk factors and risk assessment tools: A systematic review*. Washington, DC: Department of Veterans Affairs.

Hayes, L. (2010). *National study of jail suicides: 20 years later*. Washington, DC: National Institute of Corrections, US Department of Justice.

Maloney, M. P., Reitz, E., & Ward, M. P. (2001). *Prevalence of risk factors for mental illness in a large county jail*. Unpublished manuscript.

Martin, M. S., Colman, I., Simpson, A., & McKenzie, K. (2013). Mental health screening tools in correctional institutions: A systematic review. *BMC Psychiatry, 13*, 275.

Moscicki, E. (2001). Epidemiology of completed and attempted suicide: Toward a framework of prevention. *Clinical Neuroscience Research, 1*, 310–323.

National Commission on Correctional Health Care. (2008). *Standards for health services in prisons*. Chicago: National Commission on Correctional Health Care.

Prins, S. J., & Draper, L. (2009). *Improving outcomes for people with mental illness under community corrections supervision & a guide to research informed policy and practice*. New York: Council of State Governments Justice Center.

Ruiz v. Estelle, 503 F. Supp. 1265 (S.D. Tex. 1980).

Sherman, L. G., & Morschauser, P. C. (1989). Screening for suicide risk in inmates. *Psychiatric Quarterly, 60*, 119–138.

Steadman, H. J., Scott, J. E., Osher, F., Agnesa, T. K., & Robbins, P. C. (2005). Validation of the brief mental health screen. *Psychiatric Services, 56*, 816–822.

CHAPTER 12

Interviewing in correctional settings

Li-Wen Lee

Introduction

Research has shown that mental illness is disproportionately represented among incarcerated individuals as compared to the community setting (Abram, Teplin, & McClelland, 2003; Fazel & Seewald, 2012; Steadman, Osher, Robbins, Case, & Samuels, 2009; Teplin, 1994). According to the Bureau of Justice Statistics, in 2005 more than half of all jail and prison inmates had a recent history of symptoms of a mental health problem (James & Glaze, 2006). This high rate of mental illness is both an opportunity for and a source of significant challenges to the provision of much-needed treatment. Significant numbers of inmates do not present as acutely ill during intake yet have current or lifetime psychiatric disorders and may require further assessment (Trestman, Ford, & Zhang, 2007). Without adequate assessment and treatment, inmates with mental illness may harm themselves, other inmates, or correctional staff; become victimized; or disrupt facility operations (Ogloff et al., 1994). An essential component in assessment and appropriate management is the psychiatric interview.

While there are helpful standards and guidelines for mental health services in correctional settings (Hills, Siegfried, & Ickowitz, 2004; Metzner, 1997a, 1997b; National Commission on Correctional Health Care, 2008), relatively little has been written about the specific impact of the correctional setting or the specific features of the correctional population that should be understood when conducting the mental health interview. Given the importance of the interview in providing mental health treatment, the essential elements and complexities involved in conducting an effective interview in the correctional setting are presented in this chapter. This chapter assumes that the interviewer understands fundamental clinical evaluation skills (American Psychiatric Association, 2006). Aspects of the psychiatric interview are reviewed with particular attention given to how the correctional population and setting can affect the interview process. References are provided where possible; in other instances, information has been drawn from clinical experience, as there is a limited body of literature in this area.

Population factors

Presentations of mental disorders in corrections may be complicated by high rates of comorbidities, substance use, and personality disorders, in particular, that may make diagnostic clarity more difficult to achieve. An estimated 85 percent of jail and prison inmates are substance involved—they meet criteria for a history of substance use disorders or committed their offenses due to drug use or other drug-related activity (National Center on Addiction and Substance Abuse at Columbia University, 2010). Approximately 42 percent of state prison inmates and 49 percent of local jail inmates have both mental health and substance abuse problems (James & Glaze, 2006). The consequences of substance use include the more immediate effects of intoxication or withdrawal and the induction or exacerbation of symptoms of mental disorders. Inmates are at increased risk of presenting with acute consequences of substance use in jails than in prisons, as they are typically in the community before admission. Even so, interviewers should be aware that drugs and alcohol are available within prisons.

Personality disorders in prison settings have been estimated to be three times more common than in the community (Rotter, Way, Steinbacher, Sawyer, & Smith, 2002). Common disorders in the incarcerated population include antisocial and borderline personality disorders, although other diagnoses such as paranoid, schizotypal, and narcissistic personalities also pose challenges (Trestman, 2000). Interviewers should be alert to indications of a personality disorder and ensure that countertransference does not detract from the evaluation. Countertransference to severe personality disorders may lead to underdiagnosis of treatable mental illness. However, research shows that individuals with personality disorder are more likely to have worse mental health functioning and higher suicide risk (Black, Gunter, Loveless, Allen, & Sieleni, 2010).

Environmental factors

In corrections, security requirements supersede all other activities. Security staff regulates all entry, exit, and internal movement; access to inmates is dictated by security rules and institution schedules. Even with these limitations, effort should be made to ensure that there are acceptable parameters within which to conduct the evaluation. Common examples of institution schedules that limit clinicians' access to inmates include designated "count" times and meal times. Planning around institution schedules may help ensure adequate time is available; however, some situations may require established lines of communication or policy to make urgent or emergent assessments possible. In some facilities, security rules may result in interviewees remaining in restraints during an interview, or an officer may habitually remain present during the interview. In this situation, it may be appropriate to request that correctional officers wait outside the interview room but maintain safety through line-of-sight observation.

Location is another consideration. The physical space should allow for confidentiality and clear communication. It may seem logistically simpler if the evaluation is conducted cell-side. This, however, raises confidentiality issues if other inmates or officers nearby can hear the interview, and it may become difficult for the clinician and the inmate to hear one another. Interviews should occur in private, away from other prisoners and, when possible, away from correctional officers (Blaauw & van Marle, 2007).

In addition to considerations about where and when to conduct interviews, clinicians also need to be aware of their personal safety. Concerns include both the evaluee and other inmates (see Chapter 7). Assault is a possibility in many mental health settings, including community clinics and inpatient hospitals; however, clinicians understand that most mental health patients are not violent. Similarly, most patients in the correctional system are not aggressive toward clinicians, but it remains essential to be aware of the environment and to avoid exposure to vulnerable positions to the extent possible. While maintenance of confidentiality is essential, clinicians should consider whether the interview location leaves the clinician alone in a potentially dangerous situation. Clinicians should be aware of how to exit the interview area and how to obtain assistance should they need to end an interview or feel threatened.

Culture of correctional facilities

Correctional facilities have their own cultures, and understanding these cultures is an important component of assessing the interviewee (Metzner, 1998). The location where the individual is placed within the correctional setting is important. There are significant differences between minimum- and maximum-security settings and differences between general population and disciplinary segregation. There can also be notable differences between housing blocks within the general population, and prisons vary in their individual cultures. There may be differences in the level of crowding, gang presence, and the ways in which institution rules are enforced. These differences can affect symptoms and presentations during evaluation. There is also prison jargon, or slang, that carries regional variations. An interviewer's ability to understand jargon is helpful in correctly interpreting what the interviewee is saying and potentially helpful in developing rapport with the interviewee.

Ramifications of jail and prison culture extend to interactions with mental health staff and, therefore, affect the interview process. The "inmate code" discourages sharing information with staff, which may manifest as withholding information from clinicians (Rotter, McQuistion, Broner, & Steinbacher, 2005). The code places value on the appearance of strength, which may result in inmates deliberately intimidating others, including clinicians. Inmates who appear weak are more vulnerable to victimization, and identification as a mental health patient adds to the appearance of weakness, thereby motivating some inmates to avoid treatment. If mental health staff are identified with the institution's custodial administration, there may also be issues with trust. In other institutions, mental health staff may be seen as separate from security staff and, therefore, viewed as potential allies or advocates.

These perceptions may create barriers to the inmate's engagement in the evaluation and treatment process. Clinicians should be clear about the purpose of the interview, and it may help to be forthcoming about the limitations of the clinician's role. If inmates are reluctant or hostile when addressing their treatment needs, motivational interviewing (MI) may help overcome treatment resistance. MI is used to explore and resolve ambivalence toward change by using "change talk" that is empathic and supportive rather than confrontational (Hettema, Steele, & Miller, 2005). The evidence base for MI supports use in substance-abusing populations as well as those with comorbid substance abuse and schizophrenia (Barrowclough et al., 2001), and MI has been used in the forensic population (McMurran, 2009).

Confidentiality

Maintaining confidentiality is often a concern of inmates being interviewed due to the stigma and vulnerabilities associated with identification as a mental health patient. The correctional setting has additional exceptions to consider beyond dangerousness to self or others, such as information on potential security breaches at the facility. Confidentiality is also difficult to guarantee absolutely, as even lining up for medications may mark an individual as a mental health client. Acknowledging these concerns and informing interviewees when confidentiality cannot be maintained is recommended (see Chapter 8).

Communication skills

The interviewee's ability to communicate should be assessed, and the interviewer should evaluate barriers to communication and determine whether there are means of addressing those barriers (American Psychiatric Association, 2006). In-person interpreter services are often most effective; when not available, telephone interpreter services are an accepted alternative. Hearing impairment may require use of a signing interpreter and referral to medical services to assess the need for a hearing aid. In some instances, neurologic symptoms such as aphasia may be the source of the communication barrier. Psychiatric symptoms such as thought disorder may also result in difficulty communicating—assessment of symptoms is essential to appropriate diagnosis and treatment. These problems may be misinterpreted as behavioral issues with a volitional component, such as deliberately ignoring or defying instructions from officers or institutional rules. Thus, identification and understanding of communication barriers is important in this environment.

Scenario: communication skills

A recently arrested jail inmate is referred for psychiatric evaluation of psychotic symptoms. The referral describes the inmate as impulsive, irritable, having prominent word salad, and having difficulty following instructions from officers. The only known history is of epilepsy.

On interview, the inmate is indignant about the mental health referral. He speaks loudly and rapidly, and while his rhythm of speech resembles that of someone speaking in sentences, much of what he says cannot be followed. Some words sound made up. He eventually provides a history of a gunshot wound to the head six years ago, which preceded the onset of seizures. A scar is visible on the left side of his head. Prior medical records confirm brain injury with resulting Wernicke's aphasia. Due to his diagnosis, the inmate was unable to convey his history and was not psychotic.

Interview structure

The structure of the interview is similar in correctional and community settings (American Psychiatric Association, 2006). The sequence may vary, but the content typically includes the following elements: presenting illness, past psychiatric history, psychosocial and developmental history, substance abuse history, relevant medical history, legal history, review of symptoms, and mental status examination. These elements are discussed in the following paragraphs.

- Presenting illness. In exploring the chief complaint or the reason for referral, prison-specific stressors should be considered. Interpersonal stressors within corrections may involve conflict with other inmates, gangs, or correctional officers. Environmental changes can include moving to a new facility or imposition of disciplinary sanctions. Community factors can also have a role. Difficulties experienced by family may negatively affect an inmate's emotional well-being, especially when associated with frustration or guilt about inability to help loved ones due to incarceration. Incarceration can also lead to erosion of personal relationships, and a break with a significant other can be particularly difficult, as can lack of access or visitation from supports in the community.

- Past psychiatric history. A review of prior mental health treatment can provide information about the trajectory of illness, treatment options, and sources of treatment records. The interviewee's perspective on personal history can also provide an understanding of the level of insight into illness, likelihood of treatment adherence, and approaches to developing rapport. As mentioned earlier, past psychiatric history should encompass treatment while incarcerated and in the community, with review of medication history, hospitalization, outpatient care, response to treatment, and deliberate self-injury or suicide attempts.

- Psychosocial and developmental history. Developmental history may provide helpful insights into the interviewee's current difficulties. In the correctional population, assessment for developmental delay may contribute to a clearer understanding of problems with impulse control, planning, and/or comprehension, all deficits that can hinder an inmate's ability to follow institutional rules. If the history suggests intellectual disability not previously diagnosed, further cognitive testing may be indicated. Psychosocial history should include inquiry into trauma and victimization, whether from childhood abuse or adulthood experiences. Trauma may have occurred during the current or a prior incarceration. Additionally, functioning in the community should be reviewed, including histories of relationships, education, employment, and military service. In addition to contributing to the overall clinical understanding of

the individual, these areas of investigation have a specific application in corrections. Difficulties in the community may point to areas that should be addressed during treatment. The relationship history may suggest supports available to the inmate during incarceration, and an overall understanding of community functioning will assist in reentry planning.

- Substance abuse history. It is appropriate in correctional mental health interviews to conduct in-depth inquiries into substance use history. In addition to the type and extent of substance use, discussion regarding the consequences of use should be included. The possibility of ongoing use may be relevant, as drugs of abuse, while more difficult to obtain, are accessible in jails and prisons (see Chapter 24). The consequences of substance use in corrections may include debts owed to other inmates or disciplinary sanctions and may result in stressors relevant to the mental health presentation. If there is suspicion of ongoing or recent substance use, drug testing should be considered (see Chapter 24).

- Medical history. Review of relevant medical history includes a focus on brain injury, seizure disorders, and other neurologic conditions and documentation of conditions with psychiatric sequelae (see Chapter 38). In corrections, the medical service provides health screening and management of medical problems. When relevant physical health issues exist, coordination of the evaluation and subsequent treatment with the medical service may be indicated.

- Legal history. All inmates should be asked about their chronological history of arrest and conviction, including the index offense, and about the nature of the offenses and contributing factors, including violent or sexual offenses. If unsentenced, the interviewee may be unwilling to disclose details of the index defense for fear of compromising the ongoing case. It is nevertheless appropriate to obtain information about the charges, issues, and concerns the interviewee has about the pending case (see Chapter 61). Understanding the role of mental illness in prior offenses may be helpful in foreseeing potential symptom manifestations in the correctional setting and in planning reentry needs when the inmate returns to the community. Another consideration is duration of sentence and type of conviction. Certain classes of offenses, such as sexual offenses, carry stigma within the correctional population, and such offenders may be more vulnerable to interpersonal stressors if their offenses become known. They may also be at higher risk for suicide. Inmates entering the system for the first time are also more vulnerable, and inmates with lengthy sentences may face problems with hopelessness. In addition to offense history, the interviewee's experience while incarcerated should be reviewed. As mentioned earlier, trauma experienced during incarceration may affect mental disorders or cause mental health symptoms.

- Review of symptoms. The review of symptoms is similar to that in other mental health settings, with inquiry into mood, anxiety, and psychotic symptoms as well as behavioral and functional areas, including sleep, appetite, activity levels, and interest. The review may uncover additional symptoms not reported by the interviewee during discussion of the present illness.

- Mental status examination. As with other sections of the interview, the components of the mental status examination (MSE) are essentially the same as with the MSE conducted in the community, with attention to hygiene, affect, mood, thought process, hallucinations, delusions, suicidality, homicidality, insight, and judgment.

Scenario: index offense

An inmate is seen for mental health screening at intake. The index offense involved illegal gun possession and making threats to "shoot up" a college campus. He presents as calm, well spoken, and logical, and he has had no difficulties adjusting to prison. He explains the circumstances of his arrest as "a misunderstanding" and adds nothing further about what happened. Despite acknowledging a prior history of psychiatric hospitalization, he denies having mental health problems.

This scenario may not pose immediate apparent treatment needs, but the inmate's minimization of a serious offense and his unclear psychiatric history suggest that further inquiry may yield more information. Direct in-depth questioning about his history and functioning in the community and efforts to obtain prior treatment records may guide evaluation.

Additional information

As in community settings, collateral sources of information are important in interpreting interview findings. Prior treatment records, both during incarceration and in the community, should be obtained and reviewed. When possible, contacting personal supports such as family members may yield additional information. Because correctional officers typically have the most contact with inmates, they may be able to provide observations about an inmate's behavior or the context of an inmate's situation. Correctional officers may be the source of a referral for mental health evaluation. While correctional officers may be a valuable source of information, the interviewer must still exercise appropriate measures to maintain patient confidentiality.

Scenario: collateral information

An inmate is referred by a housing officer who provides little detail, saying only, "Inmate says feeling suicidal." When seen for interview, the inmate says, "I didn't mean it."

On the surface, the statement may indicate that the interviewee did not have suicidal intent or planning. The statement may have been made at the height of emotional expression and represented a fleeting thought. Even so, stopping the assessment at the point of the inmate's reassurance that he or she never made suicidal statements or that this was simply a passing feeling is premature.

Referrals from nonmental health professionals may lack relevant detail. Therefore, obtaining information on the actual statements raising concern, the context within which such statements were made, and additional environmental or situational factors can help determine whether there is legitimate concern regarding suicidality. These kinds of situations highlight the importance of obtaining and reviewing correctional and community treatment history, as this will help place the evaluation within the individual's historical context.

Telepsychiatry

The use of live two-way videoconferencing to provide correctional mental health services has steadily been increasing as a means of overcoming geographic limitations to clinician availability (Antonacci, Bloch, Saeed, Yildirim, & Talley, 2008), which is a frequent problem in correctional settings. Use of telepsychiatry has been found to be efficacious, without negative impact on clinician–patient communication, rapport, or satisfaction with treatment, at least with assessment and short-term treatment (O'Reilly et al., 2003).

The use of telepsychiatry in correctional mental health interviews simplifies safety concerns for the interviewer, but other issues remain. Scheduling and timing may be complicated by the addition of technological requirements. The same issues regarding noise and privacy during the interview also apply. An additional consideration is on-site mental health staffing. While some mental health services can be delivered effectively by video, telepsychiatry is not a substitute for on-site staff, particularly in responding to emergencies or to deliver other modalities of assessment and treatment.

Countertransference and bias

Countertransference toward inmates takes many forms. There may be the impulse to view prisoners as criminals primarily deserving punishment or who are simply untreatable. Some offenses, such as sexual offenses, or notorious offenders may engender an emotional response. There may be negative reactions to ongoing and persistent noxious behaviors in the correctional setting. The inmate may be off-putting due to strong character traits associated with a personality disorder or may have a reputation for malingering. Whatever the cause, these reactions may lead the clinician to become judgmental and lose objectivity; potential problems include failing to adequately explore relevant areas or missing diagnoses altogether. Negative countertransference may become apparent in the clinician's demeanor; clinicians may become overtly patronizing, skeptical, or judgmental. Because inmates are sensitive to being judged, this damages rapport and reduces the clinician's ability to elicit necessary information.

Clinicians may become fearful of the inmate or vicariously traumatized. If this occurs, the clinician might attempt to avoid the inmate by reducing the amount of time spent in direct interview, by withdrawing, or by interacting with the inmate in an anxious manner. This, too, can affect objectivity and therapeutic rapport and reduce diagnostic accuracy and treatment efficacy.

Positive countertransference can lead to overidentification with the inmate and overinvolvement by befriending or attraction (Hayes, Gelso, & Hummel, 2011). Boundary erosion may cloud clinical judgment and negatively affect assessment and treatment. In more severe forms, there may be serious boundary violations that place the clinician or the interviewee, or both, in vulnerable positions (Faulkner & Regehr, 2011). These can lead to professional sanctions or negatively affect personal life.

Clinicians cannot always avoid emotional responses to an inmate, but awareness enables them to appropriately manage countertransference and maintain objectivity. During the interview, clinicians should maintain a nonjudgmental attitude. Countertransference may also be a useful tool if clinicians recognize their own feelings as an opportunity to inform diagnosis and treatment (Colli, Tanzilli, Dimaggio, & Lingiardi, 2014).

Summary

Interviewing in correctional mental health is a challenging and multifaceted task that is the foundation to assessing and treating the increased numbers of incarcerated individuals with mental illness. Understanding the correctional population, environment, and culture will help the interviewer to conduct evaluations that are more nuanced and relevant to this traditionally underserved population.

References

Abram, K., Teplin, L., & McClelland, G. (2003). Comorbidity of severe psychiatric disorders and substance use disorders among women in jail. *American Journal of Psychiatry, 160*(5), 1007–1010.

American Psychiatric Association (2000). *Psychiatric services in jails and prisons: a task force report of the American Psychiatric Association.* Washington, DC: American Psychiatric Association.

American Psychiatric Association (2006). *Practice guideline for the psychiatric evaluation of adults.* Washington, DC: American Psychiatric Association.

Antonacci, D., Bloch, R., Saeed, S., Yildirim, Y., & Talley, J. (2008). Empirical evidence on the use and effectiveeess of telepsychiatry via videoconferencing: Implications for forensic and correctional psychiatry. *Behavioral Sciences and the Law, 26,* 253–269.

Barrowclough, C., Haddock, G., Tarrier, N., et al. (2001). Randomized controlled trial of motivational interviewing, cognitive behavior therapy, and family intervention for patients with comorbid schizophrenia and substance use disorders. *American Journal of Psychiatry, 158,* 1706–1713.

Blaauw, E., & van Marle, H. (2007). Mental health in prisons.In L. Moller, H. Stover, R. Jurgens, & A. Gatherer (Eds.), *Health in prison: A WHO guide to the essentials in prison health* (pp. 133–145). Copenhagen, Denmark: World Health Organization.

Black, D., Gunter, T., Loveless, P., Allen, J., & Sieleni, B. (2010). Antisocial personality disorder in incarcerated offenders: Psychiatric comorbidity and quality of life. *Annals of Clinical Psychiatry, 22*(2), 113–120.

Colli, A., Tanzilli, A., Dimaggio, G.,& Lingiardi, V. (2014). Patient personality and therapist response: An empirical investigation. *American Journal of Psychiatry, 171,* 102–108.

Faulkner, C., & Regehr, C. (2011). Sexual boundary violations committed by female forensic workers. *Journal of the American Academy of Psychiatry and the Law, 39*(2), 154–163.

Fazel, S., & Seewald, K. (2012). Serious mental illness in 33,588 prisoners: Systemic review and meta-regression analysis. *British Journal of Psychiatry, 200,* 364–373.

Hayes, J., Gelso, C., & Hummel, A. (2011). Managing countertransference. *Psychotherapy, 48*(1), 88–97.

Hettema, J., Steele, J., & Miller, W. (2005). Motivational interviewing. *Annual Review of Clinical Psychology, 1,* 91–111.

Hills, H., Siegfried, C., & Ickowitz, A. (2004). *Effective prison mental health services: Guidelines to expand and improve treatment.* Washington, DC: US Department of Justice, National Institute of Corrections.

James, D. J., & Glaze, L. E. (2006). *Mental health problems of prison and jail inmates* (NCJ 213600). Washington, DC: Department of Justice. Office of Justice Programs—Bureau of Justice and Statistics.

McMurran, M. (2009). Motivational interviewing with offenders: A systematic review. *Legal and Criminological Psychology, 14,* 83–100.

Metzner, J. (1997a). An introduction to correctional psychiatry: Part I. *Journal of the American Academy of Psychiatry and the Law, 25*(3), 375–381.

Metzner, J. (1997b). An introduction to correctional psychiatry: Part II. *Journal of the American Academy of Psychiatry and the Law, 25*(4), 571–579.

Metzner, J. L. (1998). An introduction to correctional psychiatry, part III. *Journal of the American Academy of Psychiatry and the Law, 28*(1), 107–115.

National Center on Addiction and Substance Abuse at Columbia University (2010). *Behind Bars II: Substance Abuse and America's Prison Population.* Columbia University.

National Commission on Correctional Health Care (2008). *Standards for mental health services in correctional facilities.* Chicago, IL: National Commission on Correctional Health Care.

Ogloff, J. R., Roesch, R., & Hart, S. D. (1994). Mental health services in jails and prisons: Legal, clinical, and policy issues. *Law & Psychology Review, 18,* 109–124.

O'Reilly, R., Bishop, J., Maddox, K., et al. (2003). Is telepsychiatry equivalent to face-to-face psychiatry? Results from a randomized controlled equivalence trial. *Psychiatric Services, 58*(6), 1604–1609.

Rotter, M., Way, B., Steinbacher, M., Sawyer, D., & Smith, H. (2002). Personality disorders in prison: Aren't they all antisocial? *Psychiatric Quarterly, 73*(4), 337–349.

Rotter, M., McQuistion, H., Broner, N., & Steinbacher, M. (2005). Best practices: The impact of the "incarceration culture" on reentry for adults with mental illness: A training and group treatment model. *Psychiatric Services, 56*(3), 265–267.

Steadman, H. J., Osher, F. C., Robbins, P. C., Case, B., & Samuels, S. (2009). Prevalence of serious mental illness among jail inmates. *Psychiatric Services, 60*(6), 761–765.

Teplin, L. A. (1994). Psychiatric and substance abuse disorders among male urban jail detainees. *American Journal of Public Health, 84,* 290–293.

Trestman, R. (2000). Behind bars: Personality disorders. *Journal of the American Academy of Psychiatry and the Law, 28*(2), 232–235.

Trestman, R., Ford, J., & Zhang, W. W. (2007). Current and lifetime psychiatric illness among inmates not identified as acutely mentally ill at intake in Connecticut's jails. *Journal of the American Academy of Psychiatry and the Law, 35*(4), 490–500.

CHAPTER 13

Population management

Robert L. Trestman and Kenneth L. Appelbaum

Introduction

Jails and prisons share population management challenges with hotels: What beds are available to meet requirements for which individuals? The management of large facilities and systems must recognize many safety and clinical demands in real time. Levels of security risk; medical, mental health, and addiction treatment needs; and sex offender status, among others, must all be taken into account in placement decisions (Warren, 1971). This chapter discusses such pragmatic issues, particularly in the context of the psychiatric management challenges they present.

Inmate classification

A core responsibility of correctional systems is safety and security for inmates and for staff. Several considerations affect placement decisions. Correctional systems increasingly use objective classification systems, with resources developed to help them do this (Austin, 1998; Brennan, Wells, & Alexander, 2004). In most facilities and all systems, classification requires computer support. Smaller systems integrate classification with other computerized functions. Some larger systems separate medical and mental health housing management from the security housing system. Whether integrated or separated, from a health systems perspective, the computerized inmate management system should interface with the electronic health record (when one exists). The severity and violence of the alleged offense or conviction are primary determinants of classification, but there are other considerations.

Scenario: classification challenges

BD is a 26-year-old man convicted of aiding in the rape of a 13-year-old girl. BD cooperated with authorities and testified against his codefendant. He has a history of bipolar disorder, cocaine and heroin abuse, and HIV infection. He has two prior incarcerations for nonviolent crimes but assaulted a cellmate on his previous incarceration. What are the considerations for his housing assignment?

Classification for BD presents several important considerations. His sexual offense involving a 13-year-old girl puts him at risk for assault. Other inmates often target child molesters and inmates with mental illness, both of whom tend to fall low on the status hierarchy among inmates. His cooperation with authorities and testimony against his codefendant also put him at risk of retaliation from other inmates. His prior assault on a cellmate, however, complicates the concerns about his safety. He may be a predator

as well as a potential victim during his incarceration. The classification decision needs to balance the benefits of removing him from contact with more violent inmates against the risks of housing him with more vulnerable peers. The placement decision also must consider BD's substance abuse and mental health treatment needs.

Admission and assessment

Much of the work of population management is done at the time of admission into a facility. Court documents are reviewed and prior records retrieved. Custody, medical, and (where indicated) mental health staff interview the inmate on intake. Demographics, aliases, and criminal history are detailed. In a jail, the emphasis is on safety and basic medical and mental health needs. On intake into a prison, additional concerns include educational activities, programming, and vocational needs (Motiuk, 1997).

Although more sophisticated measures are possible and may be used in selected systems (Austin & McGinnis, 2004), most correctional facilities and systems use simple five-point, graded classification scales. There is no uniformity; in some systems, 5 is the most severe, in others the most severe is represented by 1.

Typical classification scales include security; educational, vocational, medical, mental health, and addiction needs; and sex offender risk scores. Subscales are also commonly used. The unique requirements of female inmates are receiving emerging recognition (Brennan & Austin, 1997). All systems keep the genders separate, but most do not differentiate classification schemes by gender.

Security

Jails generally are designed as "one-size-fits-all" facilities; housing units range from minimum- through maximum-security levels. Prison systems generally include a range of facilities, each one designated at a specific security level. In general, inmates accused or convicted of more violent or dangerous offenses are housed in higher-security levels. Higher security comes with greater costs. Minimum-security inmates are usually housed in dormitory settings with lower correctional officer staffing ratios; maximum-security settings are generally double- or single-cell housing with limited movement and more security staff. Security scores typically are composed of several elements, including risk for violence, disciplinary history from previous incarcerations, escape risk, current offense, and gang membership (Austin & McGinnis, 2004). Inaccurate classification can create significant problems. Underclassification may place other inmates at risk;

one unintended consequence of overclassification is the potential for increased risk of rearrest and future incarcerations (Chen & Shapiro, 2007; Gaes & Camp, 2009).

Security risk group

Gang membership typically defines security risk group (SRG) identification, with status or rank in the gang reflecting level of SRG classification. SRG scoring is often defined as follows: 1, no gang affiliation; 2, prior gang affiliation successfully renounced; 3, active gang member; and 4, gang leader or threat member (Connecticut Department of Correction, 2012). The details of SRG management and concerns are discussed in Chapter 58.

Protective custody and keeping separate

Several groups require protection from other inmates during incarceration. Such groups include law enforcement personnel, inmates with low status among their peers (e.g., sex offenders and those with serious mental illness or cognitive impairment), and informants who testified against gangs, codefendants, or crime organizations. These individuals are often housed in a protective custody unit apart from the general population (Austin & McGinnis, 2004). Protective custody status raises significant concerns. Although it may protect selected individuals, it may be overused. This may occur, for example, when providing appropriate accommodations for an inmate in general population proves difficult. Protective custody also typically limits movement and precludes access to programs that would otherwise be available. This is especially problematic for inmates with special needs, such as those with mental impairments. Systems need to find ways to ensure their safety without cutting them off from beneficial programming and services.

Distinct from protective custody are individuals who must be kept apart from each other during incarceration. Such "keep-away" concerns may occur for codefendants in a trial, those who physically assaulted each other during incarceration, those known to have preexisting issues (e.g., one inmate allegedly killed the sister of another inmate), or those affiliated with opposing gangs. Keep-away issues between inmates and staff may occur, for example, when a family member of custody staff becomes incarcerated.

Education

In general, anyone under the age of 18 incarcerated in a US correctional facility without a high school diploma or a General Equivalency Degree (GED) must attend school. Those older than 18 years without a diploma or GED are generally encouraged to go to school. To do so, they must be housed in a facility with educational capacity.

Treatment needs: mental health, medical, addiction, and sex offender

Access to appropriate treatment is always a critical issue; classification helps support such access by creating a designation that allows population management staff to ensure proper inmate placement (see Chapter 22). Mental health classification, as with other classifications, should be purely functional and unrelated to diagnosis. On a five-point scale, the levels, with variability among jurisdictions, may be represented as follows: 1, no past or present treatment needs; 2, no active treatment needs; 3, needs ambulatory level of treatment; 4, requires the equivalent of supported residential housing; and 5, requires infirmary or inpatient level of care. Generally, individuals with a mental health (MH) score of MH-3 or greater will need housing in a facility with dedicated mental health clinicians and nursing staff. Functional levels are dynamic and may change frequently. Someone with bipolar disorder in remission may have MH-3 needs, become acutely manic and hospitalized for six days (during which time the score becomes MH-5), subsequently be discharged to supported housing for three weeks (with a score of MH-4), and finally return to baseline state (MH-3). Some systems also use subcodes that might assist in tracking someone who was on the active caseload of the community mental health authority and will return to the caseload on community release. Another purpose might be to record individuals with a history of suicide attempt to help alert clinical staff upon reincarceration or transfer to a new facility.

Mental health classifications have effects on inmates. In general, inmates get a week of medications for general medical conditions to hold in their cells in a process labeled KOP (keep on person). With few exceptions, nurses administer psychiatric medication individually in directly observed therapy. There are many arguments for and against this approach, but for safety concerns, this has become standard practice. That means that a patient, once placed on psychiatric medication, must be housed in a facility with nursing support. This may preclude housing in many minimum-security and prerelease facilities. As an unfortunate consequence, some patients choose to stop their medications so they can become eligible for placement in lower-security settings. This may lead to decompensation and eventual return to higher security, where they can go back on their medications. Exclusion from prerelease settings also deprives inmates on psychotropic medications of the opportunity to develop skills, under supervision, that they will need to self-monitor their medications in the community. These pragmatic concerns reflect the importance of accurate diagnosis, discussion of treatment options, and full and meaningful informed consent with the patient prior to initiating treatment (see Chapters 12 and 22).

The ways in which staff use classification systems, especially for mental health, raises concerns. For example, consider a patient currently classified as MH-3 who might benefit from a treatment program only available in a residential unit (requiring a MH-4 classification). The patient is not someone who otherwise needs a residential level of care. A clinician may, in an attempt to provide care for that patient, classify the patient as MH-4. While this may sound reasonable, such overclassification may lead to reduced availability of residential beds for those in greater need and unintended effects on parole decisions, leading to longer incarceration. Further, those placed in residential treatment units, similar to those in protective custody, may have restricted access to other programming or vocational opportunities.

Medical classification follows a similar system to mental health. Typical coding reflects the following: 1, no past or current medical treatment needs; 2, no current treatment needs; 3, active treatment well managed with medications with need for predictable access to nursing care 16 hours daily, seven days per week; 4, chronic illness requiring full-time nursing availability or disability accommodations; and 5, infirmary or inpatient level of care.

Subcodes for medical needs may include whether someone is blind or deaf, requires crutches or a sleep apnea machine, and so forth. For example, those with anaphylactic reactions to bee stings might have a subcode or designation as medical-4, with full-time access to nursing care.

Systems need to ensure proper use of their clinical beds, including residential beds for mental health needs and infirmary housing, whether for medical or mental health purposes. For example, correctional officers may want to use a designated infirmary bed to house an inmate for security purposes or use residential mental health beds for protective custody reasons or to keep inmates apart from potential enemies. Such practices need to be avoided, as they reduce the availability of limited infirmary and residential beds and complicate care delivery to patients on those units. Residential programs try to create therapeutic environments where all inmates participate in activities and programming. Boarding nonprogram inmates in these settings can undermine the therapeutic character and mission of the unit.

Addiction treatment needs include consideration of appropriate programming (see Chapter 44). These range from none through short-term psychoeducation to intensive therapeutic community placement. Given the pandemic nature of substance use treatment needs in corrections, it is a rare system that can provide treatment to all who might benefit from it.

Sex offenders are simply defined as those incarcerated for a sex-related crime (see Chapter 59) and do not necessarily include everyone with inappropriate or violent sexual behaviors. Scoring often relates to the criminal charges and history, not to treatment needs. Frequency and level of violence of the behavior are the defining characteristics. Sex offender scoring may be defined as follows: 1, no prior or current sex-offense–related charges; 2, noncontact sexual charge (e.g., voyeurism, exhibitionism); 3, one sexual offense with physical contact; 4, a pattern of two or more sexual offenses with physical contact; and 5, a pattern of repeated sexual offenses with gratuitous violence or sadism.

Internal movement

Inmates are moved within a facility and between facilities for many reasons. Changes in custody status (i.e., becoming convicted), health status, need for a specific program, or preparation for release each may trigger movement of an inmate. For security reasons, most moves are unannounced. Although this decreases the risk of escape planning, it may engender increased anxiety for the affected inmate.

Transportation

Movement in correctional systems requires planning and security. Movement to and from court, other facilities, and health care facilities for procedures or hospitalizations all require secure transportation. Movement decisions require judgment: Is an ambulance needed, or can the inmate travel to a hospital by correctional vehicle? How many officers are required for transport given the security risk of the individual? Because of security risks, inmates typically do not know the scheduled date or time of nonemergency clinical appointments outside the facility. If psychiatrists, other clinicians, or custody staff divulge this

information to an inmate, it creates an opportunity for escape planning or other safety breaches and may necessitate rescheduling of the appointment.

Respite care: interstate compacts

For many reasons, inmates in a state prison system may move to another state through an interstate compact agreement. These moves may be requested because of challenging management concerns such as repeated extreme violence or acute protective custody concerns (e.g., a high-profile and unpopular inmate), or to access resources more readily available elsewhere. Such transfers often allow for respite of exhausted staff who have dealt with a difficult inmate and may ease conflicts not easily resolved between an inmate and a correctional system (e.g., litigated demands or unresolved power struggles).

Community transition: end of sentence, halfway house, parole eligibility, and early release

Inmates often get incentives for good behavior as they progress through their incarceration. Avoiding conflict and following institutional rules allow inmates greater eligibility for job and training opportunities. Participation in appropriate programming and therapy is also often reflected in good behavior credits and progress toward rehabilitation. As inmates become eligible for early release or parole, their behavior and program participation are reviewed. If deemed adequate by the review board, the inmate may become approved for conditional release to a halfway house or other community-based parole program. Preparation for such transition opportunities may be available only at other facilities, again requiring transfer.

Often, as part of this process, the level of community supervision and support needed, on the one hand, and risk of reoffending, on the other, is assessed. This assessment process typically includes formal tools to support such determinations (Andrews & Bonta, 1995; Andrews, Bonta, & Wormith, 2004; Matiuk, 1997).

Summary

Population management is a critical component of safety and security in correctional facilities and systems. Multiple factors must be taken into account to address the at times conflicting demands of treatment, educational, vocational, and security needs. Systems have been developed to manage these complex concerns with growing efficiency. Increasing integration of evidence-based systems will likely occur in the future.

References

Andrews, D. A., & Bonta, J. (1995). *Level of service inventory—Revised.* Toronto, Canada: Multi-Health Systems.
Andrews, D. A., Bonta, J., & Wormith, S. J. (2004). *The level of service/case management inventory.* Toronto, Canada: Multi-Health Systems.
Austin, J. (1998). *Objective jail classification systems: A guide for jail administrators.* Washington, DC: National Institute of Corrections. Retrieved from https://s3.amazonaws.com/static.nicic.gov/Library/014373.pdf
Austin, J., & McGinnis, K. (2004). *Classification of high-risk and special management prisoners: A national assessment of current*

practices. National Institute of Corrections. Retrieved from https://s3.amazonaws.com/static.nicic.gov/Library/019468.pdf

Brennan, T., & Austin, J. (1997). *Women in jail: Classification issues.* National Institute of Corrections. Retrieved from https://s3.amazonaws.com/static.nicic.gov/Library/013768.pdf

Brennan, T., Wells, D., & Alexander, J. (2004). *Enhancing prison classification systems: The emerging role of management information systems.* National Institute of Corrections. Retrieved from http://nicic.gov/Library/019687

Chen, M. K., & Shapiro, J. M. (2007). Do harsher prison conditions reduce recidivism? *American Law and Economics Review, 9,* 1–29.

Connecticut Department of Correction (2012). *Objective classification manual, revised.* Retrieved from http://www.ct.gov/doc/lib/doc/PDF/PDFReport/ClassificationManualLibraryCopy.pdf

Gaes, G., & Camp, S. (2009). Unintended consequences: Experimental evidence for the criminogenic effect of prison security level placement on post-release recidivism. *Journal of Experimental Criminology, 5,* 139–162.

Motiuk, L. (1997). Classification for correctional programming: The offender intake assessment (OIA) process. In *Forum on Corrections Research* (9, 18–22). Retrieved from http://205.193.117.157/publications/forum/special/spe_e_e.pdf

Warren, M. Q. (1971). Classification of offenders as an aid to efficient management and effective treatment. *Journal of Criminal Law, Criminology and Police Science, 62,* 239.

CHAPTER 14

Disciplinary infractions and restricted housing

Mary Perrien and Maureen L. O'Keefe

Introduction

Segregation units function as the prison within a prison. Designed for the dangerous and violent offender who cannot be managed safely within the general prison environment, segregation is characterized by single-cell confinement, with minimum time out of cell for showers and exercise (e.g., 5 hours per week). Other features include highly restricted movement, limited contact with others, and few privileges and services. In 1999, King estimated that 1.8 percent of prisoners were held in segregation; however, its use has since grown, and others assert that the rate is underreported (Naday, Freilich, & Mellow, 2008).

Segregation has been criticized as an inhumane practice due to the degree of social isolation (Metzner & Fellner, 2010). Specifically, the lack of treatment, programs, and activities to engage the mind; restricted personal contact; lack of control over light and sound; lack of windows; and little or no access to the outdoors are considered to be more extreme than is required for the safe operation of prisons. The most significant issue is whether prisoners can psychologically adapt to the austere conditions for long periods, particularly those with mental illness. Because mentally ill inmates may be more prone to rule infractions due to manifestations of their illness, they are more likely to be segregated unless specific rules prohibit their placement.

Psychological impact of segregation

Numerous studies have reported on the psychological impact of segregation. A constellation of symptoms has become associated with such confinement, including perceptual changes, affective disturbances, cognitive difficulties, disturbing thought content, impulse control problems, psychological trauma, and other psychopathological features (Grassian, 1983; Haney, 2003).

Research into the impact of segregation

Segregation research has predominantly relied on cross-sectional designs. Because offenders are assessed at a single point in time, such designs are generally not suited for examining change over time; longitudinal designs are preferred. One longitudinal study found no significant changes in Canadian inmates over 60 days (Zinger, Wichman, & Andrews, 2001), and another found deterioration among Danish prisoners across a three-month period (Andersen, Sestoft, Lillebaek, Gabrielsen, & Hemmingsen, 2000).

Both had strong designs but were affected by high attrition rates (40 percent to 94 percent) resulting from shorter stays in segregation than are typically encountered in the United States.

Access issues make rigorous segregation research difficult, and the conclusions that can accurately be drawn from the literature are likewise limited. These limitations include selection bias, response bias, nonexistent or inadequate comparison groups, single assessment periods, and longitudinal designs over short time periods. Keeping these issues in mind, the Colorado study (O'Keefe, Klebe, Stucker, Sturm, & Leggett, 2010) was undertaken as a direct quasi-experimental study of the psychological effects of long-term segregation, designed to parse out the effects of segregation from those of other prison environments.

Selection bias can occur when subjects are selected nonrandomly. Without randomization, a study runs the risk of not equally representing the population from which the sample is drawn. Small sample sizes, high refusal rates, high attrition rates, and volunteer subjects are examples of selection bias that have challenged segregation research. In the Colorado study, approximately 150 inmates were targeted around the time of their segregation hearing to obtain a baseline measure at the start of solitary confinement. Because inmates with no mental illness (NMI) outnumbered those with mental illness (MI), inmates were divided into two groups so that each could be equally represented. Inmates who met study criteria were sampled to meet a testing schedule that could be conducted by a single researcher covering prisons across the entire state. Study samples appeared to represent the populations of interest as indicated by few group differences across demographic, criminal history, treatment needs, and institutional behavior measures in each of the following comparisons: study groups to eligible pool, refusers to study participants, and those who completed the entire study to those who did not.

Measurement of psychological change may be particularly susceptible to response bias whereby subjects feel compelled to respond in a way consistent with what they think is expected. Subjective measures are generally more prone to response bias than objective measures because wording of questions or nonverbal cues can subtly lead the subject to respond in the hypothesized direction; subjective measures also require clinical judgment to interpret the data. For these reasons, the Colorado study selected standardized paper-and-pencil instruments. Measures were selected for their ease of administration to inmates in noncontact visiting booths and for their strong psychometric properties (i.e., reliability, validity, normative data). Inmates completed 12 instruments (3 at baseline only); housing staff completed a prison adjustment scale; and clinical staff completed a 24-item assessment of psychological symptoms.

The Colorado study proposed to study inmates at three-month intervals over the course of one year. To limit attrition, inmates with fewer than 15 months of prison time remaining on their sentence were excluded and subjects were kept in the study even if their conditions of confinement changed. Analyses using all cases and only "pure" cases (i.e., conditions of confinement remained constant) revealed similar patterns, and thus all cases were used to increase statistical power.

Comparison groups enable researchers to separate out the effects of segregation from prison effects. The quality of a comparison group depends on its similarity to the segregation group. Where comparison groups are absent or too dissimilar (i.e., student or inmate volunteers, minimum-security inmates), it is impossible to rule out that inmates might worsen in prison overall. To match the segregation MI and NMI subjects in the Colorado study, inmates who had a segregation hearing but were returned to the general population (GP) served as comparison subjects. They met the same study criteria and selection procedures as segregated subjects. In addition, a third comparison group of behaviorally disruptive MI inmates placed in a special needs (SN) prison were selected to participate shortly after their movement into the facility. Thus, five groups were included in the study, with a total of 247 subjects.

Study hypotheses were that inmates in segregation would exhibit psychological features consistent with previous research, deterioration would be greater for MI inmates than NMI inmates, and segregated inmates would experience greater deterioration over time than comparison inmates.

Mean test scores were used to test the first hypothesis. Assessment scores were first compared to each test's published cutoff ranges. Figure 14.1 shows mean scores and cutoff ranges on the Brief Symptom Inventory (BSI; Derogatis, 1993) for each group at five testing intervals. The BSI is shown here because it

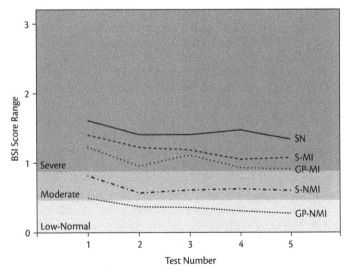

Fig. 14.1 BSI scores for each of five groups across five testing intervals. From O'Keefe et al., 2010).

BSI: Brief Symptom Inventory; SN: Special Needs; S-MI: Segregated—Mentally Ill;
GP-MI: General Population—Mentally Ill; S-NMI: Segregated—Not Mentally Ill;
GP-NMI: General Population—Not Mentally Ill.

assesses a broad range of symptoms and has a similar pattern of results to other instruments. The three MI groups scored in the severe range, with SN subjects scoring the highest and GP subjects scoring the lowest. The two NMI groups scored lower than the MI groups, with the segregated (S) inmates scoring higher than GP ones. Next, test means for each group were compared to normative means of the nearest available reference group (e.g., nonclinical males, general adult samples). On average, compared to nonclinical norms, all groups except the GP–NMI group scored significantly higher than the normative means. These findings are consistent with other research that found serious psychopathology among segregated inmates. However, this psychopathology was present around the time of placement and in the comparison groups, which suggests it was a preexisting condition and not unique to segregated inmates.

Composite scores were created from like scales across multiple instruments. For example, the anxiety composite score was derived from eight subscales across five instruments. The pattern of results for the composites was similar to that of the BSI shown in Figure 14.1. The pattern showed improvement across all composites except withdrawal–alienation, with most change occurring between the first and second testing periods, followed by relative stability for the remainder of the time. Although there were differences between the S–MI and S–NMI groups, it was not in the hypothesized direction: S–MI inmates improved more than S–NMI inmates. Comparison subjects followed the same pattern of improvement, which prevents one from concluding that segregation causes psychological improvements. Nonetheless, the results did not support the third hypothesis that segregated inmates would deteriorate relative to comparison inmates.

Limitations of current research

Several factors limit the generalizability of the Colorado study. Due to eligibility criteria, these results should not be generalized to female, illiterate, or juvenile inmates. Second, subjects may have experienced segregation previously, which could have affected their psychological functioning in this study. In fact, some may have sought segregation for their own safety or preference and, thus, perceiving it as under their control, did not experience an exacerbation of symptoms. Segregation conditions vary from system to system; this study can only be generalized to other prisons to the extent that their confinement conditions are similar to those in Colorado (see O'Keefe et al., 2010). Notably, segregated inmates had access to television and generally clean, quiet conditions, suggestive of positive inmate–staff interactions that could be a powerful protective factor. Finally, without Colorado's special needs prison, many diverted inmates would likely have been placed in segregation, which could have proven detrimental to their well-being.

The Colorado study disputes the belief that all offenders systematically worsen in segregation. However, because the researchers did not believe that no one decompensates, additional analyses were conducted to identify the rate of negative change. Seven percent of segregated inmates appeared to change negatively over the study period, a finding that Gendreau and Labrecque (in press) argue is consistent with expected effect sizes based on metaanalytic procedures on segregation research with prisoners. The Colorado findings are not intended to promote the use of segregation, as there is no evidence to suggest that it is clinically appropriate for inmates with mental illness. This study was intended to stimulate strong applied research within corrections, especially replication studies that can shed more light on inmates' mental health outcomes when conditions of confinement (i.e., services, privileges, staff, out-of-cell time) vary. Prison officials are encouraged to minimize the use of segregation and to explore means of housing offenders in the least restrictive environment possible.

Mental health treatment in segregation

Today, few would argue with the obligation to provide treatment to inmates with mental illness who are in segregation. Case law and correctional treatment standards have established that a minimum standard of care must be provided to those inmates (Cohen, 2008; National Commission on Correctional Health Care, 2008a, 2008b; Weinstein et al., 2000; see Chapter 3). Even inmates who are not believed to have a diagnosable mental illness must be monitored at regular intervals for any signs of decompensation or development of symptoms of mental illness or suicidality (National Commission on Correctional Health Care, 2008a).

The proportion of inmates with mental illness in segregation can be an indicator of the overall quality of the mental health delivery system in a facility and a correctional system (Cohen, 2008). Many agree that problematic correctional mental health systems result in more mentally ill inmates being housed in segregation (Metzner, 2002; Metzner & Fellner, 2010). Untreated or undertreated mentally ill inmates are more likely to act out. If staff do not have options (e.g., appropriate housing and treatment), there is a greater likelihood that those inmates who act out due to their mental illness will be transferred to segregation. Segregation placement does not resolve the problem; it only moves the inmate to an environment that may cause further deterioration and presents its own challenges in access to care.

Many of the characteristics that make segregation safer from a security perspective create challenges to providing care (Beven, 2005). The physical plant can present a physical barrier to adequate care, with little to no treatment or program space. Sometimes the culture can present obstacles to adequate care. Custody staff are trained with safety and security as their primary function. As a result, they may be reluctant to allow mental health staff to interview inmates alone, even handcuffed. Custodial staff may insist on being present in treatment groups for safety reasons, despite the chilling effect on the therapeutic effectiveness of those groups. It becomes increasingly difficult to establish therapeutic rapport within the segregation environment. Safety is a primary concern for all staff. As described later in this chapter, many inmates can be treated safely and confidentiality maintained, even in the highest of security settings.

Standards of care

Despite these difficulties, current standards assert that inmates in segregation are expected to have available a full range of mental health services, including comprehensive assessment, suicide risk assessment, ongoing monitoring, crisis intervention, psychotropic medication management, group and individual psychotherapy, intermediate treatment, and inpatient acute treatment (Weinstein et al., 2000). These services are developed and coordinated by the treatment team and implemented according to an individualized treatment plan. As soon as an inmate is placed in segregation, a screening review should be completed by trained, qualified health care staff and/or mental health staff to ensure there are no mental health conditions that would contraindicate such housing (National Commission on Correctional Health Care, 2008a, 2008b). When reviewing an inmate's medical record, the focus is on psychiatric symptomatology and functioning that may require a need for diversion or adaptive accommodation in segregation (National Commission on Correctional Health Care, 2008b). Accommodation may include placing the inmate in a specific segregation unit that is quieter or allowing more unstructured out-of-cell time to enhance coping.

Mental health staff are expected to monitor all inmates in segregated housing on a regular basis. The frequency and degree of monitoring vary for inmates who are on the mental health caseload and those who are not. Segregation rounds occur at minimum intervals as defined by the degree of isolation. For example, in a segregation unit with frequent periods of inmate recreation in an outdoor group yard and other "routine social contact" among themselves, mental health staff would be expected to conduct weekly rounds (National Commission on Correctional Health Care, 2008a). Often, staff will speak to each inmate in a unit during the same rounds, caseload and non-caseload alike, although caseload inmates are seen during other expected clinical contacts throughout the week. An important purpose for rounds is identification of early signs of deterioration or potential crisis, allowing for immediate intervention and improving the inmate's access to care. However, when many actual segregation rounds conducted by mental health staff were observed, the authors found that the rounds were often perfunctory, characterized by minimal interactions. There is no way that even the most skilled clinician could assess an individual and identify early decompensation from a brief glance into a darkened cell and a shouted "Hi, Mr./Ms. Smith" as he or she rushes down the tier. For segregation rounds to meet their intended goals, contact must involve some extended verbal interaction while observing the inmate at the cell front. The conditions of the cell as well as the inmate are noted. Unit security staff are also consulted for their observations regarding the inmate's functioning. Over time, these rounds and collateral data provide a valuable source of information regarding an inmate's mental status and functioning.

Treatment

Segregation inmates with mental illness must continue to receive their regular mental health treatment. Treatment in a correctional setting is primarily provided through medication management and group therapy supplemented with individual treatment. Because of the intense nature of the segregation setting, treatment contacts typically occur at least once or twice weekly, per modality, and out of the cell. The treatment team will determine the appropriate level of services based on the symptom presentation and functional level of the inmate. The goal is to allow the inmate to function as well as possible within the restricted environment and ultimately move to a less restrictive environment. For example, an inmate with a chronic mental illness and multiple functional impairments is commonly expected to receive a minimum of 10 to 15 hours per week of structured therapeutic services out of cell (Metzner & Dvoskin, 2006; see Chapter 22). An inmate who experiences an acute exacerbation of symptoms must be removed to an appropriate setting (such as an inpatient unit), treated, and stabilized until he or she can tolerate a return to segregation or general population setting (Weinstein et al., 2000).

Individual therapy can be logistically easier to provide in segregated housing than group therapy; a cuffed inmate can meet with a clinician in a small room with windows, allowing supervision by custodial staff from outside while maintaining verbal confidentiality. Group treatment can be more challenging and is often delivered under conditions that still allow custody staff to maintain visual observation from outside the room. Some facilities use treatment cubicles similar to telephone booths with bars and Lexan. As many as 10 of those cubicles may be arranged in a semicircle. Other facilities secure the inmate to a chain bolted to the floor or to the wall near the seat. There are advantages and disadvantages to each method. Clearly, treatment modules take up a significant amount of space but allow inmates to be uncuffed inside and protected from each other. It is much easier and cheaper to configure a smaller space for group treatment by cuffing the inmates to chains secured to the floor. Clinical and custody staff should jointly review the available resources and security needs for treatment, considering the impact of each of these ways of delivering treatment before reaching consensus and proceeding.

Treatment services should focus on current symptomology and functional deficits, particularly those that contributed to segregation placement. Adjustment to segregation is particularly important as an area of treatment focus. Clinically appropriate treatment groups would focus on the following areas: anger management, stress management/relaxation, social skills/interpersonal relationships, criminal thinking, managing mental illness, medication management, and adjusting to incarceration.

Treatment for inmates in segregation often begins at the most fundamental level, even if the inmate has been incarcerated for years and has previously worked with mental health staff. Because segregation is typically an adverse placement, it may be frustrating and result in a lack of cooperation with mental health staff. Consequently, initial treatment plans often focus on establishing a therapeutic relationship and engaging the inmate in treatment. When the therapeutic relationship is particularly tenuous, behavioral therapy is often the most effective at actually engaging the inmate in treatment. The inmate refusal rate to collaborate in care is often highest in segregation; it can become so common as to seem unavoidable. However, it should not be acceptable for mentally ill inmates to regularly refuse to leave their cells for necessary care. Following is an example "Scenario: Treatment Refusal". Effective behavior therapy began with custody and mental health staff working together to identify reinforcers for a particularly aggressive inmate who refused treatment. A functional analysis was completed to identify precursors to the aggressive behaviors. The inmate had not been out of his cell in five years without being handcuffed to a waist chain with mechanical restraints around his ankles. Successive approximation was used to begin to bring him out of his cell to the dayroom, with the ultimate goal being a treatment setting, using reinforcers to reward his behavior. Over a period of months, he was able to walk to the shower unrestrained. He eventually became a full participant in treatment.

When segregation is indicated for any inmate, it is important that the inmate is aware of what he or she must do to work his or her way out of segregation. In some systems, this information is very basic and minimal support is provided. The inmate is told that he or she is expected to participate in the program without any significant disciplinary infractions during the remainder of the stay (e.g., 15 days, 30 days). A number of systems have followed the lead of Ohio and Mississippi to implement structured programs designed to help inmates develop the skills necessary to function infraction-free in the general population and to reward them for their positive efforts while in segregation. These programs, often called step-down units, can greatly reduce the amount of time spent in segregation.

Kupers and colleagues (2009) described such a program in Mississippi. When the segregation population was reclassified according to more objective standards, they found that approximately 80 percent of the population had been overrestrictively classified and did not meet the new segregation criteria. This was a profound improvement in conditions of incarceration for many inmates that also yielded tremendous cost savings for the system. Successful step-down programs allow for the following: increased privileges or freedom as the inmate exhibits improved behaviors; specific treatment that has demonstrated effectiveness in reducing negative target behaviors and in increasing positive replacement behaviors (e.g., behavior therapy, cognitive-behavioral therapy); a willingness on the part of custody staff to use alternative sanctions when behavior is due to mental illness and not rely exclusively on formal disciplinary procedures; and multidisciplinary staff who can think creatively and proactively (Condelli, Dvoskin, & Holanchock, 1994; Kupers et al., 2009). These treatment programs typically use a behavior reinforcement system, often a token system, that involves all staff recognizing positive behaviors. Not only are there multiple opportunities for treatment, but there are multiple opportunities for inmates to demonstrate positive behaviors.

Training of staff

Staff training is another critical component to a successful step-down program. Custody, mental health, and nursing staff should be trained together to facilitate cohesiveness and information sharing. Initial training should focus on practical skills necessary for working with mentally ill individuals in a high-security environment. This would include information about mental health disorders and treatment, de-escalation techniques, security rules and requirements, and behavioral treatment of inmates with mental illness. Ongoing training as part of the overall quality improvement process results in continued evolution of the program and allows it to adapt to the different needs of the population over time. Treatment programs such as these are important because of their positive impact on facility safety. One study found significant decreases in disciplinary infractions, correctional discipline, suicide attempts, and use of segregation when such a program was implemented (Condelli, Dvoskin, & Holanchock, 1994).

Disciplinary process

No discussion about segregation would be complete without a discussion of the disciplinary process. The reader is directed to Cohen (2008) for a comprehensive legal review of the disciplinary process. One study (Krelstein, 2002) found that responding correctional systems typically have a policy that defines the role of the mental health clinician in the disciplinary process. Some systems assign mental health staff a role in determining whether inmates were not responsible for their infractions due to mental illness (e.g., insanity). There is disagreement regarding the utility, especially in difficult budgetary times, of requiring forensically trained psychiatrists or psychologists to evaluate all mental health caseload inmates facing serious infractions regarding the issue of responsibility (Metzner, 2002; Metzner & Dvoskin, 2006). Many systems do not have forensically trained staff and, if they do, they are better utilized. However, the clinician still has a role in the disciplinary process (Metzner & Dvoskin, 2006). The mental health professional should provide input regarding the inmate's ability to understand and participate (competency) in the disciplinary proceedings as well as the need to consider the inmate's mental illness in any disciplinary disposition for mitigation purposes.

Collaboration between mental health and custody staff is critical throughout all aspects of the disciplinary process and segregation placement. True interdisciplinary cooperation and dialogue result in improved security and mental health services. The stronger the mental health service delivery system, the safer the facility is for staff and inmates alike. Research has shown that improved treatment leads to decreases in disciplinary actions and other measures related to safety (Condelli et al., 1994).

Summary

The concern over the psychological impact of segregation on inmates, particularly those with mental illness, remains a valid one. Although the Colorado study found that few inmates were negatively affected, it cannot be assumed that these findings translate to other prison systems or even the same system over time or changing conditions. While segregation conditions vary from correctional system to system, what is constant is that conditions are austere and provide little to assist the mentally ill inmate in coping with his or her situation. As this issue becomes more prominent in the media and the courts, long-term segregation is being considered a violation of society's "evolving standards of decency." Consequently, systems must provide enhanced monitoring and services whatever the length of stay. Treatment services must be sufficient so that inmates, particularly those with mental illness, function optimally within restrictive settings, with the overarching goal of successful discharge to a less restrictive environment.

References

Andersen, H. S., Sestoft, D., Lillebaek, T., Gabrielsen, G., & Hemmingsen, R. (2003). A longitudinal study of prisoners on remand: Repeated measures of psychopathology in the initial phase of solitary versus nonsolitary confinement. *International Journal of Law and Psychiatry, 26*, 165–177.

Beven, G. (2005). Offenders with mental illness in maximum- and supermaximum-security settings. In C. Scott & J. Gerbasi (Eds.), *Handbook of correctional mental health* (pp. 209–228). Washington, DC: American Psychiatric Publishing, Inc.

Cohen, F. (2008). *The mentally disordered offender and the law* (2nd ed.). Kingston, NJ: Civic Research Institute.

Condelli, W. S., Dvoskin, J. A., & Holanchock, H. (1994). Intermediate care programs for inmates with psychiatric disorders. *Bulletin of the American Academy of Psychiatry and the Law, 22*(1), 63–70.

Derogatis, L. (1993). *Brief Symptom Inventory: Administration, scoring, and procedures manual.* Minneapolis, MN: NCS Pearson, Inc.

Gendreau, P., & Labrecque, R. M. (in press). The effects of administrative segregation: A lesson in knowledge cumulation. In J. Wooldredge & P. Smith (Eds.), *Oxford handbook on prisons and imprisonment.* Oxford, UK: Oxford University Press.

Grassian, S. (1983). Psychopathological effects of solitary confinement. *American Journal of Psychiatry, 140*, 1450–1454.

Haney, C. (2003). Mental health issues in long-term solitary and "supermax" confinement. *Crime and Delinquency, 49*, 124–156.

King, R. D. (1999). The rise and rise of supermax: An American solution in search of a problem? *Punishment and Society, 1*, 163–186.

Krelstein, M. (2002). The role of mental health in the inmate disciplinary process: A national survey. *Journal of the American Academy of Psychiatry and the Law, 30*(4), 488–496.

Kupers, T. A., Dronet, T., Winter, M., et al. (2009). Beyond supermax administrative segregation: Mississippi's experience rethinking prison classification and creating alternative mental health programs. *Criminal Justice and Behavior, 20*(10), 2–14.

Metzner, J. L. (2002). Commentary: The role of mental health in the inmate disciplinary process. *Journal of the American Academy of Psychiatry and the Law, 30*, 497–499.

Metzner, J., & Dvoskin, J. (2006). An overview of correctional psychiatry. *Psychiatric Clinics of North America, 29*, 761–772.

Metzner, J. L., & Fellner, J. (2010). Solitary confinement and mental illness in U.S. prisons: A challenge for medical ethics. *Journal of the American Academy of Psychiatry and the Law, 38*(1), 104–108.

Naday, A., Freilich, J. D., & Mellow, J. (2008). The elusive data on supermax confinement. *The Prison Journal, 88*, 69–93.

National Commission on Correctional Health Care (2008a). *Standards for health services in prisons.* Chicago: National Commission on Correctional Health Care.

National Commission on Correctional Health Care (2008b). *Standards for mental health services in correctional facilities.* Chicago: National Commission on Correctional Health Care.

O'Keefe, M. L., Klebe, K. J., Stucker, A., Sturm, K., & Leggett, W. (2010). *One-year longitudinal study of the psychological effects of administrative segregation.* Technical Report. CO Department of Corrections. Retrieved from http://www.doc.state.co.us/sites/default/files/opa/AdSegReport_2010.pdf

Weinstein, H. C., Burns, K. A., Newkirk, C. F., et al. (2000). *Psychiatric services in jails and prisons.* Washington, DC: American Psychiatric Association.

Zinger, I., Wichman, C., & Andrews, D. A. (2001). The psychological effects of 60 days in administrative segregation. *Canadian Journal of Criminology, 43*, 47–88.

CHAPTER 15

Community re-entry preparation/coordination

Henry A. Dlugacz

Introduction

When the prison gates slam behind an inmate, he does not lose his human quality; his mind does not become closed to ideas; his intellect does not cease to feed on a free and open interchange of opinions; his yearning for self-respect does not end; nor is his quest for self-realization concluded. If anything, the needs for identity and self-respect are more compelling in the dehumanizing prison environment.

Procunier v. Martinez (1974)

These words, written 40 years ago by Supreme Court Justice Thurgood Marshall, remind us that incarceration does not extinguish the prisoner's humanity. Thirty years later, President George W. Bush brought Justice Marshall's insight to its logical conclusion: "We know from long experience that if [released inmates] can't find work, or a home, or help, they are much more likely to commit crime and return to prison" (Bush, 2004).

All inmates who do not die before release—approximately 97 percent—return to the community (Council of State Governments, 2002; Travis & Waul, 2004). This simple reality makes it in society's enlightened self-interest to be concerned with the readiness of these former inmates to live a productive life. The criminal justice and correctional treatment systems affect an inmate's behavior and opportunities upon release. Was he or she treated humanely? What skills were acquired to enhance prosocial coping styles? Were educational or vocational opportunities afforded? Was mental health treatment adequate? What linkages were made prior to release to address risk factors for recidivism and the need for continued treatment, housing, or employment?

Successful re-entry planning considers these interrelated issues when building an individualized plan to address them. It begins at admission (or even sentencing) and continues after release (Petersilia, 2001). Rather than considering incarceration to be an isolated event, re-entry planning views incarceration as part of a cycle to be disrupted through targeted intervention. Correctional mental health treatment is seen as part of a continuum of care that extends to the community. Obtaining collateral information about preincarceration functioning and response to treatment aids in the accurate assessment of needs following release. Likewise, pertinent information from correctional treatment providers should be transmitted to the community programs that will provide treatment after release. These exchanges of information can be enhanced by both the nurturing of professional relationships through stakeholders' meetings and cross-training and by the creative use of technology (Dlugacz & Roskes, 2010).

Re-entry planning for people with serious mental illness should be a primary focus of correctional mental health care that is integrated into the treatment function, not an afterthought to be considered only as release is imminent—although pending discharge increases its salience in the hierarchy of treatment needs. While acceptance of personal responsibility is a critical antecedent to leading a lawful life and self-determination is a fundamental principle of recovery, it is unrealistic for service providers to rely on the individual to coordinate fragmented public systems. This is the job of those funded to provide services.

Re-entry programs develop in a complex social context

The context in which re-entry programs develop is influenced by larger societal trends. For example, the number of people in state psychiatric hospitals dropped precipitously between 1950 and the mid-2000s (Dlugacz, 2014; Hoge, Buchanan, Kovasznay, & Roskes, 2009). Enhancements to community services for these former hospital patients did not materialize. Legislators became cynical that offenders could be rehabilitated and severely limited judges' discretion to craft sentences based on individual circumstances (Weinstein & Wimmer, 2010). Restrictions on the availability of early release through parole limited the ability to manage correctional populations on the back end (Weinstein & Wimmer, 2010). Correctional populations grew at unprecedented rates. Caught in this tsunami of incarceration were many people with severe mental illness (Dlugacz, 2014; Dlugacz & Roskes, 2010).

Recently, groups such as the Council of State Governments have raised awareness about the importance of re-entry planning. It is in this context that re-entry planning for offenders with serious mental illness is evolving from a best practice to a standard of care (Dlugacz & Roskes, 2010; Metzner, 2007). All major professional organizations in correctional health care require some type of discharge planning (Dlugacz & Roskes, 2010). Physicians have an ethical duty to assist patients with continuity of care. The American Medical Association's ethical guidelines require cooperation with other treatment providers. The physician may not ethically discontinue treatment of a patient as long as further treatment is medically indicated (American Medical Association, 1990).

This suggests an ethical duty to facilitate the transition to community care for discharged inmate–patients. The overall system must provide the correctional psychiatrist with the tools needed to fulfill this duty. Following from this, professional organizations have a concomitant obligation to support systemic change so that individual clinicians can act ethically (Dlugacz, Low, Wimmer, & Knox, 2013; Metzner & Fellner, 2010).

Some US policymakers have shown a renewed confidence that treatment interventions for offenders with mental disorders are worthy of support to improve public safety outcomes. If people with mental illness are ensnared in the criminal justice system at highly disproportionate rates, the thinking goes, providing re-entry planning with connection to treatment could reduce offending among this group. Legislative initiatives signed with broad bipartisan backing appropriated funding to address obstacles faced by released inmates with serious mental illness; this marked a turning point in public attitudes (Crayton, Mukamal, & Travis, 2009; Wilson & Draine, 2006).

Scope of the problem

The United States incarcerates an immense number of people, inevitably leading to a large number of releases to the community. Annually, it is estimated that as many as 650,000 adults are released from prison (Council of State Governments, 2002) and 13 million people leave US jails (Crayton et al., 2009). Among this group are a disproportionate number of people with severe mental illness (Dlugacz, 2014; Dlugacz & Wimmer, 2013; Munetz & Griffin, 2006; Steadman, Osher, Clark Robbins, Case, & Samuels, 2009; see Chapter 32).

Despite the clear need for transitional services, they are not consistently available. A survey of US jails found that about 20 percent of inmates with mental illness received discharge planning services (Hoge, 2007; Steadman & Veysey, 1997). One survey of New Jersey jails found a large variation in prerelease efforts among facilities, with some reporting that they provided aftercare plans for fewer than 10 percent of inmates with mental illness upon release and others reporting that they did so for between 75 and 100 percent of such inmates (Wolff, Plemmons, Veysey, & Brandli, 2002). A report by the US Department of Justice indicated that 66 percent of state prisons that house adults helped released inmates obtain community mental health services (Lurigio, Rollins, & Fallon, 2004; US Department of Justice, Bureau of Justice Statistics, 2001). According to the Bazelon Center for Mental Health Law (2009), only one third of discharged inmates receive assistance with accessing benefits. When these re-entry services are provided, they vary considerably with respect to population served, approach used, and locus of administrative authority. Rather than being based on empirical data, they tend to be localized in nature (Wilson & Draine, 2006).

One survey of re-entry programs in the United States found that 74 percent were led by the criminal justice system and only 26 percent by the behavioral health system, with varying degrees of collaboration between the two. Those spearheaded by the criminal justice system were found to be more collaborative than those led by the behavioral health system (Wilson & Draine, 2006). This suggests that despite an increased focus on breaking down service "silos," improved collaboration is needed (Dlugacz, Broner, & Lamon, 2007).

Obstacles to re-entry

Inmates with serious mental illness face significant dangers when released. Within 18 months of release, two thirds are rearrested and half are hospitalized (Feder, 1991; Hartwell, 2003, 2008). One study found that inmates in general were almost 13 times more likely to die within the first two weeks of release than were other people with similar demographics (Binswanger et al., 2007a, 2007b).

Comorbid substance abuse is also a significant problem (Freudenberg, Daniels, Crum, Perkins, & Richie, 2005; US Department of Justice, Bureau of Justice Statistics, 2003). Offenders with both mental illness and substance abuse are more likely to be homeless upon release than those with just mental illness and are more likely to violate parole and recidivate (Hartwell, 2004; Mueser, Noordsy, Drake, & Fox, 2003). Overall rates of homelessness are highly elevated in the correctional population. Homeless inmates are more likely to have co-occurring mental health problems and substance abuse and may be incarcerated for longer periods of time (Freudenberg, Daniels, Crum, Perkins, & Richie, 2005; McNiel, Binder, & Robinson, 2005). The presence of either mental illness or homelessness seems to lead to an increased risk for the other (Greenberg & Rosenheck, 2008). The criminal justice population also has high levels of chronic medical conditions (Binswanger, Redmond, Steiner, & Hicks, 2012; Cuddeback, Scheyett, Pettus-Davis, & Morrissey, 2010; Regenstein & Christie-Maples, 2012) and tends to have these conditions in more advanced stages than do age-adjusted comparators.

What can be done?

While the difficulties faced by returning inmates can be daunting, they also form a template for required interventions. The interplay between mental illness and recidivism is complex and requires attention in the re-entry planning process. Noting the high rates of mental illness among the correctional population, practitioners assumed that linkage to treatment upon release would be a primary driver of improved criminal justice outcomes. While clinical interventions improved clinical outcomes, they did not appear to significantly reduce recidivism. Studies show that the specific symptoms of serious mental illness are related to arrest in fewer than 10 percent of cases, suggesting that treatment as usual across the population will not have the desired effect on recidivism (Jurginger, Claypoole, Laygo, & Crisanti, 2006; Peterson, Skeem, Hart, Vidal, & Keith, 2010; Rotter, Carr, & Frischer, 2014).

Other studies indicate that most people with mental illness have essentially the same risk factors for recidivism as do other people (Hall, Miraglia, Lee, Chard-Wierschem, & Sawyer, 2012). This suggests that the focus of treatment in jail and upon release should be on the types of cognitive-behavioral treatment that have been proven effective in reducing recidivism across the criminal justice population. Research related to the Risk–Need–Responsivity (RNR) model supports this approach (Bonta & Andrews, 2007). The RNR model uses risk assessment to identify a person's risk factors for criminal behavior so that they are specifically targeted by interventions individualized to the person's strengths, abilities, motivation, and learning style (Bonta & Andrews, 2007). In this approach, serious mental illness is only a minor risk factor (Bonta & Andrews, 2007).

However, just as the focus on standard treatment may have been overly simplistic, so, too, may be a rush to abandon it. Improving treatment outcomes has a value in and of itself and may serve to improve compliance with parole requirements. The episodic nature of psychosis may mask the relationship between mental illness and arrest (Hall et al., 2012). Because people with mental illness remain incarcerated longer than others, they may have a reduced chance to commit new crimes (Baillargeon, Binswanger, Penn, Williams, & Murray, 2009; McNiel & Binder, 2007; US Department of Justice, 1999). One large study found that inmates with major psychiatric disorders had a substantially increased risk of multiple incarcerations over a six-year period (Baillargeon et al., 2009).

However, recent studies indicate that standard mental health treatment may indeed moderate recidivism. One found that routine outpatient treatment reduced the likelihood of arrest and that medication possession in the 90-day period following hospitalization appeared to provide further protection (Van Dorn, Desmarais, Petrila, Haynes, & Singh, 2013).

Offenders with mental illness are more than a conglomeration of conditions described in the previous section. An evidence-based practice only means a greater number of people did better receiving that treatment than those who received treatment as usual (Gray, 2004), not that a particular treatment is well suited to a particular person. Matching intervention to need requires biopsychosocial–spiritual assessments of risks, needs, circumstances, and life goals.

Most studies on re-entry programs report on successful linkage to services, not whether the service, intensity, or type was adequate (Draine & Herman, 2007). While released prisoners may receive social or mental health services, one study showed that few get clinically meaningful levels of care during the first year of release (Lovell, Gagliardi, & Peterson, 2002). Also, evidence-supported services (including integrated treatment for substance abuse and mental illness; Kubiak, Essenmacher, Hanna, & Zeoli, 2011) and the types of cognitive therapies RNR research recommends may not be widely available.

Some consumers make rational decisions to reject services that do not meet their needs, an example being re-entry planning that does not address housing. One study of jail inmates found that men listed employment and education as their top priorities, while women regarded substance abuse treatment as paramount. Both adult men and women regarded housing as a high priority (Freudenberg et al., 2005). The needs identified by these inmates closely relate to known strategies that reduce recidivism. While much is made of the population's lack of insight and misguided priorities, these inmates desired exactly the type of interventions that would help them stay out of jail. A more recent study of released jail inmates with severe mental illness echoed these results, finding that housing and financial assistance were their top priorities. Only 12 percent of the group studied listed mental health treatment among their top two priorities for assistance following release (Wilson, 2013).

Successful re-entry programs tend to have certain elements in common, including the following:

- Behavioral/cognitive treatment;
- Positive reinforcement;
- Intensive services that last 3 to 12 months and that occupy between 30 and 70 percent of the person's time;
- Used with high-risk offenders;
- Target crimogenic needs;
- Use actuarial assessments of risk;
- Conduct interventions in community not institutional settings;
- Match staffing skill sets to inmates' needs and learning styles (Cullen & Gendreau, 2000; Petersilia, 2004).

The focus on high-risk offenders is supported by research demonstrating that the placement of low-risk offenders in more intensive programs often increased their failure rates (Lowenkamp & Latessa, 2004).

Treatment and rehabilitation approaches that show promise for incorporation into successful re-entry programs include peer mentoring programs (Miller, 2010), supported employment, and supportive housing (Draine & Herman, 2010). One study found that prisoners with mental illness in a work-release program had higher success rates than other prisoners in the program (Way, Abreu, Ramirez-Romero, Aziz, & Sawyer, 2007). An interim report on an expansion of supportive housing in New York City found that placement in supportive housing reduced public expenditures by approximately $10,100 during the first year for the placed group compared to the unplaced group. Savings were driven, in part, by reduced use of jails, shelters, and state-operated inpatient psychiatric hospitals (New York City Department of Health and Mental Hygiene et al., 2013).

Another promising approach is Forensic Assertive Community Treatment (FACT), which is an adaptation of traditional assertive community treatment models (Cuddeback, Wright, & Bisig, 2013). FACT attempts to close gaps in service between the mental health and treatment systems by including partnerships between the two and encouraging adherence to treatment through legal leverage (Lamberti & Weisman, 2010). Brief motivational interviewing (BMI) is an evidence-based counseling technique shown to improve motivation for treatment for a number of physical and emotional conditions (Rubak et al., 2005). BMI is well suited to corrections because it can be used by a wide array of staff. This has utility for re-entry planning because successful re-entry and retention in aftercare go hand in hand. The sustained changes in behavior promoted by BMI make it conceptually similar to a public health intervention akin to a vaccine—a brief intervention with protective benefits extending well into the future.

Benefits

No re-entry plan is likely to succeed if it is not accompanied by the means to pay for it. Entitlements such as Medicaid, Medicare, Veterans Administration benefits, and Social Security income help people to secure housing, mental health treatment, and sustenance (Bazelon Center for Mental Health Law, 2009). Because the period immediately following release poses particular risks, whenever possible inmates should be assisted with applying for benefits before they are released. When this is not achievable, appointments can be made and required documents assembled so the person is well situated to follow through promptly following release.

Correctional systems can enter into prerelease agreements with the Social Security Administration (SSA) that facilitate the submission of new applications for SSA benefits or the prompt reinstatement of suspended benefits upon an inmate's release. They standardize guidelines for communication between SSA and correctional facilities by providing point persons in each organization and establishing procedures for the submission of applications and supporting documentation (Social Security, Program Operations Manual System, 2013). Training staff to appropriately complete applications for benefits improves success rates (McCormick & Perret, 2010).

Focused attention on benefits assistance can increase access to care. One study found that a program to help inmates with serious mental illness to enroll in Medicaid increased use of mental health services by 16 percent (Wenzlow, Ireys, Mann, Irvin, & Teich, 2011). In the United States, Medicaid expansion included in the Patient Protection and Affordable Care Act could improve access to health care for released inmates (Tietelbaum & Hoffman, 2013). The act subsidizes states to provide Medicaid coverage for those whose incomes are up to 138 percent of the poverty line. The US Department of Justice estimates that former inmates and detainees will make up approximately 35 percent of the people qualifying under this provision (Kardish, 2013). Some states are aggressively working to expand coverage to former inmates (Gugliotta, 2013; Zaitz, 2013). This, together with some state statutes requiring the suspension rather than termination of Medicaid upon incarceration, could reduce the gaps in coverage that too frequently accompany even relatively brief incarcerations (Wakeman, McKinney, & Rich, 2009).

Many Western countries outside of the United States have more robust equivalence between prison and community health care (Exworthy et al., 2012; General Assembly, 1990); in countries such as the United Kingdom, universal health care reduces the concern that is so prevalent in the United States related to gaps in health coverage. Interestingly, released prisoners in the United Kingdom face many of the same obstacles to successful re-entry as do those in the United States, including lack of adequate community mental health care and difficulty securing employment and affordable housing (MacDonald, 2012). This demonstrates that while access to health benefits is a rate-limiting step in accessing needed services, it is only one part of the puzzle.

Practical suggestions

The scope of obstacles to successful re-entry can be daunting. Stakeholder meetings to create the crucial buy-in (Dlugacz et al., 2007) and interagency meetings can foster collaboration and build informal networks that can be used once programs are operational (Dlugacz et al., 2007).

In-reach by community providers prior to an inmate's release may improve the likelihood of follow-through after discharge. Where distances are prohibitive, video links can be used. Prisoners can be moved closer to home in the period leading up to their release to facilitate interaction with providers and family. Some providers are willing to meet the released prisoner at the institution's gate to assist with transportation. A supply of medications and a prescription should be provided when clinically appropriate.

Summary

The re-entry plan will be influenced by the person's illness, connection with mental health treatment while incarcerated, and ability to function in the community (Metzner, 2007), as well as the model of service delivery used and the size, location, and detention function of the facility. Re-entry planning cannot be divorced from the state of affordable housing and evidence-based

treatment available in the community to which the person will return. Difficult though it may be to create a plan to address these obstacles, it is incumbent upon those working in corrections to try.

Acknowledgment

The author thanks Emily Brouwer and Helen Haidemenos for their assistance.

References

American Medical Association (1990). *Fundamental elements of the physician–patient relationship*. Retrieved from http://www.ama-assn.org//ama/pub/physician-resources/medical-ethics/code-medical-ethics/opinion1001.page

Baillargeon, J., Binswanger, I. A., Penn, J. V., Williams, B. A., & Murray, O. J. (2009). Psychiatric disorders and repeat incarcerations: The revolving prison door. *American Journal of Psychiatry, 166*(1), 103–109.

Bazelon Center for Mental Health Law (2009). Linking to federal benefits for people exiting corrections. *Lifelines, 3*, 1–34. Retrieved from http://www.bazelon.org/News-Publications/Publications/CategoryID/7/List/1/Level/a/ProductID/6.aspx?SortField=ProductNumber,ProductNumber

Binswanger, I. A., Redmond, N., Steiner, J. F., & Hicks, L. S. (2011). Health disparities and the criminal justice system: An agenda for further research and action. *Journal of Urban Health: Bulletin of the New York Academy of Medicine, 89*(1), 98–107.

Binswanger, I. A., Stern, M. F., Deyo, R. A., et al. (2007a). Correction to release from prison: A high risk of death for former inmates. *New England Journal of Medicine, 356*, 536.

Binswanger, I. A., Stern, M. F., Deyo, R. A., et al. (2007b). Release from prison: A high risk of death for former inmates. *New England Journal of Medicine, 356*, 157–165.

Bonta, J., & Andrews, D. A. (2007). *Risk-Need-Responsivity model for offender assessment and rehabilitation*. Retrieved from www.public-safety.gc.ca/cnt/rsrcs/pblctns/rsk-nd-rspnsvty/index-eng.aspx

Bureau of Justice Statistics (2003). *Sourcebook of criminal justice statistics*. Washington, DC: Department of Justice.

Bush, G. W. (2004). *State of the Union address*. Retrieved from http://georgewbush-whitehouse.archives.gov/news/releases/2002/01/20020129-11.html

Council of State Governments (2002). *Criminal Justice/Mental Health Consensus Project*. Retrieved from http://consensusproject.org/downloads/Entire_report.pdf

Crayton, A., Mukamal, D.A., & Travis, J. (2009). A new era in inmate reentry. *Corrections Today, 71*, 38.

Cuddeback, G. S., Scheyett, A., Pettus-Davis, C., & Morrissey, J. P. (2010). General medical problems of incarcerated persons with sever and persistent mental illness: A population based-study. *Psychiatric Services, 61*, 45–49.

Cuddeback, G. S., Wright, D., & Bisig, N. (2013). Characteristics of participants in jail diversion and prison reentry programs: Implications for forensic ACT. *Psychiatric Services, 64*, 1043–1046.

Cullen, F., & Gendreau, P. (2000). Assessing correctional rehabilitation: Policy, practice, and prospects. *Criminal Justice, 3*, 109–175.

Dlugacz, H. (2014). Correctional mental health in the United States. *International Journal of Prisoner Health 10*, 3–26.

Dlugacz, H., & Wimmer, C. (2013). Legal aspects of administrating antipsychotic medications to jail and prison inmates. *International Journal of Law and Psychiatry, 36*, 213–228.

Dlugacz, H. A., & Roskes, E. (2010). Clinically oriented reentry planning. In C. L. Scott (Ed.), *Handbook of correctional mental health* (2nd ed., pp. 395–431). Washington, DC: American Psychiatric Publishing, Inc.

Dlugacz, H. A., Broner, N., & Lamon, S. (2007). Implementing reentry–establishing a continuum of care of adult jail and prison releases with mental illness. Correctional psychiatry: Practice guidelines and strategies, 12-1–12-37.

Dlugacz, H. A., Low, J. Y., Wimmer, C., & Knox, L. (2013). Ethical issues in correctional psychiatry in the United States. In N. Konrad, B. Vollm, & D.N. Weisstub (Eds.), *Ethical issues in prison psychiatry* (pp. 49–76). Netherlands: Springer.

Draine, J., & Herman, D. (2007). Critical time intervention for reentry from prison for persons with mental illness. *Psychiatric Services, 8,* 1577–1581.

Draine, J., & Herman, D. (2010) Critical time intervention. In H. Dlugacz (Ed.), *Reentry planning for offenders with mental disorders: Policy and practice* (pp. 6-1–6-11). Kingston, NJ: Civic Research Institute, Inc.

Exworthy, T., Samele, C., Urquía, N., & Forrester, A. (2012). Asserting prisoners' right to health: Progressing beyond equivalence. *Psychiatric Services, 63,* 260–275.

Feder, L. (1991). A comparison of the community adjustment of mentally ill offenders with those from the general prison population. *Law and Human Behavior, 15,* 477–493.

Freudenberg, N., Daniels, J., Crum, M., Perkins, T., & Richie, B. E. (2005). Coming home from jail: The social and health consequences of community reentry for women, male adolescents, and their families and communities. *American Journal of Public Health, 95,* 1725–1736.

General Assembly (1990). *Basic principles for the treatment of prisoners.* Retrieved from http://www.un.org/documents/ga/res/45/a45r111.htm

Gray, G. E. (2004). *Concise guide to evidence based psychiatry.* Washington, DC: American Psychiatric Publishing, Inc.

Greenberg, G. A., & Rosenheck, R. A. (2008). Jail, incarceration, homelessness, and mental health: A national study. *Psychiatric Services, 59,* 170–177.

Gugliotta, G. (2013). Michigan embraces Medicaid expansion to help inmates. *Washington Post.* Retrieved from www.washingtonpost.com/national/health-science/michigan-embracing-medicaid-expansion-to-help-inmates/2013/11/30/61a94a80-592d-11e3-ba82-16ed03681809_story.html

Hall, D. L., Miraglia, R. P., Lee, L-W. G., Chard-Wierschem, D., & Sawyer, D. (2012). Predictors of general and violent recidivism among SMI prisoners returning to communities in New York State. *Journal of the American Academy of Psychiatry and the Law, 40,* 221–231.

Hartwell, S. (2003). Short-term outcomes for offenders with mental illness released from incarceration. *International Journal of Offender Therapy and Comparative Criminology, 47,* 145–158.

Hartwell, S. (2004). Triple stigma: Persons with mental illness and substance abuse problems in the criminal justice system. *Criminal Justice Policy Review, 15,* 84–99.

Hartwell, S. (2008). *Community reintegration of persons with SMI post incarceration.* Center for Mental Health Services Research Brief. Retrieved from http://www.umassmed.edu/uploadedFiles/Brief37Reintergration.pdf

Hoge, S. K. (2007). Providing transition and outpatient services to the mentally ill released from correctional institutions. In R. B. Greifinger (Ed.), *Public health behind bars* (pp. 461–477). New York: Springer.

Hoge, S. K., Buchanan, A. W., Kovasznay, B. M., & Roskes, E. J. (2009). *Outpatient services for the mentally ill involved in the criminal justice system: Task Force report.* Washington, DC: American Psychiatric Association.

Jurginger, J., Claypoole, K., Laygo, R., & Crisanti, A. (2006). Effects of serious mental illness and substance abuse on criminal offenses. *Psychiatric Services, 57,* 879–882.

Kardish, C. (2013). *How Medicaid expansion can lower prison costs, recidivism. Governing the states and localities: Public safety & justice.* Retrieved from http://www.governing.com/news/headlines/How-Medicaid-Expansion-Lowers-Prison-Costs-Recidivism.html

Kubiak, S. P., Essenmacher, L., Hanna, J., & Zeoli, A. M. (2011). Transitions between jail and community-based treatment for individuals with co-occurring disorders. *Psychiatric Services, 62,* 679–681.

Lamberti, S. J., & Weisman, R. L. (2010) Forensic assertive community treatment: Origins, current practice, and future directions. In H. Dlugacz (Ed.), *Reentry planning for offenders with mental disorders: Policy and practice* (pp. 7-1–7-24). Kingston, NJ: Civic Research Institute, Inc.

Lovell, D., Gagliardi, G. J., & Peterson, P. D. (2002). Recidivism and use of services among persons with mental illness after release from prison. *Psychiatric Services, 53,* 1290–1296.

Lowenkamp, C. T., & Latessa, E. J. (2004). *Understanding the risk principle: How and why correctional interventions can harm low-risk offenders, topics in community corrections.* Washington, DC: National Institute of Corrections.

Lurigio, A. J., Rollins, A., & Fallon, J. (2004). The effects of serious mental illness on offender reentry. *Federal Probation, 68,* 45–52.

MacDonald, M. (2012). *Research report: United Kingdom.* Retrieved from http://www.throughcare.eu/partnerreports.html

McCormick, T. C., & Perret, Y. M. (2010). Accessing public benefits: More advocacy than entitlement. In H. Dlugacz (Ed.), *Reentry planning for offenders with mental disorders: Policy and practice* (pp. 3-2–3-20). Kingston, NJ: Civic Research Institute, Inc.

McNiel, D. E., & Binder, R. L. (2007). Effectiveness of a mental health court in reducing criminal recidivism and violence. *American Journal of Psychiatry, 164,* 1395–1403.

McNiel, D. E., Binder, R. L., & Robinson, J. C. (2005). Incarceration associated with homelessness, mental disorder, and co-occurring substance abuse. *Psychiatric Services, 56,* 840–846.

Metzner, J., & Fellner, J. (2010) A challenge for medical ethics. *Journal of the American Academy of Psychiatry and the Law, 38,* 104–108.

Metzner, J. L. (2007). Evolving issues in correctional psychiatry. *Psychiatric Times.* Retrieved from http://www.google.com/url?sa=t&rct=j&q=&esrc=s&source=web&cd=2&ved=0CDkQFjAB&url=http%3A%2F%2Fwww.psychiatrictimes.com%2Fprintpdf%2F162135&ei=_l24UqvNEefJsQTRnIDQCg&usg=AFQjCNHMP3OtpEqLFyZHyT89AZvUENbyLQ&sig2=DMG8Fut21GuMiHweVgZRtg&bvm=bv.58187178,d.cWc

Miller, L. (2010). Reentry as part of the recovery process. In H. Dlugacz (Ed.), *Reentry planning for offenders with mental disorders: Policy and practice* (pp. 10-2–10-8). Kingston, NJ: Civic Research Institute, Inc.

Mueser, K. T., Noordsy, D. L., Drake, R. E., & Fox. L. (2003). *Integrated treatment for dual disorders: A guide to effective practice.* New York: Guilford.

Munetz, M. R., & Griffin, P. A. (2006). Use of the sequential intercept model as an approach to decriminalization of people with serious mental illness. *Psychiatric Services, 57,* 544–549.

New York City Department of Health and Mental Hygiene, New York City Human Resources Administration and the New York State Office of Mental Health (2013). *New York/New York III supportive housing evaluation: Interim utilization and cost analysis.* Retrieved from https://www.health.ny.gov/health_care/medicaid/program/medicaid_health_homes/housing_and_health_homes.htm

Petersilia, J. (2001). Prisoner reentry: Public safety and reintegration challenges. *Prison Journal, 81,* 360–375.

Petersilia, J. (2004). What works in prisoner reentry? Reviewing and questioning the evidence. *Federal Probation, 68,* 4–8.

Peterson, J., Skeem, J., Hart, E., Vidal, S., & Keith, F. (2010). Analyzing offense patters as a function of mental illness to test the criminalization hypothesis. *Psychiatric Services, 61,* 1217–1222.

Procunier v. Martinez, 416 U.S. 396, 428 (1974).

Regenstein, M., & Christie-Maples, J. (2012). Medicaid coverage for individuals in jail pending disposition: Opportunities for improved health and health care at lower costs. Health Policy Faculty Publications, Paper 1. Retrieved from http://hsrc.himmelfarb.gwu.edu/sphhs_policy_facpubs/1

Rotter, M., Carr, A., & Frischer, K. (2014) The premise of criminalization and the promise of offender treatment. In H. Dlugacz (Ed.), *Reentry planning for offenders with mental disorders: Policy and practice* (vol. 2, in press). Kingston, NJ: Civic Research Institute, Inc.

Rubak, S., Sandbaek, A., Lauritzen, T., et al. (2005). Motivational interviewing: A systematic review and meta-analysis. *British Journal of General Practice, 55*, 305–213.

Social Security, Program Operations Manual System (2013). *Prerelease agreements.* Retrieved from https://secure.ssa.gov/apps10/poms.nsf/lnx/0500520910

Steadman, H. J., & Veysey, B. M. (1997). Providing services for jail inmates with mental disorders. *National Institute of Justice: Research in Brief*, 1–10.

Steadman, H. J., Osher, F. C., Robbins, P. C., Case, B., & Samuels, S. (2009). Prevalence of serious mental illness among jail inmates. *Psychiatric Services, 60*(6), 761–765.

Teitelbaum, J. B., & Hoffman, L. G. (2013). Health reform and correctional health care: How the Affordable Care Act can improve the health of ex-offenders and their communities. *Fordham Urban Law Journal, 40*, 1323–1356.

Travis, J., & Waul, M. (2004). *Prisoners once removed: The children and families of prisoners.* Washington, DC: Urban Institute.

US Department of Justice; Ditton, P. M. (1999). *Mental health and treatment of inmates and probationers.* Bureau of Justice Statistics Special Report, NCJ 172211. Retrieved from http://www.bjs.gov/index.cfm?ty=pbdetail&iid=787

US Department of Justice, Bureau of Justice Statistics; Beck, A. J., & Maruschak, L. M. (2001). Mental health treatment in state prisons, 2000. Retrieved from http://www.bjs.gov/index.cfm?ty=pbdetail&iid=788

Van Dorn, R. A., Desmarais, S. L., Petrila, J., Haynes, D., & Singh, J. P. (2013). Effects of outpatient treatment on risk of arrest of adults with serious mental illness and associated costs. *Psychiatric Services, 64*, 856–962.

Wakeman, S. E., McKinney, M. E., & Rich, J. D. (2009). *Filling the gap: The importance of Medicaid continuity for former inmates.* Retrieved from www.ncbi.nlm.nih.gov/pmc/articles/PMC2695526/

Way, B., Abreu, D., Ramirez-Romero, D., Aziz, D., & Sawyer, D. A. (2007). Mental health service recipients and prison work release: How do the mentally ill fare compared to other inmates in prison work release programs? *Journal of Forensic Sciences, 52*, 965–966.

Weinstein, J. B., & Wimmer, C. (2010) Sentencing in the United States. In H. Dlugacz (Ed.), *Reentry planning for offenders with mental disorders: Policy and practice* (pp. 1-1-1-45). Kingston, NJ: Civic Research Institute, Inc.

Wenzlow, A. T., Ireys, H. T., Mann, B., Irvin, C., & Teich, J. L. (2011). Effects of a discharge planning program on Medicaid coverage. *Psychiatric Services, 62*, 73–78.

Wilson, A. B. (2013). How people with mental illness seek help after leaving jail. *Qualitative Health Research, 23*, 1575–1590.

Wilson, A. B., & Draine, J. (2006) Collaborations between criminal justice and mental health systems for prisoner reentry. *Psychiatric Services, 57*, 875–878.

Wolff, N., Plemmons, D., Veysey, B., & Brandli, A. (2002). Release planning for inmates with mental illness compared with those who have other chronic illnesses. *Psychiatric Services, 53*, 1469–1471.

Zaitz, L. (2013). Thousands of Oregon inmates to gain health insurance as they exit prison. *The Oregonian.* Retrieved from http://www.oregonlive.com/politics/index.ssf/2013/11/thousands_of_oregon_inmates_ga.htm

SECTION IV

Common management issues

CHAPTER 16

Management of sleep complaints in correctional settings

Bernice S. Elger

Introduction

Inmates in correctional settings often seek health care for sleep and drug problems (Elger, 2004b; Feron, Paulus, Tonglet, Lorant, & Pestiaux, 2005; Kjelsberg & Hartvig, 2005; Nesset, Rustad, Kjelsberg, Almvik, & Bjorngaard, 2011). Outside correctional settings, many studies of insomnia have been conducted on the general population and various patient groups (Bixler, Kales, Soldatos, Kales, & Healey, 1979; Cunnington, Junge, & Fernando, 2013; Ford & Kamerow, 1989; Kupfer & Reynolds, 1997; Mellinger, Balter, & Uhlenhuth, 1985; Sateia & Nowell, 2004). However, studies on insomnia in correctional institutions are scarce (Elger, 2007, 2013). This chapter first outlines treatment guidelines for insomnia that apply in community settings, then presents an overview of the clinical and ethical issues of insomnia management in correctional institutions and provides evidence-based recommendations.

Insomnia management: recommendations based on studies outside prisons

According to studies on different continents, the prevalence of insomnia symptoms in the general population is high. In the United States, at least 10 percent of the population have been found to suffer from sleep problems (Kraus & Rabin, 2012; Sateia, Doghramji, Hauri, & Morin, 2000). In Australia, 13 percent to 33 percent of the adult population reported regular difficulties either getting to sleep or staying asleep (Bartlett, Marshall, Williams, & Grunstein, 2008). Similarly, between 10 percent and 50 percent of adults in western Europe complained about sleep difficulties (Chan-Chee et al., 2011; Ohayon, 2002; Ohayon & Lemoine, 2004a). Insomnia can have serious consequences, such as an increased risk of depression and hypertension (Cunnington et al., 2013) and impaired daytime functioning. The latter was reported by two thirds of the 19 percent of the general population with insomnia (Ohayon & Lemoine, 2004a). Social, psychological, and medical conditions make some individuals more vulnerable than others. Insomnia complaints are more common in women, separated or divorced individuals, people who are less educated or are unemployed, medically ill patients, those with recent stress, and those with depression, anxiety, or substance abuse (Elger, 2007; Hohagen et al., 1993; Kupfer & Reynolds, 1997; Ohayon & Lemoine, 2004b; Sateia & Nowell, 2004).

As sleep complaints are common, it is important to distinguish normal variation from sleep disorders. A well-known expert manual defines insomnia as "a repeated difficulty with sleep initiation, duration, consolidation, or quality that occurs despite adequate time and opportunity for sleep and results in some form of daytime impairment and lasting for at least one month" (American Sleep Disorders Association, 2005; Falloon, Arroll, Elley, & Fernando, 2011). While the *Diagnostic and Statistical Manual of Mental Disorders* (DSM)-IV classification (American Psychiatric Association, 2000; Elger, 2007) contained a category referred to as "primary sleep disorders," this diagnostic entity was eliminated in DSM-5 (American Psychiatric Association, 2013). Sleep–wake disorders now encompass 10 conditions characterized by disturbed sleep and "causing distress as well as impairment in daytime functioning" (American Psychiatric Association, 2013). The 10 disorder groups are insomnia disorder, hypersomnolence disorder, narcolepsy, breathing-related sleep disorders, circadian rhythm sleep–wake disorders, non–rapid eye movement sleep arousal disorders, nightmare disorder, rapid eye movement sleep behavior disorder, restless legs syndrome, and substance/medication-induced sleep disorder (Reynolds & O'Hara, 2013). DSM-5 stresses the need for "independent clinical attention of a sleep disorder regardless of mental or other medical problems that may be present" (American Psychiatric Association, 2013). Two diagnoses included in DSM-IV—sleep disorder related to another mental disorder and sleep disorder related to another medical condition—have been dropped. This permitted the provision of "greater specificity of co-existing conditions" for each of the 10 sleep–wake disorders (American Psychiatric Association, 2013).

Sateia and Novell (2004) stress that when managing insomnia complaints, physicians should be aware that in addition to the objective alterations of sleep and its pattern, the subjective perception of insomnia needs to be taken seriously. Acute (short-term) insomnia (shorter than three to four weeks) is often caused by situational stress, medical or psychological disorders, or circadian changes due to jet lag or shift work. Health care personnel need to discuss acute stress with patients and provide appropriate education. Short-term treatment strategies encompass sleep hygiene and prescription of hypnotics, usually a benzodiazepine (BZD), if necessary (Cunnington et al., 2013).

In the case of chronic insomnia (i.e., sleep problems that persist more than four weeks), two treatment strategies are supported by empirical evidence. In the past, the dominant approach was pharmacological. In general, BZD-receptor agonists were used (Morin & Benca, 2012; Sateia & Nowell, 2004). However, studies have proven that such medication alleviates symptoms only for a short time. The effectiveness of hypnotics is established for the first six weeks. After that time, treatment effects degrade in patients with chronic insomnia. Side effects of BZDs are well known and include the risk of habituation and tolerance, as well as paradoxical effects in the aging population (Kupfer & Reynolds, 1997; Lader, 2011). Despite the shortcomings of pharmacological agents, nonpharmacological treatments remain insufficiently used. Evidence shows that psychological treatments, in particular cognitive-behavioral therapy (CBT), are effective and result in long-lasting and clinically significant improvement. CBT is efficient whether used alone or in combination with pharmacological treatment, and it has similar effect sizes to those of non-BZD hypnotics (Cunnington, 2013). Nonpharmacological treatments help improve the symptoms of patients who have sleep disorders, including insomnia associated with medical or psychiatric illness. CBT does not necessarily require significant personnel resources; it can be used in individual or group therapy sessions or as self-administered written or audiovisual material. Variants of nonpharmacological treatments include stimulus control therapy, sleep restriction, sleep hygiene, paradoxical intention, progressive muscle relaxation, and cognitive therapy (Belleville, Cousineau, Levrier, & St-Pierre-Delorme, 2011; Mitchell, Gehrman, Perlis, & Umscheid, 2012; Morin & Benca, 2012; Sateia & Nowell, 2004).

Prevalence and possible causes of sleep problems in correctional settings

Most studies on sleep disturbances in correctional settings are from Europe. A study among young (average age 19 years) and juvenile (average age 16 years) detainees in the United Kingdom demonstrated differences in sleep behavior before and during prison. During detention, poor sleeping habits increased, and this increase was similar for young and juvenile detainees. Of note, the authors found an association between increased aggression and reports of impaired quantity and quality of sleep (Ireland & Culpin, 2006).

In a German prison, 54 percent of the inmates complained about sleep problems (Last, 1979). A high prevalence of insomnia complaints has also been observed in prisons in Belgium and Switzerland (Elger, 2004b; Feron et al., 2005). In a Swiss jail, 44 percent of 995 patients seen in primary care consultations were diagnosed with insomnia. Fifty-one percent of them (n = 223) were drug misusers (Elger, 2004b). Substance abuse could therefore have caused the sleep problems in half of the insomniac detainees. Overall, anxiety related to incarceration was the most frequently reported reason for sleep problems in that study. Among the insomnia patients who were not substance abusers, chronic forms of insomnia were reported more often than acute insomnia (defined as longer than three weeks). Patients who reported insomnia were more often diagnosed with anxiety or depression than prisoners without sleep complaints. The Swiss study showed that in patients who were not substance abusers, the causes for insomnia could not be attributed to transitory adaptation difficulties to incarceration. Indeed, most sleep complaints in the Swiss jail showed a chronic pattern. In the majority of cases, the sleep problems persisted longer than three weeks and were associated

with the intake of other drugs, including analgesics, and with somatic and mental disorders.

Sociologists found high prescription rates for psychotropic drugs in French prisons. Most of the psychotropic drugs were used as sleeping medications (Jaeger & Monceau, 1996). An analysis of all prescriptions distributed by the pharmacies showed that two thirds of the psychotropic drugs prescribed in French prisons were BZDs and sedating antipsychotics. The authors found significant variations in the quantity of psychotropic prescriptions when they compared different French correctional institutions. BZDs and sedating antipsychotics were prescribed more often in jails than in post-trial detention centers. Prescription rates of these hypnotic and sedative psychotropic drugs were lower in prisons where detainees had access to more activities outside the cell, including work and sports. In the United States, some detention facilities use guidelines to reduce prescriptions of BZDs. Quetiapine has been used as an alternative. However, as quetiapine has serious side effects and because many health professionals are convinced that both quetiapine and BZDs are subject to abuse (see Chapter 31), one intervention study tried to reduce those prescriptions and reported that physician education was able to decrease the numbers of inmates prescribed BZDs by 38 percent after 20 months (Reeves, 2012).

It is widely accepted that the chronic nature of sleep problems may be related to the conditions of imprisonment (Association Lyonnaise de Criminologie et d'Anthropologie Sociale, 1991). Many detainees have posttraumatic stress disorder (Crisanti & Frueh, 2011), a well-known cause of insomnia (DeViva, Zayfert, & Mellman, 2004). Other possible causes for insomnia in correctional settings are preexisting psychiatric morbidity, possibly aggravated during incarceration; drug misuse; lack of physical activity; and daytime napping (Andersen et al., 2000; Bourgeois, 1997). Incarceration frequently means that inmates have to stay in their cells during most of the day, as many international human rights regulations stipulate only a minimum of one hour outside the cell (Council of Europe, 2006). It is therefore not surprising that studies have reported immobility and boredom to be a cause of sleep problems. Long periods of inactivity, especially at night when cells are closed early, may increase the subjective impression of a need to sleep longer than physiologically required (Jaeger & Monceau, 1996; Levin & Brown, 1975; Vasseur, 2001; Zimmermann & von Allmen, 1985).

In line with more recent evidence, it seems clear that sleep–wake disorders (in the community and in correctional settings) cannot be reduced to a secondary symptom of mental disease or substance abuse. As shown in a US study, insomnia in correctional institutions seems to be a separate entity independent of disorders associated with dysphoria (Rogers et al., 2003). Rogers and colleagues suggest that the conditions of detention are a major reason for sleep disturbances, as detention may be associated with substantial fears about personal safety that, in turn, can cause hypervigilance and sleep disturbances (Rogers et al., 2003). Those responsible for the management of sleep complaints in correctional settings should keep in mind that if it is the correctional setting that causes independent "situational" insomnia, treatment of the causes would need to address the conditions of incarceration. Management should not be limited to pharmacological treatments of specific psychiatric disorders. Rather, treatment should include at least partial changes or adaptations of the prison environment wherever possible, including, for example, sufficient activities outside the cell such as work and opportunities to participate in sports that are associated with decreased prescriptions of sleep medication (see Jaeger & Monceau, 1996).

Jaeger and Monceau (1996) reported interesting additional findings about the causes of insomnia in correctional settings. They interviewed detainees and staff members. The latter reported they had observed that inmates ask for more hypnotics and sedative drugs in situations where they are under increased stress. Typical examples of such situations included life events (periods when detainees learn the final court judgment), conditions of confinement (overcrowding), and interpersonal tension (strained detainee and staff relations because of frequent conflict). An analysis of the interviews with detainees from different facilities confirmed that the conditions of incarceration seem to play a major role in the sleep complaints (Jaeger & Monceau, 1996). Detainees noted that hypnotics and tranquilizers are an important way for them to decrease the risk of suicide and to reduce violent behavior. They told the interviewers that these prescriptions not only diminish suffering but are also beneficial for survival in prison. Detainees noted that being able to sleep at night led to behavior modification, including reduction of aggressiveness and dysphoria during the day. A study in the United Kingdom 10 years later produced similar evidence (Ireland & Culpin, 2006). In the French study, about one third of prison officers were convinced that hypnotics and tranquilizers have a positive effect as they lead to more peaceful cohabitation in correctional settings, helping detainees tolerate detention (Jaeger & Monceau, 1996).

Sleep complaints in prison: a need for evidence-based management

To be effective, management of sleep complaints in prison must take into account the causes of insomnia. Medical ethics and human rights law also stipulate that health care in correctional settings should be guided by the so-called equivalence principle (Bruce & Schleifer, 2008; Elger 2008a, 2008b; Lines, 2008). Indeed, medical ethics is to be respected independently of the legal status of a patient. Detainees have the right to receive adequate treatment that is available to patients outside prisons. The principle of equivalence is enshrined in international soft law that is relevant for physicians in any country: "Health personnel, particularly physicians, charged with the medical care of prisoners and detainees have a duty to provide them with protection of their physical and mental health and treatment of disease of the same quality and standard as is afforded to those who are not imprisoned or detained. ... There may be no derogation from the foregoing principles on any ground whatsoever, including public emergency" (principles 1 and 6, United Nations, 1982). The principle of equivalence of care also applies to insomnia evaluation and treatment. However, the literature shows that the evaluation of insomnia complaints in correctional settings does not follow international standards of diligence in many cases. Treatment varies in different institutions and often remains inefficient.

While health care personnel in one correctional setting tried to implement meditation as a nonpharmacological treatment for insomnia (Sumter, Monk-Turner, & Turner, 2009), CBT is rarely used. Evidence from a retrospective study in Europe shows that the pharmacological management of insomnia complaints in

detainees who are not substance misusers is insufficient (Elger, 2003, 2004a). The study aimed to analyze the quality of medical consultation and the effectiveness of drug prescription. The evaluation for insomnia carried out by the physicians working in the correctional institution was found to be incomplete. Medical records indicated that most physicians did not question detainees about sleep habits, sleep latency, and previous hypnotic use. Information about the daytime impact of insomnia was noted in only 7 percent. In the majority of patients, insomnia improved only partially or not at all. Patients whose insomnia did not respond or responded only partially to pharmacological treatment received the highest number of hypnotic drugs (mean 2.4).

Physicians working in correctional settings should respect the principles of beneficence and nonmaleficence. An adequate evaluation of insomnia complaints is necessary to make the right diagnosis and to provide treatment that addresses the causes. Nonmaleficence (i.e., the avoidance of harm) implies vigilance and knowledge of the various consequences that result from medical decisions. Harm may result not only from side effects of pharmacological treatments but also from untreated insomnia (Cunnington et al., 2013), which include increased risks of self-harm, suicide, and aggression. Also, the principle of respect for autonomy applies in prison health care in the same way as outside prisons (see Chapter 8). Physicians should discuss potential harms and benefits with each patient (Elger, 2008a). Such management respects patient rights and can increase patient adherence and improve treatment outcomes.

While overtreatment of insomnia complaints (Reeves, 2012) is medically and ethically problematic, so, too, is undertreatment. Physicians tend to fear that detainees will misuse medication (Last, 1979; Reeves, 2012). There is a tendency to ban BZD from correctional settings and to use herbal products, antipsychotics, or antidepressants instead, although BZDs are still recognized as the evidence-based treatment of acute insomnia in the community (Cunnington et al., 2013; Morin & Benca, 2012). Moreover, antipsychotics have important side effects, while their efficiency in sleep disorders remains unclear (Maher & Theodore, 2012). If insomnia evaluation and treatment are not taken seriously in correctional settings, this is harmful to patients and may increase costs due to the possibly far-reaching consequences of undertreated insomnia. Undertreatment includes underprescription of medication and underuse of evidence-based nonpharmacological treatments. Evidence-based insomnia management in correctional institutions should include the following:

◆ *Sleep evaluation:* Insomnia complaints must be taken seriously. This requires an evaluation of the type and history of complaints, previous medication intake, and a thorough history and clinical examination to search for somatic or mental comorbidities. If the right diagnosis is not made, this may result in harm to patients and avoidable costs to the institution (Falloon et al., 2011; Sateia & Nowell, 2004).

◆ *Improvement of external factors:* Based on recommendation R (98) of the Council of Europe (1998), physicians have a duty to report public health problems (Elger, 2008b, 2011). In particular, section II states "The specific role of the prison doctor and other health care staff in the context of the prison environment," and the explanatory memorandum further asserts that health care staff must also be attentive to public health and prison conditions: "health care staff must therefore also be attentive to hygiene, food, the minimum space available to prisoners, etc.; if one or other of these criteria is not fulfilled, the doctor has a duty to inform the competent authorities in order that they may remedy the situation" (Council of Europe, 2003 Art. 23). Health care personnel should also offer adequate therapies to help detainees cope with stress.

- *Nonpharmacological treatments:* CBT and the teaching of relaxation techniques and meditation to prisoners may be the most cost-effective way to address several health problems in prison (Sumter et al., 2009). This may require such measures as sending a sufficient number of physicians who work in correctional settings to training sessions to learn CBT for insomnia and formally implementing education of detainees about sleep hygiene. Recent publications provide information and guidance on both the process and the selection and use of appropriate materials (Falloon et al., 2011).

- *Pharmacological treatments:* Pharmacological treatments should be specific and address the comorbidities associated with insomnia. Misuse of medication such as quetiapine by inmates has been observed (Reeves, 2012). Indeed, sedating antipsychotics and sedating antidepressants should not be used routinely for insomnia complaints. Patients must be informed about important side effects of most non-BZD hypnotics, such as daytime sedation, weight gain, and anticholinergic side effects. Since sedating antidepressants are more toxic and less efficient than BZDs (Falloon et al., 2011), they are justified only if special indications exist. In cases of acute insomnia, BZDs remain the first-choice drug. It is not justified to deny detainees appropriate pharmacological treatment because some of these drugs might circulate in prison and be sold on the prison black market. Different types of tranquilizers and illicit drugs enter correctional settings through many channels. Withholding BZDs from detainees if they are medically indicated is often harmful because detainees risk using more dangerous alternatives available on the black market (Elger, 2008a).

Summary

Sleep problems among detainees are common. Appropriate evaluation and treatment remain challenging in correctional settings. However, this is not primarily a problem of resources; rather, it is, to a great extent, an issue of adequate training. Correctional health professionals need appropriate education regarding insomnia evaluation and management. Guidelines should be based on the principle of equivalence of care and should take into account all evidence from research in the community and in correctional settings. Educational material from outside prisons exists and should be made available to detainees and health professionals (Falloon et al., 2011; Sateia & Nowell, 2004). Priority should be given to changes in prison conditions and to nonpharmacological treatment. There is no evidence-based justification to replace BZD prescriptions with antipsychotics or antidepressants. In correctional settings, prescriptions of antipsychotics and antidepressants for sleep problems can increase risk due to polypharmacy and higher suicide risks. Correctional physicians should monitor and document the evaluation and treatment practice concerning insomnia complaints to improve safe, evidence-based treatment.

References

American Psychiatric Association (2000). *Diagnostic and statistical manual of mental disorders, DSM-IV.* Washington, DC: American Psychiatric Association.

American Psychiatric Association (2013). *Sleep–wake disorders: Fact sheet.* Retrieved from http://www.google.ch/url?sa=t&rct=j&q=&esrc=s&source=web&cd=1&ved=0CDIQFjAA&url=http%3A%2F%2Fwww.dsm5.org%2FDocuments%2FSleep-wake%2520Disorders%2520Fact%2520Sheet.pdf&ei=krreUvr6Jsnasga6uIGAAg&usg=AFQjCNFIiWCqBWtdwL2awK9f7HUmEGEY_A&bvm=bv.59568121,d.Yms

American Sleep Disorders Association (2005). *International classification of sleep disorders, Second edition: Diagnostic and coding manual.* American Sleep Disorders Association.

Andersen, H. S., Sestoft, D., Lillebaek, T., Gabrielsen, G., Hemmingsen, R., & Kramp, P. (2000). A longitudinal study of prisoners on remand: psychiatric prevalence, incidence and psychopathology in solitary vs. non-solitary confinement. *Acta Psychiatrica Scandinavica, 102,* 19–25.

Association Lyonnaise de Criminologie et d'Anthropologie Sociale (1991). *Ouvrage collectif sous la direction de Gonin, D; commandé par le ministère de la justice. Conditions de vie en détention et pathologie somatique.* Paris: Ministère de la Justice.

Bartlett, D. J., Marshall, N. S., Williams, A., & Grunstein, R. R. (2008). Sleep health New South Wales: Chronic sleep restriction and daytime sleepiness. *Internal Medicine Journal, 38,* 24–31.

Belleville, G., Cousineau, H., Levrier, K., & St-Pierre-Delorme, M. E. (2011). Meta-analytic review of the impact of cognitive-behavior therapy for insomnia on concomitant anxiety. *Clinical Psychology Review, 31,* 638–652.

Bixler, E. O., Kales, A., Soldatos, C. R., Kales, J. D., & Healey, S. (1979). Prevalence of sleep disorders in the Los Angeles metropolitan area. *American Journal of Psychiatry, 136,* 1257–1262.

Bourgeois, D. (1997). Sleep disorders in prison. *Encephale, 23,* 180–183.

Bruce, R. D., & Schleifer, R. A. (2008). Ethical and human rights imperatives to ensure medication-assisted treatment for opioid dependence in prisons and pre-trial detention. *International Journal of Drug Policy, 19,* 17–23.

Chan-Chee, C., Bayon, V., Bloch, J., Beck, F., Giordanella, J. P., & Leger, D. (2011). Epidemiology of insomnia in France. *Revue Epidemiologie Sante Publique, 59,* 409–422.

Council of Europe (1998). *Recommendation No. R (98) 7 of the Committee of Ministers to member states concerning the ethical and organisational aspects of health care in prison.* Adopted by the Committee of Ministers on 8 April 1998. Retrived from https://wcd.coe.int/com.instranet.InstraServlet?command=com.instranet.CmdBlobGet&InstranetImage=530914&SecMode=1&DocId=463258&Usage=2

Council of Europe (2003). *Explanatory memorandum to recommendation on the ethical and organisational aspects of health care in prison.* Approved April 20, 2003. Retrieved from http://www.unav.es/cdb/ccoerec98-7exp.html

Council of Europe (2006). *Recommendation Rec(2006)2 of the Committee of Ministers to member states on the European Prison Rules.* Adopted by the Committee of Ministers on 11 January 2006 at the 952nd meeting of the Ministers' Deputies. Retrieved from https://wcd.coe.int/ViewDoc.jsp?id=955747

Crisanti, A. S., & Frueh, B. C. (2011). Risk of trauma exposure among persons with mental illness in jails and prisons: what do we really know? *Current Opinion in Psychiatry, 24,* 431–435.

Cunnington, D. (2013). Non-benzodiazepine hypnotics: do they work for insomnia? *BMJ, 346,* e8699.

Cunnington, D., Junge, M. F., & Fernando, A. T. (2013). Insomnia: Prevalence, consequences and effective treatment. *Medical Journal of Australia, 199,* S36–40.

DeViva, J. C., Zayfert, C., & Mellman, T. A. (2004). Factors associated with insomnia among civilians seeking treatment for PTSD: An exploratory study. *Behavioral Sleep Medicine, 2,* 162–176.

Elger, B. (2013). Sleep disorders. In M. Levy & H. Stöver (Eds.). *Safer prescribing of medications in adult detention.* Oldenburg: BIS-Verlag der Carl von Ossietzky Universität Oldenburg.

Elger, B. S. (2003). Does insomnia in prison improve with time? Prospective study among remanded prisoners using the Pittsburgh Sleep Quality Index. *Medicine, Science and the Law, 43,* 334–344.

Elger, B. S. (2004a). Management and evolution of insomnia complaints among non-substance-misusers in a Swiss remand prison. *Swiss Medical Weekly, 134,* 486–499.

Elger, B. S. (2004b). Prevalence, types and possible causes of insomnia in a Swiss remand prison. *European Journal of Epidemiology, 19,* 665–677.

Elger, B. S. (2007). Insomnia in places of detention: a review of the most recent research findings. *Medicine, Science and the Law, 47,* 191–199.

Elger, B. S. (2008a). Prisoners' insomnia: to treat or not to treat? Medical decision-making in places of detention. *Medicine, Science and the Law, 48,* 307–316.

Elger, B. S. (2008b). Towards equivalent health care of prisoners: European soft law and public health policy in Geneva. *Journal of Public Health Policy, 29,* 192–206.

Elger, B. S. (2011). Prison medicine, public health policy and ethics: the Geneva experience. *Swiss Medical Weekly, 141,* w13273.

Falloon, K., Arroll, B., Elley, C. R., & Fernando, A., 3rd (2011). The assessment and management of insomnia in primary care. *BMJ, 342,* d2899.

Feron, J. M., Paulus, D., Tonglet, R., Lorant, V., & Pestiaux, D. (2005). Substantial use of primary health care by prisoners: Epidemiological description and possible explanations. *Journal of Epidemiology and Community Health, 59,* 651–655.

Ford, D. E., & Kamerow, D. B. (1989). Epidemiologic study of sleep disturbances and psychiatric disorders. An opportunity for prevention? *Journal of the American Medical Association, 262,* 1479–1484.

Hohagen, F., Rink, K., Kappler, C., et al. (1993). Prevalence and treatment of insomnia in general practice. A longitudinal study. *European Archives of Psychiatry and Clinical Neuroscience, 242,* 329–336.

Ireland, J. L., & Culpin, V. (2006). The relationship between sleeping problems and aggression, anger, and impulsivity in a population of juvenile and young offenders. *Journal of Adolescent Health, 38,* 649–655.

Jaeger, M., & Monceau, M. (1996). *La consommation des médicaments psychotropes en prison.* Ramonville: Saint-Agne Editions Erès.

Kjelsberg, E., & Hartvig, P. (2005). Can morbidity be inferred from prescription drug use? Results from a nation-wide prison population study. *European Journal of Epidemiology, 20,* 587–592.

Kraus, S. S., & Rabin, L. A. (2012). Sleep America: managing the crisis of adult chronic insomnia and associated conditions. *Journal of Affective Disorders, 138,* 192–212.

Kupfer, D. J., & Reynolds, C. F., III. (1997). Management of insomnia. *New England Journal of Medicine, 336,* 341–346.

Lader, M. (2011). Benzodiazepines revisited—will we ever learn? *Addiction, 106,* 2086–2109.

Last, G. (1979). Sleep disorders in a isolation situation. Hyposomnia in older convicts. *Zeitschrift für Gerontologie Geriatrie, 12,* 235–247.

Levin, B. H., & Brown, W. E. (1975). Susceptibility to boredom of jailers and law enforcement officers. *Psychological Reports, 36,* 190.

Maher, A. R., & Theodore, G. (2012). Summary of the comparative effectiveness review on off-label use of atypical antipsychotics. *Journal of Managed Care Pharmacy, 18,* 1–20.

Mellinger, G. D., Balter, M. B., & Uhlenhuth, E. H. (1985). Insomnia and its treatment. Prevalence and correlates. *Archives of General Psychiatry, 42,* 225–232.

Mitchell, M. D., Gehrman, P., Perlis, M., & Umscheid, C. A. (2012). Comparative effectiveness of cognitive behavioral therapy for insomnia: a systematic review. *BMC Family Practice, 13,* 40.

Morin, C. M., & Benca, R. (2012). Chronic insomnia. *Lancet, 379,* 1129–1141.

Nesset, M. B., Rustad, A. B., Kjelsberg, E., Almvik, R., & Bjorngaard, J. H. (2011). Health care help seeking behaviour among prisoners in Norway. *BMC Health Services Research, 11,* 301.

Ohayon, M. M. (2002). Epidemiology of insomnia: What we know and what we still need to learn. *Sleep Medicine Reviews, 6,* 97–111.

Ohayon, M. M., & Lemoine, P. (2004a). Daytime consequences of insomnia complaints in the French general population. *Encephale, 30,* 222–227.

Ohayon, M. M., & Lemoine, P. (2004b). Sleep and insomnia markers in the general population. *Encephale, 30,* 135–140.

Reeves, R. (2012). Guideline, education, and peer comparison to reduce prescriptions of benzodiazepines and low-dose quetiapine in prison. *Journal of Correctional Health Care, 18,* 45–52.

Reynolds, C. F., III & O'Hara, R. (2013). DSM-5 sleep-wake disorders classification: overview for use in clinical practice. *American Journal of Psychiatry, 170,* 1099–1101.

Rogers, R., Jackson, R. L., Salekin, K. L., & Neumann, C. S. (2003). Assessing Axis I symptomatology on the SADS-C in two correctional samples: The validation of subscales and a screen for malingered presentations. *Journal of Personality Assessment, 81,* 281–290.

Sateia, M. J., Doghramji, K., Hauri, P. J., & Morin, C. M. (2000). Evaluation of chronic insomnia. An American Academy of Sleep Medicine review. *Sleep, 23,* 243–308.

Sateia, M. J., & Nowell, P. D. (2004). Insomnia. *Lancet, 364,* 1959–1973.

Sumter, M. T., Monk-Turner, E., & Turner, C. (2009). The benefits of meditation practice in the correctional setting. *Journal of Correctional Health Care, 15,* 47–57; quiz 81.

United Nations (1982). Principles of Medical Ethics. A37/R194. Accessed September 28, 2014 at: http://www.un.org/en/ga/search/view_doc.asp?symbol=A/RES/37/194.

Vasseur, V. (2001). *Médecin chef à la prison de la santé.* Paris: Le Livre de Poche.

Zimmermann, E., & Von Allmen, M. (1985). Medical consultation and drug use in preventive detention at the Champ-Dolon prison. *Sozial-und Praventivmedizin, 30,* 312–321.

CHAPTER 17

Detoxification or supervised withdrawal

Rebecca Lubelczyk

Introduction

Substance abuse and mental illness are frequent coexisting conditions that unfortunately complement one another. The pervasive comorbidity complicates their diagnosis, treatment, and management. This is nowhere more obvious than in correctional mental health patients. Often, psychiatric clinicians find themselves attempting to manage mental health conditions concomitant with the physical health manifestations of alcohol and drug abuse, especially in jail lockups and correctional detoxification (detox) units. According to the US Department of Justice, Bureau of Justice Statistics (2004), drugs or alcohol were used at the time of the offense by just over half of all state and federal prison inmates, necessitating screening at intake for both intoxication and risk of withdrawal. Intoxication and withdrawal can mimic signs and symptoms of an acute mental disorder or exacerbate an underlying chronic disease. One of the most difficult challenges a clinician may face is determining whether the presentation is due to a combination of intoxication/withdrawal and mental illness or mental illness alone. Using substances while on psychiatric medications can alter the pharmacology, change the effectiveness, and exacerbate the side effects of medications, potentially causing lack of response, nonadherence, or dangerous physical effects. Substance use also puts the patient at risk for trauma and exposure to infections from risky behaviors while intoxicated.

The clinician faces an imposing challenge in any attempt to accurately assess underlying psychopathology in the midst of acute detox (Wright, Cluver, Myrick, & Krishnamurthy, 2011). It is a generally accepted practice to reassess the patient's psychotropic treatment needs once detox is complete; however, individual cases may require acute intervention based on the severity of the patient's mental illness (Substance Abuse and Mental Health Services Administration, 2006). This chapter attempts to educate the correctional clinician on the common presentations of intoxication and withdrawal syndromes of various substances. The similarities to and distinctions of such syndromes with mental illnesses are discussed. Standardized medical management approaches to safeguard patients during supervised withdrawal are also presented. Following such a process allows the clinician to subsequently assess the patient's true mental health and substance abuse treatment needs.

Alcohol

Intoxication

Many psychiatric patients assert that using alcohol helps them feel better and improves their thinking or mood. This may be due to alcohol's inherent sedating effects for some, while its euphoric/amnesic effects may provide a temporary escape from unpleasant feelings or emotions for those with depression, posttraumatic stress disorder, and similar conditions. Mentally ill patients are at higher risk of having poor coping skills and may have been taught by family or peers that alcohol can make problems better when, in fact, the exact opposite is usually the case (Shivani, Goldsmith, & Anthenelli, 2002).

Signs and symptoms of alcohol intoxication vary considerably and individually. In general, disinhibition and euphoria are transitory, culminating in ataxia, nausea or vomiting, and heavy sedation (Victor & Adams, 1953). Patients who don't drink habitually may become more intoxicated with less alcohol than those who chronically drink due to the body's ability to develop tolerance. With tolerance comes dependence, and with dependence comes withdrawal. The disinhibition that occurs with intoxication all too often leads to criminal behavior, ranging from disturbance of the peace to driving violations to homicide. The subsequent process of arrest becomes a supervised, involuntary withdrawal and detox.

Detoxification

Correctional patients who come in off the street or from stays at a holding facility that are shorter than 48 hours are at high risk of withdrawal from various substances, alcohol being one of the most common and perhaps the most dangerous. By its nature, alcohol dampens the body's adrenergic system, causing it to be depressed during chronic use. Discontinuing alcohol suddenly ("going cold turkey") puts the patient at risk for a storm of norepinephrine and its metabolites, which may lead to anxiousness, tremors, tachycardia, hypertension, hallucinations, confusion, and seizures. When severe, alcohol withdrawal culminates in the syndrome of delirium tremens (the "DTs"). Patients with DTs require intensive hospitalization; mortality is about 5 percent (Hasin, Stinson, Ogburn, & Grant, 2007). Alcohol withdrawal is dangerous not only in its severity but also in its timing. The greatest risk of seizures and DTs is not at the abrupt cessation of drinking; instead, it peaks at 48 to 72 hours after cessation (Hernandez-Avila & Kranzler, 2011).

This is the time when many patients arrive at intake centers at jails or prisons.

There is a great deal of literature on the methods for safely monitoring and detoxifying a patient from alcohol. Facility protocols are primarily based on the medication and staffing resources available. The revised Clinical Institute Withdrawal Assessment for Alcohol Scale (CIWA-Ar) protocol is the most widely used and researched alcohol detox monitoring tool on which to base treatment of withdrawal (American Society of Addiction Medicine, 2001; Sullivan, Sykora, Schneiderman, Naranjo, & Sellers, 1989). The CIWA-Ar evaluates a patient's symptoms (nausea, anxiousness, tactile/auditory/visual disturbances, and headache) and signs (pulse, blood pressure, tremor, sweats, agitation, and orientation) to create the score used to guide dosing (American Society of Addiction Medicine, 2001; Sullivan et al., 1989). The CIWA is often administered by a nurse, who records the absence or severity of specific signs and symptoms of withdrawal. All patients who detoxify from alcohol need to be treated using a benzodiazepine (BZD) taper to decrease the risk of significant morbidity and mortality. BZDs are the mainstay of alcohol detox protocols as they bind the same receptors, modifying the alcohol withdrawal's adrenergic response. Dosing of BZDs is rarely needed if the CIWA score is <10. Rising CIWA scores are linked to escalating doses of BZDs. Patients' CIWA scores are reassessed frequently in intervals that can also be based on their CIWA score. This symptom-triggered protocol is the most commonly used. However, a single preset BZD taper may also be used. A preset taper prescribes every patient the same dosages of lowering-strength BZDs over a certain period of time. For either method, any BZD can be used, but those with the longest half-life are preferred, with chlordiazepoxide and diazepam being the most common. These medications are dosed less frequently and provide the patient with a more gradual detox. However, this long half-life is not optimal in patients who are cirrhotic and could become overly sedated, as their liver metabolizes BZDs more slowly. In these patients, a shorter-acting BZD such as clonazepam or lorazepam may be preferred (Carlson & Kennedy, 2006).

Since many patients who chronically abuse alcohol don't eat a well-balanced diet, nutritional deficiencies often exist. Any alcohol detox protocol must include vitamin supplementation with thiamine. Thiamine deficiency puts the patient at risk for precipitation of Wernicke's encephalopathy (ataxia, ocular weakness, nystagmus, and cognitive dysfunction). Adequate thiamine levels must be present, especially if the patient is to receive glucose. Glucose administration in the setting of thiamine deficiency increases the risk and severity of Wernicke's encephalopathy (Mayo-Smith & Krishnamurthy, 2011). Korsakoff psychosis, a permanent amnesic dementia, may remain (Devinsky, Feldmann, Weinreb, & Wilterdink, 1997). Magnesium deficiency is also common. There is no current literature suggesting that repletion of this nutrient improves the patient's clinical status; however, most protocols include a multivitamin to ensure adequate nutritional intake (Carlson & Kennedy, 2006). Even though withdrawal seizures can occur in the absence of DTs, studies do not support the use of prophylactic antiepileptic medications (Minozzi, Amato, Vecchi, & Davoli, 2010).

As the detox process progresses, underlying mental disorders may be uncovered. The patient thus becomes increasingly uncomfortable from both the symptoms of detox and the now-untreated mental illness, posing a challenge to the practitioner. The psychiatric clinician has to be wary when performing an assessment and instituting treatment if the patient has not completed detox. It is incredibly difficult to make a clear psychological evaluation while a patient is undergoing such a dramatic physical experience. The clinician should not wait until detox is complete to initiate psychiatric and substance abuse treatment. Mental health assessments on patients must begin at entry into the correctional facility and continue through the detox process as needed, with follow-up performed once the patient is medically cleared in order to determine what further psychiatric care, if any, is needed (Peters & Bekman, 2007). However, chronic psychiatric medications are not advisable during the withdrawal period unless the patient is acutely unstable and at notable risk of harm.

Although now rarely used or abused, it should be noted that barbiturates can induce a serious withdrawal syndrome similar to alcohol with delirium and seizures and should be tapered instead of abruptly stopped (Ciraulo & Knapp, 2011).

Opiates

Use and intoxication

As with alcohol, patients with mental illness may turn to opiates for various reasons. Although the "high" obtained from these substances can be the driving factor behind their use, patients may use them in an effort to manage their underlying disorder. Opiates, including heroin and narcotic pain medications, give the patient a dissociative feeling or "numbing" sensation. Patients with depression, posttraumatic stress disorder, or other disorders may use opiates to avoid memories, thoughts, feelings, or emotions that are too painful for them to reexperience. Overdoses of opiates, either alone or combined with alcohol, cause respiratory depression that can be fatal. With habitual use, the body quickly develops tolerance and craves the drug, both physically and mentally. The patient is forced to seek frequent "hits" throughout the day to avoid unpleasant withdrawal effects; this often interferes with work and relationships (National Institute on Drug Abuse, 2013a). Patients may become incarcerated either due to use or possession of the substance, as well as for the crimes committed to support the expense of the habit.

Opiate use can put patients at risk for medical problems that differ from those seen with alcohol. The stigma associated with contracting HIV or hepatitis B or C may reduce a patient's motivation to seek treatment for substance abuse. It is often during a period of incarceration that a patient discovers that he or she has been infected with HIV or hepatitis. The clinician should take this opportunity to educate the patient about the disease and offer advice on self-care and prevention of spread (Carlson & Kennedy, 2006).

Methadone (a long-acting opiate) and buprenorphine (a long-acting partial opioid agonist/antagonist) are prescription medications used to treat opioid abuse. Patients are generally unable to continue their maintenance programs during incarceration and will experience an opioid withdrawal syndrome.

Detoxification

An old adage regarding opioid withdrawal is "you won't die but you feel like you're going to die." This is fairly accurate: Opiate withdrawal is a miserable process that many try to avoid by continuing to use. The signs and symptoms include generalized deep body aches (patients may say their "bones" hurt), nausea, vomiting, diarrhea, leg cramps ("kicking"), piloerection ("skin crawling"), sneezing, yawning, watery eyes, and insomnia. This syndrome lasts two to four days and can last up to two weeks if the patient was using a long-acting preparation such as methadone (Tetrault, O'Connor, & Krishnamurthy, 2011). In a correctional setting, these substances are often discontinued, and the patient should be monitored for an abrupt detox. The majority of patients will experience some adverse effects of opiate withdrawal. Although alcohol withdrawal carries a much higher mortality risk, opioid detox can be severe, even fatal, if dehydration and electrolyte imbalances are left untreated. If the nausea prevents the patient from holding down fluids, intravenous replacement may be required. Low potassium levels and other electrolyte imbalances from vomiting and diarrhea can lead to arrhythmias or sudden cardiac death. Dehydration can precipitate rhabdomyolysis and acute renal failure (Fudala & Johnson, 2011). The Clinical Opiate Withdrawal Scale (COWS) assessment tool can be used to evaluate and medicate patients to help them feel less uncomfortable (California Society of Addiction Medicine, 2011; Wessen & Ling, 2003). Unlike alcohol detox, there is not a reliable medication taper available to most correctional facilities. Long-acting methadone tapers require facilities to have a methadone maintenance prescribing license, which most don't have. Buprenorphine is an alternate, long-acting partial opioid agonist used in detox protocols. However, many correctional programs find such protocols difficult to implement as the prescriber needs to obtain a special US Drug Enforcement Administration registration and the medication can be costly (Carlson & Kennedy, 2006). In many systems, patients who are currently in a buprenorphine program must be taken off once incarcerated. For most correctional programs, withdrawal treatment is symptomatic. Nonopioid protocols usually include an antiemetic for the nausea, an antidiarrheal agent, analgesics for aches and pains, and clonidine to mitigate some of the most uncomfortable sensations (Tetrault et al., 2011). Muscle relaxants are controversial in their medical necessity and are not ubiquitous in protocols. Sleep agents are also not standard but may be used in some practices. Many argue against both these medications in that they may introduce another addiction to a vulnerable patient.

Pregnant patients are the only individuals who should continue to receive a prescribed opiate, as any detox poses the risk of miscarriage. Methadone is the best studied and is considered as standard medication. Buprenorphine also may be effective in mitigating the withdrawal effects of opiates and decreasing the risk to the fetus; however, it is not as well studied as methadone (Carlson & Kennedy, 2006). The COWS score is often used to help dose the methadone for continuing maintenance during the pregnancy, similar to the CIWA for alcohol. Both the mother and baby undergo detox once delivery is complete. Incarcerated pregnant patients should be referred to a high-risk pregnancy obstetrician with experience in medicating addicted females.

Benzodiazepines

Intoxication

BZD intoxication is primarily manifested by varying degrees of somnolence and stupor, especially if combined with alcohol. Short-acting BZDs have the highest risk of physical and mental dependence due to their quick onset and offset. As an anxiolytic, street BZDs are popular among those with and without a diagnosed mental illness. Psychiatric patients can benefit from the sedating effects that counteract their feelings of anxiety. Unfortunately, overuse for perceived uncomfortable emotions like sadness and regret can lead to inappropriate usage, tolerance, and physical dependency (National Institute on Drug Abuse, 2011). Patients who find their prescribed dosage inadequate to manage their symptoms may use their medication more frequently or purchase more from the street market. Because BZDs are a prescribed medication, detox tends to be an adverse effect of incarceration rather than a direct cause.

Detoxification

Since BZDs stimulate the same receptors as alcohol, the withdrawal syndrome and the health risks are similar. Patients should be tapered off BZDs; abrupt discontinuation can lead to dangerous physical effects such as an unsafe rise in blood pressure, tachycardia, and seizures. As with alcohol, any BZD can be used for the tapering process. Many correctional programs use chlordiazepoxide as it is long-acting and staff are often familiar with it from its use in alcohol detox. For those patients who use BZDs and alcohol concomitantly, chlordiazepoxide is preferred since it will treat both withdrawal syndromes (Carlson & Kennedy, 2006). Short-acting BZD tapers, such as clonazepam or lorazepam, can be used if no alcohol use is suspected. These tapers are usually done over a 7- to 10-day period. However, patients may experience more emotional difficulty and anxiety during detox as they watch the effects of their prescribed medication dwindle. A long-acting medication whose dosage is unfamiliar to them may help them be less worried about how much they are getting, thus creating less anxiety about the detox process. The need for vitamin replacement is less urgent than with alcohol detox. Some facilities use vitamins as a standard in their protocols as they are inexpensive and have no adverse effects. Of note, gabapentin (Neurontin) has withdrawal syndromes similar to those for BZDs and should be given in tapered doses if it is to be discontinued (Tran, Hranicky, Lark, & Jacob, 2005).

Stimulants (cocaine, amphetamines/methamphetamine)

Intoxication

Recently incarcerated patients infrequently present with the acute high of stimulants as the effects are short-lived, lasting only a few hours. Intoxicated patients typically are in a hyperactive state, physically and mentally, characterized by tachycardia, high blood pressure, sweating, inability to focus, and, in severe cases, rhabdomyolysis or seizures. Patients may develop chest discomfort, either from cardiac or noncardiac sources. Increased cardiac demand or cocaine-induced coronary artery spasm puts patients at risk for cardiac damage. Complaints of chest discomfort should be evaluated in an emergency medical facility. Serotonin syndrome is a serious, potentially life-threatening complication of amphetamine use and overdose (Wilkins, Danovitch, Gorelick, & Krishnamurthy, 2011). Excess serotonin produces autonomic (hyperthermia, tachycardia), cognitive (agitation, hallucinations, coma), and somatic effects (clonus, myoclonus; Boyer & Shannon, 2005). Long-term, chronic methamphetamine ("meth") use has been associated with severe dental decay, mood changes, violent behavior, weight loss, anxiety, paranoia, and delusions (National Institute on Drug Abuse, 2010). Intoxication with any stimulant can resemble an acute manic episode, making it difficult to exclude mental illness as a cause of the behavior. Urine drug testing in the acute setting may be helpful in guiding management, especially if the diagnosis of intoxication is in question. Police lockups are one of the few types of facilities that might regularly deal with individuals who are acutely intoxicated with stimulants, and they are rarely prepared to managed them medically.

Detoxification

Withdrawal symptoms of cocaine and other stimulants are rarely life-threatening but they are uncomfortable. Patients may be fatigued and agitated, may have a change in appetite, or may have bad dreams. The psychological effects of dysphoria, insomnia/hypersomnia, and intense cravings are more concerning for the risk of relapse than any physical adverse effects (Hill & Weiss, 2011; Paczynski & Gold, 2011). There are no specific detox protocols and care is supportive. Increased suicide monitoring is recommended as the risk of suicidal ideation is high during the detox period. Substance-induced psychosis (not a withdrawal symptom, but it may be associated with intoxication) can continue even after the acute effects of the drug have worn off. These patients should be monitored closely. If their psychosis persists past detox, use of antipsychotic medication may be considered (Carlson & Kennedy, 2006).

3,4-Methylenedioxy-methamphetamine

Intoxication

The drug 3,4-methylenedioxy-methamphetamine (MDMA) is a popular club drug, also referred to as "Ecstasy" or "Molly." Because it is both a stimulant and a hallucinogen, the patient may experience sensations of euphoria, increased energy, emotional empathy, and warmth, while sensory perceptions are dulled. MDMA has the same cardiac risks as stimulants; in high dosages, it can interfere with temperature regulation. Teeth clenching, vision changes, and sleep or appetite disturbances are commonly seen with intoxication (National Institute on Drug Abuse, 2013b). Intoxication can be associated with serotonin syndrome as well as rhabdomyolysis and liver and kidney damage (Wilkins et al., 2011). Patients may commit criminal acts while under the influence, posing an issue for local police. The acute effects usually will have resolved by the time the patient reaches the initial evaluation by the correctional clinician.

Detoxification

There are no detox protocols for MDMA as the symptoms of withdrawal (anxiety, depression, fatigue) require no acute treatment (Carlson & Kennedy, 2006). Clinicians should evaluate patients after the acute episode for any underlying psychopathology.

Hallucinogens, PCP, ketamine, inhalants

Intoxication

Except for inhalants, these families of psychoactive drugs have few physical side effects of intoxication beyond the altered mental status. Inhalants can be damaging to the central nervous system and can cause cardiac, kidney, and liver damage (National Institute on Drug Abuse, 2012). These substances have a low risk of addiction as they do not cause the neurologic changes in the brain that produce physical dependence. Patients may want to continue to use this group of agents for the effect and may become psychologically dependent on the drug (Wilkins et al., 2011).

Detoxification

There are no specific withdrawal syndromes and no detox protocols associated with these families of substances. The patient may experience some anhedonia, fatigue, or insomnia. Rarely is medical intervention necessary. Baseline psychological health should be assessed after the acute intoxication has resolved (Carlson & Kennedy, 2006).

Complications of combining substances of abuse

Patients often combine substances of abuse. Depending on which substances are combined, the effects will vary. Alcohol and BZDs will potentiate each other's sedative effects, as well as either combined with opioids. Combinations of stimulants and depressants are often used to mitigate one another's adverse side effects, allowing the user to experience only the desired effect. Others are used in combination to give a faster, more intense high. Combining drugs puts the patient at risk for more physical injury and adverse psychological effects, complicating the clinician's attempts at treatment.

Summary

Patients with mental illness and substance abuse have a higher risk of arrest and incarceration and are more likely to serve longer custody sentences (Peters & Bekmen, 2007). For those actively using drugs, the detox protocols used in the community are effective for the incarcerated population with few modifications, depending on medication and staff resources (Wright et al., 2011). The psychiatric clinician should follow the patient from intake screening through completion of detox to determine the patient's needs for mental health treatment and psychotropic medications, if any. Early recognition and differentiation between the pathology of the intoxication/withdrawal effects and the patient's mental health disorder will help the clinician provide the most efficacious treatment and lower the patient's risk of morbidity.

References

American Society of Addiction Medicine (2001). *Addiction medicine essentials—Clinical Institute Withdrawal Assessment of Alcohol Scale, Revised* (CIWA-Ar). Retrieved from http://www.chce.research.va.gov/apps/PAWS/pdfs/ciwa-ar.pdf

Boyer, E. W., & Shannon, M. (2005). The serotonin syndrome. *New England Journal of Medicine, 352*, 1112–1120.

Bureau of Justice Statistics (2004). *Drug use and dependence, state and federal prisoners, 2004*. Retrieved from http://www.bjs.gov/index.cfm?ty=pbdetail&iid=778

California Society of Addiction Medicine (2011). *Clinical Opiate Withdrawal Scale*. Retrieved from http://www.csam-asam.org/buprenorphine-info

Carlson, H. B., & Kennedy, J. A. (2006). The treatment of alcohol and other drug withdrawal syndromes in persons taken into custody. In

M. Puisis (Ed.), *Clinical practice in correctional medicine* (2nd ed., pp. 387–399). Philadelphia: Mosby Elsevier.

Ciraulo, D. A., & Knapp, C. (2011). Sedative–hypnotics. In P. Ruiz & E. Strain (Eds.), *Lowinson and Ruiz's substance abuse: A comprehensive textbook* (5th ed., pp. 255–266). Baltimore: Lippincott Williams & Wilkins.

Devinsky, O., Feldmann, E., Weinreb, H. J., & Wilterdink, J. L. (1997). *The resident's neurology book*. Philadelphia: F. A. Davis Company.

Fudala, P. J., & Johnson, R. E. (2011). Alternative pharmacotherapies for opioid addiction. In P. Ruiz & E. Strain (Eds.), *Lowinson and Ruiz's substance abuse: A comprehensive textbook* (5th ed., pp. 494–500). Baltimore: Lippincott Williams & Wilkins.

Hasin, D. S., Stinson, F. S., Ogburn, E., & Grant, B. F. (2007). Prevalence, correlates, disability, and comorbidity of DSM-IV alcohol abuse and dependence in the United States: Results from the National Epidemiologic Survey on Alcohol and Related Conditions. *Archives of General Psychiatry, 64*, 830–842.

Hernandez-Avila, C. A., & Kranzler, H. R. (2011). Alcohol use disorders. In P. Ruiz & E. Strain (Eds.), *Lowinson and Ruiz's substance abuse: A comprehensive textbook* (5th ed., pp. 138–160). Baltimore: Lippincott Williams & Wilkins.

Hill, K. P., & Weiss, R. D. (2011). Amphetamines and other stimulants. In P. Ruiz & E. Strain (Eds.), *Lowinson and Ruiz's substance abuse: A comprehensive textbook* (5th ed., pp. 238–254). Baltimore: Lippincott Williams & Wilkins.

Mayo-Smith, M. F., & Krishnamurthy, A. (2011). Management of alcohol intoxication and withdrawal. In C. A. Cavacuiti (Ed.), *Principles of addiction medicine—The essentials* (pp. 204–211). Philadelphia: Lippincott Williams & Wilkins.

Minozzi, S., Amato, L., Vecchi, S., & Davoli, M. (2010). Anticonvulsants for alcohol withdrawal. *Cochrane Database for Systemic Review*, CD005064.

National Institute on Drug Abuse (2010). *InfoFacts: Methamphetamine*. Retrieved from http://www.drugabuse.gov/publications/drugfacts/methamphetamine (accessed on November 27, 2013.)

National Institute on Drug Abuse (2011). *InfoFacts: Commonly abused prescription drugs chart*. Retrieved from http://www.drugabuse.gov/drugs-abuse/commonly-abused-drugs/commonly-abused-prescription-drugs-chart

National Institute on Drug Abuse (2012). *InfoFacts: Inhalants*. Retrieved from http://www.drugabuse.gov/publications/drugfacts/inhalants

National Institute on Drug Abuse (2013a). *InfoFacts: Heroin*. Retrieved from http://www.drugabuse.gov/publications/drugfacts/heroin

National Institute on Drug Abuse (2013b). *InfoFacts: MDMA (ecstasy or Molly)*. Retrieved from http://www.drugabuse.gov/publications/drugfacts/mdma-ecstasy-or-molly

Paczynski, R. P., & Gold, M. S. (2011). Cocaine and crack. In P. Ruiz & E. Strain (Eds.), *Lowinson and Ruiz's substance abuse: A comprehensive textbook* (5th ed., pp. 191–213). Baltimore: Lippincott Williams & Wilkins.

Peters, R. H., & Bekman, N. M. (2007). Treatment reentry approaches for offenders with co-occurring disorders. In R. Greifinger (Ed.), *Public health behind bars—From prisons to communities* (pp. 368–384). New York: Springer.

Shivani, R., Goldsmith, R. J., & Anthenelli, R. M. (2002). *Alcoholism and psychiatric disorders-diagnostic challenges*. National Institute on Alcohol Abuse and Alcoholism. Retrieved from http://pubs.niaaa.nih.gov/publications/arh26-2/90-98.htm

Substance Abuse and Mental Health Services Administration (2006). *5 Co-occurring medical and psychiatric conditions*. Retrieved from http://www.ncbi.nlm.nih.gov/books/NBK64105/

Sullivan, J. T., Sykora, K., Schneiderman, J., Naranjo, C. A., & Sellers, E. M. (1989). Assessment of alcohol withdrawal: The revised Clinical Institute Withdrawal Assessment for Alcohol Scale (CIWA-Ar). *British Journal of Addiction, 84*, 1353–1357.

Tetrault, J. M., O'Connor, P. G., & Krishnamurthy, A. (2011). Management of opioid Intoxication and withdrawal. In C. A. Cavacuiti (Ed.), *Principles of addiction medicine—The essentials* (pp. 223–228). Philadelphia: Lippincott Williams & Wilkins.

Tran, K. T., Hranicky, D., Lark, T., & Jacob, N. J. (2005). Gabapentin withdrawal syndrome in the presence of a taper. *Bipolar Disorders, 7*, 302–304.

Victor, M., & Adams, R. D. (1953). The effect of alcohol on the nervous system. *Research Publications—Association for Research in Nervous and Mental Disease, 32*, 523–526.

Wessen, D. R., & Ling, W. (2003). The Clinical Opiate Withdrawal Scale (COWS). *Journal of Psychoactive Drugs, 35*, 253–259.

Wilkins, J. N., Danovitch, I., Gorelick, D. A., & Krishnamurthy, A. (2011). Management of stimulant, hallucinogen, marijuana, phencyclidine, and club drug Intoxication and withdrawal. In C. A. Cavacuiti (Ed.), *Principles of addiction medicine—The essentials* (pp. 229–244). Philadelphia: Lippincott Williams & Wilkins.

Wright, T. M., Cluver, J. S., Myrick, H., & Krishnamurthy, A. (2011). Management of intoxication and withdrawal: general principles. In C.A. Cavacuiti (Ed.), *Principles of addiction medicine—The essentials* (pp. 199–203). Philadelphia: Lippincott Williams & Wilkins.

CHAPTER 18

Adjustment disorders

Graham D. Glancy and Stefan R. Treffers

Introduction

For most people, becoming incarcerated and the challenges associated with incarceration are major life stressors. The development of acute adjustment disorder (AD) is very common in these settings. This chapter discusses the prevalence, presentation, assessment issues, and management concerns of AD in jails and prisons.

Prevalence of adjustment disorders in corrections

Although there are few epidemiological studies of AD, prevalence estimates in the general population have been found to be <1 percent (Patra & Sarkar, 2013). Among patients in primary care settings with psychiatric disorders, studies have indicated prevalence rates to be between 11.7 percent and 17.9 percent (Casey, 2006; Patra & Sarkar, 2013). Prevalence estimates in correctional settings are also scarce and are subject to the same diagnostic pitfalls that complicate the identification of AD in other populations. A few studies have attempted to determine prevalence rates among inmates. In a longitudinal study of mental disorder in a cohort of male prisoners on remand, AD was judged to be present in 17 (11.48 percent) newly received remand prisoners who had been identified as having a mental disorder (n = 148; Birmingham et al., 1996). In a larger study that used data on prisoners in the New Jersey correctional system, 237 inmates (7.7 percent) with an Axis I mental disorder diagnosis were identified as having AD (n = 3,073; Pogorzelski & Blitz, 2005). Another study compared the incidence of psychiatric morbidity during remand imprisonment between solitary confinement and nonsolitary confinement settings in a large Danish remand prison. AD was found to be the most common incident disorder in both settings, with 81 percent (n = 30/37) in the solitary confinement group and 93 percent (n = 13/14) in the nonsolitary confinement group (Andersen et al., 2000).

Due to a weak research foundation and what some experts perceive as "a lack of scientific interest in AD" (Jager et al., 2012), current incidence and prevalence estimates of the disorder may not accurately reflect the prison environment, especially considering that each correctional facility houses divergent populations of inmates at different stages of the judicial process and may be governed by a different set of rules and practices (Andersen, 2004). These factors are particularly relevant when AD is measured in prisoner populations remanded in custody compared to populations of long-term convicted prisoners; the two groups may have different patterns of occurrence. Factors that influence these differences between remand and convicted offenders may operate at the institutional level, such as access to psychiatric treatment, availability of offender programs and services, length of sentence exposure to serious offenders, and, at a psychological level, feelings associated with conviction, acceptance of the sentence, and coping with the prison environment. It is our experience that patients with AD represent a significant portion of those referred to psychiatric services, especially within the jail setting.

Complexity of diagnosis and identification

Given its broad classification criteria, AD has been subject to various criticisms related to validity and reliability (Jager et al., 201s). Some have challenged the classification as a "wastebasket" diagnosis (Casey, 2006), while others have pointed out the inability of the classification to appropriately distinguish between cases that require psychiatric intervention and normal adaptive reactions to stressors (Andersen, 2004; Casey, 2006; Walsh & Corcoran, 2011). Diagnosis of AD becomes further complicated by symptomatology that overlaps with other disorders, specifically mood and anxiety disorders (Andersen, 2004). Casey (2006), for example, emphasizes the difficulty in adequately distinguishing AD from major depression, especially cases of mild to moderate severity. While both disorders share a very similar set of diagnostic criteria, *the Diagnostic and Statistical Manual of Mental Disorders* precludes a diagnosis of AD when the criteria for major depression are satisfied (American Psychiatric Association, 2013). While some researchers have contended that the AD diagnosis has been subordinated to the diagnosis of other mental disorders (Jager et al., 2012), Casey (2006) suggests that research efforts have favored disorders for which specific treatments are available, thus excluding AD from more extensive clinical and academic consideration.

Despite these criticisms, individuals diagnosed with AD were seen as a distinct group compared to those without a diagnosis (Despland, Monod, & Ferrero, 1995). These diagnosed patients tended to share symptomatology with depressive disorders but were marked by differences related to age, treatment length, and type of stressor (Casey, 2006; Despland et al., 1995; Patra & Sarkar, 2013). Individuals with AD had higher quality-of-life scores than those with major depressive disorder (Patra & Sarkar, 2013). With regard to the reliability and stability of the diagnosis, studies have yielded mixed results, with varying degrees of inter-rater and predictive reliability (Casey, 2006; Jager et al., 2012; Patra & Sarkar, 2013).

Comorbidity

Diagnostic obstacles also extend to findings of comorbidity as there are no clear guidelines as to where some disorders begin and others end. Studies have found comorbidity rates to be relatively high. In a representative community sample of elderly residents in Zurich, 46.1 percent of patients were found to have one or two other mental disorders, with major depression and posttraumatic stress disorder the most common comorbidities (Maercker et al., 2008). Jager and colleagues (2012) discovered that 47.3 percent of patients had one or more comorbid mental disorders using International Classification of Diseases–10 criteria. Of those patients with comorbid diagnoses, 29.6 percent had a mental disorder resulting from psychotropic substance use and 15.4 percent from a personality disorder (Jager et al., 2012). It is likely that comorbidity is even more extensive in correctional populations. Another layer of complexity is the relationship between subthreshold symptoms of mood and anxiety disorders and a diagnosis of AD.

Guidelines for psychological treatment

Treatments of AD in the general population consist mainly of brief interventions (Casey, 2009), typically involving three broad components: removing or reducing the stressor, facilitating adaptation to the stressor, and altering the response to the stressor. Specific psychological therapies may include supportive, psycho-educational, cognitive, and psychodynamic approaches.

While none of these therapies has demonstrated therapeutic superiority in treating AD, cognitive-behavioral therapy (CBT) has become generally accepted as a treatment for a wide range of mental health problems. The clarity and brevity of this treatment make it suitable for use in a variety of settings, including correctional ones (Regehr & Glancy, 2010).

Landenberger and Lipsey (2005) have suggested that treatment effectiveness and recidivism reduction depend on the quality of the CBT provided. In environments where psychiatric resources are strained, such as prisons and especially jails, programmed treatment approaches may not be possible, although psychological therapies may be more viable in long-term correctional facilities. With high inmate turnover and a large proportion of inmates to clinicians, the fast-paced nature of remand facilities demands the symptomatic treatment and management of mental illness with limited psychiatric consultation. In addition, many inmates are admitted with little or no recorded psychiatric and medical histories, which may complicate treatment delivery.

Roberts (2000) describes a seven-stage model based on preexisting work in crisis intervention:

Initial assessment

This assessment includes a psychiatric history and mental state examination, with an emphasis on whether the patient is actively suicidal. Appropriate measures are indicated for suicidal patients (see Section 9). For patients who are not actively suicidal, the psychiatric history would include factors that would exclude the presence of a mood or anxiety disorder, a personality disorder, or a substance use disorder and withdrawal; all of these should be taken into consideration.

Establish rapport

An important skill in working in corrections is the ability to be an empathic, nonjudgmental clinician. Being empathic does not necessarily mean that the therapist is easily manipulated into doing things that would be either unethical or outside the therapeutic envelope. Nevertheless, by demonstrating concern and interest and by assisting with basic needs, it is surprising how quickly therapeutic rapport can be developed. Although the therapist's services are generally strictly rationed, the therapist is nevertheless an important figure for the patient, possibly the only person to whom he or she can ventilate safely in the situation.

Identify the major problems

It is important to attempt to delineate the various dimensions related to the patient's distress. These commonly involve not only the stresses of being in an alien and difficult environment but also absence from the usual social supports, imminent marital separation, possible job loss and resultant financial strain, and loss of reputation. Some of these problems may be chronic, likely exacerbated by the current incarceration, and others may be new. The purpose of enumerating these problems is so that the patient and therapist can work on and deal with each one in turn; the therapist should guard against becoming overwhelmed in this process.

Deal with feelings and provide support

The therapist uses active listening techniques to explore the relevant issues. This includes considering previous coping strategies and instilling hope. Positive coping strategies should be delineated and reinforced. Sometimes these are as simple as suggesting a distraction, perhaps playing cards or exercising, to reduce stress and increase involvement with others. In addition, it may be helpful to delineate supports on the outside that the patient can contact and mobilize. Some patients are ashamed to approach people; however, if encouraged to do so, friends and relatives may be accepting and supportive. Nothing is lost by the initial approach.

Explore alternatives

Some patients have limited and rigid coping strategies. Substance use and acting-out have likely been easy and quick, although maladaptive, strategies. More adaptive strategies can be suggested and worked on. It is sometimes necessary to point out that gains will be incremental, and more ambitious goals may be considered for the long term. It is necessary to gently point out alternatives and, as ever when working in corrections, to be flexible in approach, while always maintaining proper boundaries and security provisions.

Formulate an action plan

Formulating an action plan might involve specific tasks such as exercising daily and taking advantage of daily yard privileges. Suggestions such as contacting family and friends and requesting support may be helpful. Referrals to chaplaincy, social workers, and outside agencies may be considered. It is not uncommon that anticipated losses are not as bad as the patient thought they would be. For example, whereas an inmate may have heard that he was facing two to four years in jail, his lawyer may have negotiated the possibility of a plea bargain involving just a few months. Often spouses, family, and friends, who were initially rejecting, resolve their own anger and may be more accepting and accommodating to the patient.

Establish follow-up plans

The initial interventions may include seeing and working with patients on a regular basis. This can be quite reassuring to them. It is possible that after the initial period of crisis they are restored to normal equilibrium and do not require long-term support or treatment. In other cases, referrals to programs and agencies should be considered to work on long-term goals that relate to substance use disorders, antisocial peer groups, and other criminogenic factors.

In the correctional setting, CBT has reduced recidivism rates among offenders released to the community (Landenberger & Lipsey, 2005; Lipsey & Landenberger, 2001). These therapies incorporate strategies designed to manage anger, have offenders take responsibility for their behavior, improve problem-solving skills, develop life skills, and set goals (Lipsey & Landenberger, 2001). In a metaanalysis of studies that examined group-oriented CBT programs, Wilson and colleagues (2005) found that reductions in recidivism rates ranged from 20 percent to 30 percent for treated offenders compared to control groups.

Other approaches include such treatments as stress inoculation training (Meichenbaum, 1993), mindfulness-based stressed reduction (Kabat-Zinn, 1982), and mindfulness-based cognitive therapy (Segal et al., 2002). These latter approaches incorporate Eastern techniques with relaxation techniques. They have been demonstrated to be useful in various populations, and some research has suggested their utility in correctional settings (Samuelson et al., 2007).

In response to these constraints, some jails and prisons have adopted variations of crisis intervention to deal with inmates who cannot cope with a particular event and have high levels of fear, tension, confusion, and/or subjective discomfort (Dass-Brailsford, 2007). The cumulative effect of imprisonment, family disruption, strains on marriage, and the uncertainty of one's fate may cause excessive stress and lead to a crisis. Crisis intervention strategies used in a correctional context have evolved from more traditional forms practiced by frontline emergency personnel. These strategies have been tailored to deal with inmate altercations, instances of self-harm, suicidal ideation, and personal life events that can lead to conflict while in custody (French, 1981; Kulic, 2005). Research in this area has provided evidence that individuals who experience crises are somewhat more open to suggestions than they would normally be (Kulic, 2005). Crisis intervention is intended to be a short-term approach where clinicians help the offender to identify coping skills and restore precrisis functioning (Dass-Brailsford, 2007; Kulic, 2005). Through prevention and stabilization, these interventions are geared toward management of crises rather than full-fledged treatment (Dass-Brailsford, 2007; French, 1981).

Psychopharmacological approaches

In the real world of correctional psychiatry, a psychopharmacological approach to treating AD is intended to treat the symptoms of anxiety, insomnia, and possibly depression for a short duration. Another factor to be taken into consideration is that many patients are already taking medications prior to incarceration. These previous medication regimens may not be optimal (see Chapter 19). It is not uncommon to see patients who have gradually accumulated in the community redundant or multiple medications and idiosyncratic mixes of medications. Often, the first task of the correctional psychiatrist is to begin to rationalize treatment. Certain types of medications and obviously inappropriate polypharmacy should be addressed immediately, especially the chronic use of

benzodiazepines, opiates, and psychostimulants given with no clear indication. Correctional institutions tend to have restrictions on the use of these medications for a variety of reasons (see Chapter 28), such as the fact that the majority of offenders have substance use disorders, certain medications may promote aggression (Glancy & Knott, 2003), and the circulation of these medications may increase the potential for bullying and diversion (see Chapters 29 and 31).

When depressive symptoms coexist with anxiety and insomnia, sedating antidepressants may be a suitable option. These include the use of mirtazapine or trazodone (Glancy & Knott, 2003). Trazodone is particularly useful since it has antiaggressive effects, which is also useful in this population. Selective serotonin reuptake inhibitors and serotonin–norepinephrine reuptake inhibitors may also be considered for the management of anxiety. In practice, these medications appear to be useful even if prescribing them is not significantly evidence-based. Buspirone, an anxiolytic 5-HT 1 agonist with significant antiaggressive effects (Glancy & Knott 2003), also appears helpful in practice. These are generally well tolerated and helpful in the crisis period. Given that AD is typically short-lived when treated, the need for continuing pharmacological treatment should be reassessed at regular intervals. The use of sedative-hypnotic agents is discussed in more detail in Chapter 6.

These medications should ideally be given in conjunction with psychological treatments as described previously. In our experience, the crisis model is particularly applicable and can be combined with CBT on an informal or formal basis. CBT can also be given in a group format, where this is possible. Mindfulness strategies have been useful in a variety of settings, including incarceration, and should be considered if feasible given institutional resources.

Suicide risk

Many patients in correctional settings are young males, close in age to adolescents. In a study of suicidality among outpatient adolescents diagnosed with AD, Pelkonen and colleagues (2005) discovered that 25 percent showed suicide attempts, threats, or ideation. They also suggested that risk factors such as previous psychiatric treatment and severe psychosocial impairment at entry to treatment were commonly present in suicidal adolescents with major psychiatric disorders. Other findings in the adolescent sample included dysphoric mood and depressive symptoms associated with continued suicidal ideation; these symptoms were common in completed suicides by adolescents with AD (Pelkonen et al., 2005). In differentiating between suicide risks in AD patients versus those with major depression, Carta and colleagues (2009) suggested that the AD group presents a lower risk for suicide, a shorter-lived interval of suicidality, and a lower likelihood of planned suicide compared to the group with major depression.

Reported rates of suicide among inmates have varied given the diversity that exists in inmate populations (see Chapter 43). Way and colleagues (2005) suggest that AD, as a risk factor for suicide in correctional settings, should be given more attention. This is supported by their finding that 28 percent of suicide victims in a sample of prison inmates who had contact with mental health services had a diagnosis of AD. Common acute precursors to committed suicides included inmate conflict, recent disciplinary action, overall fear, physical illness, and adverse news related to one's personal circumstances (Way et al., 2005).

Clinicians must carefully assess suicidality, not only during the initial assessment period but also on an ongoing basis, especially when the patient's circumstances change. Examples of this type of change may be an adverse turn in legal proceedings (such as new charges being laid) or a change in personal circumstances (such as news that a spouse is filing for divorce or restricting access to children). Adverse life events such as these may precipitate a new crisis and decompensation, requiring the therapist to reappraise the approach to treatment.

Summary

With these complexities in mind, it is important for clinicians to use sound clinical judgment, taking into consideration the patient's personal circumstances and the context in which his or her symptoms are being presented (Casey, 2009). This chapter gives guidance to clinicians who are on the front line in very difficult circumstances. They are often dealing with patients who are overwhelmed with significant adverse life events, whose history reveals that they have dealt with emotional disturbances by acting out or who have struggled with substance abuse for many years. These patients present with complex comorbidities, often complicated by substance use disorder and withdrawal. Clinicians often have very little information at their disposal yet will have to make difficult decisions under pressure. For example, it is often impossible to collect collateral information or previous clinical records. Clinicians must take an empathic approach while maintaining clear boundaries. In addition, clinicians must bear in mind the security constraints of the institution; because of these constraints, a limited armamentarium of medications is available for use (see Chapter 28). Often clinicians work in relative isolation, without the added resources of a multidisciplinary team. In hospital practice, other professionals are available both as additional resources and as supports to the clinician, but in many correctional settings, these professionals may not be easy to access. In our view, treatment of AD in correctional settings requires a keen application of the entire complement of clinical skills.

References

American Psychiatric Association (2013). *Diagnostic and statistical manual of mental disorders* (5th ed.). Arlington, VA: American Psychiatric Publishing.

Andersen, H. S. (2004). Mental health in prison populations. A review with special emphasis on a study of Danish prisoners on remand. *Acta Psychiatrica Scandinavica, 424*, Supp, 5–59.

Andersen, H. S., Sestoft, D., Lillebaek, T., Gabrielsen, G., Hemmingsen, R., & Kramp, P. (2000). A longitudinal study of prisoners on remand: psychiatric prevalence, incidence and psychopathology in solitary vs. non-solitary confinement. *Acta Psychiatrica Scandinavica, 102*, 19–25.

Birmingham, L., Mason, D., & Grubin, D. (1996). A follow-up study of mentally disordered men remanded to prison. *Criminal Behavior and Mental Health, 8*(3), 202–213.

Carta, M. G., Balestrieri, M., Murru, A., & Hardoy, M. C. (2009). Adjustment disorder: epidemiology, diagnosis and treatment. *Clinical Practice and Epidemiology in Mental Health, 5*(15), 1–15.

Casey, P. (2006). The "afterthought" diagnosis: Rehabilitating adjustment disorders. *Expert Review of Neurotherapeutics, 6*(2), 145–151.

Casey, P. (2009). Adjustment disorder: Epidemiology, diagnosis and treatment. *CNS Drugs, 23*(11), 927–938.

Dass-Brailsford, P. (2007). Crisis interventions. In P. Dass-Brailsford (Ed.), *A practical approach to trauma: empowering interventions* (pp. 93–114). Thousand Oaks, CA: Sage.

Despland, J. N., Monod, L., & Ferrero, F. (1995). Clinical relevance of adjustment disorder in DMS-III-R and DSM-IV. *Comprehensive Psychiatry, 36*(6), 454–460.

French, L. (1981). Clinical perspectives on crisis intervention in jails. *Prison Journal, 61*(1), 43–54.

Glancy, G. D., & Knott, T. F. (2003). Psychopharmacology of violence—Part IV. *American Academy of Psychiatry and the Law Newsletter, 28*(1) 12–13.

Jager, M., Burger, D., Becker, T., & Frasch, K. (2012). Diagnosis of adjustment disorder: reliability of its clinical use and long-term stability. *Psychopathology, 45*(5), 305–309.

Kabat-Zinn, J. (1982). An outpatient program in behavioral medicine for chronic pain patients based on practice of mindfulness meditation: Theoretical considerations and preliminary results. *General Hospital Psychiatry, 4*, 33–47.

Kulic, K. R. (2005). The Crisis Intervention Semi-Structured Interview. *Brief Treatment and Crisis Intervention, 5*(2), 143–157.

Landenberger, N. A., & Lipsey, M. W. (2005). The positive effects of cognitive-behavioral programs for offenders: A meta-analysis of factors associated with effective treatment. *Journal of Experimental Criminology, 1*(4), 451–476.

Lipsey, M. W., & Landenberger, N. A. (2001). Cognitive-behavioral programs for offenders. *Annals of the American Academy of Political and Social Science, 578*, 144–157.

Maercker, A., Forstmeier, S., Enzler, A., et al. (2008). Adjustment disorders, posttraumatic stress disorder, and depressive disorders in old age: Findings from a community survey. *Comprehensive Psychiatry, 49*(2), 113–120.

Meichenbaum, D. (1993). Stress inoculation training: A twenty year update. In L. Woolfolk & P. Lehrer (Eds.), *Principles and practice of stress management* (2nd ed., pp. 373–406). New York: Guilford.

Patra, B. N., & Sarkar, S. (2013). Adjustment disorder: current diagnostic status. *Indian Journal of Psychological Medicine, 35*(1), 4–9.

Pelkonen, M., Marttunen, M., Henriksson, M., & Lonngvist, J. (2005). Suicidality in adjustment disorder: Clinical characteristics of adolescent outpatients. *European Child & Adolescent Psychiatry, 14*(3), 174–180.

Pogorzelski, W., & Blitz, C.L. (2005). Behavioral health problems, ex-offender reentry policies, and the "Second Chance Act." *American Journal of Public Health, (10)*, 1718–1724.

Regehr, C., & Glancy, G. (2010). *Mental health social work practice in Canada.* New York: Oxford University Press.

Roberts, A. R. (2000). *Crisis intervention handbook: Assessment, treatment, and research.* New York: Oxford University Press.

Segal, Z. V., Williams, J. M. G., & Teasdale, J. D. (2002). *Mindfulness-based cognitive therapy for depression: A new approach to relapse prevention.* New York: Guilford Press.

Samuelson, M., Carmody, J., Kabat-Zinn, J., et al. (2007). Mindfuless-based stress reduction I. Massachusetts Correctional Facilities. *Prison Journal, 87*(2), 254–268.

Way, B. B., Miraglia, R., Sawyer, D. A., Beer, R., & Eddy, J. (2005). Factors related to suicide in New York state prisons. *International Journal of Law and Psychiatry, 28*(3), 207–221.

Walsh, J., & Corcoran, J. (2011). A social work perspective on the adjustment disorders. *Social Work in Mental Health, 9*(2), 107–121.

Wilson, D. B., Bouffard, L. A., & Mackenzie, D. L. (2005). A quantitative review of structured, group-oriented, cognitive-behavioral programs for offenders. *Criminal Justice and Behavior, 32*(2), 172–204.

CHAPTER 19

Transition of pharmacology from community to corrections

Robert L. Trestman

Introduction

Psychopharmacology, in general, is a challenging field that includes much art as well as science. Clinicians usually depend upon self-report when making decisions regarding medication selection and dosing. When a patient becomes incarcerated, there are multiple potentially conflicting situations. Issues related to formularies, environmental stressors, changed support groups, and practice patterns all may contribute to medication management decisions. This chapter discusses both the clinical issues and pragmatic management opportunities that can lead to improved patient care and enhanced functioning.

There has been a substantial emphasis on continuity of care when people are released from correctional settings back to the community (see Chapters 15 and 47). However, much less has been written about the challenges regarding continuity of care when someone becomes incarcerated, particularly when psychotropic medications are involved. Community management of psychotropic medication is of varying standards. A patient's medication regimen may be the result of thoughtful evaluation and best practice determination over several years of careful and incremental improvement and refinement. Conversely, it may have been compromised by a range of pragmatic issues or determined in a less formal manner, and the resulting treatment regimen may be inconsistent or inappropriate for the patient's diagnosis or diagnoses (Gutheil, 2012). The patient's medications may have been determined while his or her ongoing illicit drug use confounded the diagnostic picture. Collaboration between clinician and patient may have been poor, and subsequently treatment adherence may have been marginal.

What, then, happens when a patient becomes incarcerated? The admission process is inherently stressful, filled with anxiety, uncertainty, and perhaps humiliation or fear. Such stressors may exacerbate underlying psychiatric symptoms. During this period, standard expectations include screening and an assessment interview, history taking, a release of information request, and confirmation of medications with the local pharmacy. The pharmacy will be able to confirm when and how regularly prescriptions were filled (albeit not how regularly they were taken). Contact with the treating community clinician or team, at least by obtaining copies of current, relevant treatment records (if not direct verbal communication), is very important. Unfortunately, in practice, such direct communication with the community care provider is more often the exception than the rule. When integrated into standard practice, these combined steps help support continuity of care,

particularly for patients with severe mental illness. Failures of the system through policy or implementation practices can significantly compromise patient care (Sered & Norton-Hawk, 2013). Factors to take into account at this stage of assessment include the nature and complexity of the illness or illnesses, medications being taken, co-occurrence of substance misuse, treatment adherence estimates, duration of treatment, severity of underlying illness, and fragility of the patient.

Initial clinical considerations

First and foremost, clinical considerations need to drive decisions on whether to maintain the medications the patients was taking in the community. These clinical considerations include the accuracy of the community-based diagnosis, best estimates of adherence to medication in the community, the benefits versus side-effect burden of the medications, the existence of polypharmacy, the potential effects of detoxification on the diagnosis and the effectiveness of the medication, and the appropriate duration of treatment for the underlying disorder.

The accuracy of the community-based diagnosis is a critical determinant in this process since the medications are intended to target signs and symptoms of psychiatric illness. Time pressures and constraints do not overrule the clinical and ethical obligation of the correctional psychiatrist to confirm the illness being treated. The ideal, as always, is to conduct a criterion-based assessment to determine whether specific psychiatric diagnoses, rather than nonspecific isolated symptoms, exist. Everything else follows from this. One enormous advantage of correctional psychiatry is the opportunity rarely afforded psychiatrists in the community (since the drastic reduction of community-based inpatient psychiatric lengths of stay and elevated severity thresholds for admission to inpatient units) to observe the functioning of a patient in a safe, monitored environment. When diagnostic ambiguity exists, appropriate tapering off of community medications can be conducted in many jail or prison settings with greater safety and collateral information than achievable elsewhere. This ultimately may benefit the patient far more than simply maintaining community-based medications that, in reality, may be inappropriate or unnecessary. In particular, since 60 percent to 80 percent of correctional mental health patients have co-occurring substance misuse disorders (Baillargeon et al., 2010), eliminating ready access to these illicit drugs may gradually resolve many of the anxiety, mood, and psychotic symptoms.

Adherence to medication in the community is always uncertain. Data clearly reflect that many psychiatric patients do not take their medications as prescribed. In one study that examined the treatment of schizophrenia, 29 percent of patients were nonadherent, with substance abuse a significant risk factor for nonadherence (Novick et al., 2010). Lack of response to medications that the patient was supposed to be taking in the community may have occurred simply because the patient wasn't taking them as prescribed.

A common challenge for many people with severe mental illness is that often medications are given without a specific targeted syndrome or symptom. A common response to questions about why each medication is being taken is, "I don't know." A typical scenario is that a patient may be given multiple medications, each of which is at a subtherapeutic dose. When multiple medications are used simultaneously without a clear clinical rationale and an intended purpose, the benefits diminish while the side-effect burden increases.

Polypharmacy, the simultaneous use of multiple medications, is increasing in frequency (Mojtabai & Olfson, 2010). One in three office visits to a psychiatrist results in three or more psychotropic prescriptions; the median number doubled between 1996 and 2006 (Mojtabai & Olfson, 2010). While this may be justifiable when each medication has a specific indication or is being used as a clearly defined adjuvant, there is little research evidence to support polypharmacy (Preskorn & Lacey, 2007)—but there is evidence of both attendant risks (Tiihonen, Suokas, Suvisaari, Haukka, & Korhonen, 2012) and financial costs (Valuck et al., 2007). This is notably the case where maximum therapeutic levels have not been achieved or the duration of treatment for a single medication has been insufficient (Preskorn & Lacey, 2007). On admission to a correctional setting, an assessment of such polypharmacy is an important opportunity for therapeutic improvement and harm reduction.

Chronic active substance abuse makes psychiatric diagnosis problematic at best. For example, combined opiate and cocaine abuse, with oscillating periods of intoxication and withdrawal, may readily mimic the presentation of bipolar disorder. Similarly, using psychiatric medications to treat such a presentation is very likely to be inadequate. The opportunity to observe someone, often for weeks or months, following detoxification from illicit substances may allow the clinician to make a substantially improved diagnostic assessment.

Pragmatic considerations

Multiple pragmatic considerations have an impact on continuity of care and the use of psychopharmacological agents. The first is what may be a relatively limited formulary. Correctional settings frequently have formulary restrictions that may be tighter than in many community-based environments. This may lead to a therapeutic substitution from a labeled medication to a generic that follows formulary limitations or to another agent in the same drug class upon clinical review by the psychiatrist. Virtually all institutions that have a restricted formulary do allow for nonformulary requests if the patient would clearly benefit only from a specific medication that is not on the formulary. This is particularly important for the unsentenced population who may rapidly, and unpredictably, return to the community. When an inmate is

sentenced, however, many facilities or systems will work to transition the patient to medications that are on the formulary.

In contrast to the community, the near-universal standard in correctional settings is directly observed therapy for the administration of psychiatric medications. In this context, either a nurse makes rounds with a medication cart to each housing unit or inmates present at a medication line. In either event, inmates take the medication under the observation of the nurse and/or an appropriately trained correctional officer who is expected to document whether the medication was taken and swallowed by the patient. In the community, this standard is typically met only in a hospital setting. The advantage is obvious—adherence is far more reliably determined and nonadherence may be addressed quickly. Directly observed therapy may be compromised in practice settings that limit the ability of staff to fully observe the actions of the patient. One such example is in a restricted housing unit, where medication may be administered at the cell through a small trap door. Directly observed therapy is really meaningful only when the cell door is opened to allow for full visibility of the patient. Directly observed therapy, while admittedly reducing self-empowerment on the part of the patient, does make it far easier for the correctional psychiatrist to determine the effects and benefits of prescribed medication.

In the community, only limited attention is given to the frequency and timing of medications. Twice-daily (BID) and at-bedtime (HS) frequencies are commonly used in the community. Their actual implementation in correctional settings may vary considerably from that in the community, however. Typical administration times in jails are driven by the practical needs of a facility linked to frequent court appearances. Morning medications may be administered well before 7 AM; bedtime medications may actually be administered at 6 PM. Psychiatrists in such settings must work with custody staff to provide medications at clinically appropriate times. As-needed (PRN) medications may, in fact, rarely be administered in many correctional settings, given staff limits and the fact that the medications may be housed in a part of the facility well removed from the inmate's cell. These factors may affect the patient's desire to take medications as prescribed and may also influence factors such as bioavailability and peak/trough timing.

The cost of psychotropic medications, particularly for patients with severe and persistent mental illness, is often ignored in the community, typically because the patient is on an insurance plan that traditionally covers the vast majority of medications (e.g., Medicaid; Valuck et al., 2007). Often, there is a tendency in the community to use the newest branded medication at substantial incremental cost compared to older, generic medications. With rare exception, jails are funded entirely by the county and prisons by the state, typically with tight constraints (see Chapter 10). Given limited resources and frequently capped budgets, formulary restrictions may require that medications for a new inmate undergo a review and potential replacement with generic medications of the same or a related drug class.

Consistent with growing community concerns over the abuse of prescription medication, correctional settings present with significant abuse potential, in some ways consistent with the community and in other ways substantially divergent. The main psychopharmacological challenges have to do with stimulants and with sedative-hypnotics but also include medications rarely abused in the community. Beyond ongoing community concerns with potential overprescription of psychostimulants such as dextroamphetamine or methylphenidate, in jail or prison there are concerns of diversion or extortion as well (Appelbaum, 2009). Sedative-hypnotics present similar concerns (see Chapter 29). Indeed, many correctional facilities and systems have policies prohibiting or severely limiting their use. Beyond these concerns are those consequent to the unique characteristics of jails and prisons, with the overall interdiction on illicit substances. As described in detail in Chapter 29, medications such as sedating antipsychotics (e.g., quetiapine) may be sought for their effects as sleep agents and buproprion (if crushed and inhaled nasally) for its effect as a stimulant (Phillips, 2012). In contrast, there is a growing concern that precluding such agents as psychostimulants for the treatment of attention-deficit/hyperactivity disorder may lead to negative consequences (Appelbaum, 2009), including increased (rather than reduced) criminal behavior (e.g., Lichtenstein et al., 2012).

From jail to prison or from one prison to another prison

While the foregoing has focused on the initial admission from the community into a correctional setting, many similar issues apply when a patient transfers from a jail to a prison or from one prison to another. Preparation and review of transfer summary sheets and more detailed records are just as important in these situations and should be seen as the minimum standard in policy and in practice. Ideally, continuity of care and any concerns about diagnosis or treatment are best shared through direct communication. A telephone exchange between treating psychiatrists is always better than simple written documentation.

Summary

Transition from the community to jail or prison or between correctional facilities is inherently stressful. It is also a time of significant risk of discontinuity in care management for people with serious mental illness. With thoughtful planning, however, correctional facilities and systems can develop and support policies and practices that not only minimize therapeutic disruption but also work to enhance therapeutic and functional outcomes.

References

Appelbaum, K. L. (2009). Attention deficit hyperactivity disorder in prison: A treatment protocol. *Journal of the American Academy of Psychiatry and the Law, 37*(1), 45–49.

Baillargeon, J., Penn, J., Knight, K., Harzke, A. J., Baillargeon, G., & Becker, E. A. (2010). Risk of reincarceration among prisoners with co-occurring severe mental illness and substance use disorders. *Administration and Policy in Mental Health and Mental Health Services Research, 37*(4), 367–374.

Gutheil, T. G. (2012). Reflections on ethical issues in psychopharmacology: An American perspective. *International Journal of Law and Psychiatry, 35*(5–6), 387–391.

Lichtenstein, P., Halldner, L., Zetterqvist, J., et al. (2012). Medication for attention deficit-hyperactivity disorder and criminality. *New England Journal of Medicine, 367*, 2006–2014.

Mojtabai, R., & Olfson, M. (2010). National trends in psychotropic medication polypharmacy in office-based psychiatry. *Archives of General Psychiatry, 67*(1), 26–36.

Novick, D., Haro, J. M., Suarez, D., Perez, V., Dittmann, R. W., & Haddad, P. M. (2010). Predictors and clinical consequences of non-adherence with antipsychotic medication in the outpatient treatment of schizophrenia. *Psychiatry Research, 176*(2), 109–113.

Phillips, D. (2012). Wellbutrin®: Misuse and abuse by incarcerated individuals. *Journal of Addictions Nursing, 23*(1), 65–69.

Preskorn, S. H., & Lacey, R. L. (2007). Polypharmacy: When is it rational? *Journal of Psychiatric Practice, 13*(2), 97–105.

Sered, S., & Norton-Hawk, M. (2013). Criminalized women and the health care system: The case for continuity of services. *Journal of Correctional Health Care, 19*(3), 164–177.

Tiihonen, J., Suokas, J. T., Suvisaari, J. M., Haukka, J., & Korhonen, P. (2012). Polypharmacy with antipsychotics, antidepressants, or benzodiazepines and mortality in schizophrenia. *Archives of General Psychiatry, 69*(5), 476–483.

Valuck, R. J., Morrato, E. H., Dodd, S., Oderda, G., Haxby, D. G., & Allen, R. (2007). Medicaid pharmacotherapy research consortium. How expensive is antipsychotic polypharmacy? Experience from five US state Medicaid programs. *Current Medical Research and Opinion, 23*(10), 2567–2576.

CHAPTER 20

Diagnostic review and revision

Sohrab Zahedi

Introduction

The criminalization of people with mental illness is a sad commentary on the US mental health system (Torrey, Kennard, Eslinger, et al., 2010). Yet, the phenomenon presents the field of psychiatry with an opportunity that is now scarce in civil society, that is, lengths of sentence in terms of weeks to years allow for in-depth observation and treatment of the inmate with mental illness. A few days in a hospital fails to provide the needed opportunity for a detailed and accurate evaluation. Today, people with mental illness account for more than 1 million annual arrests in the US (Hoge, Buchanan, Kovasznay, & Roskes, 2009), and many of these individuals will spend weeks to months in jail before being either transferred to a prison for sentences beyond one year or released back into the community. A mental disorder is defined as "a syndrome characterized by clinically significant disturbance in an individual's cognition, emotion regulation, or behavior that reflects a dysfunction in the psychological, biological, or developmental processes underlying mental functioning" (American Psychiatric Association, 2013). At its core, psychiatric diagnosis relies on the subjective complaints of the patient and objective signs noted on examination. Considering the chronic and fluctuating course of most psychiatric diagnoses, a thorough assessment also requires a review of past documented behaviors. When someone is hospitalized for a psychiatric condition, the first goal is often observation, followed by diagnosis, and then treatment. Psychiatric hospitals are being greatly constrained in the amount of time available for observation and accurate diagnosis; the correctional setting, as an unintended consequence of mass incarceration, provides an extended opportunity to achieve improved diagnostic accuracy. This chapter reflects on the diagnostic opportunities that a jail or prison setting affords.

Background

In the seventeenth century, Johann Weyer first theorized that deviant behavior stems from mental dysfunction that originally manifests as physical illness (Sarason & Ganzer, 1968). Cullen and Jackson later localized the source of mental dysfunction to the central nervous system (Sarason & Ganzer, 1968). Medicine's approach to assessment and treatment of dysfunctional behaviors (Ludwig & Othmer, 1977) made limited gains until the mid-twentieth century when organized attempts to classify psychiatric disorders were made and antipsychotics were discovered.

In the 1950s, hospitalization of a psychiatric patient typically spanned years. Ample opportunity existed for behavioral observation; symptoms were described in detail. The discovery of antipsychotics created an avenue, celebrated by psychiatrists, for tackling delusions, hallucinations, and agitation. In the following two decades, clinical optimism and social forces combined to push for the release of people with mental illness into communities (Brooks, 1986). Lengths of inpatient stay began to dwindle. In 1971, the average patient stay lasted 44 days. Only four years later, it was 26 days (Brooks, 1986). With fewer patient admissions, the second half of the twentieth century witnessed a rapid decline in the number of available beds in inpatient settings. In the 1950s, about 500,000 hospital beds existed in the United States (Hoge et al., 2009). Today only 44,000 beds are available. Original attempts to establish community treatment systems, while well intended, were underfunded and did not materialize (Brooks, 1986). Within a single generation, patients who previously spent years in asylums soon discovered themselves in a community with newfound liberties, including the options of refusing treatment and engaging in illicit drug use (Fisher et al., 2000). It did not help that substances of abuse were widely available. Punishment, not treatment, proved to be society's preference in tackling the problem of illicit drugs (Hoge et al., 2009).

In the 1980s, studies highlighted disproportionate rates of serious mental illness among the incarcerated compared to the general population. The Epidemiological Catchment Area Study reported one-year rates for schizophrenia and bipolar disorder of 5 percent and 6 percent, respectively, among the incarcerated. Similar numbers were found in state prisons, for example, 8 percent of New York State prisoners (Hoge et al., 2009). In the 1990s, Chicago's Cook County Jail had rates of schizophrenia, major depression, and bipolar disorder that were six times that of the national average (Fisher et al., 2000, p. 372). By 2010, jails and prisons housed three times as many mentally ill inmates as did hospitals (Stettin, Frese, & Lamb, 2013). Jails and prisons, initially flooded with individuals with severe mental illness, are now home to an increasing number of individuals with milder diagnoses (Hoge et al., 2009). In today's jails, 1 out of every 10 inmates is receiving psychotropic medications (Hoge et al., 2009).

The inmate with mental illness

Today's criminal courts are overwhelmed by the number of defendants with mental health problems. Some states have established specialized, problem-solving mental health courts (Stettin et al., 2013), with an aim to divert people with mental illness when benefits of treatment outweigh incarceration. As a rule, violent offenses are automatic exclusions from such diversion (Stettin et al., 2013). However, the magnitude of arrests has nevertheless led to more individuals with milder psychiatric conditions becoming incarcerated. In this population, the effects of drugs of abuse in circumstances that lead to an arrest cannot be overemphasized.

Once incarcerated, correctional administration is responsible for the provision of medical and mental health care. Diagnostic accuracy is essential as it guides proper treatment and should mitigate against symptoms (i.e., behaviors) that lead to violations of facility rules (Appelbaum, Hickey, & Packer, 2001). Jail and prison environments are highly stressful, even for inmates without mental health issues (Jablensky, 2012). It is not uncommon for individuals who did not require psychiatric attention at admission to eventually require care due to emergent symptoms. Considering the structured setting and decreased availability of substances of abuse that a correctional setting offers, any external evidence of dysfunctional behavior without possibility of secondary gain should be viewed as presumptive evidence of an underlying psychiatric disorder. Such diagnostic findings in the relative absence of confounders constitute one of the advantages of a correctional setting. These opportunities are absent for patients who are treated in the community where many unrecognized independent factors can color clinical presentations.

Every new inmate receives a basic medical screening as part of initial processing (see Chapter 11). The screen includes a psychiatric component so those who need monitoring and ongoing treatment are identified and referred to the mental health service. A psychiatric assessment relies on expressed, observed, or known symptoms and/or functional impairment based on previous incarcerations or documented history. Some patients arrive with the capacity to clearly convey their needs. Many, however, lack knowledge of their medications, diagnosis, or even which community clinic is responsible for their care. In such circumstances, input from a community pharmacist can inform staff about medication parameters, levels of adherence, and even contact information about community clinicians (see Chapter 19). Acute behavioral issues, when present, trigger immediate psychiatric attention and placement in a specialized housing unit with monitoring (e.g., for assessment of behavioral, neurological, and autonomic functioning). Severe medical issues, for example autonomic instability in a patient who is withdrawing from substances, may call for intensive interventions (e.g., intravascular access or continuous cardiac monitoring) and a prompt transfer to an affiliated hospital.

Three fourths of inmates with mental health issues have substance misuse comorbidities (James & Glaze, 2006). About 60 percent used drugs in the month prior to arrest (Hoge et al., 2009). Upon arrival, these inmates are often subject to the acute symptoms of substance withdrawal. A specialized psychiatric housing unit within a jail provides for initial observation of the psychiatric disease process. Medical or psychiatric housing units may be used for detoxification purposes. Such housing units are also present in prisons for intensive observation of inmates with sudden mental status changes. While the availability of drugs of abuse is reduced in a correctional environment, an inmate may still procure illicit substances and become acutely intoxicated. Psychotic symptoms, agitation, and confusion are diagnostically challenging as they can be induced by many substances and illnesses (see Chapter 17; Carpenter, 1976). Vigilance in establishing the proper diagnosis is essential as symptomatic inmates are at risk of continued in-house rule infractions, compromising the safety and order of correctional institutions (Appelbaum et al., 2001). Management of these individuals, even when they are

well known to the psychiatric service, includes assistance in the process of acclimation or adaptation to the environment and its inherent stressors (Appelbaum et al., 2001). Again, the relatively substance-free and structured environment in jails and prisons provides an opportunity for diagnostic investigation that is rarely seen in community settings. Sentenced or pretrial inmates with severe mental illness who remain compromised are further stabilized, triaged, and transferred to infirmaries or residential treatment units equipped with higher staff-to-patient ratios for further observation and treatment.

Diagnostic opportunities

Given the high rate of drug use immediately before incarceration, the initial hours and days of incarceration constitute a period of diagnostic uncertainty as intoxication or withdrawal influence the clinical picture. As a rule, newly incarcerated inmates who present with observable signs of psychosis, agitation, or confusion require intensive management. The process of initial stabilization in a specialized housing unit is followed by weeks to months of routine observation in general housing units, affording the chance to observe and develop more accurate diagnoses. If acute issues arise at regular intervals, these contribute to the appropriate recognition of conditions that are truly cyclical in nature.

Scenario: psychosis

BR is a 26-year-old woman admitted to the local jail; she is agitated and yelling that the voices are "driving her crazy." At intake, she states she is prescribed an anticonvulsant and an antipsychotic; a call to the local pharmacy confirms the prescriptions by a local clinic, but none have been filled in the past three months. The patient states she has been treated for bipolar disorder. The toxicology screen is positive for cocaine and phencyclidine. She is treated symptomatically and detoxified. Following stabilization and a few weeks of observation on a general housing unit, her medications are weaned and eventually discontinued. Routine observation during the rest of her sentence confirms an absence of symptoms and normal daily functioning with no medication. This process allows for a reconsideration of the diagnosis of bipolar disorder.

Most seriously mentally ill individuals never receive community treatment (Fisher et al., 2000). Therefore, an inmate who presents symptomatically may come to clinical attention for the first time. A lack of capacity for following orders or adhering to institutional rules is often associated with the cognitive compromise one sees with nonagitated psychotic individuals. While psychosis may signal schizophrenia (Viron, Baggett, & Hill, 2012), it is by no means pathognomonic. The differential includes a broad array of conditions including intoxication, withdrawal, delirium, infection, endocrine abnormalities, metabolic changes, electrolyte imbalance, and neurological issues (see Chapter 38). The approach to acute psychosis is pragmatic—treat the symptoms while ruling out secondary causes. This calls for observation in an infirmary health care setting where behavior and vital signs are regularly monitored.

Much like the inmate who presents with psychosis, inmates who arrive in an agitated or disoriented state cannot be relied upon to provide a coherent or complete history. Management is symptomatic as the differential diagnoses include many conditions, including delirium. In such cases and especially if the inmate is disoriented, transfer to a local hospital or an adequately staffed jail-based infirmary with frequent assessment of vital signs and neurological checks is indicated. Subsequent observation and management in less acute settings allows diagnostic clarification over a period of weeks to months.

Scenario: evolving dementia

VH is a 42-year-old man who presents on admission in a confused and euphoric state. He asks staff to give him a ride home. Due to previous arrests, he is known to staff as having a long history of intravenous heroin dependence, schizophrenia, and infection with HIV. Asked if he was recently misusing heroin, he states "of course." He complains of diffuse body aches, is seen talking to the wall, and, except for an elevated heart rate, his vital signs are within normal range. He undergoes an uneventful buprenorphine detoxification and is closely observed for the next 72 hours. Hallucinations are treated with antipsychotics and his HIV is treated with antiretrovirals. VH regains his sense of orientation, but a mild to moderate degree of cognitive compromise and active hallucinations remain. He is transferred to a subacute housing unit where several additional weeks of observation demonstrate no further improvement in cognition; hallucinations persist at a mild, less intrusive level. Neuropsychological screening confirms a dementing process. In addition to the historical diagnoses, VH is now diagnosed with HIV dementia.

For inmates with the capacity to convey subjective symptoms, efforts should be made to objectively corroborate their history. Feigning or exaggerating symptoms for secondary gain (e.g., a single cell, double meal portions, access to sedating drugs) is always a concern in correctional settings but should never lead to diagnostic cynicism (see Chapter 23). For example, the inmate who reports thoughts of suicide may need close observational status. If actively engaging in self-harm, the inmate may need a safety garment. Though resistant to use as a ligature in attempted suicide, safety garments are not very comfortable. How an individual reacts to such a status may, at times, be diagnostic; however, assessments based on just their reaction holds significant risk (see Chapter 43). Inmates who simply seek single-cell housing or other privileges may stop their self-destructive behaviors when confronted with a safety gown. Such inmates may be identified as malingerers or "behaviorally" disruptive. However, the possibility exists that someone truly at risk may behave in a similar fashion, placing him or herself at further risk. Regardless, familiarity with an inmate's behavioral responses to frustrations or triggers assists in maintaining safety. Such information requires observation that lasts weeks to months and can serve to guide the treatment approach once the individual is released back into the community.

It is not unusual in a correctional setting, especially when the mental health system is inadequate or problematic, for an inmate with a serious mental illness to exaggerate or malinger symptoms for a variety of reasons that include attempting to deal with housing issues, debts, and/or not receiving appropriate mental health treatment despite the presence of a serious mental illness. It is very common under such circumstances for the mental health clinician to focus on the malingering or "manipulative behavior" and to ignore the inmate's mental health symptoms, which often leads to poor clinical and correctional outcomes. Manipulative behavior is often a very adaptive mechanism for inmates from their perspectives; when this behavior is discussed with them in a nonjudgmental manner, a more effective means for the inmates to interact within the correctional system can be promoted.

In establishing or verifying a diagnosis, correctional clinicians should draw on all available collateral sources of information. These include local mental health authorities, pharmacies (see Chapter 19), family members, and records departments at hospitals. However, the correctional setting has additional sources of behavioral input, including an inmate's arrest report, criminal history, and behavior while in court or in their current housing unit, as well as records from previous incarcerations. The arrest report, in particular, can be very telling as it documents the patient's dysfunctional behaviors that led to incarceration. Such collateral information serves multiple purposes. Clarification of diagnosis (including influence of malingering or substances) is the primary clinical value. Recognition of maladaptive behaviors is another important purpose, with the hope of reducing recidivism risk through therapeutic rehabilitation (see Chapters 41 and 42). A proper diagnosis also holds the potential to improve quality of life.

Scenario: bipolar disorder

AC is a 30-year-old woman sentenced for assault and child endangerment who has served two years of her five-year sentence. She was admitted with a diagnosis of schizophrenia and substance use disorder (cocaine and marijuana; in current forced remission). She has been maintained on an antipsychotic, has been compliant with medication, and is functioning well. Yesterday, she began to sing loudly in her cell and tell people on her cell block that if they had sex with her, she had the power "to save them and make them holy." She was brought to the infirmary for observation; a urine toxicology screen was negative for substances of abuse. It became clear very quickly that she was experiencing mania. An anticonvulsant was added to her regimen, bringing the mania under control over the next few days. Her diagnosis was changed from schizophrenia to schizoaffective disorder, bipolar subtype. After the patient stabilized, a detailed review of her history suggested that her last manic episode was associated with the behavior that led to her arrest and conviction.

Once a preliminary working diagnosis has been determined or verified or when an inmate has been sentenced, specialized psychiatric units within a prison system that provide the level of care that is equivalent to that in a residential treatment program in the community can accommodate most chronic conditions (see Chapter 22). These settings allow for further observation and enhanced diagnostic accuracy.

Lengths of incarceration, even for some presentenced individuals, are longer than most inpatient hospital admissions. Experience shows that many individuals with mental illness who pass "under the radar" of initial processing will come to clinical attention because of in-house dysfunction, all too often in a crisis situation (see Chapter 25). Estimates point to half of inmates reporting active symptoms of mental illness during incarceration

(James & Glaze, 2006; Hoge et al., 2009). Over 40 percent note changes in appetite, psychomotor activity, feeling worthless, or excessive guilt in response to a self-report survey. One-third report persistent sadness, numbness, feelings of emptiness, or difficulty concentrating; over 10 percent affirm one or more symptoms consistent with psychosis (James & Glaze, 2006).

In most correctional facilities, individuals with milder psychiatric conditions (e.g., mild to moderate anxiety and nonsuicidal depression) can be managed at the community equivalent of an outpatient level of care with regular clinic visits. During any visit, safety risk and symptom management are universal concerns that should balance a strict reliance on the individual's report with objective data and/or collateral sources of information. The corollary is that quietly paranoid individuals often lack the insight to seek care. These individuals resist the idea of needing clinical attention. Therefore, what a patient states may poorly correlate with behavior that occurs while on a housing unit and under the watchful eye of prison staff. A healthy index of suspicion should always be present for inmates with apparent conditions that are less severe than anticipated. Many patients are able to temporarily marshal resources to minimize symptoms and enhance behavior. While this is potentially very valuable and consistent with a recovery model of care (see Chapter 40), the risk is that underreported symptoms may lead to behavioral dysfunction, violation of facility rules, or a risk of harm. In this regard, input from correctional staff may be quite valuable in diagnostic assessment, treatment adherence, and treatment response (Appelbaum et al., 2001). For the alert correctional officer, changes in an inmate's self-care or the development of irritability, bizarre behavior, or irrational speech should lead to direct communication with clinical staff. Information about treatment nonadherence or about vulnerable inmates who receive bad legal or personal news can and should be immediately communicated between services (Appelbaum et al., 2001). While clinical staff should be sensitive to the protection of clinical confidentiality, flow of information between clinical and security services cannot be effective if it is not reasonably open (Appelbaum et al., 2001).

Institutional cultures can, at times, interfere with clinical assessment because inmates with serious psychiatric issues can become labeled with perceived "behavioral" dysfunction. The "behavioral" label attaches a manipulative motivation to an inmate's dysfunction, whereas the behavior may be associated with character pathology, disinhibition secondary to traumatic brain injury, or intellectual disability (see Chapters 36, 52, and 53), all of which should be managed therapeutically. The treatment of these challenging individuals may include skill, deficit, and neuropsychological assessment as well as limit setting to curb destructive behaviors (where found). Treatment team planning that engages the inmate will help to gain the patient's trust and compliance (Appelbaum et al., 2001). A successful behavioral management approach often stems from the proper diagnosis (see Chapter 50). As the patient becomes eligible for release to the community, this information can be highly valuable to community clinicians in continuity of care.

Professional allies

The effective correctional psychiatrist has to have trusting, supportive, and collaborative relationships with medical, nursing, and correctional staffs. Irrespective of housing and throughout an inmate's stay, input by custody staff who observe patients for periods of weeks to years assists in assessment and management. Stationed officers can become very familiar with an inmate's behavioral patterns and routines. Such information can assist functionally impaired inmates with prompts to attend appointments, adhere with treatment, and alert clinicians when behavioral changes are observed. Except for a dwindling number of modern asylum beds, such levels of observation and familiarity with an individual are generally absent in community settings that provide clinical care. The ideal officer is one who is "firm but fair" in balancing security with treatment, which results in a mental health service that is both safe and therapeutic (Appelbaum et al., 2001). The correctional psychiatrist needs to establish a predictable presence within the housing units in order to establish good working relationships with the custody and nursing staffs and facilitate an effective flow of communication.

The medical primary care provider is another essential ally of the psychiatrist. The high rate of medical comorbidity among inmates with mental illness is well documented (Viron et al., 2012). The life expectancy of an adult with serious mental illness is 25 years shorter than that of the general population, with cardiovascular disease accounting for most of the mortality burden (Viron et al., 2012). Scarcity of medical resources provides a psychiatrist the opportunity to exercise discretion in tackling not just a patient's psychiatric issues but medical ones as well. For example, an inmate with schizophrenia who has come to trust the psychiatrist may be ill served by having the management of hypertension discovered during a psychiatric evaluation deferred to the primary care provider. Collaborative management of the patient's hypertension often yields improved care. Such effort calls for trust and frequent verbal consultation with the primary care provider (Jablensky, 2012).

Summary

The opportunities that correctional settings provide for diagnosis of inmates with mental illness have been reviewed in this chapter. Priorities of initial management include rapid stabilization and mitigation of the effects of situational stress and/or recent substance abuse. At this stage, establishment of an accurate diagnosis can be very challenging. Once stabilized, follow-up treatment and routine observational status provide the opportunity to fine-tune diagnosis and management. This approach calls for close coordination and communication among psychiatric, medical, nursing, and correctional staffs. Insights gained from such collaboration extend beyond establishment of an accurate diagnosis to improved management of basic medical issues and recognition of behavioral patterns of individual inmates. This opportunity depends on open and regular communication among psychiatry, medical, nursing, and custody staffs. Untreated mental illness can be disruptive to any correctional environment and detrimental to the patient's health. As physicians in the asylums of the twenty-first century, correctional psychiatrists should embrace the opportunity to properly and safely manage this highly stigmatized and vulnerable patient population.

References

American Psychiatric Association. (2013). Use of the manual. In *Diagnostic and statistical manual of mental disorders* (5th ed.). Arlington, VA: American Psychiatric Association.

Appelbaum, K. L., Hickey, J. M., & Packer, I. (2001). The role of correctional officers in multidisciplinary mental health care in prisons. *Psychiatric Services, 52,* 1343–1347.

Brooks, A. D. (1986). Law and antipsychotic medications. *Behavioral Sciences and the Law, 4,* 247–263.

Carpenter, W. T. (1976). Current diagnostic concepts in schizophrenia. *American Journal of Psychiatry, 133,* 172–177.

Fisher, W. H., Packer, I. K., Simon, L. J., et al. (2000). Community mental health services and prevalence of severe mental illness in local jails: Are they related? *Administration and Policy in Mental Health, 27,* 371–382.

Hoge, S. K., Buchanan, A. W., Kovasznay, B. M., & Roskes, E. J. (2009). *Outpatient services for the mentally ill involved in the criminal justice system: Task Force report.* Arlington, VA: American Psychiatric Association.

Jablensky, A. (2012). The disease entity in psychiatry: fact or fiction? *Epidemiology and Psychiatric Sciences, 21,* 255–264.

James, D. J., & Glaze, L. E. (2006). *Mental health problems of prison and jail inmates* (NCJ 213600). Washington, DC: Department of Justice. Office of Justice Programs—Bureau of Justice and Statistics. Retrieved from http://www.bjs.gov/content/pub/pdf/mhppji.pdf

Ludwig, A. M., & Othmer, E. (1977). The medical basis of psychiatry. *American Journal of Psychiatry, 134,* 1087.

Sarason, I. G., & Ganzer, V. J. (1968). Concerning the medical model. *American Psychologist, 23,* 507–510.

Stettin, B., Frese, F. J., & Lamb, H. R. (2013). *Mental health diversion practices: A survey of the states.* Treatment Advocacy Center. Retrieved from http://tacreports.org/storage/documents/2013-diversion-study.pdf

Torrey, E. F., Kennard, A. D., Eslinger, D., Lamb, R., & Pavle, J. (2010). *More mentally ill persons are in jails and prisons than hospitals: A survey of the states.* Treatment Advocacy Center. Retrieved from http://www.treatmentadvocacycenter.org/storage/documents/final_jails_v_hospitals_study.pdf

Viron, M., Baggett, T., & Hill, M. (2012). Schizophrenia for primary care providers: How to contribute to the care of a vulnerable patient population. *American Journal of Medicine, 125,* 223–230.

CHAPTER 21

Diversion programs and alternatives to incarceration

Merrill Rotter and Virginia Barber-Rioja

Introduction

The reported prevalence of individuals with mental illness in jails and prisons varies widely in the literature and government reports, from as low as 15% to as high as 50% (Baillargeon, Binswanger, Penn, Williams, & Murray, 2009). This variability results from both differences in settings and in definitions of what constitutes mental illness. However, even by the most stringent definitions, the prevalence of mental illness in jails and prisons is several times higher than in the general population. Individuals with mental illness are admitted to jails at approximately eight times the rate at which they are admitted to public psychiatric hospitals (Torrey et al., 1992). The causes of what has been termed "criminalization of the mentally ill" include the downsizing of state hospitals, hospitalization admission criteria that require dangerous behavior, inadequate community treatment resources, and the behaviors associated with comorbid substance use. Adding insult to the injury of criminal justice confinement is the potentially noxious and traumatizing environment that incarceration represents for individuals with mental illness—that is, the stresses typically associated with jail and prison and the frequent lack of adequate clinical care. In addressing the problem proactively, the primary approach has been to divert justice-involved individuals with mental illness into appropriate community care. This chapter includes a review of the major models used to divert those with serious mental illness from incarceration, paying attention to some of the legal and clinical issues that arise as a result of diversion initiatives.

Background

While diversion programming for justice-involved individuals with mental illness has received significant attention over the past two decades, the establishment of such programs was a recommendation of the National Coalition for Jail Reform in the 1970s (Steadman, Cocozza, & Veysey, 1999a; Steadman, Deane, Morrisey, Westcott, Salasin, & Shapiro, 1999b). Early diversion efforts were focused on individuals with substance abuse disorders with the dual goals of improving defendant functioning and protecting the public. Although many of these defendants with substance abuse probably also had mental disorders, programs that explicitly extended alternative-to-incarceration opportunities to defendants with mental illness did not develop until the 1990s.

Whether for individuals with substance abuse, mental illness, or co-occurring disorders, diversion programs all require identification of clinical eligibility and referral to clinical services in lieu of incarceration and/or continued criminal justice processing (Steadman et al., 1999a, 1999b). The potential for identification and diversion can occur at several different points in the criminal justice continuum, from initial police contact through incarceration. Jurisdictions across the United States have used the Sequential Intercept Model to identify where to best implement diversion in their systems (Munetz & Griffin, 2006).

In general, diversion programs can be classified into two broad categories: pre-booking and post-booking. Pre-booking diversion occurs before an individual is arrested or formal charges have been filed. The police officer is the primary decision maker at this point in the process. Post-booking diversion (court- or jail-based) occurs after the subject has been arrested and formal charges have been filed (Broner, Borum, & Gawley, 2002). Because charges have been filed, post-booking diversion programs require a negotiated agreement among the court, the district attorney's office, and the defense attorney. The offer includes a community treatment alternative to incarceration and a final adjudication of the criminal case. When both the instant offense and the defendant's criminal record are less serious, charges may be dropped and a referral to treatment made. More often, the defendant must plead guilty, with final sentencing (often to a lesser charge) held in abeyance until completion of mandated treatment. Mental health courts (MHCs) are diversion programs where all mentally ill defendants are handled in a single court part (Steadman, Davidson, & Brown, 2001). MHCs often use their own staff to divert and monitor clients instead of relying on an external agency.

Pre-booking diversion

Between 3% and 6% of police contacts involve individuals with mental illness (Watson, Corrigan, & Ottati, 2004). This small percentage belies the fact that large cities have a significant number of interactions that are often fraught with peril for both police officers and perpetrators. Furthermore, police officers play the pivotal role in deciding whether a person with mental illness is processed through the criminal justice system or referred for clinical care (Teplin, 2000). An intervention that does not result in arrest and the filing of charges is considered pre-booking diversion (Amrhein & Barber-Rioja, 2010). Recognizing that police are often the first responders for individuals with mental illnesses, most police departments have mental health training, and some have specialized programs to maximize the possibility of safe interactions and pre-booking diversion (Teller, Munetz, Gil, & Ritter, 2006).

The primary model for specialized pre-booking diversion from which generalized principles have been explicated is the Crisis Intervention Team (CIT). Developed initially in Memphis, TN, there are now approximately 400 programs nationwide. The model includes voluntary assignment of police officers to a specialized response team, 40 hours of mental health training for these officers, and coordination with a designated emergency psychiatry service for seamless referrals. Training is the primary intervention and consists of education about the causes, signs, symptoms, and treatment of mental illness, as well as information about relevant mental hygiene law, local treatment providers, and de-escalation techniques (Dupont & Cochran, 2002).

Studies have demonstrated that CIT programs lower arrest rates of people with mental illness (Steadman et al., 2001; TAPA Center for Jail Diversion, 2004) and increase post-referral mental health use (TAPA Center for Jail Diversion, 2004). As noted later in this chapter with reference to post-booking diversion, a critical component of success is the availability of community-based mental health services (Compton, Bahora, Watson, & Oliva, 2008).

Post-booking diversion: decentralized diversion

Despite extensive support for diversion, there are limited empirical studies of post-booking diversion programs. Further, different methodologies and outcome measures of program efficacy make direct comparisons challenging. The programs themselves also differ in the duration of court involvement, whether the person was mandated to treatment, the intensity of community outreach, incorporation of court monitoring of case management services, the capacity and quality of treatment providers, and the types of individuals identified for diversion (i.e., felony or misdemeanor, violent or nonviolent, diagnoses, and criminal justice history). Several themes, however, do emerge.

The earliest national survey of mental health diversion programs was conducted in 1995. The study estimated that only 52 programs existed in the United States and that five components were associated with the highest rates of success: all relevant mental health, substance abuse, and criminal justice agencies were involved in program development; regular meetings between key personnel from the various agencies were held; integration of services was encouraged through the efforts of a liaison; the programs had strong leadership; and nontraditional case management approaches were used (Steadman, 1995).

Since that time, several controlled longitudinal studies of program effectiveness have compared diverted offenders with offenders released to the community following adjudication of their cases without diversion. The primary outcomes shared among most of these studies are duration of time in jail, occurrence of re-arrest, type of treatment, symptom burden, presence and severity of substance abuse, and occurrence of hospitalizations (Hoff, Rosenheck, Baranosky, Buchanan, & Zonana, 1999; Lamb, Weinberger, & Reston-Parham, 1996; Shafer, Arthur, & Franczak, 2004; Steadman et al., 1999b; Weisman, Lamberti, & Price, 2004). In general, offenders who received diversion services spent less time in jail before release and were less likely to

be re-arrested (Hoff et al., 1999; Weisman et al., 2004). Clinical outcomes were more varied; some studies showed improvements in access to treatment, symptoms, and substance abuse (Steadman et al., 1999a, 1999b; Weisman et al., 2004), while others did not find symptom improvement (Shafer et al., 2004).

Interestingly, diversion was associated with an increased risk of hospitalization (Steadman et al., 1999a). This is often seen in the clinical literature as a negative outcome. With respect to jail diversion, however, this may actually be a positive indicator of closer symptom monitoring and clinical management. Factors predictive of positive outcomes included medication compliance while in jail and being mandated to treatment (Broner et al., 2002). In one large urban-based study, re-arrest rates were higher among diverted clients with histories of childhood trauma, psychopathy, and violence (Broner et al., 2002). Similarly, a large national review of more than 50 pre- and post-booking diversion programs found positive outcomes for both symptom improvement and decreased re-arrest; however, the symptom improvement was unrelated to the decreased criminal behavior. The best predictor of re-arrest in that study was the number of prior arrests (Case, Steadman, Dupuis, & Morris, 2009).

Centralized diversion: mental health courts

An alternative to incarceration programming for defendants with mental illness can be centralized in a single court docket (Steadman et al., 2001). These MHCs are one example of the more general category of problem-solving courts where the primary focus is on decreasing criminal recidivism rather than merely ensuring a fair process. The premise of problem-solving courts is that public safety goals can be met by directly addressing the problem associated with criminal activity. Examples include courts dedicated to domestic violence, trafficking (prostitution), and veterans. The most numerous of all are the drug courts: at present, there are more than 2,700 in the United States (US Department of Justice, 2013).

MHCs were created to address the problem of criminal behavior in persons with untreated or undertreated mental illness. As discussed later in this chapter, this association may be less robust than originally thought. MHCs were established due to the beliefs that mental illness may mitigate criminal behavior, that jails and prisons are especially noxious environments for individuals with mental illness, and that traditional court sanctions for mandate violations (in particular, remand to jail) are at best not effective and at worst destructive.

The first MHC was established in the late 1980s. The Broward County (Florida) Mental Health Court, which opened in 1996, was the first to be studied. Serving defendants charged with misdemeanors, the court improved access to mental health services without defendants feeling coerced into accepting the plea and treatment offered (McGaha, Boothroyd, Poythress, Petrila, & Ort, 2002).

As of 2013, there are more than 350 MHCs across the United States (Goodale, Callahan, & Steadman, 2013). It is often said, "If you've seen one mental health court, you've seen one mental health court." These courts vary widely based on clinical and legal target population, length and extent of court mandate, standard plea arrangements, makeup and responsibility of the court team, venue for identification, assessment and treatment planning, community service availability, and expectations for program completion (Redlich, 2005). The temperament and philosophy of the judge also play important roles in program and client success (Redlich, 2005).

However, successful MHCs do share several important elements, including the following: mentally ill defendants are handled on a single court docket with a specific judge and an assigned prosecutor and defense attorney; a clinical team is available that includes a clinical specialist who recommends and makes linkages to treatment; availability of appropriate clinical placement is ensured before the judge makes a ruling on diversion; and specialized court monitoring is in place with possible sanctions for noncompliance (Steadman et al., 2001). As with decentralized diversion, plea arrangements differ among jurisdictions and cases (Petrila, 2003). However, as these courts have accepted defendants with more serious charges, treatment mandates and use of criminal justice sanctions for noncompliance are increasingly part of the program (Redlich, Steadman, Monahhan, Petrila, & Griffin, 2005).

Sanctions and rewards

Sanctions and rewards in a drug court are typically prescribed and straightforward (National Association of Drug Court Professionals, 1997). Sanctions in an MHC are, as a rule, more flexible. The possibility that the violation may be the result of the underlying mental illness, rather than the flouting of judicial authority, is explicitly taken into account. Minor interventions often mimic the increased structure and support found in the clinical environment (e.g., increasing the frequency of contact with case manager or court). Remand to jail is the last resort and is reserved in most courts for situations in which immediate public safety concerns cannot be managed any other way.

Mental health court research

Studies of the efficacy of the MHC model are predominantly of two designs. A pre–post design is most common. Indices of clients' social, criminal, and clinical function before and after participation in MHC are compared. A comparison design is the alternative in which similar indices are studied between MHC participants and a matched sample of offenders who received routine criminal justice processing. The variability in actual program design, outcome measures, and length of follow-up after intervention makes it challenging to compare programs. Despite that, as with decentralized diversion, several themes emerge. Participants in MHCs receive more treatment in the community and show reductions in drug use, days spent in jail, and rates of re-arrest both while in the program and after program completion relative to either their own baseline or comparison group controls (Cosden, Ellens, Schnell, Yamini-Diouf, & Wolfe, 2003; Moore & Hiday, 2006; Steadman, Redlich, Callahan, Robbins, & Vesselinov, 2011; Trupin & Richards, 2003). Interestingly, symptomatic improvement is not always observed, despite overall programmatic success (Boothroyd, Mercado, & Poythress, 2005). This may be due, in part, to a baseline effect—that is, client clinical stability is often required prior to community placement.

As noted previously, one factor that is critical for success is the demeanor of the judge and the atmosphere in the courtroom

(Redlich et al. 2005). Rather than a dispassionate arbiter of courtroom rules, the MHC judge presents a more collaborative and even supportive persona to the defendant while maintaining ultimate authority over enforcement of the treatment mandate. MHC judges may ask defendants about treatment, school, job, family, or other areas of importance to the defendants. It is not unusual for judges to compliment defendants on their community-based successes. In such an atmosphere, defendants perceive an enhanced sense of voluntariness and fairness. The interaction with the judge has been shown to be relevant to success in previous drug court studies. In MHCs, the research in this area is scarce and results are mixed. Some studies have suggested that judges' use of praise and increased eye contact may be related to positive outcomes (Frailing, 2010; Wales & Hiday, 2010), whereas other studies found no differences in defendants' perceptions between a judge who made more supportive or praising comments versus another judge who did not (Kopelovich, Yanos, Pratt, & Hoerner, 2013).

The few studies of defendant characteristics associated with successful program completion are mostly from the drug court rather than the MHC literature. These characteristics, which overlap with one another, include race, gender, the nature of the instant offense, the extensiveness of the prior criminal history and drug use, and antisocial personality disorder (Mattson, Bardley, Halfaker, Akeson, & Ben-Porath, 2012; Stein, Deberard, & Homan, 2013). Whether a defendant's profile is indicative of program success is, of course, intimately linked to the availability of the necessary services in the community.

As noted previously, one characteristic increasingly thought not to be directly relevant to program success—at least as defined by decreased recidivism—is mental illness. That is to say, positive clinical outcomes are not associated with decreased recidivism (Jurginger, Claypoole, Laygo, & Crisanti, 2006). Past criminality is the best predictor of success in this regard. This, in turn, is in keeping with literature that suggests that serious mental illness (i.e., psychotic disorders) is a factor in less than 10% of crimes and that offenders with serious mental illness have many of the social and personality factors associated with criminality in offenders without mental illness (Peterson, Skeem, Hart, Vidal, & Keith, 2010). To this end, many MHCs and diversion programs are including the Risk-Needs-Responsivity (Andrews & Bonta, 2010) paradigm as part of their assessment for program inclusion and treatment planning. This model includes a formal evaluation of recidivism risk to adjust levels of supervision and an explicit review of recidivism-related dynamic factors as targets for intervention. Substance abuse treatment, vocational and educational support, family involvement, and the availability of prosocial activities and peers have historically been part of many programs. Antisocial factors such as antisocial personality disorder and antisocial thinking have received recent attention. Governmental grant-making bodies and diversion programs are increasingly including assessment and cognitive-behavioral interventions to address these issues. Cognitive-behavioral change programs such as Interactive Journaling (Proctor, Hoffmann, & Allison, 2012), Thinking for a Change (Golden, 2002), Moral Reconation Therapy (Little & Robinson, 1988), and Reasoning and Rehabilitation (Ross, Fabiano, & Ewles, 1988) can now be found as part of the treatment expectations for community programs affiliated with diversion projects or delivered by clinicians and case managers within the diversion team.

Jail diversion, in general, and MHCs, in particular, are not without their detractors. Among the criticisms are that diversion programs engage in "net widening." In this context, defendants who may otherwise have had the opportunity for release (after trial or plea bargain) are kept under judicial supervision with the potential for incarceration for an extended period. For example, take the situation of a case that might be difficult to prosecute and would likely result in an acquittal. This case might be referred to a mental health diversion program where a plea deal is offered. The defendant might find it difficult to refuse the deal and be subjected to longer criminal justice oversight. Defendants' interests give way to a paternalistic, clinically focused intervention that is inherently coercive. While defendants often waive privilege as a prerequisite for program participation, there may still be concerns about sharing confidential clinical information with the public at large in open court and with the judge and prosecutor. One additional concern is the potential that such information may influence criminal justice decisions.

Summary

Decreasing the number of individuals with mental illness in the criminal justice system remains a public mental health priority—one that has even reached the US Supreme Court (*Brown v. Plata*, 2011). Diverting individuals with mental illness from jail or prison decreases their exposure to that traumatic environment and addresses security concerns of corrections professionals charged with their care and management. When diversion is coupled with the court-based, problem-solving approach of monitored care and treatment in the community, public safety is improved and the clinical success of the individual is enhanced. When treatment in the community includes an explicit focus on criminogenic factors, the ability to meet public safety goals is enhanced even further. And when, as recommended, participation in the program and proposed treatment plan is truly voluntary (i.e., defendants choose to participate intelligently and competently), these programs are consistent with the mental health recovery approach critical to community stability and long-term success.

Given these goals and the considerable variability from jurisdiction to jurisdiction in court resources, treatment resources, social supports, political philosophies, and fiscal realities, the types of diversion that will work for one community may not work for another. However, most of the data are clear that diversion can be implemented with documented success in the domains described previously and that there are several beneficial models for client intercept and associated programming.

The "does diversion work?" question has been answered in the affirmative, and we are beginning to delineate better the population for whom diversion works. However, to understand what works, for whom, and how, one actually needs to define "works." Definitions include avoiding incarceration, decreasing recidivism, providing access to treatment, diminishing symptoms, improving social functioning, extracting a better criminal justice deal, saving public funds, or any combination of these. The good news is that these are achievable goals. The challenge for program developers and policymakers is to decide on the priorities and determine what is possible in their jurisdiction.

References

Amrhein, C., & Barber-Rioja, V. (2010). Jail diversion models. In S. A. Estrine, R. T. Hettenbach, H. Arthur, & M. Messina (Eds.), *Service delivery for vulnerable populations: New directions in behavioral health* (pp. 329–352). New York: Springer.

Andrews, D. A., & Bonta, J. (2010). Rehabilitating criminal justice policy and practice. *Psychology, Public Policy, and Law, 16*, 39–55.

Baillargeon, J., Binswanger, I. A., Penn, J. V., Williams, B. A., & Murray, O. J. (2009). Psychiatric disorders and repeat incarceration: The revolving prison door. *American Journal of Psychiatry, 166*, 103–109.

Boothroyd, R. A., Mercado, C.C., & Poythress, N. G. (2005). Clinical outcomes of defendants in mental health court. *Psychiatric Services, 56*, 829–834.

Broner, N., Borum, R., & Gawley, K. (2002). Criminal justice diversion of individuals with co-occurring mental illness and substance use disorders: An overview. In G. Landsberg, M. Rock, L. Berg, & A. Smiley (Eds.), *Serving mentally ill offenders: Challenges and opportunities for mental health professionals* (pp. 83–107) New York: Springer Publishing.

Brown v. Plata, 131 S. Ct. 1910 (2011).

Case, B., Steadman, H. J., Dupuis, S. A., & Morris, L. S. (2009). Who succeeds in jail diversion programs for persons with mental illness? A multi-site study. *Behavioral Sciences and the Law, 27*, 661–674.

Compton, M. T., Bahora, M., Watson, A., & Oliva, J. (2008). A comprehensive review of extant research on Crisis Intervention Team (CIT) programs. *Journal of the American Academy of Psychiatry and the Law, 36*, 47–55.

Cosden, M., Ellens, J., Schnell, J., Yamini-Diouf, Y., & Wolfe, M. M. (2003). Evaluation of a mental health court with assertive community treatment. *Behavioral Sciences and the Law, 21*, 415–427.

Dupont, R., & Cochran, S. (2002). The Memphis CIT model. In G. Landsberg, M. Rack, & L. Berg (Eds.), *Serving mentally ill offenders: challenges and opportunities for mental health professionals* (pp. 59–70). New York: Springer Publishing.

Frailing, K. (2010). How mental health courts function: Outcomes and observations. *International Journal of Law and Psychiatry, 33*, 207–213.

Golden, L. (2002). Evaluation of the efficacy of a cognitive behavioral program for offenders on probation: Thinking for a Change. Retrieved from http://www/nicic.org/pubs/2002/018190.pdf

Goodale, G., Callahan, L., & Steadman, H. J. (2013). What can we say about mental health courts today? *Psychiatric Services, 64*, 298–300.

Hoff, R. A., Rosenheck, R. A., Baranosky, M. V., Buchanan, J., & Zonana, H. (1999). Diversion from jail of detainees with substance abuse: The interaction with dual diagnosis. *American Journal of Addictions, 8*, 377–386.

Jurginger, J., Claypoole, K., Laygo, R., & Crisanti, A. (2006). Effects of serious mental illness and substance abuse on criminal offenses. *Psychiatric Services, 57*, 879–882.

Kopelovich, S., Yanos, P., Pratt, C., & Hoerner, J. (2013). Procedural justice in mental health courts: Judicial practices, participant perceptions, and outcomes related to mental health recovery. *International Journal of Law and Psychiatry, 36*, 113–120.

Lamb, H. R., Weinberger, L. E., & Reston-Parham, C. (1996). Court interventions to address the mental health needs of mentally ill offenders. *Psychiatric Services, 47*, 275–281.

Little, G. L., & Robinson, K. D. (1988). Moral Reconation Therapy: A systematic step-by-step treatment system for treatment-resistant clients. *Psychological Reports, 62*, 135–161.

Mattson, C., Bardley, P., Halfaker, D., Akeson, S., & Ben-Porath, Y. (2012). Predicting drug court treatment completion using the MMPI-2-RF. *Psychological Assessment, 24*, 937–943.

McGaha, A., Boothroyd, R. A., Poythress, N. G., Petrila, J., & Ort, T. G. (2002). Lessons from the Broward County Mental Health Court. *Evaluation and Program Planning, 25*, 125–135.

Moore, E. M., & Hiday, V. A. (2006). Mental health court outcomes: A comparison of re-arrest and re-arrest severity between mental health court and traditional court participants. *Law and Human Behavior, 30*, 659–664.

Munetz, M. R., & Griffin, P.A. (2006). Use of the Sequential Intercept Model as an approach to decriminalization of people with serious mental illness. *Psychiatric Services, 57*, 544–549.

National Association of Drug Court Professionals (1997). Defining drug courts: The key components. Retrieved from http://www.nadcp.org/sites/default/files/nadcp/KeyComponents.pdf

Peterson, J., Skeem, J., Hart, E., Vidal, S., & Keith, F. (2010). Analyzing offense patters as a function of mental illness to test the criminalization hypothesis. *Psychiatric Services, 61*, 1217–1222.

Petrila, J. (2003). An introduction to special jurisdiction courts. *International Journal of Law and Psychiatry, 3*, 3–12.

Proctor, L., Hoffmann, N. G., & Allison, S. (2012). The effectiveness of interactive journaling in reducing recidivism among substance-dependent jail inmates. *International Journal of Offender Therapy and Comparative Criminology, 56*, 317–332.

Redlich, A. D. (2005). Voluntary, but knowing and intelligent. Comprehension in mental health courts. *Psychology, Public Policy and Law, 11*, 605–619.

Redlich, A. D., Steadman, H. J., Monahan, J., Petrila, J., & Griffin, P. A. (2005). The second generation of mental health courts. *Psychology, Public Policy, and Law, 11*(4), 527–538.

Ross, R. R., Fabiano, E. A., & Ewles, C. D. (1988). Reasoning and Rehabilitation. *International Journal of Offender Therapy and Comparative Criminology, 32*, 29–35.

Shafer, M. S., Arthur, B., & Franczak, M. J. (2004). An analysis of post-booking jail diversion programming for persons with co-occurring disorders. *Behavioral Sciences and the Law, 22*, 771–785.

Steadman, H. J. (1995). The diversion of mentally ill persons from jails to community based services: A profile of programs. *American Journal of Public Mental Health, 85*, 1630–1635.

Steadman, H. J., Cocozza, J. J., & Veysey, B. M. (1999a). Comparing outcomes for diverted and nondiverted jail detainees with mental illness. *Law and Human Behavior, 23*(6), 615–627.

Steadman, H. J., Davidson, S., & Brown, C. (2001). Mental health courts: their promise and unanswered questions. *Psychiatric Services, 52*, 457–458.

Steadman, H. J., Deane, M. W., Morrisey, J. P., Westcott, M. L., Salasin, S., & Shapiro, S. (1999b). A SAMHSA research initiative assessing the effectiveness of jail diversion programs for mentally ill persons. *Psychiatric Services, 50*, 1620–1623.

Steadman, H. J., Redlich, A., Callahan, L., Robbins, P., & Vesselinov, R. (2011). Effect of mental health courts on arrest and jail days: a multisite study. *Archives of General Psychiatry, 68*, 167–172.

Stein, D. M., Deberard, S., & Homan, K. (2013). Predicting success and failure in juvenile drug treatment court: A meta-analytic review. *Journal of Substance Abuse and Treatment, 44*, 159–168.

TAPA Center for Jail Diversion (2004). *What can we say about the effectiveness of jail diversion programs for persons with co-occurring disorders.* The National GAINS Center. Retrieved from http://gainscenter.samhsa.gov/pdfs/jail_diversion/WhatCanWeSay.pdf

Teller, J. L. S., Munetz, M. R., Gil, K. M., & Ritter, C. (2006). Crisis intervention team training for police officers responding to mental disturbance calls. *Psychiatric Services, 57*, 232–237.

Teplin, L. A. (2000). *Keeping the peace: Police discretion and mentally ill persons* (NIJ Journal, 244). Washington, DC: National Institute of Justice.

Torrey, E. F., Stieber, J., Wolfe, S. M., Sharfstein, J., Noble, J. H., & Flynn, L. M. (1992). *Criminalizing the Seriously Mentally Ill: The Abuse of Jails as Mental Hospitals.* Washington, DC: National Alliance for the Mentally Ill and Public Citizens Health Research Group.

Trupin, E., & Richards, H. (2003). Seattle's mental health courts: Early indicators of effectiveness. *International Journal of Law and Psychiatry, 26*, 33–53.

US Department of Justice (2013). Drug courts. Retrieved from https://ncjrs.gov/pdffiles1/nij/238527.pdf

Wales, H. W., & Hiday, B. R. (2010). Procedural justice and the mental health court judge's role in reducing recidivism. *International Journal of Law and Psychiatry, 33*, 265–271.

Watson, A. C., Corrigan, P. W., & Ottati, V. (2004). Police responses to persons with mental illness: Does the label matter? *Journal of the American Academy of Psychiatry and Law, 32*, 378–385.

Weisman, R. L., Lamberti, J. S., & Price, N. (2004). Integrating criminal justice community healthcare and support services for adults with severe mental disorders. *Psychiatric Quarterly, 75*, 71–85.

CHAPTER 22

Levels of care

Jeffrey L. Metzner and Kenneth L. Appelbaum

Introduction

Just as in community settings, correctional systems need a continuum of mental health care. In large part, these levels of care follow the community mental health center (CMHC) model. As part of John F. Kennedy's New Frontier, the purpose of the Community Mental Health Act of 1963 (CMHA) was to provide seed funding for community-based mental health care as an alternative to institutionalization. Subsequent amendments to the CMHA (1965, 1975) mandated that a CMHC that received federal funding provide a core set of services that included the following:

◆ Outpatient mental health services, including services for specific populations, such as children, the elderly, and individuals with chronic mental illness, in addition to substance abuse services;

◆ 24-hour-a-day emergency care services;

◆ Day care that includes partial hospitalization services and other aftercare services;

◆ Access to inpatient psychiatric treatment; and

◆ Community consultation and education for caretakers.

The CMHA was intended to promote deinstitutionalization of persons with chronic mental illness and establish a model of community-based mental health treatment. It is ironic that the CMHA may have contributed to "transinstitutionalization" into the correctional mental health system (i.e., jails and prisons) due primarily to lack of adequate community-based funding. Many aspects of the CMHC model, however, can be implemented in correctional settings.

The continuum of care for inmates with mental illness includes outpatient care, emergency services, day treatment, supported residential housing, infirmary care, and inpatient psychiatric hospitalization services. This chapter describes each level of care and how they may be adapted to function in correctional settings.

Levels of care—overview

The guidelines developed by the American Psychiatric Association (APA) define mental health treatment as the use of biological, psychological, and social therapies. The goals of treatment include relief of suffering, enhancement of safety, and alleviation of symptoms that significantly interfere with an inmate's ability to function. Policies and procedures that are consistent with the standards of correctional mental health care provide a structure for offering treatment in a multidisciplinary and eclectic manner (APA, 2000; Metzner, 1998).

Mental health services are generally provided in a continuum of treatment settings or levels of care. A comprehensive system of mental health services includes the following (Metzner, 1998):

Outpatient treatment service is the least intensive level of care. In some systems, this may include a day treatment program that provides enhanced mental health services similar to a residential program, as described below. In the case of outpatient treatment, participating inmates live in a general-population housing unit with other inmates, many of whom are not in need of mental health services.

A residential program (i.e., housing unit) within the correctional setting is provided for inmates with chronic mental illness who do not require inpatient treatment but do require enhanced mental health services. Such a designated housing unit can provide a safe and therapeutic environment for those unable to function adequately within the general inmate population.

Crisis intervention services include both brief counseling and supervised stabilization. The latter, often provided in an infirmary setting, serves short-term stabilization and/or diagnostic purposes. The length of stay in such settings is usually less than 10 days.

A psychiatric inpatient program is the most intensive level of care and is often provided by the state psychiatric hospital system.

The levels of mental health care offered to inmates in jails are often limited by their short stays and the size of the facility. Essential treatment services generally emphasize psychotropic medication management by a psychiatrist and crisis intervention, which may include short-term counseling and transfer to a special needs unit or infirmary. Inmates with longer pretrial confinements or sentences might receive more extensive counseling (APA, 2000; Metzner, 1998). Other essential services include mental health screening and referral assessments (see Chapter 11), a suicide prevention program (see Chapter 43), discharge planning, and timely access to a special mental health housing unit or inpatient psychiatric bed (APA, 2000). Jails also need adequate nursing staff for medication administration and often for continuous coverage of special mental health housing units.

When it is not cost-effective to hire their own mental health staff, small jails often contract with local mental health centers, private practitioners, or for-profit mental health companies to provide services. Unfortunately, especially with private practitioners who often do not understand the needs of a correctional mental health system, the hours contracted are often not enough to provide the necessary services. Inpatient mental health services may be obtained through the forensic division of the public hospital system following negotiations with the state department of mental health or an equivalent governmental agency.

Prison mental health systems are expected to provide a more comprehensive system of mental health care than jails due to their different mission, larger inmate population, longer duration of incarceration, and greater amount of resources (see Chapter 6). Although prisons require essential mental health services that are similar to those described for jails, they are more likely to provide access to special needs housing, inpatient psychiatric care, and psychosocial rehabilitation treatment for inmates with serious mental illness.

Every inmate who receives mental health services needs a written treatment plan. Such a plan is an individualized and often multidisciplinary statement of short- and long-term goals and the methods to achieve them, including the necessary level of care and discharge planning in residential settings (National Commission on Correctional Health Care, 2008). The comprehensiveness and frequency of treatment plan reviews vary depending on the level of care and the inmate's clinical condition. Specific triggers for reviews and revisions include changes in level of mental health care and failure to achieve goals.

Outpatient mental health services

An outpatient clinic provides mental health care to most inmates who receive those services in a correctional facility. These inmates usually live in the general population and enter outpatient services via the intake mental health screening process (see Chapter 11) or by self-referral or staff referral sometime during their incarceration. The latter may occur due to changing environmental stressors, despite a negative intake screen, or following discharge from a higher level (e.g., infirmary) of mental health care. Correctional outpatient clinics have a diverse range of treatment programs and philosophies, and they require supervision and a quality improvement process to ensure provision of appropriate services (Smith & Smith, 2006).

The development of protocols for psychotropic medications by class (e.g., antidepressants, antipsychotics, mood stabilizers) helps to ensure their appropriate use. Due to the high prevalence of substance abuse among correctional populations, many clinicians discourage use of sedative-hypnotic and antianxiety medications. Other commentators advocate for close monitoring of indications for and response to these medications as part of supervised protocols (Appelbaum, 2009).

Some systems limit individual outpatient psychotherapy to crisis intervention and supportive psychotherapy for inmates with serious mental illnesses because of limited resources. However, regular monthly psychotherapy sessions are often useful for inmates with severe behavioral disorders. Group psychotherapy is a cost-effective form of treatment within a prison setting (Metzner, 1998) and may be beneficial in large jail settings as well.

Staffing for outpatient clinic services should include psychiatrists and other mental health clinicians such as psychologists, social workers, and nurses. Clerical staff provide valuable assistance with scheduling and other administrative functions (e.g., obtaining health care records) necessary to operate an effective outpatient clinic. Staffing allocations designed to ensure adequate

inmate access to needed mental health resources vary based on local differences and needs. Metzner has summarized staffing allocation guidelines developed by the state of New York and by a blue-ribbon consultation panel in Massachusetts (Metzner, 1997). The APA (2000) recommends one full-time psychiatrist for every 75 to 100 jail inmates with a serious mental illness or 150 prison inmates on psychotropic medications.

An approach for approximating discipline-specific staffing needs for a given facility that has been used by one of us (K.A.) involves determining the type of services provided by that discipline, the time required for each unit of service, and the number of units within a given period of time. For example, if a facility's social workers typically conduct 90 mental health intake assessments per week and each assessment, on average, takes 20 minutes, then the facility needs 30 hours of social work time per week for this service alone. Similar calculations can be made for other social worker services such as case management encounters and segregation rounds. Dividing the sum of all calculated service hours by the net weekly clinical time provided by a full-time equivalent (FTE) social worker will yield the approximate number of FTEs needed. This determination assumes that an FTE provides, on average, fewer than 40 hours per week of direct service (e.g., 24 hours per week) after accounting for paid time off and time spent on other functions such as meetings and training. The model does not apply to positions that require back-fill post coverage, such as infirmary nurses. A similar approach for determining psychiatric workloads in community mental health settings has been described (Bhaskara, 1999).

Sufficient suitable space, supplies, and equipment should be available for outpatient mental health services. This includes program areas that allow for confidential, private assessment and treatment of inmates; group programming; and storage of supplies and equipment (National Commission on Correctional Health Care, 2008). This principle applies equally to the outpatient programming space for high-security inmates, which generally includes those in locked-down (i.e., segregation) housing units (see Chapter 14).

Effective implementation of outpatient mental health services depends on sufficient custody staff for escorting and other security purposes within the programming areas. These positions should be established by post orders and staffed by regularly assigned officers to foster consistency of practices and compliance with pertinent policies and procedures. Effective collaboration and ongoing communication between health care and custody staff are critical for a safe and secure environment that supports meaningful and efficient treatment.

Timely access to outpatient services is an essential component of adequate mental health services. This includes a clear, easy-to-use, and readily available referral process, typically beginning with a referral form available on all housing units. The referral form should accurately identify the inmate, location of the inmate, source of referral, and date of referral and should include a brief summary of the reason for the request to be seen (Smith & Smith, 2006). The referral system may be integrated with the health services sick-call request system or may be a separate process through the mental health department. Receipt and triage of oral or written requests for nonemergency mental health services occur within 24 hours. During regular duty hours, either a qualified mental health professional or a qualified health care professional (e.g., physician,

physician's assistant, nurse, or nurse practitioner) must perform this function. On-call coverage during nonduty hours is needed. This is commonly provided on a scheduled rotating basis by the mental health staff, although other options are available depending on the system's size and resources (e.g., via a psychiatric nurse in an inpatient unit if the facility has such a unit).

Many correctional mental health systems triage referrals as emergent, urgent, or routine. Emergent referrals should be seen as soon as possible (generally within 4 hours), urgent referrals should be seen within 24 hours, and responses to routine referrals should generally occur within 5 to 10 business days. System resources often determine whether a referral is an emergent or urgent referral. For example, a referral that is triaged to require a suicide risk assessment will generally be triaged as emergent if the system does not have the staff resources to place the inmate under constant observation until the assessment occurs. The same type of referral in another system may be triaged as urgent if such resources do exist.

Continuity of care facilitates the establishment of a therapeutic alliance between the inmate and clinician, and frequent changes (e.g., more than twice in 12 months) of the inmate's psychiatrist and/or primary mental health clinician make this difficult to achieve. Frequent changes occur when there are staff recruitments, retention difficulties, and use of short-term, contract clinicians.

Residential programs for inmates with serious mental illness

A residential treatment program (often known as a residential treatment unit, intermediate care unit, supportive living unit, special needs unit, psychiatric services unit, or extended outpatient program) is a critical level of care for most prison systems and larger jails. Inmates who are appropriate for these units generally have had significant difficulty functioning in a general population environment due to symptoms of serious mental disorders (Metzner, 1998).

These programs are designed to provide supportive housing and psychosocial rehabilitation. The admission criteria and goals of these program often vary. For example, some programs are designed to teach inmates the skills they will need to eventually be mainstreamed back into the general inmate population (Lovell, Allen, Johnson, & Jemelka, 2001). Other programs attempt to mainstream but recognize that a significant percentage of inmates will need to remain in this level of care throughout their incarceration due to their inability to function in the general population.

Residential treatment programs typically house 30 to 50 inmates, which allows for cost-effective staffing. Essential features include adequate space for offices (preferably on or close to the unit), programming, individual and group therapies, indoor and outdoor recreation, a dayroom, a medication room, other nursing functions such as sick call, and designated cells near nursing or correctional officers' stations for close observation and/or therapeutic restraints. These units should be designed so that inmates can be observed from the nurses' office and the correctional officers' station. Important environmental conditions include ability to maintain reasonable room temperature, adequate ventilation, and proper acoustics to decrease the noise level in treatment and housing areas (Metzner, 1998).

The psychosocial rehabilitation model emphasizes group therapies and activities that promote socialization and productive use of time. Useful treatment modalities include psychoeducation, cognitive-behavioral therapies, socialization skills, art, music, recreation, and substance abuse and anger management groups. Weekly community meetings help to create a therapeutic milieu. Unstructured out-of-cell time for inmates in these programs should at least equal the amount of recreational time (i.e., outdoor yard) available to general-population inmates at the same security classification and should include an additional 10 hours of out-of-cell structured therapeutic programming per week for each inmate. Appropriately credentialed or supervised mental health staff conduct the therapeutic programming. Leisure activities and unstructured recreation represent additional important elements of a residential treatment program. These units also provide individual supportive counseling and access to psychotropic medications that include nonemergency, involuntary medications when appropriate and permitted, especially in high-security settings. A computerized database can help document the number of hours per week that an inmate participates in the treatment program. This information will facilitate quality improvement activities and needs assessment processes.

Staffing allocations vary based on the size of the unit and the security classification levels of the inmates. The multidisciplinary treatment team typically includes a psychiatrist, nurses, activity therapists, clerks, and other mental health professionals (e.g., psychologists, social workers, occupational therapists, mental health technicians). Staffing at one program with 97 beds, with acute care admissions occupying 22 of those beds, included 1 full-time psychiatrist and 1 psychiatric nurse practitioner, 2 clinical psychologists, 9 registered nurses, and 31 mental health counselors (O'Connor, Lovell, & Brown, 2002). Correctional officers receive enhanced mental health training for assignment to these programs, where they typically spend at least six months and serve important functions (Appelbaum, Hickey, & Packer., 2001; Dvoskin & Spiers, 2004). We recommend making them full members of the treatment team who attend team meetings, share observations, have access to clinical information, participate in therapeutic activities, and maintain confidentiality and other clinical obligations that do not conflict with security. Appropriate training to support these expectations should be provided. To facilitate a good working relationship between officers and mental health staff, the mental health director of the unit needs to have meaningful input into selection of the officers.

Providing residential treatment care for high-security inmates or those in a locked-down setting such as a supermax or segregation housing unit is staff-intensive and generally requires special physical plant modifications such as the use of "programming modules" (Metzner & Dvoskin, 2006; see Chapter 14).

Successful implementation of a residential treatment unit can enhance inmates' participation in work, school, and other programming and can reduce the need for inpatient psychiatric beds, the number of admissions to crisis beds, and the frequency of disciplinary infractions (Condelli, Dvoskin, & Holanchock, 1994; Lovell et al., 2001; O'Connor et al., 2002; Smith, Sawyer, & Way, 2004). Our own experience in consulting for and/or designing and implementing residential treatment programs confirms these benefits.

A few correctional systems have developed residential treatment programs for inmates who have significant behavior problems due to a personality disorder and are generally not appropriate for residential settings that use a psychosocial approach to treat inmates with serious mental illnesses. These programs generally use a cognitive-behavioral approach and a phase system that rewards prosocial behaviors with increasing privileges (Andrade, 2009). At least one program with a therapeutic community approach, however, has reported significant success diminishing serious incidents of violence among the system's most assaultive and disruptive inmates (Cooke, 1989).

Crisis intervention services

Crisis intervention services provide another necessary component of an adequate correctional mental health system. These services must include timely access, when clinically indicated, to housing in a crisis stabilization unit (CSU). Some systems also have an adjacent infirmary-type dormitory that serves as a transition back to general population housing (Smith & Smith, 2006). CSUs generally have single cells and 24/7 coverage by nursing and custody staffs with mental health staff on site during the usual working hours and on-call during off hours. CSUs provide observation (e.g., suicide watch), diagnosis, and treatment functions in a safe and therapeutic environment as characterized by supportive clinical interventions and a nonpunitive approach. Placing crisis cells in segregation units and routine use of strip cell status (e.g., no personal property, use of a suicide smock, no out-of-cell time) are examples of nontherapeutic milieus.

In general, CSUs have a length of stay less than 10 days. In small or resource-poor correctional facilities that have problems with access to psychiatric hospitals, a CSU often also serves as an acute care program, which results in longer lengths of stay. These valuable and scarce mental health care beds should not be used for non-health care purposes (e.g., protective custody, overflow housing) or for prolonged stays following clinical discharge.

The structure and staffing of CSUs should allow admission of inmates of any classification within the facility or catchment area for regionalized units. Clinical staff should make admission and discharge decisions with input from custody staff, especially regarding discharges. For cost-effectiveness, CSUs usually occupy a separate section of general medical infirmaries that house inmates with conditions that require 24/7 nursing care. CSUs, which almost always serve as the primary housing unit for inmates on suicide precautions or watch, need suicide-resistant cells (Metzner & Hayes, 2006) and suicide prevention policies and procedures (see Chapter 43). Because inmates in CSUs have short stays, acute symptoms, frequent need for clinical stabilization with psychotropic medications, and diagnostic uncertainty, a medical model serves as a useful operating structure. Inmates need daily contact with a psychiatrist or other appropriately credentialed mental health clinician, with continuous coverage by a psychiatrist available.

Patterns of admission to a CSU should be reviewed. Some inmates have two or more admissions to a CSU in a six-month period due to self-injurious behaviors or threats of injuring self or others. Other potentially problematic admissions include inmates who seek new housing for nonclinical reasons such as wanting to escape repayment of a debt. These inmates often precipitate

hostility and countertransference from CSU clinical and custody staff that interfere with assessment and treatment. Staff frequently, and sometimes accurately, label these inmates as malingering or having antisocial personality disorders and subsequently fail to identify other comorbid symptoms of a significant mental disorder. At times, staff inappropriately impose harsh conditions of confinement (e.g., no mattress or clothing) for such inmates in an attempt to covertly discourage them from remaining in or returning to the CSU. Inmates who have CSU stays longer than 10 days or who have multiple admissions within a six-month period should be considered for either inpatient psychiatric hospitalization or a change in their current treatment plan.

CSUs occasionally have problematic custody and clinical practices. Some correctional systems treat all CSU inmates as maximum-security inmates. This practice is based, in part, on the belief that all inmates with mental illness who need CSU care are dangerous and unpredictable. As a result, they lock down these inmates 23 to 24 hours per day, do not provide access to recreational areas, and overly restrict possession of clothing and property unrelated to clinical needs. Mental health staff need to educate custody staff regarding these misperceptions and implement policies and procedures that prevent inappropriate practices.

Other common problems include cell-front clinical contacts that lack confidentiality and absence of clinical interventions (e.g., activity/recreational therapy, individual counseling) other than observation and psychotropic medications. Chapter 25 provides more detailed information regarding crisis interventions that are well suited for correctional settings.

Psychiatric inpatient programs

Inpatient psychiatric hospitalization is the most expensive and intensive level of care and generally the least available to correctional mental health programs due to limited resources. Models used by correctional systems to provide access include the following:

An arrangement (e.g., contract or memorandum of agreement, statutory provisions) with the state department of mental health or equivalent agency to provide either an open-ended or defined number of forensic hospital beds for inmates;

A dedicated correctional system facility; and

A contract with a hospital system.

A survey of 24 European nations found that 2 provided all inmate mental health services, including hospitalizations, internally within the prison system; 4 relied entirely on the external community mental health system for services; and the remaining 18 used a mixed model of both prison-based and community-based services for inmates (Dressing & Salize, 2009).

Many correctional systems, especially jails, do not have psychiatric inpatient care directly accessible for inmates. Indirect access may be available via the court system for inmates in need of treatment or via the forensic mental health system for evaluation of competency to proceed or similar issues. Unfortunately, transfers of correctional inmates to community psychiatric hospitals tend to generate disputes between the two systems over the need for the admissions, often precipitated by security concerns on the part of the hospital (Blaauw, Roesch, & Kerkhof, 2000). Such disputes may be minimized through clear contractual language and expectations and with routinely scheduled conferences to review recent and anticipated cases.

Experience has demonstrated that the availability of CSUs and residential treatment beds has a direct bearing on the need for inpatient resources. No simple formula exists for reliably determining how many specialty psychiatric beds a system requires. However, a study in England and Wales found that 3% of sentenced prisoners needed hospital-level care (Gunn, Maden, & Swinton, 1991). A survey of 13 European nations, however, found that most of them had psychiatric beds at all levels of care available for less than 3% of their prison populations (Blaauw et al., 2000). To our knowledge, no US prison system comes close to providing inpatient psychiatric beds for 3% of its population. In the context of robust services at other levels of care, including residential treatment units and CSUs, many would contend that less than 3% inpatient beds would suffice to meet the needs of inmates with serious mental disorders.

Summary

Meeting the needs of inmates with mental disorders requires access to a range of service levels, including outpatient, residential, crisis, and inpatient care. Factors such as system size may determine the availability of these services and the extent to which external resources or programs provide them. Nevertheless, each of these four components remains essential to meet prevailing standards of care and to provide appropriate mental health services to inmates.

References

American Psychiatric Association (2000). *Psychiatric services in jails and prisons: a task force report of the American Psychiatric Association.* Washington, DC: American Psychiatric Association.

Andrade, J. T. (2009). Psychopathy: Assessment, treatment, and risk management. In J. T. Andrade (Ed.), *Handbook of violence risk assessment and treatment: New approaches for mental health professionals.* New York: Springer Publishing Company.

Appelbaum, K. L. (2009). Attention deficit hyperactivity disorder in prison: A treatment protocol. *Journal of the American Academy of Psychiatry and the Law, 37*(1), 45–49.

Appelbaum, K. L., Hickey, J. M., & Packer, I. (2001). The role of correctional officers in multidisciplinary mental health care in prisons. *Psychiatric Services, 52,* 1343–1347.

Bhaskara, S. M. (1999). Setting benchmarks and determining psychiatric workloads in community mental health programs. *Psychiatric Services, 50,* 695–697.

Blaauw, E., Roesch, R., & Kerkhof, A. (2000). Mental disorders in European prison systems. Arrangements for mentally disordered prisoners in the prison systems of 13 European countries. *International Journal of Law and Psychiatry, 23,* 649–663.

Community Mental Health Act of 1963. Public Law 88-164.

Condelli, W. S., Dvoskin, J. A., & Holanchock, H. (1994). Intermediate care programs for inmates with psychiatric disorders. *Bulletin of the American Academy of Psychiatry and the Law, 22*(1), 63–70.

Cooke, D. J. (1989). Containing violent prisoners: An analysis of the Barlinnie Special Unit. *British Journal of Criminology, 29,* 129–143.

Dressing, H., & Salize, H. J. (2009). Pathways to psychiatric care in European prison systems. *Behavioral Science and the Law, 27,* 801–810.

Dvoskin, J. A., & Spiers, E. M. (2004). On the role of correctional officers in prison mental health. *Psychiatric Quarterly, 75,* 41–59.

Gunn, J., Maden, A., & Swinton, M. (1991). Treatment needs of prisoners with psychiatric disorders. *British Medical Journal, 303,* 338–341.

Lovell, D., Allen, D., Johnson, C., & Jemelka, R. (2001). Evaluating the effectiveness of residential treatment for prisoners with mental illness. *Criminal Justice and Behavior, 28,* 83–104.

Metzner, J. (1997). An introduction to correctional psychiatry: Part II. *Journal of the American Academy of Psychiatry and the Law, 25*(4), 571–579.

Metzner, J. L. (1998). An introduction to correctional psychiatry, part III. *Journal of the American Academy of Psychiatry and the Law, 28*(1), 107–115.

Metzner, J., & Dvoskin, J. (2006). An overview of correctional psychiatry. *Psychiatric Clinics of North America, 29,* 761–772.

Metzner, J., & Hayes, L. (2006). Suicide prevention in jails and prisons. In R. Simon & R. Hales (Eds.), *Textbook of suicide assessment and management.* Washington, DC: American Psychiatric Press.

National Commission on Correctional Health Care (2008). *Standards for mental health services in correctional facilities.* Chicago: National Commission on Correctional Health Care.

O'Connor, F. W., Lovell, D., & Brown, L. (2002). Implementing residential treatment for prison inmates with mental illness. *Archives of Psychiatric Nursing, 16,* 232–238.

Smith, H., Sawyer, D. A., & Way, B. B. (2004). Correctional mental health services in New York: Then and now. *Psychiatric Quarterly, 75,* 21–39.

Smith, H., & Smith, L. D. (2006). Correctional-based mental health services: Designing a system that works. In M. Puisis (Ed.), *Clinical practice in correctional medicine.* Philadelphia: Elsevier Inc.

CHAPTER 23

Evaluation of malingering in corrections

James L. Knoll, IV

Introduction

Malingered mental illness in the correctional setting poses a complicated dilemma. Many factors change the typical presentation and detection strategies, and inaccurate determinations have serious consequences. Detection requires a thorough knowledge of the characteristics of genuine psychiatric illness, a systematic approach to evaluation, identification of objective indicators, and use of scientifically validated psychological tests when necessary (Heilbronner, Sweet, Morgan, Larrabee, Millis, & Conference Participants, 2009).

Malingering

Malingering is a condition not attributable to a mental disorder. The *Diagnostic and Statistical Manual of Mental Disorders* (DSM-5) defines it as the intentional production of false or grossly exaggerated physical or psychological symptoms, motivated by an external incentive (American Psychiatric Association, 2013). Malingering often requires differentiation from a factitious disorder in which the patient simulates illness with a motive to assume the sick role, which can be thought of as an internal (i.e., psychological) incentive (Kanaan & Wessely, 2010).

Malingering may be further divided into three categories: pure malingering, partial malingering, and false imputation (Resnick, West, & Payne, 1997). In pure malingering, an individual feigns a disorder that does not exist. Partial malingering involves conscious exaggeration of actual symptoms. False imputation refers to ascribing genuine symptoms to a cause that the individual consciously recognizes as unrelated.

Motives to malinger always involve external incentive and fall into two general categories: avoiding difficult situations or punishment (avoiding pain) and obtaining compensation or medications (seeking pleasure). In civilian settings, external incentives include financial gain or psychiatric admission to obtain room and board or social services (Knoll & Resnick, 2006). In criminal courts, malingerers may seek to avoid punishment by feigning insanity or incompetence to stand trial (Soliman & Resnick, 2010).

DSM-5 cautions that "under some circumstances, malingering may represent adaptive behavior—for example, feigning illness while a captive of the enemy during wartime" (American Psychiatric Association, 2013, pp. 726–727). Many correctional facilities remain harsh, dangerous, and underresourced, causing difficulty when distinguishing malingering from adaptive coping strategies. Exaggeration of symptoms may be an adaptive response by mentally ill inmates to sparse or difficult-to-obtain mental health resources (Kupers, 2004). For example, staff might ignore requests for treatment unless symptoms are amplified.

Inmates with serious mental illness may exaggerate symptoms to avoid toxic and stressful environments such as punitive isolation. Some inmates may malinger to seek the relatively protected environment of a mental health unit, particularly if general-population inmates harass them. Not all inmate patients malinger for adaptive reasons. Some have motives such as obtaining medications to abuse, avoiding appropriate disciplinary actions, or gaining transfer to other living situations. Inmates nearing the end of their sentence may malinger to obtain disability benefits in the community.

Difficulties detecting malingering in corrections

The assessment of malingering (McDermott, 2012) requires a comprehensive evaluation (i.e., testing, unstructured evaluation, behavioral observations, collateral information, review of records) to avoid false-positive attribution (DeClue, 2002). The rate of malingered mental illness by inmates is unclear. One study found that 32% of prisoners referred to forensic mental health services fabricated or exaggerated symptoms of mental illness (Pollock, Quigley, Worley, & Bashford, 1997). A study of jail inmates confirmed malingering in more than 66% of suspected cases (McDermott & Sokolov, 2009).

Most studies of malingering in corrections rely on structured tests developed for settings with clear external incentives, such as avoiding incarceration. In prison the incentives to malinger become more complex. Thus, commonly used detection strategies may not be as reliable after conviction. Further, Vitacco and Rogers (2005) noted that DSM screening indices for suspected malingering do not apply in a correctional setting.

Although tests such as the Structured Interview of Reported Symptoms (SIRS) may help, a conclusion of malingering cannot be made solely on their basis (Drob, Meehan, & Waxman, 2009; Green & Rosenfeld, 2011). Currently available tests cannot identify the motivation to malinger and thus cannot distinguish between external and internal motives. For example, individuals with factitious disorder, or Ganser syndrome, may appear to be malingering, but tests cannot distinguish factitious and hysterical pathology from malingering.

An incorrect diagnosis of malingering may have seriously detrimental and long-lasting effects for an inmate with genuine mental illness. A label of malingering may be difficult to overcome and lead to adverse outcomes. In addition to denial of needed treatment, an improper diagnosis of malingering can result in disciplinary actions in some prisons and lead correctional staff to disregard genuine complaints by that inmate.

A finding of malingering also does not rule out the presence of true mental illness and genuine psychopathology. Such either/or dichotomies are best avoided. Therefore, a determination of malingering should not exclude the inmate from receiving mental health services. Table 23.1 lists clinical factors to consider prior to reaching a conclusion of malingering (Knoll, 2006, 2009; Kupers, 2004).

Punitive isolation might also produce atypical or transient psychotic symptoms that could be mistaken for malingering. The psychological effects of punitive isolation remain unclear (O'Keefe, Klebe, Metzner, Dvoskin, Fellner, & Stucker, 2013), but it might exacerbate symptoms of mental illness or even produce them de novo (Haney, 2008; Kupers, 2008).

Some experts have referred to a "SHU (special housing unit) syndrome" (*Jones' El v. Barge*, 2001; *Madrid v. Gomez*, 1995) to describe symptoms such as pervasive anxiety, agitation, perceptual distortions (e.g., hallucinations), aggressive fantasy, and suicidal ideation (Abramsky & Fellner, 2003; Ferrier, 2004; Smith, 2006) experienced by some inmates, especially those with preexisting mental illness, after prolonged confinement. This phenomenon may have features of an atypical psychosis, leading an evaluator to incorrectly conclude that malingering is present.

Finally, the challenges of detecting malingering may increase when inmate patients have intellectual disabilities. Few studies have addressed the efficacy of forensic assessment in this population (Weiss, Rosenfeld, & Farkas, 2011). Patients with intellectual disabilities might be falsely identified as showing poor effort, particularly on cognitive tests (Salekin & Doane, 2009). When they were administered the SIRS, many individuals with intellectual disabilities were misclassified as malingering (Ferrier, 2004). These findings were most frequent when subjects had comorbid psychiatric diagnoses, which is common in corrections.

Table 23.1 Clinical factors warranting caution before diagnosing malingering in a correctional setting

- No clear external incentive
- Extensive history of psychiatric treatment
- Not self-referred
- Defensive, minimizes illness, or opposes treatment
- Shows improvement on psychiatric medications
- Does well or improves in a mental health unit
- Intellectual disability
- Frequently requires special observations
- High number of objective suicide risk factors
- History of serious traumatic brain injury

Clinical detection of malingering

Detection of malingering requires a thorough knowledge of genuine psychiatric symptoms and how they usually present. This enables more accurate differentiation of malingered symptoms from genuine symptoms. Genuine psychopathology and feigned/exaggerated symptoms commonly co-occur, and the clinician must delineate the relative presence of each (Heilbronner et al., 2009).

Hallucinations

Patients should be questioned in great detail about atypical hallucinations with nonleading questions about content, vividness, and other characteristics of the hallucinations (Resnick & Knoll, 2008). Genuine hallucinations are usually associated with delusions (Lewinsohn, 1970) and are typically intermittent instead of continuous (Goodwin & Rosenthal, 1971). Olfactory and tactile hallucinations commonly have general medical causes. Auditory hallucinations are rarely vague or inaudible. They are usually heard clearly and in both ears simultaneously.

Approximately one third of auditory hallucinations are accusatory, and most persons feel worried or upset by their hallucinations (Carter, Mackinnon, & Copolov, 1996). Auditory hallucinations in schizophrenia are usually persecutory or instructive (Small, Small, & Andersen, 1966). The voices are often threatening, obscene, accusatory, or insulting (Sadock & Sadock, 2007). Hallucinations of music are rare (Fischer, Marchie, & Norris, 2004) and often related to organic brain pathology, aging, or sensory impairment.

Command auditory hallucinations are particularly easy to malinger. However, persons who experience them usually also have noncommand hallucinations and delusions (Thompson, Stuart, & Holden, 1992). Further, command hallucinations are rarely obeyed in the absence of other psychological variables (e.g., beliefs about the voices, coexisting delusions; Braham, Trower, & Birchwood, 2004). Isolated command hallucinations without other psychotic symptoms should raise concerns about malingering.

Persons with schizophrenia typically develop coping strategies. For example, hallucinations tend to diminish when patients engage in activities (Goodwin & Rosenthal, 1971). Thus, patients should be asked what they do to make the voices go away or diminish in intensity. Common strategies include taking medications, exercising, or listening to music. Malingerers may report hallucinations consisting of stilted or implausible language or even language that provides justification for illegal activity. For example, an inmate charged with smuggling contraband into the prison claimed to hear voices that said, "Tell your girlfriend to smuggle in a cell phone."

Dramatic or otherwise atypical visual hallucinations should arouse suspicions (American Psychiatric Association, 2013; Powell, 1991). Malingerers report visual hallucinations more often than do genuinely psychotic persons (Cornell & Hawk, 1989). Visual hallucinations are usually of normal-sized people and seen in color (Green & Rosenfeld, 2011). Hallucinations of small people (Lilliputian hallucinations) may occur with alcohol use, organic disease (Cohen, Alfonso, & Haque, 1994), or toxic psychosis such as anticholinergic toxicity (Asaad, 1990). On one occasion, the author diagnosed genuine Lilliputian hallucinations in an inmate patient with verified complex partial seizures whose antiepileptic medications had been erroneously discontinued.

Genuine visual hallucinations in psychosis do not usually change if the eyes are closed or open. In contrast, drug-induced hallucinations are more readily seen with the eyes closed or in darkened surroundings (Asaad & Shapiro, 1986). Unformed hallucinations, such as flashes of light, shadows, or moving objects, are typically associated with neurologic disease or substance use (Cummings & Miller, 1987; Mitchell & Vierkant, 1991).

Delusions

Most genuine delusions involve the following themes: somatic, grandiose, jealous, erotomanic, persecutory, and religious (Spitzer, 1992). Persecutory delusions are more likely to be acted on than other types of delusions (Wessely, Buchanan, Reed, Cutting, Everitt, Garety, & Taylor, 1993). Genuine delusional systems will reflect the intelligence level of the individual in terms of complexity and sophistication. Delusions of nihilism, poverty, disease, and guilt are commonly seen in depressive psychoses. Delusions with technical content (e.g., computer chips, electronic devices) occur seven times more frequently in men than women (Kraus, 1994).

Malingerers are more likely to claim a sudden onset or disappearance of a delusion. In contrast, genuine delusions usually take weeks to develop and much longer to disappear. The resolution of genuine delusions follows a course of gradual surrender. First, the delusion will become somewhat less relevant. Later, the individual will slowly relinquish the belief over time after adequate treatment (Sacks, Carpenter Jr., & Strauss, 1974).

The more bizarre the content of the reported delusions, the more disorganized the individual's thinking is likely to be. Individuals with genuine psychotic disorders who demonstrate disordered thought and bizarre beliefs also have disordered speech and odd behavior (Harrow, O'Connell, Herbener, Altman, Kaplan, & Jobe, 2003). Thus, when suspect delusions are alleged, associated behavior and speech patterns should be carefully considered.

With genuine delusions, the individual's behavior is usually consistent with the content of the delusions. Observations of the inmate should confirm behavior that is in accord with the delusions. Allegations of persecutory delusions without any corresponding paranoid behaviors should arouse suspicion. One exception to this principle is the inmate patient with chronic schizophrenia who has grown accustomed to the delusions and may no longer behave in a corresponding manner. An inmate patient who alleges a firm conviction about a delusion should be carefully assessed for impaired work performance, leisure activities, programming, and functioning among peers (Harrow, Herbener, Shanklin, Jobe, Rattenbury, & Kaplan, 2004).

Cognitive symptoms

Malingerers' strategies generally follow two approaches: exaggeration and/or reducing cognitive capability. Malingerers may believe that faking intellectual deficits, in addition to psychotic symptoms, will make them more believable (Bash & Alpert, 1980; Schretlen, 1988). Thus, malingerers may give incorrect answers to patently obvious questions that an individual with a genuine, serious cognitive disorder could answer correctly. Malingerers may also believe that they must demonstrate serious memory deficits inconsistent with their level of functioning. They may claim impairment discordant with typical patterns seen in genuine memory impairment, such as claiming long-term memory impairment greater than short-term impairment (Soliman & Resnick, 2010).

Malingerers are more likely to give vague or hedging answers to straightforward questions (Resnick & Knoll, 2008). For example, when asked whether an alleged voice was male or female, a malingerer may reply, "It was *probably* a man's voice." Malingerers may also answer, "I don't know" to detailed questions about psychotic symptoms. The individual with genuine hallucinations could easily give an answer; the malingerer who has never experienced the symptoms "doesn't know" the correct answer, nor what the evaluator should be told.

Persons with genuine intellectual disability have been known to exaggerate their cognitive deficits, and persons of normal intellectual ability may successfully feign low IQ scores on intelligence tests (Graue, Berry, Clark, Sollman, Cardi, Hopkins, & Werline, 2007). Multiple tests of effort are recommended for accuracy and to decrease the number of false positives, in addition to collateral data (Victor, Boone, & Boone, 2007). In particular, the Test of Memory Malingering (TOMM) has demonstrated a high rate of success in detecting malingering in groups of intellectually disabled subjects (Shandera, Berry, Clark, Schipper, Graue, & Harp, 2010).

Clinical indicators of malingering

Malingerers may be detected clinically when they have inadequate knowledge of the illness they are faking or when they overact their part in a mistaken belief that it will be more convincing (Wachspress, Berenberg, & Jacobson, 1953). Conversely, "successful" malingerers are more likely to endorse fewer symptoms and avoid endorsing bizarre or unusual symptoms (Edens, Guy, Otto, Buffington, Tomicic, & Poythress, 2001). Malingerers give a greater number of evasive answers and may repeat questions or answer slowly to give themselves time to think about how best to deceive the evaluator or to observe the evaluator for nonverbal clues to the correct response (Knoll & Resnick, 2006).

Malingerers are more likely to call attention to their illness; this is in contrast to patients with genuine schizophrenia, who are often reluctant to discuss their symptoms (Ritson & Forrest, 1970). An important caveat in the correctional setting is that symptom amplification may be used to ensure needed psychiatric attention. Malingerers may attempt to take control of the interview or behave in an intimidating manner so that the psychiatrist will prematurely terminate the interview. Malingerers are unlikely to be able to successfully imitate the subtle signs of schizophrenia, such as deficit symptoms (e.g., flat affect, alogia), digressive speech, or peculiar thinking. Exceptions to this include inmate patients with a history of genuine schizophrenia or those who have become familiar with these symptoms by observing others with genuine serious mental illness.

Special attention should be given to rare or improbable symptoms, as they are almost never reported even in severely disturbed persons (Rogers, Bagby, & Dickens, 1992; Thompson, LeBourgeois, & Black, 2004). Malingerers may be asked about improbable symptoms to see if they will endorse them. For example, a suspected malingerer may be asked, "When people talk to you, do you see the words they speak spelled out?" (Miller, 2001). For alleged auditory hallucinations, a suspected malingerer may be asked, "When you hear the voices, do they ever speed up or sound like they are on 'fast forward'?" In the case of alleged visual hallucinations, the suspected malingerer may be asked, "When you see things other people can't see, do they ever appear to be upside down or vibrating?"

Malingerers may give a false or incomplete history, so it is critical to compare their current self-reports with descriptions in the psychiatric or correctional mental health records (Heilbronner et al., 2009; Soliman & Resnick, 2010). Inconsistencies or disparities between self-report and behavioral observations should be investigated. Inconsistencies may be conceptualized as either internal or external to the individual's presentation. Internal inconsistencies exist when a malingerer reports severe symptoms such as mental confusion or memory loss but can give multiple examples of confusion and memory loss. External inconsistencies occur between the reported level of functioning and the level of functioning observed by others. For example, malingerers may allege debilitating hallucinations, while staff observations confirm they are undefeated in card games on the unit.

Comprehensive malingering evaluation

Because of the complexities involved, a comprehensive malingering evaluation is recommended in difficult cases (Heilbronner et al., 2009; McDermott, 2012; Rogers, Vitacco, & Kurus, 2010). An outline for the comprehensive evaluation of malingering is given in Table 23.2. Records and collateral data should be reviewed prior to the interview.

Data supporting or refuting alleged symptoms should be carefully reviewed (e.g., prior records, offender files, correctional staff observations). The interview may need to be prolonged since fatigue can diminish a malingerer's ability to maintain fake symptoms (Anderson, Trethowan, & Kenna, 1959). In difficult cases, inpatient assessment should be considered because feigned psychotic symptoms are difficult to sustain under daily observation.

Interview technique is critical in the detection of malingering. It is important to refrain from verbal or nonverbal communications of suspicion (McDermott & Sokolov, 2009). The evaluation should begin with open-ended questions that allow the inmate patient to report symptoms without prompting. Open-ended questions provide less direction or data for a malingerer to use (Soliman & Resnick, 2010).

Inquiries about symptoms should initially be phrased to avoid giving clues to the correct responses. Later in the interview, the evaluator can proceed to more detailed questions about specific symptoms. In particularly difficult cases, evaluators can use a technique called "set shifting," which involves interspersing malingering detection questions with history-taking, distractor

Table 23.2 Comprehensive malingering evaluation

- ◆ Review psychiatric records
- ◆ Review relevant sources of collateral information (offender files, staff observations)
- ◆ Identify plausible external incentive
- ◆ Behavioral observations (over time and/or on inpatient unit)
- ◆ Forensic psychiatric evaluation(s) (may require several and/or extended length)
- ◆ Analyze clinical indicators of malingering
- ◆ Psychological testing if necessary (e.g., MMPI-2, SIRS-2, M-FAST, PAI, TOMM)
- ◆ Support conclusion of malingering with multiple factual bases

questions, or even informal conversation. This may cause the malingerer to momentarily forget the malingering role and reveal important data (Drob & Berger, 1987).

Challenging clinical scenarios

Two common clinical challenges related to malingering in the correctional setting are faked mental wellness and so-called manipulative suicide threats.

Dissimulation

A longstanding maxim in correctional mental health contends that inmates who seek inpatient admission may be "faking bad," whereas those wishing to avoid inpatient admission may be "faking good." Dissimulation is the concealment of genuine symptoms of mental illness to portray psychological health. The denial of psychiatric symptoms has been reported anecdotally in persons who have committed crimes (Diamond, 1994), but there is little research on individuals who suppress signs of mental illness (Rogers, 2008b).

Reasons inmate patients may dissimulate include denial of illness to avoid the stigma and consequences of a mental illness diagnosis. It is not uncommon for inmates with mental illness to be the target of harassment, humiliation, and coercion. Some may feel a greater sense of control over their illness by alleging that they faked past symptoms. Other reasons include negative cultural views about mental illness and fears surrounding involuntary treatment. Some individuals conceal symptoms voluntarily, while others may do so due to lack of insight into their illness (Caruso, Benedek, Auble, & Bernet, 2003).

"Manipulation" versus suicide

Until recently, little was known about the prevalence of self-injurious behavior in corrections. A study of 51 state and federal prison systems found that a very small percentage (<2%) of inmates engage in self-injurious behavior each year. However, the acts occurred at least weekly in 85% of systems and were disruptive and necessitated a disproportionate amount of resources (Appelbaum, Savageau, Trestman, Metzner, & Baillargeon, 2011). From a clinical standpoint, self-injurious behavior in an inmate patient is very challenging and raises concerns about suicide risk, personality disorder, and manipulative intent (see Chapter 49). These factors must be considered carefully to avoid making a premature conclusion of manipulation or malingering.

The term "deliberate self-harm" has been used to describe the willful self-infliction of painful, destructive, or injurious acts without the intent to die. However, there is no universally accepted definition (Mangnall & Yurkovich, 2008). An individual may simultaneously possess a desire to self-harm *and* a desire to commit suicide. There is also the risk of accidental death while the inmate patient engages in deliberate self-harm.

"Manipulative" may be an inaccurate description of the behavior seen in some inmate patients who come to psychiatric attention (Hamilton, Decker, & Rumbaut, 1986). Avoidable risk may arise when persons with "recent instrumental suicide-related behavior" are dismissed "as manipulative or attention seeking" (Berman, 2006; Skeem, Silver, Appelbaum, & Tiemann, 2006). Self-mutilation and suicide attempts cannot be easily differentiated, even in cases where patients are questioned about suicidal intent (Konrad, Daigle, Daniel,

Dear, Frottier, Hayes, Kerkhof, Liebling, & Sarchiapone, 2007). This fact underscores the importance of the systematic suicide risk assessment on a case-by-case basis (Simon, 2004; see Chapter 43).

Correctional mental health staff often struggle with the conundrum of whether an inmate patient is feigning suicidal intent. Unfortunately, there is no evidence that feigned suicidal intent can be reliably distinguished from genuine suicidal intent (Freedenthal, 2007). The DSM considers suicidal ideation a symptom; however, in the final analysis, the act of suicide is a behavior. A symptom is observed or reported, while a behavior is performed. While psychiatry has tools for detecting feigned symptoms (Rogers, 2008a), there are no reliable tools for predicting low-base-rate behaviors such as suicide. This is precisely why the standard of care is to assess risk, not predict behavior (Simon, 2002).

Summary

The detection of malingering in corrections is necessary to ensure the judicious use of limited resources and to bring diagnostic accuracy to assessments. A comprehensive, systematic approach is required. The clinician must assemble evidence from a thorough evaluation, clinical records, collateral data, and psychological testing when necessary. A conclusion of malingering is best supported with multiple factual bases.

The correctional setting provides many unique challenges to detecting malingered mental illness. The finding that an inmate patient has malingered symptoms does not rule out the presence of true mental illness, and a determination of malingering should not exclude the inmate from receiving needed mental health services.

References

Abramsky, S., & Fellner, J. (2003). *Ill-equipped: US prisons and offenders with mental illness* (pp. 145–168). New York: Human Rights Watch.

American Psychiatric Association (2013). *Diagnostic and statistical manual of mental disorders (DSM-5)*. Washington, DC: American Psychiatric Association.

Anderson, E. W., Trethowan, W. H., & Kenna, J. C. (1959). An experimental investigation of simulation and pseudo-dementia. *Acta Psychiatrica Scandinavica Supplementum, 34*(132), 1–42.

Appelbaum, K. L., Savageau, J. A., Trestman, R. L., Metzner, J. L., & Baillargeon, J. (2011). A national survey of self-injurious behavior in American prisons. *Psychiatric Services, 62*(3), 285–290.

Asaad, G. (1990). *Hallucinations in clinical psychiatry: A guide for mental health professionals*. New York: Brunner/Mazel.

Asaad, G., & Shapiro, B. (1986). Hallucinations: Theoretical and clinical overview. *American Journal of Psychiatry, 143*(9), 1088–1097.

Bash, I. Y., & Alpert, M. (1980). The determination of malingering. *Annals of the New York Academy of Sciences, 347*(1), 86–99.

Berman, A. L. (2006). Risk management with suicidal patients. *Journal of Clinical Psychology, 62*(2), 171–184.

Braham, L. G., Trower, P., & Birchwood, M. (2004). Acting on command hallucinations and dangerous behavior: A critique of the major findings in the last decade. *Clinical Psychology Review, 24*(5), 513–528.

Carter, D. M., Mackinnon, A., & Copolov, D. L. (1996). Patients' strategies for coping with auditory hallucinations. *Journal of Nervous and Mental Disease, 184*(3), 159–164.

Caruso, K. A., Benedek, D. M., Auble, P. M., & Bernet, W. (2003). Concealment of psychopathology in forensic evaluations: a pilot study of intentional and uninsightful dissimulators. *Journal of the American Academy of Psychiatry and the Law Online, 31*(4), 444–450.

Cohen, M. A. A., Alfonso, C. A., & Haque, M. M. (1994). Lilliputian hallucinations and medical illness. *General Hospital Psychiatry, 16*(2), 141–143.

Cornell, D. G., & Hawk, G. L. (1989). Clinical presentation of malingerers diagnosed by experienced forensic psychologists. *Law and Human Behavior, 13*(4), 375–383.

Cummings, J. L., & Miller, B. L. (1987). Visual hallucinations: Clinical occurrence and use in differential diagnosis. *Western Journal of Medicine, 146*(1), 46.

DeClue, G. (2002). Feigning malingering: A case study. *Behavioral Sciences & the Law, 20*(6), 717–726.

Diamond, B. (1994). The Psychiatrist in the Courtroom: Selected Papers of Bernard L. Diamond, M. D. J. Quen (Ed.). Hillsdale, NJ: The Analytic Press, Inc.

Drob, S. L., & Berger, R. H. (1987). Determination of malingering: A comprehensive clinical-forensic approach. *Journal of the American Academy of Psychiatry and the Law, 15*, 519.

Drob, S. L., Meehan, K. B., & Waxman, S. E. (2009). Clinical and conceptual problems in the attribution of malingering in forensic evaluations. *Journal of the American Academy of Psychiatry and the Law Online, 37*(1), 98–106.

Edens, J. F., Guy, L. S., Otto, R. K., Buffington, J. K., Tomicic, T. L., & Poythress, N. G. (2001). Factors differentiating successful versus unsuccessful malingerers. *Journal of Personality Assessment, 77*(2), 333–338.

Ferrier, R. M. (2004). Atypical and significant hardship: The supermax confinement of death row prisoners based purely on status—A plea for procedural due process. *Arizona Law Review, 46*, 291.

Fischer, C., Marchie, A., & Norris, M. (2004). Musical and auditory hallucinations: A spectrum. *Psychiatry and Clinical Neurosciences, 58*(1), 96–98.

Freedenthal, S. (2007). Challenges in assessing intent to die: Can suicide attempters be trusted? *OMEGA—Journal of Death and Dying, 55*(1), 57–70.

Goodwin, D. W., & Rosenthal, R. (1971). Clinical significance of hallucinations in psychiatric disorders: A study of 116 hallucinatory patients. *Archives of General Psychiatry, 24*(1), 76.

Graue, L. O., Berry, D. T., Clark, J. A., Sollman, M. J., Cardi, M., Hopkins, J., & Werline, D. (2007). Identification of feigned mental retardation using the new generation of malingering detection instruments: Preliminary findings. *Clinical Neuropsychologist, 21*(6), 929–942.

Green, D., & Rosenfeld, B. (2011). Evaluating the gold standard: A review and meta-analysis of the structured interview of reported symptoms. *Psychological Assessment, 23*(1), 95.

Hamilton, J. D., Decker, N., & Rumbaut, R. D. (1986). The manipulative patient. *American Journal of Psychotherapy, 40*(2), 189–200.

Haney, C. (2008). A Culture of Harm: Taming the Dynamics of Cruelty in Supermax Prisons. *Criminal Justice and Behavior, 35*(8), 956–984.

Harrow, M., Herbener, E. S., Shanklin, A., Jobe, T. H., Rattenbury, F., & Kaplan, K. J. (2004). Follow-up of psychotic outpatients: Dimensions of delusions and work functioning in schizophrenia. *Schizophrenia Bulletin, 30*(1), 147.

Harrow, M., O'Connell, E. M., Herbener, E. S., Altman, A. M., Kaplan, K. J., & Jobe, T. H. (2003). Disordered verbalizations in schizophrenia: A speech disturbance or thought disorder? *Comprehensive Psychiatry, 44*(5), 353–359.

Heilbronner, R. L., Sweet, J. J., Morgan, J. E., Larrabee, G. J., Millis, S. R., & Conference Participants 1. (2009). American Academy of Clinical Neuropsychology Consensus conference statement on the neuropsychological assessment of effort, response bias, and malingering. *Clinical Neuropsychologist, 23*(7), 1093–1129.

Jones' El v. Barge (W.W. Wis. 2001). (164 F. Supp. 2d 1096, 1101-1102 ed.).

Kanaan, R. A., & Wessely, S. C. (2010). The origins of factitious disorder. *History of the Human Sciences, 23*(2), 68–85.

Knoll, J. L. (2006). *Real world challenges in correctional psychiatry*. Presentation at the American Academy of Psychiatry and the Law 2006 Annual Meeting, Chicago, Illinois.

Knoll, J. (2009). Malingering—Are you really, really sure? *Correctional Mental Health Report, 11*(2), 1–22, 30.

Knoll, J., & Resnick, P. J. (2006). The detection of malingered post-traumatic stress disorder. *Psychiatric Clinics of North America*, 29(3), 629–647.

Konrad, N., Daigle, M. S., Daniel, A. E., Dear, G. E., Frottier, P., Hayes, L. M., Kerkhof, A., Liebling, A., & Sarchiapone, M. (2007). Preventing suicide in prisons, part I: Recommendations from the international association for suicide prevention task force on suicide in prisons. *Crisis: The Journal of Crisis Intervention and Suicide Prevention*, 28(3), 113.

Kraus, A. (1994). Phenomenology of the technical delusion in schizophrenics. *Journal of Phenomenological Psychology*, 25(1), 51–69.

Kupers, T. (2004). Malingering in correctional settings. *Correctional Mental Health Report*, 5(6), 81.

Kupers, T. A. (2008). What to do with the survivors? Coping with the long-term effects of isolated confinement. *Criminal Justice and Behavior*, 35(8), 1005–1016.

Lewinsohn, P. (1970). An empirical test of several popular notions about hallucinations in schizophrenic patients. In W. Keup (Ed.), *Origin and mechanisms of hallucinations* (pp. 401–403) New York: Plenum Press.

Madrid v. Gomez, 889 F. Supp. 1146 (N. D. Cal. 1995).

Mangnall, J., & Yurkovich, E. (2008). A literature review of deliberate self-harm. *Perspectives in Psychiatric Care*, 44(3), 175–184.

McDermott, B. E. (2012). Psychological testing and the assessment of malingering. *Psychiatric Clinics of North America*, 35, 855–876.

McDermott, B. E., & Sokolov, G. (2009). Malingering in a correctional setting: The use of the Structured Interview of Reported Symptoms in a jail sample. *Behavioral Sciences & the Law*, 27(5), 753–765.

Miller, H. (2001). *M-FAST interview booklet*. Lutz, FL: Psychological Assessment Resources.

Mitchell, J., & Vierkant, A. D. (1991). Delusions and hallucinations of cocaine abusers and paranoid schizophrenics: A comparative study. *Journal of Psychology*, 125(3), 301–310.

O'Keefe, M. L., Klebe, K. J., Metzner, J., Dvoskin, J., Fellner, J., & Stucker, A. (2013). A longitudinal study of administrative segregation. *Journal of the American Academy of Psychiatry and the Law Online*, 41(1), 49–60.

Pollock, P. H., Quigley, B., Worley, K., & Bashford, C. (1997). Feigned mental disorder in prisoners referred to forensic mental health services. *Journal of Psychiatric and Mental Health Nursing*, 4(1), 9–15.

Powell, K. E. (1991). *The malingering of schizophrenia*. Unpublished manuscript, University of South Carolina, Columbia.

Resnick, P., & Knoll, J. (2008). Malingered psychosis. In R. Rogers (Ed.), *Clinical assessment of malingering and deception* (3rd ed., p. 51). New York: Guilford Press.

Resnick, P. J., West, S., & Payne, J. W. (1997). Malingering of posttraumatic disorders. *Clinical Assessment of Malingering and Deception*, 2, 130–152.

Ritson, B., & Forrest, A. (1970). The simulation of psychosis: A contemporary presentation. *British Journal of Medical Psychology*, 43(1), 31–37.

Rogers, R. (2008a). *Clinical assessment of malingering and deception*. New York: Guilford Press.

Rogers, R. (2008b). Current status of clinical methods. In R. Rogers (Ed.), *Clinical assessment of malingering and deception* (3rd ed., p. 401). New York: Guilford Press.

Rogers, R., Bagby, R. M., & Dickens, S.E. (1992). *SIRS, Structured Interview of Reported Symptoms: Professional manual*. Lutz, FL: Psychological Assessment Resources.

Rogers, R., Vitacco, M. J., & Kurus, S. J. (2010). Assessment of malingering with repeat forensic evaluations: Patient variability and possible misclassification on the SIRS and other feigning measures. *Journal of the American Academy of Psychiatry and the Law Online*, 38(1), 109–114.

Sacks, M. H., Carpenter,W. T.,Jr, & Strauss, J. S. (1974). Recovery from delusions: Three phases documented by patient's interpretation of research procedures. *Archives of General Psychiatry*, 30(1), 117.

Sadock, B. J., & Sadock, V. A. (2007). Chapter 13: Schizophrenia, in *Kaplan and Sadock's synopsis of psychiatry: Behavioral sciences/Clinical psychiatry* (10th ed.), Philadelphia, PA: Lippincott, Williams & Wilkins, p. 482.

Salekin, K. L., & Doane, B. M. (2009). Malingering intellectual disability: The value of available measures and methods. *Applied Neuropsychology*, 16(2), 105–113.

Schretlen, D. J. (1988). The use of psychological tests to identify malingered symptoms of mental disorder. *Clinical Psychology Review*, 8(5), 451–476.

Shandera, A. L., Berry, D. T., Clark, J. A., Schipper, L. J., Graue, L. O., & Harp, J. P. (2010). Detection of malingered mental retardation. *Psychological Assessment*, 22(1), 50.

Simon, R. I. (2002). Suicide risk assessment: What is the standard of care? *Journal of American Academy of Psychiatry Law*, 30(3), 340.

Simon, R. I. (2004). *Assessing and managing suicide risk: Guidelines for clinically based risk management*. Arlington, VA: American Psychiatric Publishing.

Skeem, J. L., Silver, E., Aippelbaum, P. S., & Tiemann, J. (2006). Suicide-related behavior after psychiatric hospital discharge: Implications for risk assessment and management. *Behavioral Sciences & the Law*, 24(6), 731–746.

Small, I. F., Small, J. G., & Andersen, J. M. (1966). Clinical characteristics of hallucinations of schizophrenia. *Diseases of the Nervous System*, 27(5), 349–353.

Smith, P. (2006). The effects of solitary confinement on prison inmates: A brief history and review of the literature. *Criminal Justice and Behavior*, 34, 441–568.

Soliman, S., & Resnick, P. J. (2010). Feigning in adjudicative competence evaluations. *Behavioral Sciences & the Law*, 28(5), 614–629.

Spitzer, M. (1992). The phenomenology of delusions. *Psychiatric Annals*, 22(5), 252–259.

Thompson, J., LeBourgeois, H., & Black, F. (2004). Malingering. In R. Simon & L. Gold (Eds.), *Textbook of forensic psychiatry* (pp. 427–448). Washington, DC: American Psychiatric Press.

Thompson, J. S., Stuart, G. L., & Holden, C. E. (1992). Command hallucinations and legal insanity. *Forensic Reports*, 5, 29–43.

Victor, T. L., & Boone, K. B. (2007). Identification of feigned mental retardation. In Boone, K. B. (Ed.), *Assessment of feigned cognitive impairment: A neuropsychological perspective* (pp. 310–345). New York: Guilford Press.

Vitacco, M. J., & Rogers, R. (2005). Malingering in corrections. In C. Scott (Ed.), *Handbook of correctional mental health*. Washington, DC: American Psychiatric Publishing, Inc.

Wachspress, M., Berenberg, A. N., & Jacobson, A. (1953). Simulation of psychosis. *Psychiatric Quarterly*, 27(1), 463–473.

Weiss, R. A., Rosenfeld, B., & Farkas, M. R. (2011). The utility of the structured interview of reported symptoms in a sample of individuals with intellectual disabilities. *Assessment*, 18(3), 284–290.

Wessely, S., Buchanan, A., Reed, A., Cutting, J., Everitt, B., Garety, P., & Taylor, P. J. (1993). Acting on delusions: I. Prevalence. *British Journal of Psychiatry*, 163(1), 69–76.

CHAPTER 24

Intoxication and drugs in facilities

Jason D. Ourada and Kenneth L. Appelbaum

Introduction

Active abuse of substances by inmates poses a challenge for correctional psychiatrists. Substance use disorders (SUDs) are common among inmates, with higher prevalence usually found in those with general psychiatric conditions (see Chapter 32). Correctional psychiatrists assess and treat these inmates and provide consultations for other staff. Issues addressed include mental status changes, intoxication, detoxification in infirmaries, withdrawal, protracted abstinence syndromes, psychiatric prescribing, motivational interviewing and assessment of stages of change, and general treatment and discharge planning. Knowledge about substance use in correctional facilities fosters competent clinical intervention and enhances management at all levels.

Psychiatrists who work in jails and prisons have the challenging task of maintaining therapeutic alliances with patients who have co-occurring SUDs and also may be actively using substances. Patients might not spontaneously report use during incarceration because they fear retribution by correctional staff or not receiving needed treatment for medical and mental health problems. Psychiatrists need to remain aware of this and to screen for SUDs and active substance use as part of comprehensive treatment planning. The clinical challenges in jails and prisons differ, and the substances found in facilities vary geographically. This chapter highlights these differences, outlines clinical management, and describes an interdisciplinary approach to intervention.

Substances commonly found in correctional settings

Although psychiatrists may know the commonly used substances in their facilities, no formal systems exist for collecting this data (Rowell et al., 2012). In 2000, the US Department of Justice reported on drug use, testing, and treatment in 3,328 jails but did not address specific substances (Wilson, 2000). Some studies have used interviews and inmate self-report in gathering data such as a 2002 Canadian study of inmate use of cocaine, cannabis, and hallucinogens (Plourde & Brochu, 2002). Most studies have focused on classes of illicit substances such as opiates, stimulants, cannabis, and alcohol. Opiate use was shown to continue at higher rates than cocaine and methamphetamine in a study of persistent substance use in correctional facilities (Strang et al., 2006). External factors, such as economic forces, may account for this, but the opioid withdrawal syndrome itself causes enough physical

and mental suffering to perpetuate drug-seeking behavior. Several studies have examined the efficacy of methadone maintenance programs and potential reduction of injection drug use and spread of infectious disease such as HIV and viral hepatitis in correctional facilities (Stallwitz & Stover, 2007). Nevertheless, systematic data collection is lacking, and prison administrators sometimes restrict researchers from collecting data about substance use (Rowell et al., 2012).

A 2010 Spanish study quantitatively examined drugs in the wastewater of a Catalonian prison using liquid chromatography–tandem mass spectrometry. Among the illicit substances and prescribed medications tested for, methadone (prescribed by medical staff for treatment of opioid dependence) was the most prevalent, followed by alprazolam, ephedrine, cannabis, heroin, cocaine, Ecstasy, methamphetamine, and amphetamine (Postigo, de Alda, & Barcelo, 2011). Although costly, this method could provide useful monitoring data for clinicians and correctional systems.

Most state departments of corrections ban indoor tobacco and many also prohibit tobacco on outdoor grounds (Cork, 2012). Even in systems that have bans, however, tobacco products manage to enter facilities.

The illicit substances available in correctional facilities may closely resemble those in the local community; therefore, understanding geographic differences is important. For example, methamphetamine use in the United States has been most prevalent in the West, Midwest, and South (Hunt et al., 2006). Psychiatrists who work in facilities in these regions may encounter methamphetamine addiction more frequently than psychiatrists in other regions.

Origins of substances in facilities

SUDs among inmates fuel demand for illicit substances and create economic forces that can lead to gang activity, staff complicity in smuggling, and the presence of contraband such as cell phones and drug paraphernalia. Cell phones can aid coordination of smuggling; novel and creative methods that evade detection continually challenge staff efforts to curb the flow of substances into facilities. Visitation provides a common means of entry (*Washington Times*, 2010). One technique involves passing balloons filled with drugs from mouth to mouth when kissing (Ferranti, 2013; Malcolm, 1989). The recipient swallows the balloon and later recovers it by vomiting or collection from feces. If suspicion of such behavior exists, inmates may be housed in a cell with no running water until the material passes. Other techniques include passing small packages during visits and concealment in oral, vaginal, or anal cavities to evade normal search procedures (Malcolm, 1989). Media reports describe smuggling of buprenorphine by dissolving it on papers and mailing them to inmates (Goodnough & Zezima, 2011). Recent attempts to drop drugs and tobacco into recreation yards from drones have occurred in correctional facilities in the United States and Canada, and paint guns and catapults have been used to send drugs over perimeter fences (Doyle & Williams, 2013; Ernst, 2013; *Washington Times*, 2010).

In contrast to opiates and other illicit substances that must be brought into facilities, alcohol is typically manufactured within correctional facilities. Alcohol brewed in prison, known as "pruno," is usually made from fruit, water, ketchup, and sugar mixed in a plastic bag and allowed to ferment over several days (Centers for Disease Control and Prevention, 2012, 2013). Hand sanitizers provide another source of alcohol (Doyon & Welsh, 2007).

Clinical presentation and assessment of substance use in correctional facilities

A thorough intake history of substance use, including prior overdoses and complicated withdrawal syndromes such as delirium tremens, will inform treatment staff about the likelihood of continued use and associated risks during incarceration. Inmates, however, may underreport their history in order to bypass confinement to an infirmary for medical observation. Some want to avoid detection of their problem by detoxifying themselves in general population with smuggled substances. Other helpful components of the intake assessment include collateral information and findings on physical examination, toxicology screens, and general laboratory tests. Some factors found to have a positive association with drug abuse inside prison include young age, white race, greater number of years incarcerated, nonparticipation in religious services, drug-related activities in the community, negative attitudes toward correctional rules, and facility overcrowding (Gillespie, 2005). In the absence of a knowledgeable and comprehensive diagnostic assessment, correctional psychiatrists may fail to detect an inmate's SUD (Fazel, Bains, & Doll, 2006).

Laboratory specimens used in drug testing include urine, blood, hair, saliva, sweat, and nails (toenails and fingernails). They provide different levels of specificity, sensitivity, and accuracy (Moeller, Lee, & Kissack, 2008). Drug screening by immunoassay requires confirmation of positive results with more sensitive methods such as gas or liquid chromatography coupled with mass spectrometry. Detection times for specific substances and means of collection differ. Urine and hair samples (especially head and body hair) have the advantages of long detection windows and ease of collection. Blood and saliva samples offer narrower windows of detection. Oral fluid samples may require longer collection times and yield lower volumes, which can necessitate collection of another type of sample (Drummer, 2006).

Many psychiatric and nonpsychiatric medications can cause false-positive immunoassay results. Such medications include bupropion, trazodone, and chlorpromazine on amphetamine screens; venlafaxine on phencyclidine screens; diphenhydramine, clomipramine, chlorpromazine, quetiapine, and thioridazine on methadone screens; and sertraline on benzodiazepine screens (Brahm et al., 2010).

An inmate's substances of choice on the street may shift to different and more available substances during incarceration. Therefore, a prior diagnosis of a particular SUD should not deter consideration of current use of other, or multiple, substances. Similarly, injection drug use may continue or commence while an inmate is incarcerated. Imprisonment favors high-risk behavior with drugs because of concentrated at-risk populations and risk-conducive conditions such as overcrowding and increased prevalence of violence. The potential consequences of drugs in jail or prison include deaths, suicide attempts, and self-harm. Drug use tends to be more dangerous inside correctional facilities than outside because of the scarcity of drugs and sterile injecting equipment. Although 45.7 percent of individuals shared needles outside prison, 70.5 percent of injection drug–using individuals reported sharing needles while incarcerated (Stover & Michels, 2010).

Because of the many substances found in correctional facilities, psychiatrists should consider a broad differential diagnosis when evaluating altered mental status. Intoxication or withdrawal can present with acute anxiety, perceptual changes, delusions, suicidal or homicidal thinking, and other signs and symptoms associated with mental and medical illnesses (see Chapter 17). For example, the black market for tobacco in facilities with bans warrants consideration of nicotine withdrawal in inmates who present with irritability, difficulty concentrating, anxiety, depression, restlessness, or insomnia (Hughes, 2007).

General psychiatric disorders often accompany SUDs, and the transition into correctional facilities can affect the expression of both conditions. When thrust into an environment with restricted access to substances and, in some cases, restrictive formularies, symptoms of psychiatric disorders and of SUDs (including withdrawal and craving) may appear. Understanding how this transition period affects an inmate's mental health helps guide treatment planning.

The following review of intoxication and withdrawal syndromes focuses on the most commonly abused substances in correctional settings: cannabis, stimulants, alcohol, and opiates. More extensive discussions of withdrawal management, addiction programming, medication-assisted therapies, and community re-entry can be found in Chapters 17, 44, 46, and 47 respectively.

Cannabis

Cannabis was found to be the drug most commonly used by inmates in one Canadian study (Plourde & Brochu 2002). Users experience relaxation, euphoria, slowed time perception, altered sensory perception, increased awareness of the environment, and increased appetite. Adverse effects include impaired concentration, anterograde amnesia, and motor dyscoordination. Higher doses and stressful conditions may result in hypervigilance, anxiety, paranoia, derealization and depersonalization, panic attacks, hallucinations, and delirium. Management of cannabis intoxication occasionally requires benzodiazepines and/or antipsychotic medications (Wilkens, Danovitch, & Gorelick, 2009) and, more rarely, infirmary observation. The most recent *Diagnostic and Statistical Manual of Mental Disorders* (DSM-5) recognizes cannabis withdrawal as a clinical syndrome with irritability, nervousness, sleep difficulty, decreased appetite, restlessness, depressed mood, and physical symptoms and discomfort (Hesse & Thylstrup, 2013). In contrast to the potential mortality associated with opiates and alcohol, correctional staff might not view cannabis intoxication and withdrawal as requiring treatment. Therefore, the correctional psychiatrist can offer guidance and education about these potential consequences.

Stimulants

Stimulants, including cocaine, amphetamine, and methamphetamine, may be snorted, inhaled, injected, or inserted rectally by inmates. Stimulants increase catecholamine neurotransmitter and sympathetic nervous system activity and may cause physiologic changes, including mydriasis, tachycardia, palpitations, tremor, hyperreflexia, and mild fever (Wilkens et al., 2009). Intoxication is associated with increased energy, alertness, and euphoria and decreased fatigue, need for sleep, and appetite. With chronic use, stimulant intoxication can cause anxiety, panic, irritability, hypervigilance, grandiosity, impaired judgment, stereotyped behavior, paranoia, and hallucinations (including tactile ones, such as formication). Severe intoxication may produce a potentially fatal excited delirium. Cocaine intoxication sometimes requires hospitalization because of asthma exacerbation, arrhythmia, myocardial or cerebral infarction, rhabdomyolysis, acute renal failure, or seizures. Other adverse effects include psychosis and agitation that require treatment with benzodiazepines and/or antipsychotic medications. Care should be taken if using antipsychotics, however, as they may exacerbate cardiovascular effects, lower the seizure threshold, and increase the risk of hyperthermia.

Alcohol

Psychiatric evaluation may be crucial to the detection of alcohol withdrawal, especially with prominent perceptual disturbances and delusional thinking. Autonomic instability, diaphoresis, and tremor provide clues to alcohol withdrawal as the etiology of mental status changes. Complicated withdrawal syndromes can cause acute mental status changes among patients who have been in the general population for extended periods but have developed physiological dependence on alcohol manufactured within the facility. In prisons, in particular, where inmates serve long sentences and alcohol production may be sophisticated, psychiatrists should consider the possibility of regular drinking, intoxication, and physiological dependence by inmates. In a 2007 case, an inmate's intoxication and agitation from ethyl alcohol in a hand sanitizer required haloperidol and fluid repletion in an emergency department (Doyon & Welsh, 2007). Chapter 17 discusses alcohol and benzodiazepine withdrawal in greater detail.

Cases of botulism from the use of raw potatoes in the production of pruno have been reported (Centers for Disease Control and Prevention, 2012; Vugia et al., 2009). The second and third largest botulism outbreaks in the United States since 2006 occurred in a Utah prison in 2011 and an Arizona prison in 2012 consequent to the use of raw potatoes in manufacturing pruno. The Utah outbreak cost an estimated $500,000 and involved many hours of investigation and prompt hospital treatment (Centers for Disease Control and Prevention, 2012). In the Arizona outbreak, seven of the eight affected inmates were intubated for 11 to 14 days before receiving tracheostomies (Centers for Disease Control and Prevention, 2013). The patients in these cases presented with common signs and symptoms of botulism, including blurry vision, dysarthria, dysphagia, shortness of breath, and generalized muscle weakness (Vugia et al., 2009). Complicating diagnostic assessment is the fact that the onset of botulism may follow the consumption of pruno by several hours, when the inmate no longer has slurred speech, motor incoordination, and mental status changes associated with alcohol intoxication.

Opiates

Opiate use by inmates presents medical and mental health staff with significant challenges. Given the typical frequency of injections, the potential exists for the transmission of infectious disease and for overdose (intended and unintended). Several medications prescribed by psychiatrists ameliorate opioid withdrawal symptoms. Medications that patients may request for this reason include clonidine (for anxiety; Gold et al., 1980), sedatives, antiemetic agents, and analgesics (Kosten & O'Connor, 2003). Abrupt cessation of opiates, as commonly occurs at the time of incarceration, can cause sleep disturbance that can last for weeks to months. Withdrawal symptoms limit the efficacy of medications such as antidepressants and mood stabilizers in improving insomnia. Buprenorphine suppresses opioid withdrawal symptoms in opioid-tolerant individuals, and inmates not tolerant to opiates can get high by taking buprenorphine sublingually, intranasally, or intravenously. Chapter 17 includes a detailed discussion of the presentation and management of opioid withdrawal.

An outpatient in a British addiction clinic with several incarcerations told his addiction providers about his motivation for smuggling opiates and other substances into correctional facilities. The patient, who took methadone in the community, had his dose routinely reduced from 110 mL to 40 mL (1 mL = 1 mg of methadone) when incarcerated. This predictably led to intense opioid withdrawal symptoms. The patient reduced the intensity of this problem by using a smuggled supply of illicit substances (George et al., 2009).

The risk of overdose and death from opiate abuse makes detection, rapid triage, and medical intervention crucial. Opioid overdose may present with altered level of consciousness, respiratory depression (rate <12/minute), and miotic pupils. Patients often have needle track marks, fresh injection sites, drug paraphernalia, and positive toxicology screens.

Consultative roles of the correctional psychiatrist

Correctional psychiatrists play important roles in educating other staff about SUDs, consulting in clinical situations, and crafting policies. Each task enhances clinical care and safety.

All correctional, medical, and mental health staff need a basic understanding of SUDs. Psychiatrists can provide education about the nature of SUDs, especially signs of intoxication and overdose and factors that contribute to substance use by inmates. Educational activities include formal presentations, case conferences, and day-to-day interactions with other staff about specific cases and situations.

As clinical consultants, psychiatrists help with diagnosis, including assessing for the presence and contribution of coexisting medical or mental disorders. They also assist with the interpretation of toxicology screens and with general treatment planning.

Consultations can involve direct clinical evaluation of inmates with mental status changes potentially caused by substance use or withdrawal. Delirium tremens from alcohol or benzodiazepine withdrawal, for example, may resemble psychosis or intoxication. In these cases, consultation with medical staff supports coordination of care and informs decisions about transfer to an emergency department. Chapter 45 reviews in more detail coordination of care for patients with dual diagnoses of mental disorders and substance abuse.

All facilities need policies on screening for, detecting, and treating SUDs. By playing an active role in developing these policies, psychiatrists enhance the provision of appropriate services and care. Administrative support for this and similar activities may require adjustment of psychiatrists' schedules and caseloads.

Disciplinary issues related to substance use by inmates

Data from the 2000 US Department of Justice report on drug use, testing, and treatment in jails (Wilson, 2000) illustrate how custody and administrative staff view substance use differently from psychiatrists and other health providers. Potential legal sanctions for inmates found using substances include new charges (39.3 percent of jurisdictions) and time added to current sentence (20.3 percent of jurisdictions). Administrative sanctions, by the percentage of jurisdictions that impose them, include loss of privileges (69.9 percent), loss of time credited for early release for "good time" (52.2 percent), reclassified security level (48.9 percent), increased testing (25.4 percent), and mandatory treatment (8.0 percent). Custody staff have understandable concerns about the presence of controlled substances or other contraband, especially because of the increased risk of violence or disruptive behaviors associated with inmates who possess these items (Friedmann et al., 2008). The relatively low percentages of jurisdictions that respond with increased drug testing and mandatory treatment, however, suggest an opportunity for enhanced education among correctional administrators. Such education may focus on the nature of SUDs and the treatments that could promote positive disciplinary outcomes.

Punitive administrative sanctions such as loss of privileges or "good time" (i.e., earned credit for early release through good behavior) may have a deterrent effect, but they do not address the clinical symptoms (e.g., craving, anxiety, mood instability) that drive substance use. In addition to its therapeutic benefits, treatment may decrease demand for illicit substances in correctional facilities. Correctional psychiatrists can inform their custody counterparts about the advantages of a clinical approach that might, for example, include contingency management strategies (e.g., re-earning good time and privileges).

Security staff monitor for illicit substances and other contraband with pat-downs, drug-sniffing dogs, radiography, metal detectors, and similar methods. They also collect blood, urine, or other specimens to test for recent substance use by inmates. Medical and mental health providers, however, do not participate in drug analyses done for nonclinical reasons. Nevertheless, custody staff might seek psychiatric input to help them understand the general use and interpretation of toxicology screening. Psychiatrists provide a service to the system and inmates by ensuring that custody administrators understand the accuracy and limitations of testing.

Inmates could receive unwarranted sanctions if custody administrators lack adequate information about drug testing. Penalties after false-positive drug test results caused by legitimately prescribed medications (as noted earlier in this chapter) are only one example. In other cases, inmates have received undeserved punishment for an inability to provide urine samples. Paruresis, sometimes referred to as shy bladder or psychogenic urinary retention, involves difficulty initiating or sustaining urination while being observed or potentially observed by others. Symptoms range from mild to severe and can vary for individuals at different times and under different circumstances (Boschen, 2008; Vythilingum, Stein, & Soifer, 2002; Zgourides, 1987). Sometimes it is impossible for affected individuals to provide a witnessed urine sample or an unwitnessed sample under time pressure. The recognizably situational and psychogenic nature of the condition makes physiological evaluation fruitless and unnecessary. Instead, inmates who claim to have this difficulty need accommodation by allowing them to void unobserved in a room without water or, when necessary, to provide alternative samples such as blood or saliva. Attempts at fluid loading or prolonged observation until an inmate voids risk bladder damage and water intoxication (Klonoff & Jurow, 1991). In addition, courts in the United States have recognized paruresis as a condition covered by the Americans with Disabilities Act [42 U.S.C. sec. 12132]. Correctional systems risk successful litigation if they sanction inmates who cannot provide urine samples instead of offering them reasonable accommodations (*Dwyer v. Dubois,* 1998). Consultation and guidance from a well-informed psychiatrist can avoid potentially serious physical harm to inmates while sparing a system from litigation.

Summary

Active substance abuse by inmates presents clinical and systemic challenges for correctional psychiatrists. The interplay among mental health, medical, and custody staff regarding screening, detection, triage, management, and treatment lies at the heart of these challenges. Correctional psychiatrists make important contributions by providing direct assessment and treatment to inmates and by offering educational, clinical, and policy consultations to other staff. These contributions help prevent potentially life-threatening complications of intoxication and withdrawal, ensure integrated and evidence-based care, and avoid misguided or ill-informed disciplinary or other institutional practices.

References

Boschen, M. J. (2008). Paruresis (psychogenic inhibition of micturition): Cognitive behavioral formulation and treatment. *Depression and Anxiety, 25,* 903–912.

Brahm, N. C., Yeager, L. L., Fox, M. D., et al. (2010). Commonly prescribed medications and potential false-positive urine drug screens. *American Journal of Health System Pharmacy, 67,* 1344–1350.

Centers for Disease Control and Prevention (2012). Botulism from drinking prison-made illicit alcohol—Utah 2011. *Morbidity and Mortality Weekly Report, 61,* 782–784.

Centers for Disease Control and Prevention (2013). Notes from the field: Botulism from drinking prison-made illicit alcohol—Arizona, 2012. *Morbidity and Mortality Weekly Report, 62,* 88–88.

Cork, K. (2012). *Tobacco behind bars: Policy options for the adult correctional population.* St. Paul, MN: Public Health Law

Center at William Mitchell College of Law. Retrieved from http://publichealthlawcenter.org/sites/default/files/resources/phlc-policybrief-tobaccobehindbars-adultcorrections-2012.pdf

Doyle, J., & Williams, D. (2013). *Gang foiled as they fling drugs and mobiles to inmates over prison wall with 8ft catapult.* Retrieved from http://www.dailymail.co.uk/news/article-2389469/Gang-foiled-fling-drugs-mobiles-inmates-Midlands-prison-wall-8ft-CATAPULT.html

Doyon, S., & Welsh, C. (2007). Intoxication of a prison inmate with an ethyl alcohol-based hand sanitizer. *New England Journal of Medicine, 356,* 529–530.

Drummer, O. H. (2006). Drug testing in oral fluid. *Clinical Biochemist Reviews, 27,* 147–159.

Dwyer v. Dubois. (1998). Massachusetts Superior Court Civil Action No. 95-05162-G.

Ernst, D. (2013). *Special delivery: Drone drops contraband into Georgia prison yard.* Retrieved from http://www.washingtontimes.com/news/2013/nov/27/drone-drops-contraband-georgia-prison-yard/

Fazel, S., Bains, P., & Doll, H. (2006). Substance abuse and dependence in prisoners: a systematic review. *Addiction, 101,* 181–191.

Ferranti, S. (2013). *Inside the Aryan Brotherhood's prison heroin empire.* Retrieved from http://www.salon.com/2013/03/19/inside_the_aryan_brotherhoods_prison_heroin_empire_partner/

Friedmann, P. D., Melnick, G., Jiang, L., et al. (2008). Violent and disruptive behavior among drug-involved prisoners: relationship with psychiatric symptoms. *Behavioral Sciences and the Law, 26,* 389–401.

George, S., Clayton, S., Namboodiri, V., et al. (2009). "Up yours": smuggling illicit drugs into prison. *BMJ Case Reports,* doi:10.1136/bcr.06.2009.1935

Gillespie, W. (2005). A multilevel model of drug abuse inside prison. *Prison Journal, 85,* 223–246.

Gold, M. S., Pottash, A. C., Sweeney, D. R., et al. (1980). Opiate withdrawal using clonidine. A safe, effective, and rapid nonopiate treatment. *Journal of the American Medical Association, 243,* 343–346.

Goodnough, A., & Zezima, K. (2011). *When children's scribbles hide a prison drug.* Retrieved from http://www.nytimes.com/2011/05/27/us/27smuggle.html?pagewanted=all&_r=0

Hesse, M., & Thylstrup, B. (2013). Time-course of the DSM-5 cannabis withdrawal symptoms in poly-substance abusers. *BMC Psychiatry, 13,* 258.

Hughes, J. R. (2007). Effects of abstinence from tobacco: Valid symptoms and time course. *Nicotine and Tobacco Research, 9,* 315–327.

Hunt, D. E., Kuck, S., Truitt, L., et al. (2006). *Methamphetamine use lessons learned.* Cambridge, MA: Abt Associates. Retrieved from http://purl.access.gpo.gov/GPO/LPS123253

Klonoff, D. C., & Jurow, A. H. (1991). Acute water intoxication as a complication of urine drug testing in the workplace. *Journal of the American Medical Association, 265,* 84–85.

Kosten, T. R., & O'Connor, P. G. (2003). Management of drug and alcohol withdrawal. *New England Journal of Medicine, 348,* 1786–1795.

Malcolm, A. H. (1989). *Explosive drug use creating new underworld prisons.* Retrieved from http://www.nytimes.com/1989/12/30/us/explosive-drug-use-creating-new-underworld-prisons.html?pagewanted=print&src=pm

Moeller, K. E., Lee, K. C., & Kissack, J. C. (2008). Urine drug screening: Practical guide for clinicians. *Mayo Clinic Proceedings, 83,* 66–76.

Plourde, C., & Brochu, S. (2002). Drugs in prison: A break in the pathway. *Substance Use and Misuse, 37,* 47–63.

Postigo, C., de Alda, M. L., & Barcelo, D. (2011). Evaluation of drugs of abuse use and trends in a prison through wastewater analysis. *Environment International, 37,* 49–55.

Rowell, T. L., Wu, E., Hart, C. L., et al. (2012). Predictors of drug use in prison among incarcerated Black men. *American Journal of Drug and Alcohol Abuse, 38,* 593–597.

Stallwitz, A., & Stover, H. (2007). The impact of substitution treatment in prisons—a literature review. *International Journal of Drug Policy, 18,* 464–474.

Stover, H., & Michels, II. (2010). Drug use and opioid substitution treatment for prisoners. *Harm Reduction Journal, 7,* 17.

Strang, J., Gossop, M., Heuston, J., et al. (2006). Persistence of drug use during imprisonment: relationship of drug type, recency of use and severity of dependence to use of heroin, cocaine and amphetamine in prison. *Addiction, 101,* 1125–1132.

Vugia, D. J., Mase, S. R., Cole, B., et al. (2009). Botulism from drinking pruno. *Emerging Infectious Diseases, 15,* 69–71.

Vythilingum, B., Stein, D. J., & Soifer, S. (2002). Is "shy bladder syndrome" a subtype of social anxiety disorder? A survey of people with paruresis. *Depression and Anxiety, 16,* 84–87.

Washington Times (2010). Drugs inside prison walls. January 27, 2010. Retrieved from http://www.washingtontimes.com/news/2010/jan/27/drugs-inside-prison-walls/print/

Wilkens, J., Danovitch, I., & Gorelick, D. (2009). Management of stimulant, hallucinogen, marijuana, phencyclidine, and club drug intoxication and withdrawal. In R. Ries, D. Fiellin, S. Miller, et al. (Eds.). *Principles of addiction medicine* (4th ed., pp. 607–628). Philadelphia, PA: Lippincott Williams and Wilkins.

Wilson, D. J. (2000). *Drug use, testing, and treatment in jails.* Washington, DC: US Department of Justice, Bureau of Justice Statistics.

Zgourides, G. D. (1987). Paruresis: Overview and implications for treatment. *Psychological Reports, 60,* 1171–1176.

SECTION V

Emergencies

CHAPTER 25

Crisis assessment and management

Reena Kapoor

Introduction

Crisis calls occur frequently in correctional settings, so much so that they can begin to seem routine. Psychiatrists are regularly called away from scheduled assignments such as diagnostic interviews or medication clinics to respond to a wide array of concerns, including suicide attempts, acute psychosis, seizures, destruction of property, self-injury, smearing of bodily waste, fire setting, flooding, and many others. Requests for urgent intervention with inmates can range from the informal, "Doc, I need you to take a look at Jones . . ." to the formal system of color-coded emergency response after violence or suicide attempts. Regardless of the psychiatrist's formal work assignment, handling crises—almost always in conjunction with security staff—is an expected part of the job. This chapter reviews the pragmatics of evaluating and managing many common correctional events that lead to mental health crisis calls.

Background

Although psychiatrists can be asked to respond to crises anywhere within a correctional institution, some settings and subpopulations of inmates are more likely to require crisis intervention. Inmates who have a history of mental illness frequently use emergency care; almost 70% of inmates requiring crisis intervention in one state correctional system had at least one mental health diagnosis (Center for Health Policy, Planning, and Research, 2007). Inmates who are housed in high-security settings such as restrictive housing units and supermax facilities are also likely to require emergency intervention (Knoll & Beven, 2010). A disproportionate number of prison suicides occur in isolation units (Patterson & Hughes, 2008), and inmates are also more likely to display evidence of behavioral disturbances in those settings (Lovell, 2008). Finally, psychiatrists in jails may be called to respond to suicide attempts more frequently than those assigned to prisons, as both attempts and completed suicides are more common in jail settings (Bureau of Justice Statistics, 2012).

For psychiatrists new to corrections, emergency responses can be unfamiliar and even frightening. In contrast to other health care settings, a crisis response in prisons and jails often involves the use of chemical agents, riot gear, and video cameras. These features of the emergency response can be intimidating. In addition, psychiatrists must adjust to the idea that they are not leading the response team, but instead must collaborate with security staff.

The medical model of crisis intervention takes a back seat to safety and security in correctional settings, and psychiatrists must adapt accordingly.

Despite the tension that sometimes arises between security officers and mental health professionals, an effective crisis response that involves both disciplines can result in significantly improved facility safety. Several studies have found a decrease in violence in facilities where officers were trained to recognize and respond appropriately to mental illness (Dupont, Cochran, & Pillsbury, 2007). Use of force by officers during crises decreased by approximately 70%, and "battery [of officers] by bodily waste" decreased by approximately 50% after corrections staff underwent mental health training (Hicks, 2011; Parker, 2009). In addition, officers referred many more inmates for mental health evaluation after the crises instead of disciplining them (Center for Health Policy, Planning, and Research, 2007). Because of these substantial benefits, collaboration between mental health and security professionals in crisis response is rapidly becoming a best practice.

Common types of crisis evaluations in correctional settings

Correctional psychiatrists receive requests for urgent consultations from many sources, including security staff, other physicians, other mental health staff, and even persons outside the facility such as family members, court personnel, and attorneys. Table 25.1 lists common types of urgent evaluations in correctional settings.

Although these evaluations address a wide variety of problems, some features are common to all types of crisis assessments. Therefore, the correctional psychiatrist can use a relatively standardized approach to handling crises that serves both to improve patient care and to decrease the psychiatrist's anxiety in these challenging situations.

Approach to crisis assessment and management

Maintaining a therapeutic role and appropriate boundaries

When collaborating with security staff in crisis situations, psychiatrists can be tempted to prioritize security concerns over health concerns. This temptation can be particularly acute when an

Table 25.1 Common requests for urgent psychiatric evaluation

Requesting Party	Type of Evaluation
Security staff	◆ Suicide attempts ◆ Other self-injury ◆ Clearance for placement in segregated housing ◆ Destruction of property ◆ Smearing of bodily waste ◆ Bizarre behavior observed in housing unit ◆ Homicidal statements (usually in conjunction with other signs of mental illness)
Other physicians and medical providers	◆ Management of acute drug or alcohol withdrawal ◆ Refusal of medical care ◆ Swallowing or insertion of foreign bodies ◆ Mental status and competence to engage in hunger strike
Other mental health professionals	◆ Ordering of therapeutic restraints ◆ Emergency medication ◆ Discharge from treatment setting or transfer to less therapeutic environment
Courts	◆ Bizarre behavior observed during court appearance ◆ Suicide assessment after imposition of long sentence
Families and attorneys	◆ Suicidal statements made during visit with family or attorney ◆ Suicidal or threatening letters written by inmate

inmate has engaged in behavior that repeatedly disturbs the officers, such as banging on doors or smearing bodily waste. Security officers often see punishment as the most effective method of stopping this behavior, and they seek the psychiatrist's approval or collaboration in moving forward with this plan. The psychiatrist may also feel exasperated by the inmate's behavior, viewing it as an attempt to manipulate the conditions of confinement rather than as a symptom of mental illness.

Despite these pressures to ally with security staff, correctional psychiatrists must remember that their primary role is therapeutic, and therefore they must focus on the inmate's best interest. Even if the inmate displays evidence of antisocial traits, psychiatrists must complete a thorough and independent evaluation. When deciding on a course of action, they must not allow their desire to maintain collegial relationships with security staff to supersede their concern for the well-being of the patient. Furthermore, they must recognize their own feelings of frustration and ensure that they are not acting out against the patient or reflexively jumping to a diagnosis of malingering. Maintaining a therapeutic stance when working with severely disturbed individuals can be challenging but is nevertheless essential to creating an effective treatment relationship.

Some mental health professionals, however, may inadvertently distort the concept of a therapeutic relationship. They may feel pressure to engage in boundary violations on behalf of the inmate. For example, inmates often ask psychiatrists to intervene in areas

that are traditionally managed by security staff, such as phone calls or cellmate decisions. In addition, some inmates make romantic overtures toward mental health professionals and view their relationship as more than strictly professional. While psychiatrists should feel free to advocate for the health of their patients, they must also take care to maintain appropriate boundaries and avoid developing personal relationships with inmates. In crisis situations, psychiatrists should also be careful not to promise more assistance to inmates than they are capable of providing. Inmates may attempt to apply pressure on the psychiatrist by promising to end the crisis if their demands are met; such negotiations are usually counterproductive in the long term. Maintaining appropriate boundaries and clear role definitions between security and psychiatry is consistently a better approach.

Confidentiality and communication with the requesting party

In emergencies, psychiatrists need as much information about the crisis as possible. Therefore, rapid and open communication with security staff about the events leading up to the psychiatrist's intervention is essential. Psychiatrists should obtain information about who first identified the problem with the inmate, what steps were taken to address the matter, and what the inmate's response was. In addition, psychiatrists should clarify what the party requesting the evaluation expects of the psychiatrist; this can range from informal assessments—"just take a look at him"—to involuntary medication and transfer to a psychiatric hospital.

In most cases, all of this preliminary information is best shared openly, with the inmate's confidentiality a secondary concern to safety. However, if at all possible, mental health and security staff should discuss this information in a private setting away from other inmates. Psychiatric emergencies, and sometimes just the presence of an unfamiliar face on the housing block, can attract many curious onlookers from other cells. As any information that inmates (or even other staff members) gain about the crisis may be used to taunt or harass the involved inmate at a later time, maintaining confidentiality should not be taken lightly.

In addition to the concern about future harassment by inmates or officers, psychiatrists should evaluate the inmate in a confidential setting (whenever feasible) for the usual therapeutic reasons; people are more likely to share their true feelings if not fearful of being overheard. Psychiatrists should make clear to the inmate that they are there in a therapeutic capacity and are not trying to punish the inmate. They should also explain that, except in cases that involve an immediate threat to the safety and security of the facility, the conversation will be kept confidential and details of the encounter will not be shared with security staff.

Environmental factors

During crises, correctional psychiatrists are often asked to evaluate inmates through the cell door, in a cage, or while being video recorded. The inmate may be restrained with handcuffs and in some instances a chemical agent has already been sprayed in the area. All of these environmental factors can influence the quality of the psychiatrist's assessment. A quiet, confidential setting is always preferable when conducting a psychiatric evaluation but cannot always be achieved in a crisis. In some situations, such as when an inmate is acutely agitated or possesses a weapon, a psychiatrist would be foolish to interview him alone or without restraints. In other situations, inmates may simply refuse to come out of the cell. Although not ideal, a cell-side psychiatric evaluation may be required in these circumstances.

In addition to security concerns, recording devices can also play a role in shaping the psychiatrist's assessment during a crisis. In many emergencies, particularly those that are formally designated by a color-coded response system, corrections officers will videotape the actions of staff and the inmate for use in clinical review and potential subsequent litigation. Psychiatrists who are new to corrections may be unaccustomed to conducting an assessment while being filmed. They may be anxious about omitting part of the evaluation or about how their actions will be perceived by those reviewing the tape. However, psychiatrists must quickly become familiar with the process of recording their actions during crisis, and they should do their best to behave as they would when not being filmed. Ultimately, the video recording should serve to protect psychiatrists against future claims of negligence. As long as the intervention is conducted in a professional, therapeutic manner, subsequent review is not a concern (see Chapter 3).

De-escalation

Psychiatrists responding to crises can use several de-escalation techniques to help inmates calm themselves and avoid the use of force (Richmond, Berlin, Fishkind, Holloman Jr., Zeller, Wilson, Rifai, & Ng, 2012). First, psychiatrists should respect the personal space of the inmate, trying to stand at least two arms lengths away. When approaching the inmate, psychiatrists should introduce themselves and state their role clearly. Multiple persons responding to a crisis can be perceived as threatening, so only one person at a time should talk to the inmate to minimize fear and distress. Body language is important; psychiatrists should avoid gestures like clenched fists or crossed arms, which can be interpreted as provocative.

Psychiatrists and security officers should listen attentively and allow inmates to express the concerns that led to the crisis. Repeating the inmate's words back to him and using statements such as, "Tell me if I have this right . . ." can help him to feel heard. If the inmate is delusional, psychiatrists should avoid actively challenging the delusions, instead focusing on the emotions expressed by the inmate in response to the delusions. Similarly, psychiatrists should avoid making accusations of lying or malingering in the crisis situation, as these accusations can heighten tensions and prolong the crisis. The goal is to allow the inmate to express wishes and emotional distress without feeling attacked or demeaned.

To the extent possible, offering choices to the inmate can also be helpful. For example, sometimes the inmate can be allowed to choose which officer or mental health staff member attends to the crisis. This technique makes use of preexisting therapeutic alliances and can help the inmate maintain some control over the situation. In another example, a choice between different forms of oral medication (liquid, pill, or dissolving strip) can be offered as an alternative to intramuscular injection. While de-escalation may not be successful in all cases, making an effort to avoid the use of force can be beneficial both in the short term and long term.

Inmates see that the psychiatrist is compassionate enough to help them avoid traumatic experiences such as cell extractions and restraints, and officers can learn more therapeutic and effective approaches to crisis management.

Elements of the psychiatric evaluation

While maintaining a relatively standardized approach, the specific elements of a psychiatric evaluation in a crisis can vary greatly based on the circumstances. For example, the assessment of an inmate who has just attempted suicide can be very different, both in its focus and its duration, from the assessment of an inmate who has declared a hunger strike. In the former circumstance, the initial focus may be on getting the inmate appropriate medical treatment for asphyxiation or lacerations. The psychiatrist may only briefly assess the inmate before making arrangements for hospital transport. In the latter circumstance, the psychiatrist may conduct an extended evaluation, carefully documenting the inmate's history of any mental illness, stated rationale for engaging in the hunger strike, formal mental status exam, and a determination of mental capacity to refuse food. Both situations require urgent assessment, but the psychiatrist's approach is tailored to the needs of the inmate and the requesting party.

In all cases, psychiatrists should conduct as thorough an evaluation as circumstances require, without regard for external pressures such as staff shift changes or desires to transfer the inmate to another facility quickly. The inmate's health and stability are the psychiatrist's primary concern. In general, psychiatrists should attempt to interview the inmate, gather information from relevant collateral informants, perform necessary elements of the mental status exam, and discuss any changes to the treatment plan with the inmate during a crisis evaluation. If any of these elements are omitted, psychiatrists should ensure that they are not omitted for the sake of convenience or because of inadequate resources. All elements of the assessment performed and the rationale for the chosen course of action must be documented.

Disposition options

When psychiatrists intervene in crisis situations, they are often asked to recommend a particular course of action to security staff. If an inmate has made a serious suicide attempt, the course of action is usually clear—stabilize the inmate medically and then admit him to an intensive psychiatric treatment setting. However, many types of crises allow mental health and security staff to use more discretion to resolve the situation. Changes in housing placements, privilege levels, medication, and frequency or type of therapy are all possible. In some cases, transfer to a psychiatric or medical hospital may be necessary. With so many options, psychiatrists may find it difficult to make recommendations, particularly when facing time pressure.

Many correctional systems alleviate this confusion in non-emergency situations or subsequent to a crisis by creating multidisciplinary teams to review decisions about inmates' mental health treatment and conditions of confinement. This approach can be very helpful to ensure that all relevant factors are considered before making a decision. The review team can consider the inmate's psychiatric stability, interpersonal relationships, history of violence, and coping skills before implementing recommendations. During the emergency, however, psychiatrists do not typically have the luxury of working through this supportive process and must reach a decision about immediate concerns quickly.

If the evaluating psychiatrist is concerned about the inmate's safety, he or she should advocate for placing the inmate in a secure and therapeutic setting such as an inpatient psychiatric unit or a psychiatric observation cell. This measure should be taken even if the inmate engages in repetitive, nonlethal acts of self-injury and staff are growing tired of frequent transfers. If questioned about the need for emergency transfer, psychiatrists can refer to the literature about the high risk of completed suicide in patients who have made prior attempts, particularly by hanging, strangulation, or suffocation (Runeson, Tidemalm, Dahlin, Lichtenstein, & Lanstrom, 2010; Tidemalm, Langstrom, Lichtenstein, & Runeson, 2008). Of course, crisis response is only one part of a comprehensive treatment plan for suicidal patients; psychiatrists should also advocate for a better long-term treatment plan for the inmate so as to avoid repeated inpatient placements. However, in an emergency situation (in the absence of an existing long-term plan), psychiatrists should act cautiously and place the inmate in a safe setting.

In the most severe cases of violence or self-injury, emergency medication or therapeutic restraints may be necessary. When considering whether to order chemical or physical restraints, psychiatrists should use criteria consistent with the community standard—for example, Is the patient an acute danger to self or others? Have less restrictive interventions failed? (Metzner, Tardiff, Lion, Reid, Recupero, Schetky, Edenfield, Mattson, & Janofsky, 2007; National Commission on Correctional Health Care, 2008). Four-point therapeutic restraints, similar to those found in the community, should be used. In almost all circumstances requiring therapeutic restraints, the inmate should be transferred to a health care setting to be monitored (Metzner et al., 2007). Therapeutic restraints should be used for the shortest duration of time possible to ensure the patient's safety (Metzner et al., 2007).

Many correctional systems use different types of restraints for security purposes, such as shackles, belly chains, or restraint chairs. A psychiatrist should never order these for a therapeutic purpose. The use of so-called custody restraints is governed by many factors unrelated to mental illness, such as seriousness of charge, gang affiliation, and history of institutional violence. The restraints are used to incapacitate inmates in a wide variety of circumstances, from acute assaults to routine transportation between areas of the facility. While some of these considerations may be relevant to an emergency psychiatric assessment, in general they are less important than the inmate's current mental status and intent for harm to self or others. The psychiatrist should focus on the inmate's acute safety and health, using the same narrow criteria and therapeutic techniques used in the community to respond to the dangerous behaviors of individuals with mental illness.

Finally, crises often involve disciplinary actions against an inmate, either as a precipitant to a mental health crisis or as a consequence of engaging in crisis-generating behavior. Psychiatrists frequently are asked to give opinions regarding the inmate's suitability for discipline in these situations. These evaluations are challenging, as psychiatrists are unaccustomed to answering questions about how much punishment a person can or should endure. Nonetheless, psychiatrists play an important role in the inmate disciplinary process, and their opinions are given considerable weight. Security staff typically ask two questions of psychiatrists: Is the inmate stable enough to proceed with the disciplinary process? and Did mental illness play a role in the events leading to the disciplinary infraction? Psychiatrists should consider these questions carefully and answer them honestly, giving the inmate the benefit of the doubt in areas of uncertainty (see Chapter 14).

Documentation

After a crisis has been diffused, the psychiatrist must document the encounter in the medical record. Progress notes should contain all relevant information about the crisis and its resolution, including how the psychiatrist became involved in the situation, what information was obtained from collateral informants, the inmate's version of events, the inmate's mental status, and the psychiatrist's assessment and plan. Psychiatrists should carefully articulate why they chose a particular course of action and why they rejected alternatives. In addition to protecting against litigation, this information guides mental health professionals who subsequently work with the inmate to understand the treatment history.

Depending on the nature and severity of the crisis, documentation in addition to the clinical record may also be required. Most correctional systems require documentation to keep track of serious incidents of self-injury, use of restraints, and use of cell extraction teams. In addition, a clinical review of every completed suicide (or serious suicide attempt) should be conducted, and recommendations about policy or procedure changes resulting from this review should be documented (National Commission on Correctional Health Care, 2008).

Summary

Crisis calls are common in correctional settings, and psychiatrists play an integral role in crisis management. Requests for urgent psychiatric evaluations can come from many sources, including security staff, nonpsychiatric physicians, mental health staff, courts, attorneys, and family members. Psychiatrists responding to these requests for evaluation may feel tremendous pressure to reach a conclusion that is consistent with the opinions of the requesting party. However, it is crucial to maintain an independent and therapeutic stance when conducting crisis evaluations.

Some aspects of psychiatric evaluations in crisis situations are unique to the correctional environment, including cell-side evaluations, video recording, and leadership by security staff rather than medical professionals. Nonetheless, correctional psychiatrists should be guided by the same principles of medical ethics that apply to patient care in the community, placing the patient's well-being above all other concerns. They should strive, when possible, to conduct a thorough assessment in a confidential setting. In considering how best to resolve the crisis and care for the patient, psychiatrists should err on the side of caution and recommend placement in a safe and therapeutic setting, at least until a multidisciplinary team can consider other options. Finally, they should document the encounter carefully, articulating the rationale for the chosen course of action.

References

Bureau of Justice Statistics (2012). Mortality in local jails and state prisons, 2000–2010—Statistical. Retrieved from http://www.bjs.gov/content/pub/pdf/mljsp0010st.pdf

Center for Health Policy, Planning, and Research (2007). Crisis intervention team (CIT) training for correctional officers. Retrieved from http://www.une.edu/chppr/upload/nami_cit_eval_report.pdf

Dupont, R., Cochran, S., & Pillsbury, S. (2007). Crisis intervention team core elements. Retrieved from http://www.nami.org/Template.cfm?Section=CIT&Template=/ContentManagement/ContentDisplay.cfm&ContentID=150242

Hicks, E. (2011). Crisis intervention in a correctional setting. Retrieved from http://www.correctionsone.com/jail-management/articles/4206236-Crisis-intervention-in-a-correctional-setting/

Knoll, J. L.,IV & Beven, G. E. (2010). Supermax units and death row. In C. L. Scott (Ed.), *Handbook of correctional mental health* (pp. 435–475). Washington, DC: American Psychiatric Publishing.

Lovell, D. (2008). Patterns of disturbed behavior in a supermax prison. *Criminal Justice and Behavior, 35*, 985–1004.

Metzner, J. L., Tardiff, K., Lion, J., Reid, W. H., Recupero, P. R., Schetky, D. H., Edenfield, B. M., Mattson, M., & Janofsky, J. S. (2007).

Resource document on the use of restraint and seclusion in correctional mental health care. *Journal of the American Academy of Psychiatry and the Law, 35*, 417–425.

National Commission on Correctional Health Care (2008). *Standards for mental health services in correctional facilities.* Chicago: National Commission on Correctional Health Care.

Parker, G. F. (2009). Impact of a mental health training course for correctional officers on a special housing unit. *Psychiatric Services, 60*(5), 640–645.

Patterson, R. F., & Hughes, K. (2008). Review of completed suicides in the California Department of Corrections and Rehabilitation, 1999 to 2004. *Psychiatric Services, 59*, 677–681.

Richmond, J. S., Berlin, J. S., Fishkind, A. B., Holloman G. H., Jr., Zeller, S. L., Wilson, M. P., Rifai, M. A., & Ng, A. T. (2012). Verbal de-escalation of the agitated patient: Consensus statement of the American Association for Emergency Psychiatry Project BETA de-escalation workgroup. *Western Journal of Emergency Medicine, 13*, 17–25.

Runeson, B., Tidemalm, D., Dahlin, M., Lichtenstein, P., & Langstrom, N. (2010). Method of attempted suicide as predictor of subsequent successful suicide: National long term cohort study. *British Medical Journal, 341*, c3222.

Tidemalm, D., Langstrom, N., Lichtenstein, P., & Runeson, B. (2008). Risk of suicide after suicide attempt according to coexisting psychiatric disorder: Swedish cohort study with long term follow-up. *British Medical Journal, 337*, a2205.

CHAPTER 26

Use of restraint and emergency medication

Gerard G. Gagné, Jr.

Introduction

The use of seclusion and/or restraint (S/R) in mental health settings has long been fraught with legal and ethical concerns; the practice can be dangerous. This is perhaps accentuated in the more punitive environment of jails and prisons within the United States. As a result, there is a national movement to reduce the use of S/R of mentally ill patients both in the community and within jails and prisons. However, S/R remains an effective intervention when less invasive interventions to maintain the safety of an inmate or others have failed. While some may perceive S/R as an intervention ultimately to be eliminated, facilities that use S/R for mentally ill patients, be they hospitals, jails, or prisons, should not eliminate it; in limited cases, S/R is an appropriate option, particularly for acutely aggressive, agitated patients who require immediate intervention. The use of S/R preserves the safety of the patient, other patients and inmates, and staff. This, in turn, supports a safer milieu.

Appropriately established and closely followed guidelines in the community in many cases have led to an overall reduction in the use of S/R. When discussing guidelines for the use of S/R in jails and prisons, it is important to acknowledge several issues. First, critical differences from community settings exist that need to be addressed in establishing such guidelines for jails and prisons. Second, while national guidelines emphasize common themes, the specifics of correctional systems can vary considerably between jurisdictions.

In 1999, the Health Care Financing Administration, now the Center for Medicare and Medicaid Services (CMS), defined rules for the use of S/R for facilities that participate in Medicare and Medicaid (42 C.F.R. § 482.13). While CMS regulations do not govern correctional facilities, these rules nevertheless heavily influenced subsequent guidelines, including the American Psychiatric Association's resource document (APA RD) on the use of S/R in correctional health care (Metzner, Tardiff, Lion, Reid, Recupero, Schetky, Edenfield, Mattson, & Janofsky, 2007) and that of the American Bar Association (2011).

This chapter reviews both the APA RD on the use of S/R in correctional managed health care (2006) and the CMS Conditions of Participation, Patient's Rights (42 C.F.R. § 482.13) and discusses the pragmatic issues of implementation and management of S/R. The RD was designed, in part, to address the significant inconsistencies and variability in the use of S/R throughout the United States (Appelbaum, Savageau, Trestman, Metzner, & Baillargeon,

2011). Of note, the focus is solely on the use of S/R for mentally ill inmates and not their use by custody staff for safety or security reasons. It also highlights the differences between seclusion and restraint in the community compared to jails and prisons.

Location

In jails and prisons, S/R may occur in corrections-based hospitals, infirmaries, or other special housing. If an inmate is transferred out of a jail or prison into a community hospital for care, CMS rules typically guide the placement and monitoring of the inmate in S/R. When S/R occurs in jail or prison, a health care setting with 24-hour nursing coverage, such as an infirmary, should be used. While guiding principles of CMS should still apply, the specific security needs of the correctional environment will shape the physical characteristics of the seclusion room and the restraint.

In most minimum-security settings, congregate dormitory environments are common. In medium- or maximum-security jails and prisons, inmates may have limited contact with others except for meals, work, or programs. At other times, they will be confined to their cells, or "locked down." This confinement could last as long as 23 hours a day for administrative or disciplinary reasons. Given that many special needs units within jails and prisons lack 24-hour nursing care, the APA RD (Metzner et al., 2007) specifies that if S/R is to be used, 24-hour nursing care must be available. It is not appropriate to use locked-down housing units for inmates with mental illness who require S/R for clinical reasons. Not only are these units typically not supportive or therapeutic, but they likely will exacerbate the clinical condition for which the S/R is indicated in the first place. They also typically lack the health care staff necessary for treatment and monitoring.

Indications

There are several indications for S/R. They are appropriate when less restrictive forms of treatment have not proven effective or are not appropriate for the gravity of the clinical situation (Table 26.1).

Just as there are indications for S/R, so, too, there are situations in which S/R is not appropriate: patients who have a marked fear of being restrained; patients who have marked claustrophobia in a seclusion room; lack of trained, qualified mental health and/or medical staff to monitor the S/R; lack of a seclusion room

Table 26.1 Indications for the Use of Seclusion and/or Restraint in the Correctional Setting

- ◆ Signs and symptoms of significant danger to others that cannot be managed by less restrictive means
- ◆ Severe agitation for which emergency medication is inadequate or unavailable (e.g., allergy or known previous adverse effect) or has not yet taken effect
- ◆ Significant disruption of the clinical or residential milieu that threatens the rights or safety of patients or staff and for which less restrictive interventions are inadequate or not feasible
- ◆ Dangerous, agitated, or disruptive behavior whose origins are unclear and for which restraint and seclusion are likely to be safer than medication or other measures because of insufficient knowledge about the inmate's medical condition

sufficiently free of ways in which a patient may self-injure; and staff requests for S/R that the ordering physician believes reflect neglect, abuse, or simply staff convenience. Restraint should not be used if a patient's medical status is unknown, restraint is likely to cause harm, or the restraint position is contraindicated. As noted previously, health care staff should never order S/R for punitive purposes. Behaviors such as obnoxiousness, rudeness, or public masturbation are not reasons for S/R.

The decision to initiate S/R requires the careful consideration of factors that reflect the unique characteristics of each patient. Carefully formulating a treatment plan and consistently following that plan likely will lead to reduced reliance on S/R or may eliminate its use altogether. Once the circumstances that led to the use of S/R have been resolved, careful follow-up of the patient may uncover the motivation behind the aberrant behavior. The patient should be a part of this discussion.

Prior to the use of S/R, less restrictive interventions (reflecting verbal, environmental, or pharmacological aspects) should be used when appropriate. Staff should be adequately trained to address the underlying psychopathology before and after S/R, and the patient's housing unit should have sufficient staffing and treatment programs to address the patient's mental illness.

Restraints

Custody restraints (usually metal handcuffs) should not be used for mental health purposes. Typically, soft, adjustable restraints are applied to both wrists and ankles. While "restraint chairs" are available in some jails and prisons, allowing for ease of transport and application, their use should be discouraged because the threshold for using S/R is more likely to be lowered and it may occur in a suboptimal environment (i.e., in a place where 24-hour nursing care is not available).

Seclusion room design

The safe practice of S/R includes design of the seclusion room. The National Association of Psychiatric Health Systems (Sine & Hunt, 2007) has published seclusion room design guidelines that address the type of fixtures, temperature controls, lighting, and patient visibility, among others. While these factors (and others) might sound esoteric or inconsequential, they play a role both in treatment and in preventing self-injury or staff assault.

It is not uncommon to have constant, full-room lighting, particularly for several hours after the patient is placed in seclusion, to allow for easy staff visualization of the patient to assess ongoing aggressive behavior. The walls should be made of materials that cannot be picked apart or gouged for use in self-injury or as a weapon against staff. The room should be free of sharp corners and fixtures that jut out from the walls or ceiling. Windows should be made of shatterproof material, and the door should open outward so that the inmate cannot barricade the room. Only staff should control locks. Furniture should be limited to a mattress. Toilet and sink, if included, should be of unitary metal construction with no sharp edges. If not available in the room, toileting provisions must be made: a simple hole in the floor for toileting is inappropriate, as it is unsanitary and dehumanizing.

Restraint rooms are very similar in design to seclusion rooms, the one major difference being the inclusion of a restraint bed. Given the limited resources in many jails and prisons, it is not uncommon for a single room to be used both for seclusion and restraint, in which case the restraint bed should be made of a resilient, durable material and should be a single, unitary platform; it should be secured to the floor. Recessed attachments for restraints should be an integral feature of a restraint bed.

Property

Unless specifically contraindicated, inmates who are being secluded and/or restrained should have access to clothing (preferably made of tear-resistant materials to prevent their use for new or additional self-injury), a blanket (also made of tear-resistant materials), and a mattress (preferably one made of foam, which is harder for patients to use for self-injurious behavior).

Emergency medications

Emergency medication is sometimes used prior to or in conjunction with S/R. In acute psychosis, drug intoxication or withdrawal, or similar situations, emergency medication may be appropriate. CMS guidelines consider medication to be a restraint if it is not being used for standard therapy. Medication used as a form of restraint is not being prescribed for the patient's medical or psychiatric illness; it results in controlling the patient's acute behavior and/or restricting his acute freedom of movement. Naturally, the individual circumstances and the inmate's needs should be considered before a medication is used to treat acute episodes of patient agitation. Whether in an emergency department, jail, or prison, use of any medication should have a clearly defined medical indication that is documented in the chart; it may not be used as punishment.

Time frame

CMS guidelines specify that S/R should be ordered by a physician or "licensed independent practitioner" (LIP) and that the initial face-to-face interview must occur within 1 hour of making the order. The APA RD uses a 4-hour time frame, which may still be reasonable as the correctional setting, in most cases, is not a hospital. The only exception is the need to protect the patient or staff from imminent, substantial harm (e.g., an acutely psychotic patient who is attempting to assault a custody officer). If the LIP is not a physician, consultation with the physician should occur within 4 hours. The physician's order for S/R should be obtained within 1 hour of the LIP initiating the S/R.

A face-to-face assessment during seclusion should occur no less frequently than every 12 hours after the initial assessment by a trained LIP, physician, or registered nurse. In certain cases, these face-to-face assessments should occur more frequently, particularly when patients present with comorbid medical conditions, dementia, significant intoxication, or withdrawal.

Prolonged seclusion and, in particular, restraint can lead to adverse events and even death from medical complications such as deep vein thrombosis and pulmonary embolism, even in healthy persons. This and other reasons dictate that time limits should be placed on S/R. Initial orders for S/R should be limited to 4 hours for adults and 2 hours for children and adolescents (aged 9–17 years). The APA RD requires consultation (at least by phone) with a physician (preferably a psychiatrist) when the face-to-face assessment is not performed by a physician. After the first set of orders, renewal orders for further S/R are required, which may be based on information conveyed by telephone or face-to-face evaluation. These renewal orders may, if required, be repeated for up to 24 hours. The duration of each renewal should follow the previously mentioned guidelines based on age (i.e., 4 hours for adults, 2 hours for children and adolescents).

Monitoring and patient protection

Once S/R is initiated, medical and mental health staff need to carefully monitor the patient. During restraint, the inmate is at risk for asphyxiation or compromised circulation, especially when the period of restraint is lengthy. The inmate is also more vulnerable to abuse by other patients. Medical and mental health staff should consider continuous monitoring for patients who are intoxicated or withdrawing from substances, are actively engaged in self-injurious behavior, or are unfamiliar to staff.

Custody and medical/mental health staff should carefully document their observations of the inmate during S/R. Notes should be taken at regular intervals. Staff may tend to complete observation checklists prematurely or to fill them in retrospectively, particularly during prolonged S/R; this practice must be prevented.

Many facilities have closed-circuit television monitoring. This may be a useful supplement but alone does not constitute adequate monitoring. While a different staff member may be assigned to monitor a single screen, direct observation is the standard.

Documentation of visual observation does not constitute a full assessment; it should include date and time along with comments about the patient's behavior. Some facilities have custody officers and nursing staff assigned to monitor inmates on S/R status. Checklists designed to facilitate regular (frequently staggered 15-minute intervals) observation of patients while in seclusion are typically used. Checklists typically include a coding system for monitoring appearance and behavior along with written prompts for regular observation.

During the first 2 hours of restraint, a nurse should repeatedly assess the condition of all four extremities, noting pulses, circulation, and evidence of injuries caused by the inmate or the restraint. This ensures that the restraints were applied appropriately and that no injuries have been overlooked. Every 2 hours, the nurse should perform a more complete assessment of the patient that includes the circulation and integument examinations mentioned

previously. In addition, the patient's behavior, general physical condition, and responses to interactions/treatment should be noted; this more complete examination should be documented. Every 2 hours, the nurse should perform range-of-motion exercises with each limb in sequence, ideally without the restraints in place on that limb, unless this is contraindicated. This assessment, like the previously mentioned assessments, should be performed based on the patient's level of cooperation to avoid unnecessary risks for staff or patient. For example, if an inmate remains highly agitated and threatening, safety dictates that range-of-motion exercises should not be performed. The rationale for the deferral of any portion of an assessment should be clearly documented.

Other staff responsibilities that are conducted at least every 2 hours include appropriate toileting and hygiene; nourishment needs should be addressed every 4 hours. Inmates can be escorted to nearby bathrooms if they are available and it is safe to do so. The alternative is to offer a urinal or bed pan (along with privacy). Vital signs should be assessed no less frequently than once every 8 hours, again assuming it is safe to do so. Fluids and meals should be offered regularly, the former more regularly than the latter. Meal times should be the same as the rest of the facility; sharp utensils that could serve as a weapon or for self-injury must not be provided. In addition to the concerns noted, careful attention should be paid to patients who are susceptible to exhaustion or patients at high risk of adverse reactions to S/R (e.g., obese patients, older patients, or medically compromised patients).

Policy

Written policies and procedures for S/R should be part of the institution's formal health care policy and procedures manual. Initial training and annual retraining of medical, mental health, and custody staff who are involved in S/R is essential. Where applicable, photographs and videotapes to augment regular training should be available. For example, the mechanical restraints typically used for medical restraint are not the same as those used for custody restraint. Staff should be familiar with the different types of restraints to optimize comfort and proper fit and to avoid injury or assaultive behavior. Training and retraining should focus on, but not be limited to, techniques of restraining inmates and the required follow-up assessments and interventions (e.g., range-of-motion exercises, vital signs checks, and observation of the patient's mental state). All staff should receive annual documented recertification. Ideally, training should include an experiential portion led by seasoned instructors so that techniques can be practiced and critiqued. Benefits of training include improved patient outcomes and decreased staff-related costs. Specifically, reduced staff and patient injuries result from the proper initiation and monitoring of S/R and training that reduces the need for S/R (Recupero, Price, Garvey, Daly & Xavier, 2011).

Orders for S/R should be time- and behavior-specific. For example, "please initiate four-point therapeutic restraints, not to exceed 3 hours, for agitation and self-injurious behavior." It is never appropriate to make S/R a standing order. The patient's medical record should reflect the indication for S/R, the less restrictive/invasive interventions that were considered before initiating S/R, and why those interventions failed or were not appropriate. Each increment of continued S/R should be documented in a similar fashion, including the risks, benefits, and alternatives to extending S/R.

Clear documentation of each S/R episode provides an opportunity for rigorous review, ensuring policy compliance and providing meaningful feedback for potential policy modification. As many correctional systems have multiple facilities, such data support quality assurance and quality improvement programs and allow insight into site-specific challenges that can be ameliorated before adverse events occur.

Technique

Once the LIP or physician decides to initiate S/R, an S/R "leader" should be identified. The leader coordinates with custody staff to jointly inform the patient of the decision. To maximize efficiency and reduce potential harm, the team should present to the patient, in a calm, controlled manner, a simple, clear, united statement. The S/R leader should clearly state the purpose of the S/R, identifying the target behaviors that are driving the decision to initiate S/R and that will need to stop before S/R is terminated. This interaction is not a time for psychodynamic formulation, negotiation, or decision reversal; to do so is not clinically indicated and can exacerbate an already fragile situation.

Whenever possible, the patient should be led by calm and quiet staff to the S/R room. If the patient will not go to the designated room, the leader uses a predetermined signal to inform staff members that they should quickly secure a preassigned extremity or the head and bring the patient to the S/R room. If restraints and medication are required, emergency medication may be administered once the patient is secured to the restraint bed. It should be offered orally; if clinically indicated but refused, it may be administered intramuscularly.

Proper positioning of the inmate in restraints is critical. Prone positioning during brief containment is common. While there are risks if a patient is restrained in a supine position (e.g., aspiration, spitting, or biting), the patient should rarely be restrained in a prone position given the risk of asphyxiation. Specific justification for the use of prone restraint should be provided and medical clearance (e.g., not obese, no cardiac or pulmonary compromise) should be documented.

Just as important as the decision to initiate S/R is the decision to terminate it. When the patient has achieved the defined goals (e.g., agitation or aggression under control) and when the safety of the patient and staff is reasonably ensured, the patient should be released. This information is gathered through ongoing assessment and interaction with the patient (e.g., "How are you feeling right now? Do you feel in control of your behavior?") and can be inferred from direct observation (e.g., a once-agitated patient is no longer pacing the seclusion room; a once-threatening patient is calmly engaging staff and following directions).

Releasing S/R may be a graded process, titrated appropriately to follow the progressive improvement of a patient or to test a once highly threatening one. For example, it might be reasonable to release one or two extremities from a four-point therapeutic restraint to assess the patient's tolerance of gradually increasing levels of freedom. Likewise, while still being monitored closely by staff, an inmate might remain in the seclusion room with the door ajar. It is important to explain the rationale of the tapering in advance to the patient whenever possible; some patients might misinterpret a gradual taper versus completely terminating S/R as threatening or as staff "toying" with them.

Following the placement of a patient on S/R, the staff should debrief as a group. This affords a review of the techniques used and allows staff to release tension and emotion related to initiating and completing the S/R process. A specific discussion of what interventions might have prevented the need for S/R should also be held. Follow-up with the patient is critical to review the rationale for S/R and the subsequent behavior that led to release. It is helpful to elicit the patient's impressions about the usefulness of the procedure, as this may provide insight into what he or she identifies as triggers that led to the problematic behavior. This information can be incorporated into the patient's treatment plan. Naturally, the process of S/R should be well documented in the medical record.

Reducing the use of seclusion and restraint

Jails and prisons are being challenged to do more to limit the use of S/R as an intervention and to increase the therapeutic milieu of admittedly stark environments for mentally ill patients (Appelbaum, 2007; Champion, 2007; Metzner et al., 2007). Acknowledgment of the inherent risks associated with S/R as a tool for managing inmates with mental illness and the ethical dilemmas it poses have given momentum to the development of guidelines. Public health intervention models in the community have reduced the use of S/R by as much as 75%, with no increase in injuries to staff and patients (Lewis, Taylor, & Parks, 2009). Lion (2011) suggests that part of the solution to optimizing S/R is first acknowledging that it is an effective intervention that should be used in only rare situations and that it might require clinical certification.

In reflecting on the document developed by Metzner and colleagues (2007), Appelbaum (2007) questioned whether even these detailed guidelines go far enough, given that inmates with mental illness generally fare worse than inmates without mental illness, are at increased risk of sexual victimization while incarcerated, are more likely to receive disciplinary reports for rule infractions, and thus are more likely to spend time in segregation units. Although many correctional staff do their best to provide compassionate supervision, they generally are not trained mental health providers, and compassionate supervision often is subservient to their primary mission—that is, the safe and secure operation of facilities designed with a punitive component.

Ulrich and colleagues (2013) found that a hospital designed with integral stress-reducing features decreased the use of S/R, including chemical restraint, compared to an older hospital that cared for comparable psychiatric patients without similar environmental features. To that end, the authors proposed a tentative theory for designing psychiatric environments that foster reduced aggression. Such an environment would reduce crowding and noise, keep group sizes small, minimize noise with good acoustics, provide external window views, and maximize normal daylight exposure. The intent is to reduce the factors that contribute to aggression and to enhance staff outcomes (e.g., reduce job strain and injuries, foster higher job satisfaction). Ulrich and colleagues (2013) commented specifically on the factors involved in reducing environmental stressors, many of which are germane to jail and prison settings. The authors found that the stress of crowding is likely more affected by the layout of dorms (e.g., number of rooms, number of patients per room, privacy access) than spatial density per se. There is lower perceived crowding and more helping behavior with smaller numbers of people on floors, corridors, or units. Also, while there are no specific studies regarding the effect of noise on aggression in psychiatric patients, Ulrich and colleagues (2013) pointed to evidence that reduced noise in nonpsychiatric inpatient hospital settings led to reduced blood pressure and lower staff stress, annoyance, and perceived work demands, which, in turn, are likely to lower patient stress.

Summary

The judicious use of S/R, including emergency medication, can yield positive results for inmates who are at an imminent risk of self-injury or injury to others and where other interventions have failed or are inappropriate. The process is optimized with appropriate legal and ethical safeguards and with maintenance of a culture and environment that seek to decrease the incidence of distress and aggression. Before initiating S/R, the clinician must carefully weigh the clinical and ethical concerns of doing so. The ideal situation is one in which S/R is used as a tool of last resort as part of a more comprehensive, individualized treatment plan that seeks to ultimately ameliorate the behaviors and circumstances for which S/R is indicated.

References

American Bar Association (2011). *Treatment of prisoners* (3rd ed., p. 391). Washington, DC: American Bar Association. Retrieved from http://www.americanbar.org/content/dam/aba/publications/criminal_justice_standards/Treatment_of_Prisoners.authcheckdam.pdf

Appelbaum, K. L. (2007). Commentary: The use of restraint and seclusion in correctional mental health. *Journal of the American Academy of Psychiatry and the Law, 35,* 431–435.

Appelbaum, K. L., Savageau, J. A., Trestman, R. L., Metzner, J. L., & Baillargeon, J. (2011). A national survey of self-injurious behavior in American prisons. *Psychiatric Services, 62*(3), 285–290.

Champion, M. K. (2007). Commentary: Seclusion and restraint in corrections—A time for change. *Journal of the American Academy of Psychiatry and the Law, 35,* 426–430.

Lewis, M., Taylor, K., & Parks, J. (2009). Crisis prevention management: A program to reduce the use of seclusion and restraint in an inpatient mental health setting. *Issues in Mental Health Nursing, 30,* 159–164.

Lion, J. R. (2011). Commentary: On regulation, wishfulness, and denial. *Journal of the American Academy of Psychiatry and the Law, 39,* 477–479.

Metzner, J. L., Tardiff, K., Lion, J., Reid, W. H., Recupero, P. R., Schetky, D. H., Edenfield, B. M., Mattson, M., & Janofsky, J. S. (2007). Resource document on the use of restraint and seclusion in correctional mental health care. *Journal of the American Academy of Psychiatry and the Law, 35,* 417–425.

Recupero, P. R., Price, M., Garvey, K. A., Daly B., & Xavier, S. L. (2011). Restraint and seclusion in psychiatric treatment settings: Regulation, case law, and risk management. *Journal of the American Academy of Psychiatry and the Law, 39,* 465–476.

Sine, D. M., & Hunt, J. M. (2007). *Design guide for built environment of behavioral health facilities.* Washington, DC: National Association of Psychiatric Health Systems.

Ulrich, R. S., Bogren, L., & Lundin, S. (2013). Toward a design theory for reducing aggression in psychiatric facilities. Retrieved from ARCH 12: ARCHITECTURE/RESEARCH/CARE/HEALTH. 42 C.F.R. § 482.13 http://www.gpo.gov/fdsys/pkg/CFR-2010-title42-vol5/pdf/CFR-2010-title42-vol5-sec482-13.pdf; reviewed 12/10/2013

CHAPTER 27

Hospitalization

Michael A. Norko, Craig G. Burns, and Charles Dike

Introduction

In its Task Force Report on Psychiatric Services in Jails and Prisons, the American Psychiatric Association (APA) noted the fundamental principle that "timely and effective access to mental health treatment is the hallmark of adequate mental health care" (APA, 2000, p. 2). Appropriate and adequate access to mental health care involves the entirety of the correctional mental health service delivery system. For many individuals with mental health needs in these settings, such access requires a therapeutic milieu. The APA report specifies the details of a correctional therapeutic milieu, including a humane environment, sufficient resources and mental health staff, social interactions, and transfer to a mental health facility when these conditions cannot be met (APA, 2000, p. 18). The last item in this list includes models for delivering mental health care across institutional boundaries. This chapter explores the role of hospitalization in such models, along with other relevant considerations.

Prevalence of mental illness in jails and prisons

The need for hospitalization of inmates and detainees is a product of the prevalence and acuity of mental illness and the availability of mental health services in correctional environments compared to the therapeutic milieu of a hospital. The Substance Abuse and Mental Health Services Administration (SAMHSA) reported the prevalence of any mental illness as 56% in state prisons, 45% in federal prisons, 64% in local jails, and 20% in the nonincarcerated general population (SAMHSA, 2012).

For serious mental illness, data regarding prevalence span a wide range of findings due to varying methodologies among the studies (Baillargeon, Hoge, & Penn, 2010). For example, studies reviewed in 1998 placed the rate of schizophrenia in jails at between 6% and 75% of the population (Metzner, Cohen, Grossman, & Wettstein, 1998). A 2002 review of 62 surveys in Western countries concluded that 3% of men and 4% of women in prison had psychotic illness, with 10% of men and 12% of women diagnosed with major depression (Fazel & Danesh, 2002). The APA report noted that the rate of serious mental illness in jails and prisons is approximately 20% (APA, 2000, p. xix), which is consistent with other authors' estimates of 16% to 24% (Lamb & Weinberger, 2005) or 11% to 26% (National Commission on Correctional Health Care [NCCHC], 2002). In contrast, SAMHSA reported that the rate of serious mental illness in the nonincarcerated general population varies among the states from 3.5% to 7%, with a 4.8% rate in a national sample (SAMHSA, 2012).

The much higher rates of serious mental illness in correctional settings may not be related so much to the direct effects of mental illness on criminal behavior as to a higher level of criminogenic needs (e.g., antisocial attitudes, substance abuse, lack of problem-solving and self-control skills) in this population. This is due to their lower social status, poverty, inactivity, decreased social effectiveness and economic productivity over the life course, and frequently changing life circumstances (Fisher, Silver, & Wolff, 2006; Skeem, Manchak, & Peterson, 2011). A study of offense patterns among people with mental illness demonstrated that criminal behavior was related to psychosis in 5% of cases (Peterson, Skeem, Hart, Vidal, & Felicia, 2010). Estimates of acute symptoms of serious mental illness range from 5% among inmates and detainees (APA, 2000) to 6% for males and 15% for females at booking (NCCHC, 2002).

Several studies have looked at rates of hospitalization or need for hospitalization among inmates and detainees with identified mental health problems. Hospitalization rates in the year prior to arrest were 3.2% for federal prisoners, 5.8% for state prisoners, and 6.6% for jail detainees. After incarceration, the rates of hospitalization were slightly lower at 2.7% for federal prisoners, 5.4% for state prisoners, and 2.2% for jail detainees (James & Glaze, 2006). These data give some indication of the subpopulation for whom hospitalization might be reasonably considered.

Prison and jail management of acute disorders

The acutely psychiatric ill inmate poses unique challenges. Given the number of inmates who have a history of psychiatric impairment, acute illness will frequently arise when the inmate is in custody. We refer here to those inmates whose symptoms, dangerousness, or grave disability make them inappropriate for either the general population or a specialized mental health block for nonacute mentally ill inmates (where such environments are available). Decisions about whether to seek outside hospitalization require consideration of potential advantages and risks in the custody and hospital environments for such individuals.

Acutely ill offenders may be identified at any time while they are in the criminal justice system. Each custody environment or experience has its own stressors that can move otherwise dormant illness into manifest impairment. Unpredictable community-based events such as the death of loved ones, reports of grave illness in family members, divorce, loss of child custody, and other issues can contribute to an inmate's rapid decompensation. Some seriously ill inmates can remain undetected for most of an incarceration but come to the awareness of staff as the stress of returning to the community results in acute decompensation (Felthous, 2013b).

Acutely decompensated inmates may act out, generating disciplinary issues before mental health interventions are instituted. Mechanisms for mitigation of disciplinary response to infractions, through consultation with mental health services, aid in effective management of acutely mentally ill offenders. This is best accomplished when mental health and custody staff engage in collaborative efforts to maintain safety and security while also attending to the health care needs of inmates. Custody staff will often mirror mental health staff's approach to decompensated inmates. If good boundary management is mixed with a compassionate, understanding approach, custody staff will often adopt this behavior. It can be extremely validating for custody staff if the psychiatrist takes the time to solicit opinions from officers and to include these observations in mental health formulations. Such efforts often serve as the roots of mutual appreciation and collaboration. This supports the safe, effective management of acutely mentally ill inmates; the critical nature of this approach cannot be overstated.

Biological responses to medications will generally be the same no matter where they are administered. Reducing offender stress by increasing the understanding and humanity shown to inmates will aid adaptation and lead, as much as possible, to a correctional environment that operates more like that in a community setting. The absence of a thoughtful, inclusive approach, as described previously, in the care of the acutely mentally ill inmate will generally lead to undesirable results.

The care of acutely mentally ill offenders in jails and prisons may have some advantages over care in forensic psychiatric hospitals. Security can often be better managed for unpredictable and dangerous mentally ill offenders in corrections. Part of this advantage is mediated by elements of the physical plant. Correctional housing design routinely inhibits the movement of inmates, while hospitals are prohibited from such restrictions except for brief periods of emergency management. Individual custody cells can be monitored by camera, and locks and utilities can be remotely operated. Cell traps offer a safe way of passing medication and food to highly aggressive and acutely ill individuals. Custody staff have extensive training and experience in secured movement, coordinated response to violent behavior, and crisis negotiation, and they operate within a clear chain of command that facilitates accountability and organization.

Even severely impaired and potentially violent inmates will often respond to the regulation and structure provided in prison. Set times for waking up, eating, hygiene, recreation, medication administration, and other interventions create predictability. Even an inmate experiencing severe psychosis will often respond appropriately to uniformed officers and the commanding presence of an officer in a leadership position who is directing interactions. These factors help manage dangerous inmates in acute decompensation of mental illness, at least as long as appropriately enhanced clinical care is also available.

It is possible to generate enhanced clinical psychiatric care in a correctional environment by following the standards and guidelines provided by the NCCHC and APA, among others. For example, many relevant sections are presented in the NCCHC's *Standards for Mental Health Services in Correctional Facilities*, including those on safety, personnel and training, health care services and support, inmate care and treatment, special mental health needs and services, and medicolegal issues (NCCHC, 2008).

Systems that can offer both the essential and important elements described may have less of a need to rely on outside hospitals than those that struggle to meet even essential standards (see Chapter 63 for a more extensive discussion). However, even correctional systems that expend significant human and capital resources to approximate specialized hospital settings must acknowledge that, in the end, they are still jails and prisons. To provide a full range of services for inmates, collaborative relationships with area psychiatric hospitals should be developed, with the ability to transfer inmates to those facilities for specialized care.

Collaboration with hospitals

Custody environments that meet these standards should have a reduced need for outside psychiatric hospital care. Different models may be used to provide care through state agencies, private vendors, medical institutions, and partnerships that combine two or more of these entities (Daniel, 2007). Development of full-service psychiatric care units within correctional settings remains an important consideration. Custody environments without dedicated, internal, specialized psychiatric care will have a greater reliance on outside psychiatric or forensic psychiatric hospitals (Vogel, Lanquillon, & Graf, 2013). While states vary in the degree to which they use transfers to internal special mental health units or to external psychiatric hospitals, no outcome data support the choice of one model over the other (Phillips & Caplan, 2003).

Most inmates with mental illness survive the transition from community to custody. In fact, many states have more mentally ill inmates than psychiatric hospital patients (Torrey, Kennard, Eslinger, Lamb, & Pavle, 2010). Mentally ill offenders, however, are more likely to have maladaptive responses to custody, often resulting in management problems, longer periods of incarceration secondary to disciplinary infractions (periodically rooted in untreated symptoms), and the loss of appropriate community supervision when full sentences are served. These inmates also have higher rates of suicide than inmates who are not psychiatrically impaired (Lamb & Weinberger, 1998; Lurigio, Rollins, & Fallon, 2004; Torrey et al., 2010).

Court orders for hospitalization (e.g., for competency restoration) early in the adjudication process can have a protective effect on mentally ill offenders. Movement to an inpatient hospital can provide a more supportive transition to custody while symptoms are remediated. Even when mentally ill offenders are hospitalized for other than court-ordered reasons, they are still likely to return to prison, and adaptation to prison life remains an important goal.

Even with fully informed consent, voluntary transfers of mentally ill offenders to hospitals can have unintended legal consequences. Prosecutors and defense attorneys may be wary of transfering pretrial detainees to psychiatric hospitals for reasons other than those ordered by the court for fear of influencing the trial process. Prosecutors may be concerned about the generation of mitigating factors that may weaken their case, and defense attorneys may be concerned about the detection of malingered symptoms that may influence the court. Ultimately, a physician's responsibility is to the needs of the patient, which should be the driving force that determines where an inmate receives care (Vogel et al., 2013).

To assist with that determination, Vogel and colleagues (2013) proposed the concept of "fitness for imprisonment." They offered an algorithm for the decision about hospital transfer based on European prison experience that consists of assessments and analyses of whether the needed treatment is practicable in the correctional setting. They suggest evaluating four criteria, in this order: psychiatric diagnosis, acute need for treatment, danger to self and others, and inability to comply with treatment. In their suggested scheme, if all are present, the inmate is not "fit" for prison and should be transferred. If only some of the four criteria are present, additional criteria should be reviewed, including first clinical manifestation of a psychological disorder, prognosis in prison versus hospital, need for special monitoring with the initiation of complex medication regimens, diagnostic uncertainty, and lack of trained staff (Vogel et al., 2013).

Also, other inmates may victimize mentally ill inmates (Phillips & Caplan, 2003). These vulnerabilities and risks may be temporarily better managed in a hospital. On a case-by-case basis, consideration of individual inmate needs and risks, especially if formalized as protocols between correctional facilities and area psychiatric hospitals, will help clinical decision makers choose the best place to meet offenders' needs.

Under British Columbia's Temporary Absence model, if a treating physician feels that an inmate's clinical needs would be better served in a hospital, a second physician's evaluation is required prior to continuing with the application for Temporary Absence (Olley, Nicholls, & Brink, 2009). Another approach considers whether the inmate can be ethically managed in prison. Such an analysis may consist of several considerations: the gravity of the inmate's condition, the severity of the clinical and other risks involved, and the necessity of involuntary medication administration (Felthous, 2012).

Involuntary medication

An acutely psychiatrically ill offender may have a temporary risk of violence while symptoms remain untreated. Pharmacological treatment may be instituted more quickly in some correctional settings than in hospitals located in jurisdictions that have more complex procedural protections for hospitalized patients.

The process of involuntarily medicating inmates in some custody settings is accomplished via a *Harper* panel (*Washington v. Harper*, 1990). This involves an administrative hearing before a panel (including a psychiatrist who is not involved in the prisoner's care, as described in *Washington v. Harper*, where clinical rather than judicial determinations were preferred), notice of the hearing and right to attend the hearing and present evidence and witnesses, right to cross-examine witnesses, right to an advocate, and right to appeal. The hearing must conclude that the individual has a serious mental illness and is "dangerous to self or others and the treatment is in the inmate's medical interest" (*Washington v. Harper*, 1990, p. 1040). In some jurisdictions, this process can be accomplished more quickly than in forensic hospitals, if required procedures in the latter setting are more complex. In other jurisdictions, the same procedural requirements may apply equally to individuals in either setting, and thus the rapidity of instituting pharmacological treatment is not a relevant consideration in the

decision about hospitalization versus management within corrections. Thus, clinicians involved in this work need to be aware of the procedural requirements within their jurisdiction, recognizing that states may impose more restrictions on involuntary treatment than constitutionally required.

The APA report does not specifically mention involuntary medication use in correctional settings but does emphasize the principle of providing the same level of service in prison as in the community (APA, 2000; Felthous, 2012). Use of the *Harper* process appropriately requires attention to significant inmate protections. This helps staff to know that their actions and decisions, despite the environment, are still based on the highest standards of patient care. Clinicians must also be aware that *Harper* procedures may not be legally adequate in all jurisdictions.

Some authors have argued that when medications are given involuntarily in prisons, the treatment should occur in acute-care psychiatric units to ensure safe and proper administration within a therapeutic milieu (Daniel, 2007; Felthous, 2013a). Involuntary medication use within nonmedical prison units can raise multiple concerns, including that medical staff may not be fully informed about the success of the administration of medication (Felthous, 2012). The use of involuntary medications when an inmate is unwilling or unable to give consent also raises concerns about the voluntariness of inmate decisions within an inherently coercive environment (28 CFR 549, 2011; Dlugacz & Wimmer, 2013; Metzner et al., 1998).

Although the due process elements of *Harper* are constitutionally sound, state laws may also raise the bar on the necessary components of that due process (28 CFR 549, 2011; Dlugacz & Wimmer, 2013; NCCHC, 2008, MH-I-02). Emergency situations may not require *Harper* procedures but usually require a determination of dangerousness and mental illness. The NCCHC requires written administrative protocols for this purpose in order for a facility to achieve accreditation (NCCHC, 2008, MH-I-02). Interestingly, the federal code views seclusion and restraint as an alternative to consider before giving medications (28 CFR 549, 2011, 549.46(b)(1)(i)), although this is not generally how these procedures are ranked from a clinical perspective. For example, medical staff in a hospital would be unlikely to consider seclusion or restraint as a first alternative before administering involuntary medication in an emergency situation. Hospitals are restricted in the use of seclusion and restraint and have limits on staff's physical response and management of unpredictably violent individuals.

The need for involuntary medications may be one indication for hospital transfer in a subset of inmates (Felthous, 2012). Historically, medication refusal has been found to be the second most common cause of hospitalization of prison inmates (Smith, 1989). Inmates transferred involuntarily to a hospital will need to be provided with the minimum due process articulated in *Vitek v. Jones*, including effective and timely notice, a hearing with an independent decision maker, the right to testify and examine other witnesses, and a written statement by the fact-finder noting the reasons for a decision to transfer (*Vitek v. Jones*, 1980). This minimum due process will not be sufficient in jurisdictions that require other or more expansive procedures by statute or case law. In some jurisdictions, a *Vitek* hearing may also be used to facilitate an involuntary medication order; however, this may not provide sufficient procedure to accomplish that goal without further due process (Dlugacz & Wimmer, 2013; Metzner et al., 1998,

p. 249). Even in a hospital setting, the evaluation of capacity to give informed consent requires enhanced sensitivity.

Forensic hospitals have some distinct advantages over correctional environments for the care of acutely psychiatrically ill inmates. However, truly secure care and the speed with which the use of involuntary medications may be authorized are areas in which some correctional environments may offer advantages.

Hospitalization for acute or refractory disorders

Although some prisons have excellent mental health services, they still prioritize security. Further, prisons have no obligation to adhere to the provisions of the federal Patient Bill of Rights (42 USC § 9501) or state versions of the same for mentally ill patients. This bill was promulgated to protect and enhance the interests and recovery of patients in the least restrictive environment. Because of their different primary goals, the milieu of mental health units in prisons is not the same as that of a hospital. Hospitals are increasingly directed toward recovery and rehabilitation (Prince, 2006), while prisons focus on punishment and security. Consequently, it is more difficult for correctional institutions to provide care in an environment that is equivalent to a community hospital milieu, which is why the APA Task Force required transfer to a hospital when needed (APA, 2000).

A supportive hospital milieu by itself fosters recovery. For some severely mentally ill individuals with refractory illness, such a milieu augments the effect of psychotropic and psychotherapeutic interventions. The milieu should, therefore, be part of the analysis in considering hospital transfer for inmates with serious acute or refractory illness. The same applies to the increasing population of mentally ill elderly inmates and to all seriously mentally ill inmates with additional physical or emotional attributes that make them more vulnerable to victimization. These include prisoners with a significant history of trauma, intellectual or physical disabilities, gender identity issues, or low-level psychosis that impairs their ability to follow prison rules, provide for themselves, or defend themselves as necessary.

The discussion is further complicated by the observation that for some dangerous psychiatrically ill inmates, transfer to a hospital could lead to markedly increased restrictions in their freedom; hospital staff might feel they have to place these patients on close observation, sometimes by more than one staff member, for safety. These patients could require frequent use of restraints to manage their aggressive behavior. In these highly restrictive situations, the hospital might not be the least restrictive environment for providing treatment to the patient who could be more easily managed in a standard prison cell. The US Supreme Court has acknowledged similar concerns in concluding that prisoners retain a "residuum of liberty that would be infringed by a transfer to a mental hospital without complying with minimum requirements of due process" (*Vitek v. Jones*, 1980, p. 491).

The admission of prisoners to a forensic hospital unit is not without notable challenges. A major hurdle is getting front-line staff of the facility to view the transferred prisoners as they do other patients on the unit, not as criminals. The criminal history profile of many psychotic prisoners is similar to those of their nonpsychotic fellow prisoners (Coid & Ulrich, 2011); they are at higher risk of exhibiting behaviors associated with psychopathy (such as violence, intimidation, and exploitation of others) and substance abuse and may be perceived to have a higher risk of escaping from the hospital. In one study, 75% of prisoners referred to a hospital due to medication refusal had been convicted of serious violent offenses compared to 50% in the general prison population (Smith, 1989). The presence of prisoners on a hospital unit may also disrupt the therapeutic program and place lower-functioning hospital patients at risk of victimization (Phillips & Caplan, 2003).

Accordingly, these patients present significant safety and security risks that should be managed with as much care and attention as in prison. Areas of vulnerability for the hospital include access to materials that could be fashioned into sharp objects; the mix of dangerous prisoners with the usual public-sector patient population; safe and secure transportation of these patients to medical or other appointments outside of the hospital; and the limited ability of staff to closely monitor patient phone calls. Hospitalized patients have a right to converse with others privately, to have convenient and reasonable access to the telephone and mail, and to see visitors during regularly scheduled hours (42 USC § 9501). Hospital staff need to be particularly alert to the potential for these patients to conspire with accomplices outside or inside the hospital in an attempt to escape from the hospital or to cause a disruption in the hospital, respectively. Careful attention should be paid to the increased staffing needs of hospitals that house transferred prisoners and the need for other resources to engage them in therapeutic and rehabilitation activities; keeping these patients busy for a significant portion of each day is useful for providing structure, improving coping skills, and decreasing opportunities for mischief.

Management of prison inmates in a hospital would be nearly impossible without an easy process for their transfer back to prison when their aggressive or criminal behaviors overwhelm the hospital's resources. Therefore, interagency collaboration between the correctional agency and the psychiatric facility is key to successful management of mentally ill prisoners.

Stigma and the hospitalization decision

The US Supreme Court has recognized that the consequences of involuntary hospitalization are "qualitatively different" from the usual effects of punishment (*Vitek v. Jones*, 1980, p. 493). But whether prisoners receive intensive mental health care in prison or a hospital, they are subject to the same stigma, at least in terms of the attitudes of other inmates (Edwards, 2000). Of course, with respect to the general public, such individuals are stigmatized by both their imprisonment and their mental illness. Thus, prison officials and clinicians confronted with an acutely psychiatrically ill prisoner or detainee must choose between treatment environments that each have advantages and disadvantages. Such considerations may be aired in a *Vitek* hearing; however, the clinical principles described previously should drive these decisions. The unique circumstances of each case warrant individual analysis in deciding how the inmate or detainee is to be best managed. Clinical concerns must always be paramount in such decisions, but matters of security and safety cannot be ignored.

Summary

A significant number of people with serious mental illness are found in correctional settings and must be provided with clinical care commensurate with their needs. Many of those needs may be met within the mental health care systems established in jails and prisons. When clinical conditions are more complex and require more intensive management, the availability of hospital-level care becomes important. While the decision to pursue hospitalization for an acutely ill inmate is driven chiefly by clinical considerations, it is also influenced by security and safety concerns. These factors need to be considered on an individual basis, weighing the advantages and disadvantages of treatment in an outside hospital versus management in the prison or jail with available resources.

Involuntary medication and involuntary hospital transfer are situations that involve important legal rights, the protection of which requires due process established by federal and state laws and case precedents. Clinicians who work in corrections and hospital settings that admit inmates and detainees must be aware of the relevant procedures required for these involuntary treatment modalities. In all jurisdictions, hospital-level care is necessary for a subset of sentenced inmates and jail detainees and must therefore be made available when appropriate.

References

28 CFR 549.46 (2011). Procedures for involuntary administration of psychiatric medication. Retrieved from http://federal.eregulations.us/cfr/section/title28/chapterv/part549/sect549.46?selectdate=11/1/2011

42 USC § 9501—Mental Health Rights and Advocacy—Bill of Rights. Retrieved from http://www.gpo.gov/fdsys/pkg/USCODE-2006-title42/pdf/USCODE-2006-title42-chap102.pdf

American Psychiatric Association. (2000). *Psychiatric services in jails and prisons: a task force report of the American Psychiatric Association.* Washington, DC: American Psychiatric Association.

Baillargeon, J., Hoge, S. K., & Penn, J.V. (2010). Addressing the challenge of community reentry among released inmates with serious mental illness. *American Journal of Community Psychology, 46,* 361–375.

Coid, J., & Ullrich, S. (2011). Prisoners with psychosis in England and Wales: Diversion to psychiatric inpatient services. *International Journal of Law and Psychiatry, 34,* 99–108.

Daniel, A. E. (2007). Care of the mentally ill in prisons: Challenges and solutions. *Journal of the American Academy of Psychiatry and the Law, 35,* 406–410.

Dlugacz, H., & Wimmer, C. (2013). Legal aspects of administrating antipsychotic medications to jail and prison inmates. *International Journal of Law and Psychiatry, 36,* 213–228.

Edwards, K. A. (2000). Stigmatizing the stigmatized: a note on the mentally ill prison inmate. *International Journal of Offender Therapy and Comparative Criminology, 44,* 480–489.

Fazel, S., & Danesh, J. (2002). Serious mental disorder in 23000 prisoners: a systematic review of 62 surveys. *Lancet, 359,* 545–550.

Felthous, A. R. (2012). The involuntary medication of Jared Loughner and pretrial jail detainees in nonmedical correctional facilities. *Journal of the American Academy of Psychiatry and the Law, 40,* 98–112.

Felthous, A. R. (2013a). The Ninth Circuit's *Loughner* decision neglected medically appropriate treatment. *Journal of the American Academy of Psychiatry and the Law, 41,* 105–113.

Felthous, A. R. (2013b). Prisons and mental health: Introductory editorial: Hospitalizing mentally ill patients. *International Journal of Law and Psychiatry, 36,* 185–187.

Fisher, W. H., Silver, E., & Wolff, N. (2006). Beyond criminalization: Toward a criminologically informed framework for mental health policy and services research. *Administration and Policy in Mental Health and Mental Health Services Research, 33,* 544–557.

James, D. J., & Glaze, L. E. (2006). *Mental health problems of prison and jail inmates* (NCJ 213600). Washington, DC: Department of Justice. Office of Justice Programs—Bureau of Justice and Statistics.

Lamb, H. R., & Weinberger, L. E. (1998). Persons with severe mental illness in jails and prisons:A review. *Psychiatric Services, 49,* 483–492.

Lamb, H. R., & Weinberger, L. E. (2005). The shift of psychiatric inpatient care from hospitals to jails and prisons. *Journal of the American Academy of Psychiatry and the Law, 33*(4), 529–534.

Lurigio, A. J., Rollins, A., & Fallon, J. (2004). The effects of serious mental illness on offender reentry. *Federal Probation, 68,* 45–52.

Metzner, J. L. Cohen, F., Grossman, L. S., & Wettstein, R. M. (1998). Treatment in jails and prisons. In R. W. Wettstein (Ed.), *Treatment of offenders with mental disorder* (pp. 211–264). New York: Guilford Press.

National Commission on Correctional Health Care (2002). *The health status of soon-to-be-released inmates. A report to Congress* (vol. 2). Retrieved from https://www.ncjrs.gov/pdffiles1/nij/grants/189736.pdf

National Commission on Correctional Health Care (2008). *Standards for mental health services in correctional facilities.* Chicago: National Commission on Correctional Health Care.

Olley, M. C., Nicholls, T. L., & Brink, J. (2009). Mentally ill individuals in limbo: Obstacles and opportunities for providing psychiatric services to corrections inmates with mental illness. *Behavioral Sciences and the Law, 27,* 811–831.

Peterson, J., Skeem, J., Hart, E., Vidal, S., & Keith, F. (2010). Analyzing offense patters as a function of mental illness to test the criminalization hypothesis. *Psychiatric Services, 61,* 1217–1222.

Phillips, R. T. M., & Caplan, C. (2003). Administrative and staffing problems for psychiatric services in correctional and forensic settings. In R. Rosner (Ed.), *Principles and practice of forensic psychiatry* (2nd ed., pp. 505–512). London: Arnold.

Prince, J. D. (2006). Incarceration and hospital care. *Journal of Nervous and Mental Disease, 194,* 34–39.

Skeem, J. L., Manchak, S., & Peterson, J. K. (2011). Correctional policy for offenders with mental illness: Creating a new paradigm for recidivism reduction. *Law and Human Behavior, 35,* 110–126.

Smith, L. D. (1989). Medication refusal and the rehospitalized mentally ill inmate. *Hospital and Community Psychiatry, 40,* 491–496.

Substance Abuse and Mental Health Services Administration (2012). *Mental health, United States, 2010.* HHS Publication No. 12–4681. Rockville, MD: Substance Abuse and Mental Health Services Administration. Retrieved from http://store.samhsa.gov/product/Mental-Health-United-States-2010/SMA12-4681.

Torrey, E. F., Kennard, A. D., Eslinger, D., Lamb, R., & Pavle, J. (2010). *More mentally ill persons are in jails and prisons than hospitals: A survey of the states.* Treatment Advocacy Center and National Sheriffs' Association. Retrieved from https//www.treatmentadvocacycenter.org/storage/documents/final_jails_v_hospitals

Vitek v. Jones (1980). 445 U.S. 480.

Vogel, T., Lanquillon, S., & Graf. M. (2013). When and why should mentally ill prisoners be transferred to secure hospitals: A proposed algorithm. *International Journal of Law and Psychiatry, 36,* 281–286.

Washington v. Harper (1990). 110 S. Ct. 1028.

SECTION VI

General pharmacology issues

CHAPTER 28

Formulary management/ pharmacy and therapeutics committees

Robert H. Berger, Robyn J. Wahl, and M. Paul Chaplin

Introduction

While the cost of health care rises in all public health care organizations, budgets for that care have remained the same or have decreased. Because pharmaceutical expenditures are a substantial percentage of a health care organization's budget, medication use is closely scrutinized. This is most certainly true in correctional health care delivery systems with fixed budgets, increasing patient populations, serious medical needs, and rising costs of health care and medication (Douglas & Mundey, 1995).

Clinicians must consider the appropriateness, effectiveness, and safety of medications prescribed to incarcerated patients. The abundance of available drugs and the complex issues about their safe and effective use make a sound program for maximizing rational drug use critical (Lundquist & Becker, 2010). This is a challenging task in jails and prisons, where clinicians are required to reexamine the treatments provided and improve prescribing patterns. This is not a process of arbitrarily limiting prescribers' choices or their decision-making authority solely based on cost-saving incentives: We believe that evidence-based best practices that inform the development of, and adherence to, disease management guidelines and a preferred, restricted medication formulary enhance the quality, safety, and effectiveness of the care provided.

This chapter details the process and procedures for developing, implementing, and monitoring prescription practice change by establishing an effective Pharmacy and Therapeutics Committee (P&TC). The chapter addresses the roles and responsibilities of a P&TC, P&TC decision-making processes, formulary development and modification, formulary process decision making, medication therapy management guidelines, prescriber education, and data analytics to assist in monitoring outcomes, medication use, and prescriber adherence to P&TC policies. Prescribing challenges specific to the incarcerated population are also addressed.

The pharmacy and therapeutics committee: membership and committee organization

As early as 1965, the Joint Commission on the Accreditation of Hospitals included an active P&TC in its accreditation requirements. For more than two decades, these P&TCs operated primarily as ad hoc committees, meeting infrequently and without a defined mission. The typical product was no more than a formulary that listed drugs stocked by the pharmacy (Tyler, Cole, May, Millares, Valentino, Vermeulen, & Wilson, 2008). More recently, the only reference to a P&TC in the requirements for accreditation promulgated by the National Commission on Correctional Health Care (NCCHC) 2008 Standards for Mental Health Services in Correctional Facilities is that "there is a formulary for prescribers" and that "a psychiatrist, pharmacist, or therapeutics committee should be involved in developing a formulary" (NCCHC, 2008).

Developing, managing, reviewing, and updating the formulary are key roles of the P&TC. With the introduction of many new medications, approval by the US Food and Drug Administration (FDA) of additional indications, and advances in clinical trials, the P&TC must devote considerable time to making formulary decisions; this process is discussed in greater detail later in the chapter. The role of the P&TC should not, however, be limited to formulary development and management. The World Health Organization has identified and promoted drug and therapeutics committees as one of the pivotal models for promoting the rational use of medicines to improve patient care. P&TC decisions and policies aim to elicit change (Tan, Day, & Brien, 2005). To meet such a key responsibility, the P&TC should be formalized in the organization's policies, supported by the executive leadership, and granted the authority to implement its policies and decisions.

The mental health P&TC is typically organized and chaired by the chief of psychiatric services (or comparable position). In correctional organizations that contract for health services, the P&TC might be cochaired by the department of correction director/chief of psychiatric services and that of the contracted agency. The director of pharmacy or designated clinical pharmacist is cochair in many correctional and community health care systems. While not an essential assignment, a senior pharmacy department representative is expected to serve on the P&TC. The importance of a close working relationship between the P&TC and the agency's pharmacy department cannot be overstated.

The P&TC is not a *pro forma* committee; it convenes on a consistent schedule. Meetings should be held at least quarterly; given the dynamic activity of the system, monthly meetings are generally necessary. Some correctional system facilities and staff are spread out over great distances, so it might not be possible for all members to be physically present at every meeting. When necessary, teleconferencing or videoconferencing is feasible, but face-to-face meetings enhance communication, discussion, and effective decision making. An option is to rotate the site of meetings to accommodate members, facilitate the process, and maximize member attendance. Members who miss many meetings should be replaced (Quintiliani & Quercia, 2003).

The P&TC chairperson(s) selects the core committee members, who, apart from the pharmacist, are usually psychiatrists. They are chosen based on their demonstrated competence and expertise in psychopharmacology and prescribing practice. They should represent a broad range of the organization's facilities and populations served. Current P&TCs are, to an increasing extent, multidisciplinary and include nursing staff, midlevel prescribers, and psychologists. Members should be able to work collaboratively, be open to evaluating evidence-based data, and contribute their specific practice experiences. Committee membership should be time-limited (perhaps two or three years) and with staggered rotation schedules. All members should confirm in writing any conflicts of interest (e.g., being a paid pharmaceutical consultant or speaker, holding substantial pharmaceutical stock, or being the recipient of a large pharmaceutical industry–sponsored research grant). While those individuals may be appropriate P&TC members, they should not be allowed to vote on any products produced or marketed by the relevant company (Quintiliani & Quercia, 2003).

The P&TC should consult specialists (including ethicists) on an advisory basis for issue-specific discussions (Loorand-Striver, 2011) or convene subcommittees to address issues that require special expertise, knowledge, or skills (Hatton, Gonzolez-Rothi, Smith, & Knudsen, 2005). Additional front-line clinicians should be invited to P&TC meetings on a rotating basis. Such an inclusive process helps the committee learn facility-specific concerns and achieve buy-in from front-line staff who observe first-hand the committee process.

Committee meeting minutes are taken and formalized in a document that is distributed to committee members and made available to all staff by, for example, being posted on the organization's web portal. The minutes should include all relevant discussion topics, decisions made regarding medication use and prescribing practice, and an agenda for the next meeting, including any issues identified for follow-up. New or modified forms are included as attachments as well as peer-reviewed articles that informed committee discussion. Such articles might bear on decisions to add or remove medications from the formulary based on research findings of risks and side effects, as well as guidelines and suggestions for medication monitoring. The previous meeting's minutes are reviewed by the members prior to the next meeting with feedback, corrections, and/or additions provided by the members to the secretary or chairperson(s). These minutes are reviewed at the next meeting; acceptance (with modifications as required) of those minutes is documented. Requests are taken for additions to the current meeting's agenda. New forms or form revisions are reviewed and finalized. Broadcast memos that are to be distributed to clinical staff regarding P&TC decisions are discussed, drafted, reviewed, and finalized. The success of a P&TC depends on multidisciplinary members who have technical and clinical competence, whose decisions rely on evidence-based resources, who work collaboratively in a consistent direction, and whose process and decisions are transparent to the organization as a whole (Holloway & Green, 2003).

Pharmacy and therapeutics committee: Roles, responsibilities, and committee process

The roles and responsibilities of the P&TC have become increasingly challenging. In addition to preparing, updating, managing, and supervising the implementation of the drug formulary (i.e., process; Tan et al., 2005), the P&TC must continuously evaluate whether medication prescribing is safe, effective, ethical, and fiscally responsible (i.e., outcomes). Current practice requires P&TCs to enhance evidence-based prescribing practices and develop clinical protocols, disease management programs, and guidelines. Through extensive data analysis, the committee monitors drug budget impact, prescribing practices, and clinicians' compliance with committee directives and medication use guidelines, and monitors outcomes of committee initiatives and policies. Working closely with the committee's clinical pharmacist, the P&TC develops protocols for additions to and deletions from the formulary, procedures for nonformulary requests (NFRs), and processes for assessing the validity, effectiveness, and safety of off-label indication prescribing. Because the risks associated with psychotropic medication use must be identified and minimized or avoided when possible, the P&TC develops risk management strategies for monitoring side effects. With the support of the clinical pharmacist, the P&TC conducts medication use evaluations, monitors adverse drug reactions, and alerts staff of black-box warnings. The P&TC directs the pharmacy to report deviations from recommended prescribing cautions and ensures that all protocols required for the prescribing of medications with a risk evaluation mitigation strategy (REMS) designation have been satisfied (Loorand-Striver, 2011). Furthermore, the P&TC is responsible for developing and implementing medication use policies and procedures that are consistent with state or county correctional policies and administrative directives (Marcoux, Simeone, Colavita, & Larrat, 2012).

Although the roles and responsibilities of the P&TC are extensive, demanding, and time-consuming, they are paramount in promoting safe, effective, and cost-efficient patient care. Engaging all health care professionals involved in the medication use process throughout the organization is also critical to the success of P&TC initiatives, obligations, and goals. This is achieved by a communication plan that allows staff access to P&TC members and alerts the committee to the actual problems, obstacles, and issues confronting individual prescribers in their day-to-day patient encounters (Fijn, van Epnhuysen, Peijnenburg, Brouwers, & de Jong-van den Berg, 2002). P&TC members are responsible for providing education, supervision, advice, and consultations to staff that are consistent with the member's expertise and licensure. This may include providing facility-based case presentations, organizing statewide trainings, providing individual and group supervision, sending informational broadcast emails, disseminating pertinent articles, and providing training regarding drug use policies and P&TC initiatives. The combination of these will gain support for, and compliance with, critical formulary modifications, changes in prescribing practices, and evolving evidence-based treatment guidelines (Reddan, Sheehan, Eskew, & Elmes, 2004).

Principles of formulary management and the decision-making process

In correctional health care organizations, a mental health medication formulary is a list of preferred drugs approved for the treatment of psychiatric disorders. Formulary medications do not require preauthorization by the P&TC. The formulary is restricted to specific medications chosen following a rigorous selection process to identify the most medically appropriate, effective, safe, and cost-efficient drugs that best serve the health needs of the incarcerated population. A medication is considered for formulary inclusion only when there are ample, reliable data from clinical studies on its safety and efficacy and it is appropriate for administration in a correctional setting.

For a medication to be selected for formulary inclusion, the P&TC, in consultation with pharmacy and relevant experts, conducts an evidence-based evaluation of its risks and benefits, a review of published clinical trials, a cost analysis, and a comparison study with medications of the same class that already exist on the formulary. The P&TC should minimize duplication of the same basic drug type or product. Pharmacoeconomic assessments, while critical to the decision-making process, should be factored in only after questions of efficacy, effectiveness, availability, and safety have been considered (Johnson & Friesen, 1998).

This formulary selection process provides opportunities to advance and monitor appropriate medication prescribing practices; support compliance with disease management guidelines; educate and inform clinicians; and, identify, assess, and (when indicated) limit the prescribing of high-risk, expensive, and newly released medications as well as medications with a high potential for misuse, abuse, and diversion in the correctional setting (Lyles, Luce, & Rentz, 1997).

Newly admitted inmates to jail who were prescribed and adherent with psychotropic medication in the community may present unique challenges for prescribers. Such challenges include nonformulary medications; the medications prescribed in the community are not indicated for the mental disorder (or lack thereof) diagnosed by the intake clinician; a history of polysubstance abuse and dependence; prescription of inordinately high doses of benzodiazepines; prescription of stimulants; and demands by an inmate that each of the medications prescribed in the community be continued while incarcerated (see Chapter 19). Intake facility prescribers can apply guidelines and policies, analyze the situation, and make safe, clinically appropriate, and cost-effective prescribing decisions. Drug tapers and detoxification protocols may be initiated for those medications with a high potential for misuse, abuse, and diversion in jails and prisons, including benzodiazepines (Reeves, 2012), stimulants (Burns, 2009), quetiapine (Reeves, 2012; Tamburello, Lieberman, Baum, & Reeves, 2012), and bupropion (Hilliard, Barloon, Farley, Penn, & Koranek, 2013; see Chapter 29 and 31). Therapeutic substitution (Hoover, White, & Weiner, 1990) may be applied by cross-tapering a high-cost antipsychotic nonformulary medication with a low-cost formulary medication of equal efficacy and a safer side-effect profile (Ducate & Pondrom, 2003; Rosenheck, Leslie, Busch, Rofman, & Sernyak, 2008). Nonformulary brand--name medications may be switched for pharmacologically equivalent generic formulary medications. Tapers may be initiated for sedating antipsychotic and antidepressant medications prescribed for chronic sleep disturbances (American Psychiatric Association, 2013b; see Chapter 16). The patient should be fully informed of the logic and rationale for any changes. The patient should be scheduled for a series of frequent follow-up visits to monitor the effects of any medication changes and to clarify the diagnosis(es); this new information will guide further medication adjustments in accordance with established disease management guidelines.

Prescribers working in intake facilities frequently ask whether it is the clinician's obligation to continue all medications prescribed in the community. It is not. The clinician's obligation is to competently use clinical judgment to ensure that psychotropic medications are prescribed appropriately and safely in accordance with evidence-based disease management protocols (American Psychiatric Association, 2013b). While use of a formulary does not alone restrict correctional use of medications prescribed in the community, medications should be prescribed only when they are clinically indicated; generics or other equivalent substitutions may be made (NCCHC, 2008; Rucker & Schiff, 1990).

The formulary must be dynamic, reviewed at least annually, and revised as clinically indicated. It must be readily available and accessible from all facilities. Current evaluations and studies that dispute or contradict earlier studies continually appear in the literature. New information regarding efficacy, therapeutic profile, and frequency and severity of hepatotoxic, neurotoxic, metabolic, and other side effects of formulary-approved medications is a P&TC agenda priority. "In recent years," a prominent clinical researcher warns, "many treatments once thought to be highly advantageous, have been revealed by new independent research to be substantially less so" (Rosenheck et al., 2008). P&TC members must stay well informed.

Formulary management

Nonformulary requests

More than a decade ago, the American Psychiatric Association expressed concerns regarding formulary restrictions and considered it to be the treating clinician's ethical responsibility to advocate for the use of a nonformulary medication when indicated. The organization recommended that psychiatrists be able to override restrictions for a patient's benefit and that administrative processes should be reasonable (Moffic, 2006). We believe that the purpose of a formulary is not to restrict prescribing choices but to guide appropriate, effective, safe, and cost-efficient prescribing, which, in our experience, leads to better patient care. Medications included on the formulary should be vetted through a stringent, evidence-based selection process. Nonformulary medications should not be prohibited, but the P&TC does typically require the prescribing clinician to complete an NFR and to justify the use of the requested medication. It is routinely the clinician's responsibility to provide appropriate information explaining why formulary medications are not appropriate and to identify patient-specific or disease- or symptom-specific factors that would likely benefit from a specific nonformulary medication. The P&TC should have a formal process for submitting and reviewing NFRs, rendering a decision quickly, and notifying the prescriber and the pharmacy of the decision. If a reviewing P&TC member requires additional information, he or she should directly contact the requesting prescriber to expedite the process.

Formulary additions and deletions

A documented protocol for formulary additions and deletions is the responsibility of the P&TC. The protocol should specify a mechanism by which any prescribing clinician in the organization can make suggestions for formulary additions and deletions. The clinician requesting that a medication be added to the formulary must first provide reasoning that is based on safety, efficacy, and published studies. The second phase of the protocol requires clinical pharmacists to conduct a standardized process where the available literature on each drug considered for formulary addition or deletion is researched and compared to any formulary agents in the same drug class. A summary of the findings is prepared, including the quality of any supporting data, and a recommendation made to the committee (Quintiliani & Quercia, 2003). As the third and final phase of the protocol, P&TC members vote on the request, document the reasoning for their decision, and inform the requesting clinician.

Medication risk management and black-box warnings

Risk management principles apply to the decision-making process for evaluating a new agent for formulary inclusion or when reevaluating an agent's formulary status (Raber, 2010). Once a drug is included in the formulary, the clinical pharmacist working with the P&TC ensures that all necessary precautions, prerequisites, and monitoring are followed. Staff are informed of drugs with black-box warnings, drugs with REMS, and drugs requiring guided-use strategies (FDA, 2011; Raber, 2010). The clinical pharmacist strictly monitors the use of these drugs and ensures clinician compliance with registration required for prescribing REMS medications and ongoing monitoring of blood values at the required intervals. The pharmacist enforces dose-related requirements of medications with black-box warnings and reports critical findings or deviations to the P&TC. Any action or prescriber supervision necessary to ensure patient safety and eliminate deviation from these practice requirements is the shared responsibility of the P&TC chairperson and pharmacist.

Off-label prescribing

The use of a drug prescribed for an indication not specifically approved by the FDA is referred to as an off-label use. It is an accepted and not uncommon prescribing practice to use medications for indications other than those approved by the FDA. It is the responsibility of the P&TC to evaluate evidence for off-label use and either permit prescribing of these medications for mental health and behavioral indications or restrict the medication to use only for FDA-approved indications. A relevant example of this is when our mental health P&TC found insufficient clinical research studies to demonstrate gabapentin's effectiveness for mood stabilization; its use was subsequently restricted to neuropathic pain.

When considering approval of a medication for off-label use, the P&TC must rely on the scientific evidence, and the committee's decision must be supported by multiple sources of published evidence. Safety and efficacy are primary considerations. If a drug is approved and it is anticipated that multiple clinicians will be prescribing the medication for off-label indications, the P&TC should prepare guidelines for that use (Tyler et al., 2008).

Influencing prescribing practices: evidence-based disease management guidelines and treatment algorithms

The effectiveness of P&TC approaches to optimize medication management and ensure effective and safe treatment while controlling the quality and cost of medication use is largely dependent on the ability to alter prescribing behavior (Schumock, Walton, Park, Nutescu, Blackburn, Finley, & Lewis, 2004). One good measure of the P&TC's effectiveness is the extent to which prescribing practices evolve throughout the organization. Initiatives that generally promote the greatest change include an evidence-based formulary and disease management guidelines (also referred to as clinical practice guidelines, medication management guidelines, or standard treatment guidelines), medication use policies, data analysis and individual supervision, dissemination of information, and training and education. Patient outcome measures and cost-savings analysis are equally important. Sustained impact on prescribing patterns is maximized when these strategies are used in combination (Reeves, 2012).

Evidence-based medicine uses the best clinically relevant research obtained from a systematic review of the published literature along with clinical expertise to guide clinical practice and medication management decisions. Peer-reviewed clinical studies provide an evidence-based foundation for developing disease management guidelines and decision-support algorithms (Hatton et al., 2005; Kamath, Zhang, Kesten, Wakai, Shelton, & Trestman, 2013). Evidence-based disease management guidelines promote quality patient care by encouraging medication use that is consistent with nationally recognized treatment standards. Adhering to a formulary list alone will not improve prescribing practices; even medications chosen from an evidence-based formulary can be used inappropriately if there are no guidelines for disease management. For disease management guidelines to be successful, they must be chosen or adapted collaboratively with the prescribing staff, be clear and concise, and be introduced formally in the context of training and supervision of all pertinent clinicians (Holloway & Green, 2003).

Disease management guidelines and treatment algorithms should have a consistent format; provide decision support for first-, second-, and third-line medications; and specify the factors that would lead the clinician to discontinue one medication and move to the next. These factors should be clear and include sequence, dose, and duration. The decision-support algorithm should rank medications in a rational sequence, maximizing the efficacy, safety, and simplicity of the regimen. Medications should be prescribed at the lowest effective dose; a trial at maximum tolerated therapeutic doses should be reached before switching to another medication. Medications should be continued for adequate time to properly evaluate efficacy (typically four to six weeks). If there is an inadequate response to the medication after an appropriate duration, it should be discontinued and another medication selected (Finnerty, Altmasberger, Bopp, Carpinello, Docherty, & Fisher, 2002).

There are several guideline resources to consider, the largest of which is the federal government's National Guideline Clearinghouse (http://www.guideline.gov). The *Manual of Forms and Guidelines for Correctional Mental Health* includes evidence-based guidelines with algorithms for psychiatric disorders generally encountered in correctional settings (Lundquist & Becker, 2010). Evidence suggests that such algorithms may be successfully adapted for use in correctional settings (Kamath et al., 2013).

The American Psychiatric Association defines practice guidelines as "systematically developed documents in a standardized format that present patient care strategies to assist psychiatrists in clinical decision making." Each practice guideline follows a standardized format that includes goals of treatment, efficacy data, side effects and safety, and implementation issues (American Psychiatric Association, 2013a).

The NCCHC further underscores the importance of disease management guidelines by noting in Standard MH-D-02, "The responsible physician and the responsible mental health clinician shall develop facility-specific guidelines regarding prescribing practices for psychotropic medications" (http://www.ncchc.org/guidelines). The NCCHC's guidelines for disease management (http://www.ncchc.org/guidelines) "encourage total disease management . . . with a focus on the challenges and special considerations inherent in correctional settings, they are designed to help health care providers improve patient outcomes."

Evidence-based disease management guidelines are not intended to constrain prescribers but rather to advise and guide best practices and quality patient care. Prescribers retain their decision-making autonomy, but that comes with the obligation to make appropriate and responsible medication use decisions.

Summary

Throughout the United States, correctional health care systems rely on a variety of models for pharmaceutical management and care delivery. We suggest that the most effective model is one in which an active, empowered, multidisciplinary P&TC is at the center of and responsible for system-wide medication-related management decisions. Using evidence-based medicine as its core philosophy, the P&TC advances policies and strategies that drive clinically effective, safe, and fiscally responsible medication use and prescribing practice. Our P&TC accomplished this by carefully devising an evidence-based formulary of preferred medications, implementing evidence-based disease management guidelines, and using these in conjunction with educational strategies, supervision, and a data-informed medication use evaluation process. We found that ongoing feedback to prescribers, open lines of communication between P&TC members and our clinical staff, continuous dissemination of information, and training are integral to optimized prescribing. This resulted in increased compliance, improved patient care outcomes, and decreased pharmaceutical expenditures. The role of the P&TC, its policies, disease management guidelines, and the formulary will each need to evolve to incorporate new evidence-based data and new medication management models.

References

American Psychiatric Association (2013a). Clinical practice guidelines. Retrieved from http://psychiatryonline.org/guidelines.aspx

American Psychiatric Association (2013b). Choosing wisely: What not to prescribe. Retrieved from www.psychiatry.org/choosingwisely

Burns, K. A. (2009). Commentary: The top ten reasons to limit prescription of controlled substances in prisons. *Journal of American Academy of Psychiatry and the Law, 37,* 50–52.

Douglas, T., & Mundey, L. (1995). Making managed care principles work in a correctional setting. *Corrections Today, 57*(6), 99–102.

Ducate, S., & Pondrom, M. (2003). Ziprasidone reduces pharmacy costs in correctional in-patient psychiatric facilities. *International Congress on Schizophrenia Research, 21,* 335.

Food & Drug Administration (2011). Guidance medication guides—Distribution requirements and inclusion in risk evaluation and mitigation strategies (REMS). Retrieved from http://www.fda.gov/downloads/Drugs/GuidanceComplianceRegulatoryInformation/Guidances/UCM244570.pdf

Fijn, R., van Epnhuysen, L. S., Peijnenburg, A. J. M., Brouwers, J. R. B. J., & de Jong-van den Berg, L. T. W. (2002). Is there a need for critical ethical and philosophical evaluation of hospital drugs and therapeutics (D&T) committees? *Pharmacoepidemiology and Drug Safety, 11,* 247–252.

Finnerty, M., Altmasberger, R., Bopp, J., Carpinello, S., Docherty, J. P., & Fisher, W. (2002). Using state administrative and pharmacy data bases to develop a clinical decision support tool for schizophrenia guidelines. *Schizophrenia Bulletin, 28*(1), 85–94.

Hatton, R. C., Gonzolez-Rothi, R. J., Smith, W. D., & Knudsen, A. K. (2005). The use of virtual expert panels: formulary decision-making in the 21st century. *Formulary, 40,* 78–85.

Hilliard, W. T., Barloon, L., Farley, P., Penn, J. V., & Koranek, A. (2013). Bupropion diversion and misuse in the correctional facility. *Journal of Correctional Health Care, 19*(3), 211–217.

Holloway, K., & Green, T. (2003). *Drug and therapeutics committees: A practical guide.* Geneva: World Health Organization.

Hoover, S. E., White, L. J., & Weiner, J. (1990). Therapeutic substitution and formulary systems. *Annals of Internal Medicine, 113*(2), 160–163.

Johnson, J. A., & Friesen, E. (1998). Reassessing the relevance of pharmacoeconomic analysis in formulary decisions. *Pharmacoeconomics, 5* (PT 1), 479–485.

Kamath, J., Zhang, W., Kesten, K., Wakai, S., Shelton, D., & Trestman, R. L. (2013). Algorithm-driven pharmacological management of bipolar disorder in Connecticut prisons. *International Journal of Offender Therapy and Comparative Criminology, 57*(2), 251–264.

Loorand-Striver, L. (2011). Hospital-based pharmacy and therapeutics committees: evolving responsibilities and membership. *Environmental Scan: Canadian Agency for Drugs and Technologies in Health, 23,* 1–15.

Lundquist, T., & Becker, T. (2010) Medication management in correctional settings. In A. Ruiz, J. Dvoskin, C. Scott, & J. Metzner (Eds.), *Manual of forms and guidelines for correctional mental health* (pp. 83–111). Washington, DC: American Psychiatric Publishing, Inc.

Lyles, A., Luce, B. R., & Rentz, M. (1997). Managed care pharmacy, socioeconomic assessments and drug adoption decisions. *Society of Science and Medicine, 45*(4), 511–521.

Marcoux, R. M., Simeone, J. C., Colavita, M., & Larrat, E. P. (2012). An innovative approach to pharmacy management in a state correctional system. *Journal of Correctional Health Care, 18*(i), 53–61.

Moffic, H. S. (2006). Ethical principles for psychiatric administrators: the challenge of formularies. *Psychiatry Quarterly, 77,* 319–327.

National Commission on Correctional Health Care (2008). *Standards for mental health services in correctional facilities.* Chicago: National Commission on Correctional Health Care.

Quintiliani, R., & Quercia, R. A. (2003). How to create a therapeutics committee that is scientifically and economically sound. *Formulary, 38,* 594–602.

Raber, J. H. (2010). The formulary process from a risk management perspective. *Pharmacotherapy, 30,* 42S–47S.

Reddan, J. G., Sheehan, A. H., Eskew, J., & Elmes, G. (2004). Integration of a medication management infrastructure in a large, multihospital system. *American Journal of Health- System Pharmacists, 61,* 2557–2561.

Reeves, R. (2012). Guideline, education, and peer comparison to reduce prescriptions of benzodiazepines and low-dose quetiapine in prison. *Journal of Correctional Health Care, 18*(1), 45–52.

Rosenheck, R. A., Leslie, D. L., Busch, S., Rofman, E. S., & Sernyak, M. (2008). Rethinking antipsychotic formulary policy. *Schizophrenia Bulletin, 34*(2), 375–380.

Rucker, T. D., & Schiff, G. (1990). Drug formularies: Myths-in-formation. *Medical Care, 28*(10), 928–939.

Schumock, G. T., Walton, S. M., Park, H. Y., Nutescu, E. A., Blackburn, J. C., Finley, J. M., & Lewis, R. K. (2004). Factors that influence prescribing decisions. *Annals of Pharmacotherapy, 38,* 557–562.

Tamburello, A. C., Lieberman, J. A., Baum, R. M., & Reeves, R. (2012). Successful removal of quetiapine from a correctional formulary. *Journal of the American Academy of Psychiatry and the Law, 40,* 502–508.

Tan, E. L., Day, R. O., & Brien, J. E. (2005). Perspectives on drug and therapeutics committee policy implementation. *Research in Social and Administrative Pharmacy, 1,* 526–545.

Tyler, L. S., Cole, S. W., May, J. R., Millares, M., Valentino, M. A., Vermeulen, L. C. Jr., & Wilson, A. L. (2008). ASHP guidelines on the pharmacy and therapeutics committee and the formulary system. *American Journal of Health-System Pharmacists, 65,* 1272–1283.

CHAPTER 29

Hypnotic agents and controlled substances

Ingrid Li, Arthur Brewer, and Rusty Reeves

Introduction

Sleep medications are among the most frequently prescribed medications in the community. Many other class II controlled substances, such as benzodiazepines and opiate medications, have become a major public health concern through overuse and abuse. Within correctional settings, these concerns are heightened, and special considerations must be included in any treatment decision. This chapter evaluates best practices in this arena of prescription practice.

Background

Any prescription of a controlled substance in a correctional institution must attend to this crucial fact: most inmates abuse drugs, perhaps as many as 70 to 90 percent (American Psychiatric Association, 2000; Fazel, Bains, & Doll, 2006; Mumola & Karberg, 2004). This abuse is many times greater than in the general population (Fazel, 2006). With limited access to contraband drugs, inmates often turn to abuse of prescription medications. They may exaggerate or feign symptoms in order to obtain controlled substances. Aside from substance abuse per se, there is a culture among prisoners of taking pills to relieve uncomfortable feelings. Then there is diversion of medications. Medications can be used as currency to buy or trade items or favors. Inmates may intimidate or victimize other inmates in order to obtain controlled substances. This inappropriate use of medications wastes staff time and resources in prison (Burns, 2009). Chapter 31 further addresses the endlessly creative misuse of prescribed medications in prisons.

Given this well-known abuse of medications in prison, controlled substances are universally prescribed with caution, if at all, in correctional settings in the United States. Prescribers recognize they have a responsibility not only to treat the individual patient in the prison but also to protect the safety and security of the prison environment. State departments of corrections often have internal guidelines for the prescription of controlled substances. However, there has been little published as to the best correctional practices for prescription of these medications. Currently, England has the most complete national prescribing guidelines for correctional clinicians, published by the Royal College of General Practitioners (RCGP; 2011). The correctional psychiatric community in the United States may similarly wish to adopt formal national practice guidelines for the use of controlled substances in the correctional setting.

This chapter takes steps in that direction. The authors surveyed attendees at a conference of the National Commission on Correctional Health Care (NCCHC). The 38 respondents, representing both jails and prisons in the United States, completed a survey on availability of and guidelines for opiates, benzodiazepines, and hypnotic medications. The survey was not scientific. The authors of this chapter have grouped jail and prison respondents together. Based on these surveys, a review of the literature, and their own experience in corrections, the authors offer suggestions for best practices in the prescription of opiates, benzodiazepines, and sleep medications in correctional settings.

Opiates

Opiates have been used for centuries and remain to this day the most potent and reliable analgesic agents (Pasternak, 2011). They are used for the treatment of acute, chronic, and terminal pain. In time-limited circumstances, the efficacy of opiates has been extensively documented and broadly accepted (Fields, 2011). Opiates used long-term, however, run the risk of abuse and diversion. The previously mentioned survey indicated that opiates are commonly prescribed in correctional institutions; only one respondent stated that opiates were not available in their facility or system. However, respondents also expressed concern about misuse, especially in treatment of chronic pain. Slightly fewer than half of the respondents indicated that their system or facility used a guideline for the prescription of opiate medication. Chapter 39 includes a more extensive discussion of pain management in correctional settings.

When used for the treatment of acute pain, opioid medications should only be used when the severity of the pain warrants the use of opioids and after determining that nonopioid pain medications will not provide adequate pain relief. If opioid medications are prescribed, the duration of therapy clearly must be limited based on the condition being treated. Long-acting opioids should not be used in the treatment of acute pain, including postoperative pain, except in circumstances where adequate monitoring can be conducted (Rolfs, Johnson, Williams, & Sundwall, 2010).

Given their risk for abuse and diversion in corrections and the availability of suitable alternatives, opiates should not be used as first-line medications for the treatment of chronic noncancer pain (CNCP; National Commission on Correctional Health Care, 2012). The International Association for the Study of Pain (IASP) has defined CNCP as "pain that persists beyond the normal tissue healing time, which is assumed to be three months. It should be of sufficient intensity to adversely affect a patient's well-being, level of function, and quality of life." Cancer pain and end-of-life pain are not addressed in this chapter. CNCP is a challenge in the community as well as in corrections. The IASP has identified the following five major challenges in pain management today: lack of evidence-based information of most things provided to patients by health care providers, insufficient education of primary care providers about patients and treatment of pain, the largely unproven value of opioid treatment of patients with CNCP, resources for providers of pain management, and access to multidisciplinary care (Loeser, 2012).

According to the NCCHC (2012) guideline for the treatment of CNCP, the best practice for the treatment of chronic pain includes a thorough history of the pain, physical examination, review of records, and judicious testing. Assessment of psychiatric and substance abuse histories are essential. According to one study (Edlund et al., 2007), a nonopioid substance abuse history was the strongest predictor of opioid abuse/dependence. In this same study, a psychiatric disorder was a moderate predictor of opioid abuse/dependence. The state's prescription monitoring registry should be reviewed. The patient's functional status should be clearly documented and must include staff observation as well as the patient's self-report.

Treatment should start with nonpharmacological efforts, including patient education, physical therapy evaluation, exercises, stretches, psychological support, relaxation, and perhaps cognitive–behavioral therapy. Preferred initial nonopioid medications are acetaminophen, aspirin, or a nonsteroidal anti-inflammatory drug. Anticonvulsant and noradrenergic antidepressant medications are second-line alternatives. According to the NCCHC (2012), opioids should be considered only when all alternatives have failed to improve pain and function; there is objective evidence of disease; there is evidence of significant impaired function; the patient provides written, informed consent; and strict monitoring of use of the drug is feasible. Measures of success must be determined before an opioid is started. If those goals are not met, the drug should be tapered and discontinued (see Chapter 39).

Benzodiazepines

Benzodiazepines are controlled substances used to treat anxiety, agitation, insomnia, and withdrawal from alcohol. More than half of the survey respondents stated that benzodiazepines were formulary medications. Only two respondents stated that benzodiazepines were unavailable in their facility or system. Half of the respondents stated they used a guideline for the prescription of benzodiazepines. In their comments, many of the respondents indicated that benzodiazepines were used primarily for detoxification or that other restrictions were placed on their use (e.g., crushed pills, use limited to two weeks). None of the respondents indicated that benzodiazepines were used for the treatment of insomnia or long-term treatment of anxiety.

The authors' survey and recommendations from the literature (Burns, 2010; Royal College of General Practitioners, 2011) confirm the authors' experience that benzodiazepines are subject to abuse and diversion in prisons and should not be prescribed as a first-line treatment of insomnia or anxiety. (Chapters 16 and 35 more comprehensively address treatment of insomnia and anxiety, respectively, in corrections.)

Safer first-line treatments of anxiety should initially be considered, including psychotherapy or medications such as selective serotonergic reuptake inhibitors, venlafaxine, or mirtazapine (Ciraulo & Nace, 2000). Alternatives include nonbenzodiazepine anxiolytics such as buspirone or hydroxyzine. A second-line agent for the autonomic manifestations of anxiety is propranolol (Royal College of General Practitioners, 2011; Lundquist & Becker, 2010).

Benzodiazepine prescribing in correctional psychiatry should generally be limited to detoxification from benzodiazepines or alcohol and treatment of acute and severe agitation (as from psychosis or mania). Treatment should be for a short period, generally, less than two weeks. The treatment of insomnia with benzodiazepines should be rare. It should be reserved for severe and observed insomnia, after an alternative less abuse-prone medication has failed, and then only for a short period of time. The risk–benefit ratio beyond short-term use is unestablished but can certainly result in dependence or withdrawal symptoms (Lader, 2011). Prior to prescribing benzodiazepines, the clinician should have a clear discussion with the inmate that the medication is time-limited and will be discontinued on a set date. Unless absolutely indicated, inmates should be tapered off benzodiazepines by the time they are released from prison to prevent withdrawal or abuse.

Specific methods to reduce the potential for diversion include direct observation of pill administration by custody and nursing staff, prescribing medication in liquid form, or crushing and dissolving medication in liquid (crush and float). Use of toxicology screens can also help limit the abuse of benzodiazepines (Ciraulo & Nace, 2000). Patients who are prescribed a benzodiazepine should have a toxicology screen to confirm that they are, in fact, taking the medication rather than diverting it.

A practical and effective method used by one of the authors (Reeves, 2011) to reduce the prescription of benzodiazepines in the New Jersey Department of Corrections involved physician-to-physician comparison (i.e., peer pressure). The New Jersey Department of Corrections established a guideline for the treatment of insomnia that discouraged the use of benzodiazepines for sleep. Staff physicians received education on the guideline. The author then ranked each physician on a graph in the order of frequency of prescriptions. The ranking was done anonymously; each physician knew where he or she ranked among colleagues but did not know the identities of the colleagues. This technique reduced the number of benzodiazepine prescriptions by 38 percent after 20 months. The reductions were seen in the high-frequency prescribers; low-frequency prescribers did not change their prescribing practice.

Another, and perhaps more effective, way to reduce the prescriptions of benzodiazepines in prisons is simply to make these medications nonformulary. (Jails routinely use benzodiazepines for alcohol detoxification.) A clinician who wishes to prescribe a nonformulary medication must apply to a supervisor for permission to prescribe. In addition to the "hassle" of applying, a nonformulary process reduces prescriptions by allowing a second opportunity to say no. The nonformulary process can also alleviate the burden of those prescribers who lack the fortitude to say no. A useful technique in prison for a physician who has difficulty saying no is to say, "I took an oath not to harm anyone. Given your history, if I prescribed this medication, it could harm you. I won't do that." This quiets most objectors. The downside of making a medication nonformulary is that, unless an exception is made, it is not available for use in an emergency. Benzodiazepines are effective when used appropriately and can even be life-saving in cases of severe agitation and withdrawal. Thus, the authors recommend—and their survey substantiates—that at least one benzodiazepine remain on a psychiatric formulary.

The most certain way to reduce the use of benzodiazepines—to reduce the use of any medication—is to simply make them unavailable. For the reason described, the authors discourage this maneuver.

Sleep medications

The inmate quest for medications to treat sleep complaints is ubiquitous in corrections, and anecdotes abound about the dubiousness of these complaints. In the survey of correctional providers, sleep medications were commonly prescribed, but the concern about inappropriate use or overuse was apparent in most systems. The most commonly prescribed medications were diphenhydramine and hydroxyzine. Whether sleep medications were formulary or not did not prevent clinicians from prescribing these medications. Indeed, one respondent who worked in a system in which sleep medications ostensibly were unavailable wrote that prescribers "get around it" by writing for a sedating medication purportedly used for another reason. The authors are not surprised by the comment. Trying to entirely eliminate sleep medications in corrections is like squeezing a balloon—it pops out somewhere no matter what you do. Very few of the facilities or jails had a prescribing guideline for sleep medications. The most intriguing comment was that sleep issues were managed by direct observation, which "eliminates 99% of the problem."

In light of this comment that direct observation resolved almost all complaints of insomnia, it is perhaps surprising that there have been few published studies investigating the percentage of accurate inmate complaints of insomnia. Studies are absent despite the known disruptions to a good night's sleep in jails and prisons, which include clanging doors, obstreperous inmates, a sedentary lifestyle, lack of exposure to a normal day/night light cycle, and damage to sleep architecture caused by use of illicit drugs.

Inmate patients with a history of substance abuse often turn to pharmacological rather than psychosocial interventions. These individuals can have unrealistic expectations of sleep during periods of sobriety while incarcerated. In particular, they may have a distorted perception of normal sleep latency and disruption, as they are accustomed to sleeping while under the influence of benzodiazepines, opiates, or alcohol (Royal College of General Practitioners, 2011). Heroin abusers experience a reduced sleep period, which may not resolve when the patient ceases heroin use (Staedt et al., 1996). One review article, noting that sleep medications did not relieve insomnia complaints in a sizable number of inmates, suggested that nonpharmacological treatments should be used more frequently to treat insomnia in prisons (Elger, 2007). This recommendation accords with general insomnia research. Nonpharmacological treatments of insomnia have been shown to achieve long-lasting, clinically significant improvement (Elger, 2004). Hypnotic drugs are most effective in treating short-term acute insomnia; long-term effectiveness is not proven.

If an inmate presents with the chief complaint of insomnia, he or she should first be evaluated to assess if there is obvious evidence of a mental disturbance. During the initial evaluation, the inmate should be asked to complete a sleep diary. A more objective alternative to a sleep diary would be confirmation of the reported sleep pattern by custody officers during rounds. Such observations may tax the limited resources of custody staff and, in any case, are routinely resisted by officers whose primary goal is to maintain safety, security, and control at the institution. Such observation, if it were to be successful, would likely require the cooperation and support of the facility's administration—just as most successful correctional health initiatives do. Some institutions in Pennsylvania move inmates to the infirmary to conduct a "sleep study" where nursing staff record the patient's sleep patterns for one or two nights. If the evaluation determines that the inmate suffers transient insomnia related to adjustment to incarceration, then a nonpharmacological intervention should be pursued.

Nonpharmacological interventions are also known as cognitive behavioral treatments for insomnia (CBT-I). One component of CBT-I includes sleep hygiene education. A list of sleep hygiene techniques (e.g., reduce caffeine, increase exercise during the day, wear ear plugs) should be discussed and provided to the inmate when he or she reports difficulty sleeping. Sleep hygiene groups are one approach. In New Jersey and Pennsylvania, according to the authors' experiences, attempts at sleep groups were short-lived, if not futile. Inmates did not want to attend, and overcommitted therapists were not interested in providing the education. Other CBT-I include stimulus control therapy, relaxation techniques, paradoxical intention, sleep restriction, and cognitive therapy to change maladaptive or irrational thoughts. These skills can be taught in either individual or group sessions by mental health staff. Cognitive behavioral treatments may lower health care costs, do not have the side effects of medications, avoid interactions with other drugs, and avoid perpetuating drug abuse. Nonpharmacological treatments have been shown to improve sleep and have long-lasting effects (Elger, 2007).

If a major mental disorder underlies the insomnia, then a referral should be made to a psychiatrist. The psychiatrist should obtain a sleep history. An assessment should be taken of pertinent associated symptoms such as heightened arousal or excessive daytime sleepiness; sleep/wake schedule disorders; restless legs; snoring and other symptoms of sleep apnea; depression, anxiety, or other mental disorder; drug or alcohol abuse; and medical problems or current medications. If the psychiatrist suspects a medical condition underlies the insomnia, the psychiatrist can make a referral to the internist.

If the inmate fails behavioral approaches for a primary sleep disturbance, a brief, 14-day trial of medication, such as hydroxyzine, trazodone, or mirtazapine, can be considered to restore the sleep–wake cycle (Lundquist & Becker, 2010). The length of the short-term treatment should be discussed with the inmate at the outset. Hypnotic medications are effective in short-term treatment of insomnia but have not been proven in long-term treatment (Elger, 2007). Medications should be given under direct observation by nursing staff to prevent diversion or hoarding of the medication. Low-dose antidepressants or antipsychotics that offer the side effect of sedation should not be prescribed long term to treat insomnia. Using these medications off label to treat insomnia taxes limited psychiatric resources in prisons (Burns, 2010).

Summary

The prevalence of inmate drug abuse is many times higher than in the general population. A survey of practitioners in jails and prisons in the United States expresses the concern that sleep, opiate, and benzodiazepine medications can be abused or diverted. There has been little published as to the best correctional practice for the prescription of these medications. In general, sleep medications and controlled substances should be prescribed cautiously in a correctional setting and should be avoided as first-line treatment and as long-term treatment, if possible. Sleep medications are the most difficult to control since the quest for medications to treat sleep complaints is ubiquitous in corrections. Guidelines, thoughtful use of formulary controls, and a measure of flexibility will assist in the appropriate prescription of these medications.

References

American Psychiatric Association. (2000). *Psychiatric services in jails and prisons* (2nd ed.). Washington, DC: American Psychiatric Association.

Burns, K. A. (2009). Commentary: The top ten reasons to limit prescription of controlled substances in prisons. *Journal of American Academy of Psychiatry and the Law, 37,* 50–52.

Burns, K. A. (2010) Pharmacotherapy in correctional settings. In C. Scott (Ed.). *Handbook of correctional mental health* (2nd ed., pp. 321–344). Washington, DC: American Psychiatric Publishing.

Ciraulo, D. A., & Nace, E. P. (2000). Benzodiazepine treatment of anxiety or insomnia in substance abuse patients. *American Journal on Addictions, 9,* 276–284.

Edlund, M. J., Steffick, D., Hudson, T., et al. (2007). Risk factors for clinically recognized opioid abuse and dependence among veterans using opioids for chronic non-cancer pain. *Pain, 129,* 355–362.

Elger, B. S. (2004). Management and evolution of insomnia complaints among non-substance-misusers in a Swiss remand prison. *Swiss Medical Weekly, 134,* 486–499.

Elger, B. S. (2007). Insomnia in places of detention: a review of the most recent research findings. *Medicine, Science and the Law, 47,* 191–199.

Fazel, S., Bains, P., & Doll, H. (2006). Substance abuse and dependence in prisoners: a systematic review. *Addiction, 101,* 181–191.

Fields, H. L. (2011). The doctor's dilemma: Opiate analgesics and chronic pain. *Neuron, 69*(4) 591–594.

Lader, M. (2011). Benzodiazepines revisited—will we ever learn? *Addiction, 106,* 2086–2109.

Loeser, J. D. (2012). Five crises in pain management. *Pain Clinical Updates,* 20(1). Retrieved from http://www.iasp-pain.org

Lundquist, T., & Becker, T. (2010) Medication management in correctional settings. In A. Ruiz, J. Dvoskin, C. Scott, & J. Metzner (Eds.). *Manual of forms and guidelines for correctional mental health* (pp. 83–111). Washington, DC: American Psychiatric Publishing, Inc.

Mumola, C., & Karberg, J. Drug use and dependence, state and federal prisoners, 2004. Bureau of Justice Statistics—Special Report. October 2006. Retrieved from http://www.bjs.gov/content/pub/pdf/dudsfp04.pdf

National Commission on Correctional Health Care. (2012). Guideline for disease management in correctional settings: Chronic noncancer pain management. Retrieved from http://ncchc.org

Pasternak, G. W. (2011). *The opiate receptors.* New York: Humana Press/Springer.

Reeves, R. (2012). Guideline, education, and peer comparison to reduce prescriptions of benzodiazepines and low-dose quetiapine in prison. *Journal of Correctional Health Care, 18,* 45–52.

Rolfs, R. T., Johnson, E., Williams, N. J., & Sundwall, D. N. (2010). Utah clinical guidelines on prescribing opioids for treatment of pain. *Journal of Pain and Palliative Care Pharmacotherapy, 24*(3), 219–235.

Royal College of General Practitioners, Secure Environments Group. (2011). Safer prescribing in prisons. Retrieved from http://www.rcgp.org.uk/news/2011/november/~/media/Files/News/Safer_Prescribing_in_Prison.ashx

Staedt, J., Wassmuth, F., Stoppe, G., et al. (1996). Effects of chronic treatment with methadone naltrexone on sleep in addicts. *European Archives of Psychiatry and Clinical Neuroscience, 246,* 305–309.

CHAPTER 30

Medication administration and management
Directly observed therapy

Catherine M. Knox

Introduction

The courts and professional organizations recognize access to clinically appropriate and timely treatment with psychotropic medication as an essential element of an adequate correctional mental health system (Cohen, 2008; Hills, Siegfried, & Ickowitz, 2004; Metzner, 2009). While receiving treatment, incarcerated patients must be monitored and supervised clinically so that optimal patient outcomes are achieved (Anno, 2001; Hills et al., 2004). For many mentally ill inmates, incarceration is an opportunity to receive treatment that was not accessible in the community. In the analysis by Wilper, Woolhandler, Boyd, Lasser, McCormick, Bor, and Himmelstein (2009) of the health and health care of inmates in prison and jail, only one third of those diagnosed with schizophrenia or bipolar disorder were receiving medication at the time of arrest compared to two thirds during incarceration. This chapter addresses the processes involved in the mechanics of medication dispensing, distribution, and administration and speaks to opportunities to enhance therapeutic adherence in correctional settings.

Components of medication delivery

There are many steps, people, and processes involved in getting medication to the patient within a correctional facility. The major components of pharmacy services are prescribing, dispensing, distribution, and continuity (Table 30.1).

Prescribing

Any correctional facility that houses inmates with serious mental illness has several types of antipsychotic, antidepressant, mood-stabilizing, and anxiolytic medications on the formulary, available in oral and injectable forms and both short- and long-acting preparations. In addition, pharmacy consultation should be available to prescribers either at the site via phone or other means. A pharmacist should review each order in relation to the patient's medication profile before medication is dispensed. Access to medication that is not on the formulary is obtained by completing a nonformulary request (Appelbaum, 2010; Burns, 2010; Schwartz-Watts & Frierson, 2006). Policy and practice should allow continuance of a nonformulary medication

for a newly admitted inmate who was being treated with such a medication while in the community (National Commission on Correctional Health Care [NCCHC], 2014a, 2014b; Burrow, Knox, & Villanueva, 2006).

Decisions about the choice of drug, dosing, and monitoring should factor in the inmate's program assignments and how medication is administered in the correctional facility. The patient's adherence to medication is affected by the prescriber's decisions and facility practices (Burns, 2010; Harmon, 2013). For example, ordering a noontime dose is ineffective if the inmate has a job or program assignment that makes him or her unable to attend the noon medication pass. Further, patient adherence may be enhanced by communicating the order and its intended effects to other members of the treatment team for use in patient coaching and support (Ruiz, 2010).

Medication administration is costly in terms of nursing and correctional staff time. If the volume of medication prescribed exceeds the time available or staffing capacity, medications will be missed or given at inappropriate intervals. Use of evidence-based practice guidelines and strategies regarding dosage, strength, and frequency in prescribing are ways to manage the volume of medication to be administered each day (Appelbaum, 2010; Burns, 2010; Burrow et al., 2006). If an order cannot be written to accommodate the inmate's availability or the program's staffing capacity, the psychiatrist should have the inmate transferred to a location that can carry out the intended treatment plan.

Dispensing

Medication delivery is a high-volume and high-risk activity. The Institute of Medicine (2006) reports that medication error is the reason for 19% of all adverse patient safety events and that prescribing and administration account for 75% of all medication errors. Advances in dispensing, such as electronic ordering, patient medication profiles, unit-dose packaging, and patient-specific labeling, improve patient safety. These improvements in patient safety have required changes in longstanding but less safe practices. The change process can cause delays in treatment initiation as staff adjust to newer processes for ordering, dispensing, and delivering medication.

Table 30.1 Components of medication delivery

Prescribing	◆ The formulary includes several forms of each class of drug.
	◆ Medications not on the formulary are accessed via nonformulary request.
	◆ Orders for medication administration do not conflict with inmate program and facility schedules.
	◆ Medication is administered consistent with the time it is ordered.
Dispensing	◆ Patients receive the first dose of new medications in a timely manner.
	◆ Medications are available if treatment must be administered before the pharmacy dispenses.
	◆ The physician and pharmacist jointly determine stock and starter medications.
Distributing	◆ Medications are delivered in a timely, safe, and clinically effective manner.
	◆ Security procedures prevent medication misuse.
	◆ Patient questions, absences, and refusals are addressed but do not delay medication delivery.
	◆ Medication administration is documented and used to guide clinical care.
Continuity	◆ Medication treatment is uninterrupted.
	◆ Problems that contribute to medication discontinuity are resolved.
	◆ Reminders for refills and renewals are used to prevent medication misses.
	◆ Medications are continued upon release from the facility.

It is important for prescribers to know how long it will take for the patient to receive the first dose after an order is written. Depending on the location and staffing of the pharmacy, this may be less than an hour or as long as a week if stock medications are unavailable. Another potential delay is the time it takes for nursing staff to verify medications received from the pharmacy and to prepare them for administration. It may take another day or two before the medication is available to the patient, especially if large deliveries are received from the pharmacy and staffing levels are not adjusted to handle the influx. Although less satisfactory from a patient safety standpoint, arrangements must be made to administer from stock medications or for the psychiatrist to dispense a starter packet for the nursing staff to administer if the medication needs to be started before the pharmacy can dispense it. The pharmacy and physician should mutually determine clinically acceptable dispensing turnaround times and identify what medications need to be available at the site to initiate treatment (Burrow et al., 2006).

Distribution

In contrast to the community, the majority of psychotropic medications in correctional facilities are administered to each patient dose by dose (Burns, 2010). These medications have great potential for misuse because of their sedative effects. Hoarding, overdose, trading, and intimidation leading to noncompliance are forms of misuse in the correctional environment that can lead to adverse events (Burns, 2010; Burrow et al., 2006; Harmon, 2013). An unintended advantage of this practice is the ability to directly observe the patient receiving treatment. Some argue that this also contributes to nonadherence if inmates feel, for example, they have no choice about when to take the medication, the time spent waiting in line is too long, or the medication is administered at an inconvenient time (Burns, 2010; Ehret, Shelton, Barta, Trestman, Maruca, Kamath, & Golay, 2013; Harmon, 2013; Shelton, Ehret, Wakai, Kapetanovic, & Moran, 2010). When correctional facilities do allow inmates to self-administer medications, it is in preparation for release, since the individual will be expected to do this when residing in the community, or it is because the medication has low potential for misuse (Burrow et al., 2006; Harmon, 2013; Hills et al., 2004).

Medication is individually administered either by having inmates come to a designated location (i.e., medication cart or pill window) at a specified time or by delivering the medication to each individual in his or her housing unit or cell. In medium- and minimum-security housing areas, medication administration may be handled in a centralized location such as the clinic. On inpatient treatment units (e.g., mental health units, infirmary, and step-down programs), medication administration takes place on the unit. In segregation or high-security areas, medication is administered at the cell or in the pod. Each approach carries an operational burden. Decentralized medication administration is staff-intensive, while centralized medication lines are challenging for correctional facilities to manage safely. Most facilities use several methods based on the amount of inmate movement that is allowed (Burns, 2010; Burrow et al., 2006).

The time, methods, and location for medication delivery are a joint decision of the facility administrator and the health authority (Burrow et al., 2006; NCCHC, 2014a, 2014b). The primary objective is to administer medication in a manner that is timely, safe, and optimally therapeutic (Anno, 2001; Burrow et al., 2006). Either nursing or correctional staff may observe inmates to ensure that medication is not "cheeked"; observation should be based on whether the patient has cheeked medication previously and whether there is the potential to misuse the drug. Medication administration should not interfere with meals, sleep, visitation, recreation, and work or program assignments. The potential for stigma or victimization associated with centralized pill call and long waiting times should also be minimized (Ehret et al., 2013; Harmon, 2006; Shelton et al., 2010). Sometimes, due to staffing issues at the facility or schedules for inmate activities, doses are given too early (primarily morning and/or nighttime doses), requiring providers to advocate for more clinically appropriate times for medication administration (Burns, 2010).

Correctional officers manage inmate movement to and from the medication area or escort health care personnel cell to cell to administer medication. Officers assist inmates to get ready to take their medications (e.g., getting off the bunk, getting water, being dressed appropriately), eliminate distractions (e.g., loud television or games, crowding the medication area), and observe the inmate ingest the medication (Anno, 2001; Burrow et al., 2006). Basic training for correctional officers should include the purpose of psychotropic medications in treatment as well as important precautions and side effects. Officers with this knowledge and skill can provide valuable information to health care providers about how an inmate is tolerating medication and play a key role in the prevention, early identification, and management of negative side effects (Burns, 2010; Hills et al., 2004; Shelton et al., 2010).

Questions, requests, and refusals can cause delays that contribute to conflict and untimely medication delivery. The nurse who administers medication can answer simple questions while the medication is being prepared. If it is complicated, the inmate should be asked to wait until after the medication pass is over or can be seen by the nurse later in the day. If medication is not taken, the reason should be ascertained (e.g., the patient was at court or a medical appointment, had a visitor, was transferred, or had not been let out of the cell). An inmate who refuses a dose should be asked why to determine if there is a simple remedy to the problem (Burrow et al., 2006; NCCHC, 2014a, 2014b).

Continuity

Continuity of medication is a challenge in correctional facilities. For example, when an inmate is transferred from one housing location to another, his or her medication may not be moved to the corresponding medication cart or pill line. Housing assignments are a function of institutional operations. If the facility does not communicate this information to the health care program, patients miss doses until the medication catches up or the pharmacy dispenses a new supply. Medication discontinuity can also occur when the pharmacy is inconsistent in processing refills or delivering supplies. Finally, discontinuity occurs if medication refills and renewals are not timely. Instances of medication discontinuity should be reported, tracked, and reviewed to identify ways to correct or prevent the problem.

Continuity of medication upon admission prevents potential crisis or relapse. Incarceration is also an opportunity to assess the medical necessity of medication prescribed while the patient was in the community (Appelbaum, 2010; see Chapter 19). Inmates who report taking psychotropic medication on admission should be referred to a psychiatrist to assess their need for medication at the next available appointment. In the meantime, a prescriber should be contacted to determine whether interim medication orders are needed. If possible, intake staff should contact the community pharmacy to verify the prescription before the patient is seen by a provider (Burrow et al., 2006). Some correctional systems have established interagency agreements with the mental health system that facilitate verification of this information (Smith & Smith, 2006).

The standard of care is to arrange for continuity of psychotropic medication in the transition to community mental health providers (Baillargeon, Hoge, & Penn, 2010; Dlugacz & Roskes, 2010; Hills et al., 2004). The correctional prescriber writes a prescription for release medication based on a clinical evaluation of the patient when informed of the pending release. Patients are given a supply of medication at the time of release or arrangements are made to fill the prescription in the community (Dlugacz & Roskes, 2010; Smith & Smith, 2006). Methods to enhance the likelihood of medication continuity include stabilizing patients on medications prior to release, using medications that are available and not cost-prohibitive in the community, and considering the use of long-acting forms of medication (Lee, Connolly, & Dietz, 2005; Velligan, Weiden, Sajatovic, Scott, Carpenter, Ross, & Docherty, 2010b).

Adherence

Adherence is defined as the extent to which a person's behavior corresponds with the recommendations for treatment to which he or she agreed. Taking 80% of recommended doses is generally considered the standard for adherence (Brown & Bussell, 2011; Shelton et al., 2010; Velligan, Weiden, Sajatovic, Scott, Carpenter, Ross, & Docherty, 2009). Adherence with psychotropic medication among prisoners is essentially the same as that estimated among persons in the community (Ehret et al., 2013; Gray, Bressington, Lathlean, & Mills, 2008; Shelton et al., 2010). In a review of the literature, low rates of psychotropic medication adherence among prisoners were associated with relapse, violent behavior resulting in crime, conviction for more serious felonies, and increased frequency of hospitalization (Shelton et al., 2010). Interventions with evidence to support medication adherence among prisoners with mental illness are summarized in Table 30.2.

Addressing adherence as part of treatment

Adherence should be addressed as a regular part of the patient's treatment plan. Community-based adherence is measured most often by self-report, which tends to be an overestimate (Julius, Novitsky, & Dubin, 2009; Osterberg & Blaschke, 2005; Velligan et al., 2010b). In correctional settings, a more objective assessment of medication-taking behavior is possible by reviewing the patient's medication administration record. If patients are nonadherent, this information should be reviewed weekly; adherent patients should be reviewed monthly (Velligan, Weiden, Sajatovic, Scott, Carpenter, Ross, & Docherty, 2010a). The patient may also be asked to keep a self-reporting tool or medication diary and to bring it to his or her appointments (Ehret et al., 2013; Shelton et al., 2010; Velligan et al., 2010b).

Adherence is complex and dynamic, involving the patient's knowledge, beliefs, and attitudes as well as his or her relationship with health care providers (Brown & Bussel, 2011; Julius et al., 2009; Velligan et al., 2010b). Fifty percent of inmates report past nonadherence to psychotropic medication. Some of the reasons offered for nonadherence include the following (Bressington, Gray, Lathlean, & Mills, 2008; Mills, Lathlean, Forrester, Van Veenhuyzen, & Gray, 2011):

◆ Feeling better, so did not need the medication anymore

◆ Medication not as important as other priorities

◆ Forgetfulness

◆ Did not think the medications worked

◆ Side effects were too distressing

Mistrust of health care professionals, lack of time with providers, impeded access to psychotherapy, and a passive patient role reduce medication adherence among prisoners (Bressington et al., 2008; Ehret et al., 2013; Gray et al., 2008; Mills et al., 2011). Other variables associated with adherence/nonadherence among prisoners who take psychotropic medication are listed in Table 30.3.

Consideration of demographics and use of a structured interview to evaluate the patient's attitude and experience with treatment can help identify those at greater risk for nonadherence. This information is valuable in selecting the most effective interventions to support adherence (Shelton et al., 2010; Velligan et al., 2010b). Adherence has also been associated with the use

Table 30.2 Supporting medication adherence among prisoners with mental illness

Treatment objective	Interventions
Devote time to address adherence as part of treatment	◆ Identify the patient's motivation and goals for treatment. ◆ Link treatment interventions to the patient's motivation and goals. ◆ Assess the patient's perspective about the importance of treatment and confidence in and satisfaction with treatment. ◆ Explore past and present reasons for nonadherence. ◆ Use active listening and acknowledge the patient's experience, motivation, and goals for treatment. ◆ Develop and/or use structured interview tools to identify patients at high risk for poor adherence. ◆ Use decision-support protocols that assess adherence and promote patient involvement.
Facilitate development of insight and self-care ability	◆ Provide access to psychotherapy and psychoeducational programming. ◆ Provide information and education about the medication, reasons why it is prescribed, expected side effects, and self-care. ◆ Use motivational interviewing techniques to discuss direct and indirect benefits of treatment in relation to the patient's goals and motivation for treatment. ◆ Use cognitive-behavioral approaches to link adherence to symptom reduction. ◆ Discuss reasons for nonadherence with the patient. ◆ Embed medication taking into the patient's daily routine. ◆ Provide the patient choice of time to take medication. ◆ Provide reminders such as daily diaries, visual clues, and calendars. ◆ Assign a medication buddy to help the patient remember to take medication.
Optimize treatment efficacy	◆ Monitor impact of medication on symptoms. ◆ Anticipate side effects; provide guidance about how to manage them. ◆ Acknowledge and explore the patient's distress with side effects. ◆ Train staff in early identification and management of side effects. ◆ Increase visit frequency to facilitate development of insight and self-care ability. ◆ Simplify or alter medication regimen to coincide with patient experience, motivation, and goals; consider dose-forgiving or long-acting formulas. ◆ Eliminate or modify facility routines or culture that cause disruption or are disincentives to adherence (i.e., transfers, schedule conflicts, distance to walk, potential vulnerability and long waiting times at pill line, and countertherapeutic administration times).

Adapted from Bressington et al., 2008; Ehret et al., 2013; Gray et al., 2008; Mills et al., 2011; and Shelton et al., 2010.

Table 30.3 Variables associated with psychotropic medication adherence and nonadherence

Medication adherence	Medication nonadherence
Older age	Younger age
Male gender	Hispanic race
Personal motivation	Physical barriers to taking medication
Inmate involvement in care	Adverse effects of medication
Therapeutic relationship with health care providers	Impaired cognition
Assigned guardian	
Positive outcomes of treatment	
Prior experience with psychiatric treatment	

Source: Shelton et al. (2010). Reprinted with permission from John Wiley and Sons © Blackwell Publishing.

of structured decision support tools to guide treatment (Ehret et al., 2013).

Insight and self-care

The second objective in supporting adherence is to facilitate development of insight and capacity for self-care. Ehret and colleagues (2013) found that adherence improved as symptoms decreased among female prisoners with bipolar disorder. Other studies have reported that adherence among prisoners who take antipsychotic medication is most strongly associated with patients' perception of treatment efficacy (Bressington et al., 2008; Gray et al., 2008; Mills et al., 2011). Access to psychotherapy, use of motivational interviewing, and cognitive-behavioral therapy can increase insight regarding the benefits of treatment, support development of a therapeutic alliance, and link adherence to symptom reduction (Bressington et al., 2008; Ehret et al., 2013; Shelton et al., 2010). Inmates who are passive participants in their treatment are also less adherent (Bressington et al., 2008). Offering patients some choice about their medication and when to take it promotes patient involvement and helps to develop a therapeutic alliance (Brown & Bussell, 2011; Julius et al., 2009).

Inmates report that they are not given enough information or explanation about medications, their side effects, and their purpose (Bressington et al., 2008; Mills et al., 2011). Therefore, education is a key component of adherence improvement when used in conjunction with behavioral and affective strategies (Brown & Bussell, 2011; Chong, Aslani, & Chen, 2011; Haynes, Ackloo, Sahota, McDonald, & Yao, 2008; Julius et al., 2009; Velligan et al., 2010b).

The structure of the correctional setting can enable inmates to take medication regularly; however, the inflexibility of the routine can be a disincentive as well (Bressington et al., 2008; Ehret et al., 2013; Mills et al., 2011). Discussing the reasons for nonadherence with the patient provides information to tailor interventions. Such interventions may include visual reminders or a medication buddy. The patient's experience may also identify problems such as long wait times that can be addressed systemically (Bressington et al., 2008; Ehret et al., 2013; Shelton et al., 2010).

Treatment efficacy

The third and most important objective in supporting adherence is to optimize treatment efficacy. Lack of response to treatment is associated with poor adherence and was given as one of the reasons inmates are nonadherent (Gray et al., 2008; Velligan et al., 2010b). Ehret and colleagues (2013) found that female inmates with more severe symptoms had lower rates of adherence and that as symptoms improved, adherence also improved. In a qualitative study, nearly all prisoners interviewed about their experiences taking psychotropic medication had side effects; 20% reported that this reduced adherence (Mills et al., 2011). In another study, only one third of males who took antipsychotic medication while in prison said that the benefits of treatment were worth tolerating the side effects (Bressington et al., 2008; Gray et al., 2008).

An advantage in treating mental illness in the correctional setting is the ability to closely and objectively observe the effects of prescribed medication, both intended and unintended. With this information, it is possible to increase visit frequency and adjust interventions to address symptoms quickly (Bressington et al., 2008; Ehret et al., 2013). The treating psychiatrist should

communicate to appropriate staff the thresholds for referring nonadherent patients. For high-risk patients, this could be defined as missing a single dose; for other patients, it might be three missed doses. The patient's clinical situation should guide referral instructions (Harmon, 2013; Velligan et al., 2010a). Inmates report having good relationships with their mental health providers but felt they had trouble accessing supportive and counseling services (Bressington et al., 2008; Mills et al., 2011). Access is increased when correctional officers and nurses are considered members of the treatment team who are trained to recognize symptoms and side effects associated with psychotropic medications, and on when to refer inmates to mental health staff, and can coach inmates in self-care (American Correctional Association, 2002; Hills et al., 2004; NCCHC, 2014a, 2014b; Shelton et al., 2010).

The structural aspects of medication administration can also be altered to improve adherence (Bressington et al., 2008; Ehret et al., 2013; Gray et al., 2008; Mills et al., 2011; Shelton et al., 2010). These include simplifying the medication regimen by reducing the number of doses each day, changing to a long-acting preparation, and administering medication at times and in ways that are safer and more convenient for the patient but are still clinically acceptable. Reducing the reasons for medication discontinuity, as discussed earlier in this chapter (e.g., transfers and schedule conflicts), also reduces the incidence of adverse events and optimizes treatment efficacy (Hills et al., 2004; Shelton et al., 2010).

Summary

Psychopharmacology is a keystone in the treatment of mental illness. The prescription, preparation, delivery, and monitoring of psychotropic medication use is a complex process and involves many personnel from health, mental health, and correctional services. In addition to the patient's clinical condition, the correctional environment and facility practices should be taken into account when making decisions about treatment. To support patient adherence, the psychiatrist should explain why medication has been prescribed, should instruct the patient on its intended effects, and should discuss how to address side effects. Adherence is assessed at each follow-up visit, and reasons for nonadherence are explored with the patient (Ehret et al., 2013). The psychiatrist provides information and education to other members of the treatment team so that they can participate in the effort to achieve better patient outcomes (Appelbaum, 2010; Shelton et al., 2010).

In addition to ordering medications for treatment of individual patients, psychiatrists are involved in the development of policies, procedures, and clinical guidelines concerning medication treatment at the correctional facility. They also are involved in decisions about medications to be included on the formulary and management of nonformulary requests (Burns, 2010). Psychiatrists review prescribing practices as well as the accuracy, timeliness, and efficacy of medication delivery. The prescription and provision of psychotropic medication should be monitored as part of the facility's continuous quality improvement program (Metzner, 2009; Ruiz, 2010; Smith & Smith, 2006). Quality indicators for medication services based on the content reviewed in this chapter are summarized in Table 30.4.

Table 30.4 Quality improvement indicators

Psychotropic medications per inmate per month
Cost of psychotropic medication per inmate per month
Number of prescriptions for high cost and/or high risk medications
Medication errors and adverse events
Number and types of non-formulary requests
Turnaround time for review of non-formulary requests
Number of inmates in general population receiving medications three or four times a day
Turnaround time from prescription to first dose
Incidence of missing medications
Patient knowledge of what medication they are taking and why
Patient satisfaction with medication treatment

References

American Correctional Association (2002). *Performance-based standards for correctional health care in adult correctional institutions.* Alexandria, VA: American Correctional Association.

Anno, B. J. (2001). *Correctional health care: Guidelines for the management of an adequate delivery system.* Chicago: National Commission on Correctional Health Care.

Appelbaum, K. L. (2010). The mental health professional in a correctional culture. In C. L. Scott (Ed.), *Handbook of correctional mental health* (2nd ed., pp. 91–118). Washington, DC: American Psychiatric Press.

Baillargeon, J., Hoge, S. K., & Penn, J. V. (2010). Addressing the challenge of community reentry among released inmates with serious mental illness. *American Journal of Community Psychology, 46,* 361–375.

Bressington, D., Gray, R., Lathlean, J., & Mills, A. (2008). Antipsychotic medication in prisons: satisfaction and adherence to treatment. *Mental Health Practice, 11*(10), 18–21.

Brown, M. T., & Bussell, J. K. (2011). Medication adherence: WHO cares? *Mayo Clinic Proceedings, 86*(4), 304–314.

Burns, K. A. (2010). Pharmacotherapy in correctional settings. In C. L. Scott (Ed.), *Handbook of correctional mental health* (2nd ed., pp. 321–344). Washington, DC: American Psychiatric Press.

Burrow, G. F., Knox, C.M., & Villanueva, H. (2006). Nursing in the primary care setting. In M. Puisis (Ed.), *Clinical practice in correctional medicine* (2nd ed., pp. 426–459). Philadelphia: Elsevier Inc.

Chong, W. W., Aslani, P., & Chen, T. F. (2011). Effectiveness of interventions to improve antidepressant medication adherence: a systematic review. *International Journal of Clinical Practice, 65*(9), 954–975.

Cohen, F. (2008). *The mentally disordered offender and the law* (2nd ed.). Kingston, NJ: Civic Research Institute.

Dlugacz, H. A., & Roskes, E. (2010). Clinically oriented reentry planning. In C. L. Scott (ed.), *Handbook of correctional mental health* (2nd ed., pp. 395–431). Washington, DC: American Psychiatric Publishing, Inc.

Ehret, M. J., Shelton, D., Barta, W., Trestman, R., Maruca, A., Kamath, J., & Golay, L. (2013). Medication adherence among female inmates with bipolar disorder: results from a randomized controlled trail. *Psychological Services, 10*(1), 106–114.

Gray, R., Bressington, D., Lathlean, J., & Mills, A. (2008). Relationship between adherence, symptoms, treatment attitudes, satisfaction, and side effects in prisoners taking antipsychotic medication. *Journal of Forensic Psychiatry and Psychology, 19*(3), 335–351.

Harmon, R. E. (2013) Mental health. In L. Schoenly & C. M. Knox (Eds.), *Essentials of correctional nursing* (pp. 221–245). New York: Springer Publishing Company LLC.

Haynes, R. B., Ackloo, E., Sahota, N., McDonald, H. P., & Yao, X. (2008). Interventions for enhancing medication adherence. *Cochrane Database of Systematic Reviews,* issue 2.

Hills, H., Siegfried, C., & Ickowitz, A. (2004). *Effective prison mental health services: Guidelines to expand and improve treatment.* Washington, DC: US Department of Justice, National Institute of Corrections.

Institute of Medicine (2006). *Preventing medication errors: Report brief.* Washington, DC: Institute of Medicine. Retrieved from http://www.iom.edu/~/media/Files/Report%20Files/2006/Preventing-Medication-Errors-Quality-Chasm-Series/medicationerrorsnew.pdf

Julius, R. J., Novitsky, M. A., & Dubin, W. R. (2009). Medication adherence: A review of the literature and implications for clinical practice. *Journal of Psychiatric Practice, 15*(1), 34–44.

Lee, C., Connolly, P. M., & Dietz, E. O. (2005). Forensic nurses views regarding medications for inmates. *Journal of Psychosocial Nursing and Mental Health, 43*(6), 32–39.

Metzner, J. L. (2009). Monitoring a correctional mental health care system: The role of the mental health expert. *Behavioral Sciences and the Law, 27,* 727–741.

Mills, A., Lathlean, J., Forrester, A., Van Veenhuyzen, W., & Gray, R. (2011). Prisoners' experiences of antipsychotic medication: influences on adherence. *Journal of Forensic Psychiatry and Psychology, 22*(1), 110–125.

National Commission on Correctional Health Care (2014a). *Standards for health services in jails.* Chicago: National Commission on Correctional Health Care.

National Commission on Correctional Health Care (2014b). *Standards for health services in prisons.* Chicago: National Commission on Correctional Health Care.

Osterberg, L., & Blaschke, T. (2005). Adherence to medication. *New England Journal of Medicine, 353*(5), 487–497.

Ruiz, A. (2010). Continuous quality improvement and documentation. In C. L. Scott (Ed.), *Handbook of correctional mental health* (2nd ed., pp. 149–166). Washington, DC: American Psychiatric Publishing, Inc.

Schwartz-Watts, D. M., & Frierson, R. L. (2006). Crisis stabilization in correctional settings. In M. Puisis (Ed.), *Clinical practice in correctional medicine* (2nd ed., pp. 306–316). Philadelphia: Elsevier Inc.

Shelton, D., Ehret, M. J., Wakai, S., Kapetanovic, T., & Moran, M. (2010). Psychotropic medication adherence in correctional facilities: A review of the literature. *Journal of Psychiatric and Mental Health Nursing, 17,* 603–613.

Smith, H., & Smith, L. D. (2006). Correctional-based mental health services: Designing a system that works. In M. Puisis (Ed.), *Clinical practice in correctional medicine* (2nd ed., pp. 292–305). Philadelphia: Elsevier Inc.

Velligan, D. I., Weiden, P. J., Sajatovic, M., Scott, J., Carpenter, D., Ross, R., & Docherty, J. P. (2009). The expert consensus guideline series: adherence problems in patients with serious and persistent mental illness. *Journal of Clinical Psychiatry, 70*(suppl 4), 1–48.

Velligan, D. I., Weiden, P. J., Sajatovic, M., Scott, J., Carpenter, D., Ross, R., & Docherty, J. P. (2010a). Assessment of adherence problems in patients with serious and persistent mental illness: Recommendations from the Expert Consensus Guidelines. *Journal of Psychiatric Practice, 16*(1), 34–45.

Velligan, D. I., Weiden, P. J., Sajatovic, M., Scott, J., Carpenter, D., Ross, R., & Docherty, J. P. (2010b). Strategies for addressing adherence problems in patients with serious and persistent mental illness: Recommendations from the Expert Consensus Guidelines. *Journal of Psychiatric Practice, 16*(5), 306–324.

Wilper, A. P., Woolhandler, S., Boyd, J. W., Lasser, K. E., McCormick, D., Bor, D. H., & Himmelstein, D. U. (2009). The health and health care of US prisoners: A nationwide survey. *American Journal of Public Health, 99*(4), 666–672.

CHAPTER 31

Prescribed medication abuse
Limitless creativity

Anthony C. Tamburello

Introduction

Substance use disorders are common among inmates and are not reliably interrupted by a period of incarceration. Controlled medicines, such as opiates and benzodiazepines, by definition carry risk for abuse and dependence. Even if not classified as controlled by the US Drug Enforcement Agency (DEA), other prescribed medications may also be misused or abused by inmates. For the purpose of this chapter, the word "abuse" is used to describe the taking of medication for reasons unintended by the prescriber (including recreational use), either without a prescription or by not following instructions in terms of dosing, timing, or route of administration.

Although preferred by those with a substance use disorder, illegal drugs are difficult to obtain in a correctional facility. When purchased from peers or staff, their cost in correctional facilities (reflecting the time, effort, and risks associated with this criminal activity) is often prohibitively expensive. By comparison, prescription medications are either stocked on site within the jail or prison or easily obtained by the correctional health care system from community pharmacies. When prescribed, inmates receive them at little or no cost and can expect them to be dispensed in a reliable and timely manner. Even if caught using such medication inappropriately, the risk to the inmate of legal consequences, beyond institutional sanctions, is remote.

While prescription medications are sometimes used to achieve a "high," they may also be sought to ease discomforts commonly experienced in a jail or prison (e.g., insomnia, subclinical anxiety, or simply boredom). Some may seek stimulating medications to counteract the effects of prescribed sedatives to allow them to be "on point" (i.e., ready to respond to real or perceived dangers in the facility). Stimulants may also be sought to manage real or perceived symptoms of attention-deficit/hyperactivity disorder. Institutional policies and the practice of individual prescribers may make it difficult to acquire medicines for these reasons through legitimate channels. Thus, inmates may feign or exaggerate mood, anxiety, psychotic, or somatic symptoms with the goal of being prescribed medications with the desired effects.

More insidious is the diversion of prescribed medications to a third party. Many prescribed medicines have a "street value" in correctional settings. They may be sold or bartered for items of interest. A patient with a legitimate need for medication, who may already have poor illness insight, may be enticed or coerced into transferring his or her medication to a peer. This creates several dangerous problems. The source inmate may worsen or fail to improve, which may lead to dose escalation, an incorrect conclusion about a treatment failure, poor functioning, and behavioral sequelae, including disruptive or violent conduct. Meanwhile, the recipient is exposed to medication risks without the benefits of informed consent or medical supervision.

Community trends

The abuse of prescription medications is increasing in the community (Substance Abuse and Mental Health Services Administration, 2011). Emergency room visits for toxicity from nonsuicidal "nonmedical use of pharmaceuticals" rose 132 percent between 2004 and 2011. Excluding controlled drugs, the top prescription medications implicated in the need for emergency care were antidepressants (7.1 percent), antipsychotics (5.0 percent), and anticonvulsants (3.6 percent). Both prudence and clinical experience suggest that abuse of medications traditionally thought to have a low abuse potential is just as (or even more) likely to occur among inmates. Therefore, when available, data from the community on the abuse of medications may be presented in this chapter.

Methods of abuse of prescribed medications

The inmate who intends to abuse or divert medicine must obtain it without arousing suspicion from staff, move it to an unmonitored area, alter it if desired, then either transfer it to a third party or store it for later use. Almost universally, psychiatric medications are administered by directly observed therapy. Commonly, this occurs in a medication line. Here, the inmate must give the impression of having taken the medication while not actually ingesting it. Common methods for this include "cheeking," where the medication is placed into the mouth but not swallowed, and "palming," where the medicine is kept in the hand without putting it into the mouth. The powder from crushed tablets may be recovered by patients who hold it in the mouth between the jaw and an area of dried mucosa.

When staff are no longer directly observing the individual, he or she may expectorate or vomit the pill and (optionally) wash it. The inmate may then crush the tablet using available hard objects and surfaces in preparation for intranasal (or intravenous) use, if desired. If a larger dose is required to achieve an anticipated effect, the product is accumulated and hidden to avoid detection.

Specific medications of abuse in a prison setting
Antipsychotics

Quetiapine, a second-generation antipsychotic well known for its sedative and anxiolytic properties, has achieved notoriety as a medication abused in prison. Some have observed the practice of prescribing low-dose quetiapine to manage insomnia in prison (Reeves, 2012). Quetiapine is known colloquially as "quell," "Suzie Q," "Q," "squirrel," or "baby heroin" (Del Paggio, 2005; Waters & Joshi, 2007; Wen, 2009) and has been cited in rap lyrics that describe its use for recreational purposes. Case reports in the community have been published documenting evidence for the misuse and abuse of quetiapine, including feigning or exaggerating serious psychiatric symptoms, preference for quetiapine versus an effective alternative agent, withdrawal and use to mitigate the symptoms of withdrawal from other substances, tolerance, self-dosing, combining it with illicit substances to achieve a hallucinatory effect, obtaining it from multiple sources, and theft and selling (Erdoğan, 2010). Some of the earliest case reports of quetiapine abuse involved prisoners, including descriptions of intranasal (Pierre, Shnayder, Wirshing, & Wirshing, 2004), smoked (Royal College of General Practitioners [RCGP], 2011), and intravenous (Hussain, Waheed, & Hussain, 2005) consumption.

These concerns have led to the removal of quetiapine from medication formularies in various correctional settings (Del Paggio, 2005). When quetiapine was removed from the medication formulary of the New Jersey Department of Corrections (DOC), nearly 45 percent of inmates whose quetiapine was stopped (n = 161) did not require an alternative antipsychotic medication at a six-month follow-up (Tamburello, Lieberman, Baum, & Reeves, 2012).

Community case reports exist on the abuse of olanzapine for relaxing or euphoric effects (Kumsar & Erol, 2013). One patient admitted to combining olanzapine with alcohol or benzodiazepines for an improved effect. Second-hand information in that report indicated that olanzapine was a "popular drug at parties," with an informal name of "Zy," and could be used intravenously by dissolving an oral-disintegrating tablet in water and then injecting it (Reeves, 2007). In addition to quetiapine, olanzapine was the only other antipsychotic that was "repeatedly named" as a psychotropic medication of abuse by providers within the Santa Rita Jail (Del Paggio, 2005).

A South Dakota DOC study on institutional disciplinary reports found evidence for the abuse of risperidone by inmates (Harlow & Davidson, 2010). To date, there are no published case reports of the abuse of other antipsychotic medications; however, expert opinion cautions about the risk of abuse and diversion of lower-potency antipsychotics such as chlorpromazine (Gunter & Antoniak, 2010).

Antidepressants

The abuse of tricyclic antidepressants (TCAs) in the community has been well reported. Of 346 persons enrolled in a methadone program, 86 admitted to using amitriptyline for euphoric effects (Cohen et al., 1978). In a case series that informally reviewed 15 years of community hospital records, 14 cases of TCA abuse were identified. All of these were prescribed tertiary TCAs (e.g., amitriptyline, doxepin, and/or imipramine). Patients reported a sedative or euphoric effect from these medicines. All but one patient had a preexisting substance disorder diagnosis and only one had a current diagnosis of major depressive disorder. Four admitted to obtaining the TCA from a community drug dealer (Shenouda & Desan, 2013).

TCAs are also prescribed by general medical practitioners for indications such as neuropathic pain. Most TCAs are inexpensive and, thus, may escape the attention of pharmacy and therapeutics committees (P&TCs). The likelihood of QT prolongation is considered higher with tertiary TCAs than with secondary TCAs (Goodnick, Jerry, & Parra, 2002). The greater anticholinergic and antihistaminergic properties of tertiary TCAs may explain both their greater toxicity and their greater incidence of abuse.

Bupropion has known stimulant properties that are similar to, although milder than, methylphenidate, likely related to its inhibition of the reuptake of norepinephrine and dopamine (Chevassus et al., 2013). The abuse of bupropion in both the community and correctional systems has been described. Published case reports of such abuse in the community were, in most cases, prompted by serious complications, including seizures. A euphoric effect is more easily obtained when bupropion is crushed and then insufflated (snorted) or smoked, which are routes of administration that bypass first-pass metabolism (Reeves & Ladner, 2013).

Colloquial terms for bupropion in correctional settings include "wellies," "dubs," and "'Barnies." Bupropion was the most frequently cited prescription drug of abuse in disciplinary charges in the South Dakota DOC (Harlow & Davidson, 2010). When removed from the correctional formulary for the Texas correctional system, prescriptions for bupropion diminished from 1,966 to less than 100 from 2005 to 2013. The clinical effects of this formulary change are unknown (Hilliard, Barloon, Farley, Penn, & Koranek, 2013).

Other antidepressants cited in disciplinary reports in the South Dakota DOC were venlafaxine, fluoxetine, mirtazapine, trazodone, and citalopram (Harlow & Davidson, 2010). Referred to as "red dragon" by some inmates, venlafaxine inhibits the reuptake of norepinephrine and serotonin and weakly inhibits the reuptake of dopamine. In community case reports, an "amphetamine-like" high was achieved by patients who took venlafaxine (Quaglio, Schifano, & Lugoboni, 2008; Sattar, Grant, & Bhatia, 2003). Higher doses, crushed tablets, and immediate-release forms of venlafaxine are purportedly more euphorogenic. Community case reports of misuse and abuse of fluoxetine began to appear in the literature in 1987 when a woman with anorexia nervosa reported using high doses as an appetite suppressant (Wilcox, 1987). Since then, other reports indicate its recreational use and potential for dependence, apparently driven by the experience of euphoria from higher doses (Taïeb, Larroche, Dutray, Baubet, & Moro, 2004). While no case reports to date have emerged regarding the recreational use of mirtazapine or trazodone, their sedating properties suggest their potential for abuse in correctional systems. The RCGP Guidance for Clinicians on Safer Prescribing in Prisons warns that for citalopram, "euphoria is a recognized side effect," although [it is] "less alerting than fluoxetine" (RCGP, 2011).

Tranylcypromine, a monoamine oxidase inhibitor with a chemical structure similar to that of D-amphetamine, has been cited in numerous community case reports as being abused by patients for its stimulant effects (Haddad, 1999). The prescription of tranylcypromine is rare, especially in correctional settings, where the required tyramine-free diet may be difficult to enforce.

Antiepileptic drugs

Antiepileptic drugs (AEDs) may be prescribed by either psychiatrists or general medical providers for epilepsy, neuropathic pain, and bipolar disorder or off-label for various indications. Although case reports on AED abuse are variable, their sedating properties confer a risk for abuse within the prison system (RCGP, 2011).

Numerous community case reports exist regarding the abuse of and even dependence on gabapentin (Kruszewski, Paczynski & Kahn, 2009; Pittenger & Desan, 2007; Victorri-Vigneau et al., 2007). In a Florida DOC intake facility, only 19 of 96 bottles of gabapentin remained with the inmate to whom it had been prescribed. Five inmates admitted to abusing gabapentin, reporting a feeling of euphoria from it (Recoppa et al., 2004). Some inmates informally refer to gabapentin tablets as "Johnnies" (Ourada, 2013). The abuse of gabapentin has been linked in a curious manner to the abuse of bupropion in correctional settings (Del Paggio, 2005). "Preclinical data" support the use of gabapentin as a topical anesthetic (Prommer, 2008), and anecdotal reports exist about prisoners using its powder to numb nasal passages in order to prevent nasal irritation from the insufflation of bupropion (E. Hamel, personal communication, October 30, 2013).

In two community case reports, patients achieved a euphoric effect from combining carbamazepine with alcohol, a practice reportedly learned from the "street drug scene" in Austria and Germany (Sullivan & Davis, 1997). In another report, a patient obtained the same effect from carbamazepine alone (Stupaeck, Whitworth, & Fleischhacker, 1993).

While similar pharmacologically to gabapentin, pregabalin is classified as schedule V by the DEA. Despite that classification, community case reports of pregabalin abuse are readily found (Grosshans et al., 2013; Skopp & Zimmer, 2012). In a study of opiate-dependent individuals in Germany, 12.1 percent (n = 124) has a urine test positive for pregabalin, despite none of these patients having been prescribed it (Grosshans et al., 2013). The cost of pregabalin limits its present availability for abuse in a correctional environment.

Anticholinergics

Case reports of the abuse of anticholinergic/antiparkinsonian medications, including in patients with and without a mental illness, abound in the literature (Dilsaver, 1988; Land, Pinsky, & Salzman, 1991). Purported effects include euphoria, hallucinations, mood elevation, and relaxation. According to the RCGP Guidelines for Safer Prescribing in Prisons (2011), "Misusers report that anticholinergic antihistamines are used to boost opiate highs." Some persons show evidence of tolerance to desired effects. Withdrawal symptoms of dysphoria and anxiety have been observed with abrupt discontinuation of anticholinergic medicines (Dilsaver, 1988).

A psychiatrist wrote that at San Quentin Prison in 1963, trihexyphenidyl "was widely enjoyed by the inmates as a drug of abuse." According to a patient there, "If I take five Artanes, I can see my mother. If I take 10 Artanes, I can see my girlfriend" (Lowry, 1977). Psychiatrists in a Louisiana prison learned that inmates were crushing trihexyphenidyl tablets, mixing them with tobacco, and smoking them for a euphoric effect. They were using these tablets as currency with which to gamble (Rouchell & Dixon, 1977). In another report, both inmates with and without mental illness housed in a maximum-security prison hospital admitted to abusing trihexyphenidyl, adding that drinking large amounts of coffee augmented the "high" from it. Some who took trihexyphenidyl recreationally said that they needed antipsychotic medication to prevent them from "going psychotic" (Weinstock, 1978). Two individuals in the community reported preferring to use trihexyphenidyl (which they obtained on the streets) intravenously (Rubinstein, 1978).

In a community treatment center in Australia, of 22 patients suspected of abusing anticholinergic medications (including trihexyphenidyl, benztropine, and orphenadrine), 17 admitted to using it not as prescribed in the prior month. The most frequent explanations were using it "to get high" or "to increase pleasure." The authors suggested that "peer pressure" in their system played a role in the "culture" of anticholinergic medication abuse (Buhrich, Weller, & Kevans, 2000).

Although its antihistaminergic properties have been speculated to counteract potentially reinforcing anticholinergic effects (Dilsaver, 1988), diphenhydramine abuse and dependence has been described in the community (Roberts, Gruer, & Gilhooly, 1999; Thomas, Nallur, Jones, & Deslandes, 2009).

Promethazine is an antiemetic with antihistaminic, anticholinergic, and weak antidopaminergic properties. In patients in a methadone clinic in San Francisco, 26 percent (n = 334) had a urine test positive for promethazine, with only 13 percent of these having a valid prescription for it (Shapiro et al., 2013). While promethazine is purported to augment an opiate high, its value in correctional settings may also be related to its sedating properties. Some inmates refer to promethazine tablets as "Finnigans" (Ourada, 2013).

Others—antihypertensives, muscle relaxants, and cold preparations

In a study of 90 nonhypertensive women in a methadone clinic, one third either admitted to abusing clonidine or had a positive urine test for it (Anderson et al., 1997). In a survey of 1,320 current or former intravenous drug users in Baltimore, 11 percent admitted to the "nonmedical" use of clonidine (Khosla, Juon, Kirk, Astemborski, & Mehta, 2011). Users report desired effects including anxiolysis, sedation, and augmentation of the effects of other drugs (Anderson, Paluzzi, Lee, Huggins, & Svikis, 1997; Lauzon, 1992; Schaut & Schnoll, 1983; Schindler, Tirado-Morales, & Kushon, 2013). Some inmates informally refer to clonidine tablets as "Deans" (Ourada, 2013).

The abuse of muscle relaxants has been reported in the community, particularly those with more sedating properties, including baclofen (May, 1983; McDonald, Festa, & Wilkins, 2001; Perry, Wright, Shannon, & Woolf, 1998; Weißhaar et al., 2012) and cyclobenzaprine (Harden & Argoff, 2000). Baclofen overdose has been associated with serious morbidity and mortality, including coma and nonconvulsive status epilepticus (Weißhaar et al., 2012). Reports of abuse of and dependence on carisoprodol were considerable enough for the DEA to reclassify it from noncontrolled to a schedule IV controlled substance in 2011 (Department of Justice, 2011).

Prison physicians in Poland discovered six inmates who were caught (or admitted to) inhaling xylometazoline nasal drops by heating them on a metal surface and inhaling the vapor. These individuals reported stimulant effects from this compound, which they obtained by malingering symptoms of rhinitis, sinusitis, or allergic reactions (Anand, Salamon, Habrat, Scinska, & Bienkowski, 2008). Xylometazoline is an alpha-adrenergic decongestant not available in the United States. Whether this feat may be accomplished with similar and more readily available nasal decongestants (e.g., phenylephrine, oxymetazoline, or midodrine) is unknown.

Methods to counter and manage abuse or diversion of prescribed medications

Concerns about the abuse or diversion of medications should never prevent the treatment of legitimate medical and mental illnesses. A measured approach to this problem, balancing clinical acumen and environmental sensitivity, is both necessary and appropriate when prescribing in a jail or prison.

Inappropriate prescribing is best avoided by accurate diagnosis. Avoid making reflexive decisions solely based on symptom reporting. Place greater weight on objective signs of illness or dysfunction and collateral information (e.g., staff observations, outside records). Awareness of and sensitivity to an inmate patient's history of substance disorders is important, as prescribed medications may be sought as a substitute for the drug of choice. If the diagnosis is unclear and the situation is nonemergent, consider delaying pharmaceutical intervention to allow time for further observations and data collection. Consider using clinician-rated symptom scales, referral to a mental health tier, or referral for psychological testing to aid in diagnostic clarification.

Consider evidence-based psychotherapies as first-line treatment for primary insomnia, uncomplicated adjustment disorders, and mild depression or anxiety symptoms. When pharmacotherapy is required, certain prescribing strategies may reduce, although not eliminate, the risk for abuse or diversion. Whenever appropriate, avoid medications known to present a higher risk for such in a correctional setting. Do not prescribe medication without an indication, avoid prescribing off-label, and avoid prescribing sedating medications on a PRN basis. Prescribe the lowest effective dose. If a patient requires repeated dose escalation, carefully reevaluate the diagnosis and treatment. It is appropriate to include treatment of substance disorders in inmate patients' treatment plans; this may reduce the demand for diverted medications (Gunter & Antoniak, 2010).

Although highly motivated inmates may defeat these strategies, prescribing medication in liquid form or crushing tablets and "floating" them in water will increase the difficulty of diverting medications and should reduce the demand. Although consultation with a pharmacist is advisable, most pills (with extended-release formulations being notable exceptions) can be dispensed in crushed form. If available, serum levels may show evidence of noncompliance or partial compliance. Screening of the urine or blood is of limited value for the detection of unauthorized use of noncontrolled prescription medication, although testing for a specific substance may be appropriate on a case-by-case basis. For patients who require antipsychotic medication, a long-acting injectable virtually eliminates the risk of covert nonadherence. Anticholinergic medication is not always required for the prophylaxis of extrapyramidal symptoms, even for those prescribed first-generation agents (World Health Organization, 2012). If prescribed as a precaution for a patient on antipsychotic medication, consider a taper of anticholinergic medication to establish its necessity.

Systematic approaches to this problem include staff training, medication administration policy, and formulary controls. Anyone responsible for administering or monitoring medication (including nursing and custody staff) should receive training on the detection of cheeking and similar techniques. Physicians and physician extenders, regardless of discipline, should receive orientation and ongoing in-service training on this issue. Controlled medications and those with psychotropic properties are best administered as directly observed therapy. If institutional policy requires that a medication be dispensed as keep-on-person, the smallest practicable quantity should be allowed. As medical or mental health providers may prescribe higher-risk medications, interdisciplinary collaboration and communication are important. P&TCs should preferentially include medications with lower risk for abuse and diversion in the formulary and should promulgate guidelines to limit requests for higher-risk medicines to carefully selected cases.

Summary

The landscape of prescription medication abuse is likely to change with new medications, the increased availability of established medications (as may follow a patent expiration), and creative developments by inmates in terms of methods of abuse and experimentation with endless potential combinations of licit and illicit substances. Prescribers must therefore have an "ear to the ground" and make reports on developments in this regard. P&TCs should solicit and respond to information regarding emerging trends in prescription medication abuse and diversion.

References

Anand, J. S., Salamon, M., Habrat, B., Scinska, A., & Bienkowski, P. (2008). Misuse of xylometazoline nasal drops by inhalation. *Substance Use and Misuse, 43,* 2163–2168.

Anderson, F., Paluzzi, P., Lee, J., Huggins, G., & Svikis, D. (1997). Illicit use of clonidine in opiate-abusing pregnant women. *Obstetrics and Gynecology, 90*(5), 790–794.

Buhrich, N., Weller, A., & Kevans, P. (2000). Misuse of anticholinergic drugs by people with serious mental illness. *Psychiatric Services, 51*(7), 928–929.

Chevassus, H., Farret, A., Gagnol, J. P., et al. (2013). Psychological and physiological effects of bupropion compared to methylphenidate after prolonged administration in healthy volunteers. *European Journal of Clinical Pharmacology, 69*(4), 779–787.

Cohen, M. J. (1978). Abuse of amitriptyline. *Journal of the American Medical Association, 240*(13), 1372–1373.

Del Paggio, D. (2005). Psychotropic medication abuse in correctional facilities. *Bay Area Psychopharmacology Newsletter, 8,* 1–6.

Dilsaver, S. C. (1988). Antimuscarinic agents as substances of abuse: A review. *Journal of Clinical Psychopharamacology, 8*(1), 14–22.

Department of Justice, Drug Enforcement Administration (2011). Schedules of controlled substances: Placement of carisoprodol into schedule IV. *Federal Register, 76*(238), 77330–77360.

Erdoğan, S. (2010). Quetiapine in substance use disorders, abuse and dependence possibility: A review. *Turk Psikiyatri Derg, 21*(2), 167–175.

Goodnick, P. J., Jerry, J., & Parra, F. (2002). Psychotropic drugs and the ECG: Focus on the QTc interval. *Expert Opinion on Pharmacotherapy*, 3(5), 479–498.

Grosshans, M., Lemenager, T., Vollmert, C., et al. (2013). Pregabalin abuse among opiate addicted patients. *European Journal of Clinical Pharmacology* [published online August 30, 2013].

Gunter, T. D., & Antoniak, S. K. (2010). Evaluation and treating substance use disorders. In C.L. Scott (ed.), *Handbook of correctional mental health* (2nd ed., p. 170). Washington, DC: American Psychiatric Publishing, Inc.

Haddad, P. (1999). Do antidepressants have any potential to cause addiction? *Journal of Psychopharmacology*, 13(3), 300–307.

Harden, R. N., & Argoff, C. (2000). A review of three community prescribed skeletal muscle relaxants. *Journal of Back and Musculoskeletal Rehabilitation*, 15, 63–66.

Harlow, M. C., & Davidson, C. M. (2010). Suzy Q, Barney, and the Red Dragon: A tale of correctional addiction. Poster presentation at the American Academy of Psychiatry and the Law, 2010 Annual Meeting.

Hilliard, W. T., Barloon, L., Farley, P., Penn, J. V., & Koranek, A. (2013). Bupropion diversion and misuse in the correctional facility. *Journal of Correctional Health Care*, 19, 211–217.

Hussain, M. Z., Waheed, W., & Hussain, S. (2005). Intravenous quetiapine abuse. *American Journal of Psychiatry*, 9, 1755–1756.

Khosla, N., Juon, H. S., Kirk, G. D., Astemborski, J., & Mehta, S. H. (2011). Correlates of non-medical prescription drug use among a cohort of injection drug users in Baltimore City. *Addictive Behaviors*, 36, 1282–1287.

Kruszewski, S. P., Paczynski, R. P., & Kahn, D. A. (2009). Gabapentin-induced delirium and dependence. *Journal of Psychiatric Practice*, 15(4), 314–319.

Kumsar, N. A., & Erol, A. (2013). Olanzapine abuse. *Journal of Substance Abuse*, 34, 73–74.

Land, W., Pinsky, D., & Salzman, C. (1991). Abuse and misuse of anticholinergic medications. *Hospital and Community Psychiatry*, 42(6), 580–581.

Lauzon, P. (1992). Two cases of clonidine abuse/dependence in methadone-maintained patients. *Journal of Substance Abuse Treatment*, 9, 125–127.

Lowry, T. P. (1977). Trihexyphenidyl abuse. *American Journal of Psychiatry*, 134(11), 1315.

May, C. R. (1983). Baclofen overdose. *Annals of Emergency Medicine*, 12(3), 171–173.

McDonald, N. J., Festa, M. S., & Wilkins, B. (2001). Instructive case: Teenage coma. *Journal of Paediatrics and Child Health*, 37, 395–396.

Ourada, J. (2013). Illicit substance use in correctional facilities. Presented at the 44th Annual Meeting of the American Academy of Psychiatry and the Law, San Diego, October 25 2013.

Perry, H. E., Wright, R. O., Shannon, M. W., & Woolf, A. D. (1998). Baclofen overdose: drug experimentation in a group of adolescents. *Pediatrics*, 101(6), 1045–1048.

Pierre, J. M., Shnayder, I., Wirshing, D. A., & Wirshing, W. C. (2004). Intranasal quetiapine abuse. *American Journal of Psychiatry*, 9, 1718.

Pittenger, C., & Desan, P. H. (2007). Gabapentin abuse, and delirium tremens upon gabapentin withdrawal. *Journal of Clinical Psychiatry*, 68(3), 483–484.

Prommer, E. E. (2008). Topical analgesic combinations for bortezomib neuropathy. *Journal of Pain Symptom Management*, 37(3), e3–5.

Quaglio, G., Schifano, F., & Lugoboni, F. (2008). Venlafaxine dependence in a patient with a history of alcohol and amineptine misuse. *Addiction*, 103, 1572–1574.

Recoppa, L., Malcolm, R., & Ware, M. (2004). Gabapentin abuse in inmates with prior history of cocaine dependence. *American Journal on Addictions*, 13, 321–323.

Reeves, R. (2012). Guideline, education and peer comparison to reduce prescriptions of benzodiazepines and low-dose quetiapine in prison. *Journal of Correctional Health Care*, 18(1), 45–52.

Reeves, R. R. (2007). Abuse of olanzapine by substance abusers. *Journal of Psychoactive Drugs*, 39(3), 297–299.

Reeves, R. R., & Ladner M. E. (2013). Additional evidence of the abuse potential of bupropion. *Journal of Clinical Psychopharmacology*, 33(4), 584–585.

Roberts, K., Gruer, L., & Gilhooly, T. (1999). Misuse of diphenhydramine soft gel capsules (Sleepia): A cautionary tale from Glasgow. *Addiction*, 94(10), 1575–1578.

Rouchell, A. M., & Dixon, S. P. (1977). Trihexyphenidyl abuse. *American Journal of Psychiatry*, 134(11), 1315.

Royal College of General Practitioners (2011). *Safer prescribing in prisons*. Retrieved from http://www.rcgp.org.uk/news/2011/november/~/media/Files/News/Safer_Prescribing_in_Prison.ashx/

Rubinstein, J. S. (1978). Abuse of antiparkinsonism drugs: feigning of extrapyramidal symptoms to obtain trihexyphenidy. *Journal of the American Medical Association*, 240, 2365–2366.

Sattar, S. P., Grant, K. M., & Bhatia, S. C. (2003). A case of venlafaxine abuse. *New England Journal of Medicine*, 348(8), 764–765.

Schaut, J., & Schnoll, S. H. (1983). Four cases of clonidine abuse. *American Journal of Psychiatry*, 140(12), 1625–1626.

Schindler, E. A. D., Tirado-Morales, D. J., & Kushon, D. (2013). Clonidine abuse in a methadone-maintained clonazepam-abusing patient. *Journal of Addiction Medicine*, 7(3), 218–219.

Shapiro, B. J., Lynch, K. L., Toochinda, T., Lutnick, A., Cheng, H. Y., & Kral, A. H. (2013). Promethazine misuse among methadone maintenance patients and community-based injection drug users. *Journal of Addiction Medicine*, 7, 96–101.

Shenouda, R., & Desan, P. H. (2013). Abuse of tricyclic antidepressant drugs: a case series. *Journal of Clinical Psychopharmacology*, 33(3), 440–442.

Skopp, G., & Zimmer, G. (2011). [Pregabalin—a drug with abuse potential?]. *Archiv fur Kriminologie*, 229(1–2), 44–54.

Stuppaeck, C. H., Whitworth, A. B., & Fleischhacker, W. W. (1993). Abuse potential of carbamazepine. *Journal of Nervous and Mental Disease*, 181(8), 519–520.

Sullivan, G., & Davis, S. (1997). Is carbamazepine a potential drug of abuse? *Journal of Psychopharmacology*, 11(1), 93–94.

Substance Abuse and Mental Health Services Administration, Drug Abuse Warning Network (2011). *National estimates of drug-related emergency department visits*. HHS Publication No. (SMA) 13-4760, DAWN Series D-39. Rockville, MD: Substance Abuse and Mental Health Services Administration.

Taïeb, O., Larroche, C., Dutray, B., Baubet, T., & Moro, M. R. (2004). Fluoxetine dependence in a former amineptine abuser. *American Journal of Addictions*, 13(5), 498–500.

Tamburello, A. C., Lieberman, J. A., Baum, R., & Reeves, R. (2012). Successful removal of quetiapine from a correctional formulary. *Journal of American Academy of Psychiatry and the Law*, 40(4), 502–508.

Thomas, A., Nallur, D. G., Jones, N., & Deslandes, P. N. (2009). Diphenhydramine abuse and detoxification: a brief review and case report. *Journal of Psychopharmacology*, 23(1), 101–105.

Victorri-Vigneau, C., Guerlais, M., & Jolliet, P. (2007). Abuse, dependence and withdrawal with gabapentin: a first case report. *Pharmacopsychiatry*, 40, 43–44.

Waters, B. M., & Joshi, K. G. (2007). Intravenous quetiapine-cocaine use ("Q-ball"). *American Journal of Psychiatry*, 164(1), 173–174.

Weißhaar, G. F., Hoemberg, M., Bender, K., et al. (2012). Baclofen intoxication: a 'fun drug' causing deep coma and nonconvulsive status epilepticus—a case report and review of the literature. *European Journal of Pediatrics*, 171(10), 1541–1547.

Weinstock, R. (1978). Interactive effects of trihexyphenidyl and coffee. *American Journal of Psychiatry*, 135(5), 624–625.

Wilcox, J. A. (1987). Abuse of fluoxetine by a patient with anorexia nervosa. *American Journal of Psychiatry*, 144(8), 1100.

Wen, P. (2009). Psychiatric drug sought on streets. *Boston Globe*, July 13, 2009.

World Health Organization (2012). *Role of anticholinergic medications in patients requiring long-term antipsychotic treatment for psychotic disorders*. Retrieved from http://www.who.int/mental_health/mhgap/evidence/resource/psychosis_q6.pdf

SECTION VII

Disorders and syndromes

CHAPTER 32

Diagnostic prevalence and comorbidity

Stuart D. M. Thomas

Introduction

Prisons and jails remain a growth industry, with many countries increasing correctional services to cope with the ever-burgeoning inmate population. One longstanding issue in the literature and popular press across many jurisdictions has been the perceived prevalence of mental disorders in prisons. This chapter outlines the best available evidence pertaining to the correctional prevalence of common mental disorders and considers the key challenges involved in ascertaining the rates of these different diagnoses.

Setting the scene

Studies of the prevalence of mental disorders in prisons and jails have been prevalent in the literature for more than two decades. Early commentators argued that people with mental disorders were, in fact, overrepresented in our criminal justice system because we have been "forced" to criminalize behaviors exhibited by these individuals, largely due to the distinct lack of viable community-based options (e.g., Gunn, Maden, & Swinton, 1991; Teplin, 1984). However, more recent commentators assert that a range of factors, including the social disadvantage that accompanies mental disorders, and not the mental disorders per se lead to imprisonment (e.g., Draine, 2002; Engel & Silver, 2001).

A review of the international literature on diagnostic prevalence reveals considerable heterogeneity, with considerable study-to-study variability. Apart from untangling the reasons behind these apparent discrepancies, it is also necessary to consider with whom or where comparisons are being made to assert that mental disorders are over- or underrepresented. For example, a control/comparison population should ideally be as similar to those (in this case) in the prison setting where mental disorders are being assessed (with respect to age, gender, and similar characteristics) and to those who have been assessed for the presence of mental disorders using the same approach—whether that be screening instrument, assessment, or diagnostic test—to ensure that comparisons are "like with like." Therefore, to make and/or substantiate the claim that mental disorders (and more specifically individual mental illnesses such as schizophrenia, depression, and substance use disorders) are disproportionally represented in prisons, a comparison needs to be made between the estimated rates of these disorders in prison with those in the general community.

Research findings report either point prevalence (i.e., the number of people with the disorders of interest as a proportion of the total number of individuals being considered) or period prevalence, which considers the number of "cases" that are counted/identified over a specified timeframe. Other studies have contrasted "current" rates of mental disorder (cross-sectional at one point in time, in the last month, or over the last 12 months) with lifetime history of mental disorder to not only capture a snapshot of the current psychiatric morbidity but also to consider a broader vulnerability for those not currently symptomatic but potentially requiring a different approach to their rehabilitative and psychosocial needs.

To contextualize the available data on rates of mental disorders in prisons, and noting that there are some differences in prevalence estimates between different countries, overall 12-month prevalence estimates suggest that between 8.4% and 29.1% of people in the community experience mental illness and that between 12.2% and 48.6% of people experience mental illness across their lifetimes. The most commonly diagnosed disorders, affecting more than one third of people across their lifespan, are anxiety disorders, mood disorders, and substance use disorders. Lifetime comorbid disorders are also common, varying from 26.7% (in Mexico) to 56.3% (in the United States; World Health Organization International Consortium in Psychiatric Epidemiology, 2000).

How common are mental disorders in prisons?

While there have been a number of very persuasive commentaries documenting the rise of mental disorders in prisons (e.g., Torrey, Kennard, Eslinger, et al., 2010), a very poignant observation, made more than 30 years ago, still has considerable contemporary significance. It stated that prisons have been left to deal with inmates whose behavior, while being "marked enough to interfere with discipline and communication," was not sufficient to satisfy admission criteria to psychiatric services (Walker & McCabe, 1973). This powerful statement has been supported more recently in a review of mental health care in prisons, which stated that actually only a minority of prisoners experienced mental disorders of sufficient severity and longevity to require detention under the relevant mental health legislation and that, in fact, the majority of those in prison actually have common mental health problems, albeit commonly complicated by substance use problems (Senior & Shaw, 2008, p. 175). The question therefore becomes one of service provision and the degree to which prisons can cater to the needs of those with different mental disorders. While it is clear that prisoners should have access to the same quality and range of mental health services as they would be able to access in the community (Reed, 2003) and that prisons have a legal obligation to provide this (Steadman, Scott, Osher, et al., 2005), recent research has found that prisoners present with significant ongoing needs across a wide range of domains (Thomas, McCrone, & Fahy, 2008). Many prisoners also present with symptoms that are best treated in mental health settings (Earthrowl, O'Grady, & Birmingham, 2003; Torrey et al., 2010).

One additional consideration in interpreting the literature is that studies operationalize and/or report their prevalence estimates according to idiosyncratic, practical, or financial reasons, which leads to the inclusion and/or exclusion of various mental disorders. This, in turn, has an impact on prevalence estimates and helps explain the variability reported across studies. So, for example, a recent French study reported that in excess of one in four male prisoners had a clinically significant mental disorder at the time they were interviewed (Falissard et al., 2006). While this point-prevalence study included alcohol and drug dependence disorders, it excluded substance use disorders and personality disorders, arguably missing substantial psychiatric morbidity. A US study that compared the gender-based prevalence of current major depressive, bipolar, and psychotic disorders noted that female prisoners had double the prevalence of male prisoners (31% versus 14.5%, respectively; Steadman, Osher, Clark Robbins, et al., 2009). An Australian study that included male and female prisoners noted that 43% of their sample screened positive for psychotic, anxiety, or affective disorders in the last 12 months (Butler, Allnutt, Cain, et al., 2005). Of note, reception (unsentenced) prisoners recorded higher rates than sentenced prisoners, and females had substantially higher psychiatric morbidity overall than males (61% versus 39%). An additional national study published the following year reported that four of five reception prisoners met diagnostic criteria for at least one psychiatric disorder in the previous year (including anxiety, affective, substance abuse, and personality disorders; Butler et al., 2006); this rate was substantially higher than that in the community. The higher rates of psychiatric morbidity among female prisoners have been supported in findings from a US study that considered mental health problems generally (James & Glaze, 2006), as well as a more nuanced study that reported that 69.7% of prisoners surveyed met criteria for a lifetime mental disorder (77% females versus 69.4% males) when substance disorders and personality disorders were additionally considered (Trestman, Ford, Zhang, & Wiesbrock, 2007).

One of the most extensive publications in the area remains a systematic review that pooled 62 studies from 12 countries to estimate rates of serious mental disorders among just short of 23,000 prisoners (Fazel & Danesh, 2002). The authors included studies that captured diagnoses in the last six months, while personality was considered across the lifespan. It found that personality disorder (predominantly antisocial personality disorder) was the most common mental disorder among prisoners, accounting for 65% of male and 42% of female prisoners. Estimated rates of psychosis were 3.7% for males and 4.0% for females, while major depressive disorders were found among 10% of male and 12% of female prisoners. The authors concluded that the rates of psychosis and major depression were several times higher than those found in the general community, but that antisocial personality disorder had

the most marked overrepresentation—roughly 10 times higher among prisoners than in the general community.

Specific mental disorders have also been investigated in certain "high-risk" prison populations. For example, a study of homicide offenders found that 8.7% of a sequential series of homicide offenders in the State of Victoria, Australia, had a diagnosis of schizophrenia. This rate was more than 13 times higher than that found in the general community (Bennett et al., 2011) and more than double the pooled estimate for psychotic disorders reported by Fazel and Danesh (2002).

A mental disorder that has recently received increasing attention in relation to criminality and imprisonment is problem and/or pathological gambling. Several recent reports have indicated that it is an increasing and significant problem, leading to imprisonment and presenting continued problems for correctional staff due to gambling and related activities among inmates (McEvoy & Spirgen, 2012). While studies suggest that the prevalence of problem and pathological gambling is between 0.5% and 4% in community samples, one recent international review of offender populations posited that one in three prisoners met criteria for problem gambling (Williams, Royston, & Hagen, 2005). This is additionally important in this context because pathological gambling commonly co-occurs with antisocial personality disorder, substance use disorders, and mood disorders (Crockford & el-Guebaly, 1998). The additive effects of gambling in prison can lead to additional vulnerability and distress.

Substance use problems dominate the correctional mental disorder literature; the association with criminal activity is noted at all stages of the justice system. An Australian study by Heffernan and colleagues (2003) found that, at the front end, 86% of police arrestees had at least one substance use disorder, many had multiple disorders, and 80% were classified as substance dependent. Similar proportions of their sample had significant psychological distress, with rates proportionate to the number of substance-related disorders. A British study of remand and sentenced prisoners reported similarly high rates of substance use prior to imprisonment, with high rates of comorbidity between mental and substance abuse disorders. Furthermore, those who were dependent on stimulants or opioids were more than six times more likely to also present with a personality disorder (Singleton, Farrell, & Meltzer, 2003).

A systematic review that examined the prevalence of substance dependence and abuse among male and female prisoners reported substantial heterogeneity between studies; estimated point-prevalence rates for alcohol abuse and dependence varied between 18% and 30% for male prisoners and between 10% and 24% for female prisoners. These estimates were between 10% and 48% for males and 30% and 60% for female prisoners with respect to drug dependence and abuse (Fazel, Bains, & Doll, 2006). The authors commented that the rates were dramatically higher than those found in the general population and particularly high with respect to the female prisoner population. These consistently high prevalence estimates have led some influential commentators to press for prison to be considered as a distinct substance abuse "treatment opportunity" (Brooke, Taylor, Gunn, & Maden, 2002).

While the majority of the available literature has focused on rates of mental disorder in male prisons, several studies that solely focused on female prisoners have also been reported. For example, Parsons and colleagues (2001) found that more than half of a sample of females remanded to prison had at least one mental disorder (which did not include those with substance dependence) and that 11% of the females were psychotic. An Australian study (Tye & Mullen, 2006) reported similar rates but highlighted the dramatic increase in prevalence (up to 84%) when substance use and dependence were included. This study found that more than one third of the females were diagnosed with drug-related disorders, major depression, and posttraumatic stress disorder.

Comorbidity of disorders

The added complexity of the increased rates of comorbid mental disorders found among prisoners serves to define a prison subgroup that places additional demands on prison health care services (Thomas et al., 2008). Studies suggest that comorbid mental health and substance use disorders are common (e.g., DiCataldo, Greer, & Profit, 1995) and of particular concern (Brinded, Simpson, Laidlaw, et al., 2001). A study conducted across the jails in Connecticut reported high rates of comorbid Axis I disorders (39.3%); nearly one in four prisoners met *Diagnostic and Statistical Manual of Mental Disorders*–IV (DSM-IV) criteria for multiple Axis II disorders and one in three had at least one Axis I and one Axis II disorder (Trestman et al., 2007). This supports findings from an earlier study that almost all male prisoners with lifetime histories of severe disorders (schizophrenia, bipolar disorder, and major depression) met criteria for comorbid antisocial personality disorder or substance use disorders (Côte & Hodgins, 1990).

Of concern is the compelling evidence that prisoners with comorbid mental health and substance-related disorders have worse criminal justice outcomes (e.g., Baillargeon, Binswanger, Penn, et al., 2009; Forsythe & Gaffney, 2012; Trestman et al., 2007). For example, a recent Australian report by the New South Wales Bureau of Crime Statistics and Research found that prisoners diagnosed with both mental health and substance-related disorders (in excess of 40% of a sample of 1,208 prisoners) re-offended at a higher rate than those who were diagnosed with solely a substance use disorder or a nonsubstance use mental disorder (Smith & Trimboli, 2010). Abram and colleagues (2003) specifically highlight the importance of screening for comorbid substance-related disorders and contend that prisons must facilitate pathways into treatment for this group.

How are mental disorders identified?

A central explanation for the variability in the estimated prevalence of mental disorders relates to the means and method used for case ascertainment. Many studies have sought to consider mental disorders through very general means such as through answers to simple questions from the broad health screens routinely administered upon reception to prison. Such screening questions record self-reported histories of contacts with mental health services and/or self-reported diagnoses and are generally used on entry to prison to screen for placement associated with identified inmate vulnerability. Large-scale prison surveys that have been reported commonly in the literature generally adopt a similar approach, with relatively generic questions about mental health used to gain a general sense about the extent of psychiatric morbidity (among other things) in prison. These studies are useful in that they can provide a cost-efficient "snapshot" of the rates of psychiatric morbidity in prisons; however, they are also limited in detailing the extent, nature, and severity of the presenting conditions.

There is a strong human rights argument about the need to adequately identify and treat inmates with mental disorders and ample evidence that the reception screening process misses a considerable proportion of those with mental illnesses (e.g., Teplin, 1990). More detailed screening tools have been developed—for example, the Brief Jail Mental Health Screen (Steadman et al., 2005), the Correctional Mental Health Screen (Ford, Trestman, Weisbrok, & Zhang, 2009), and the Jail Screening Assessment Tool ((Nicholls, Lee, Corrado, & Ogloff, 2004). Chapter 11 includes an extensive discussion on this topic. While they have shown some promise in related environments (Baksheev et al., 2012a), their utility, as tested through replication studies, remains largely unknown (Martin, Colman, Simpson, & McKenzie, 2013). Other authors have suggested a short checklist suitable for use by correctional officers later during imprisonment; this checklist focuses on behavioral and visual cues indicative of mental health concerns (Birmingham & Mullee, 2005). Birmingham (1999) has noted the general ability of correctional officers to recognize major signs and symptoms of mental disorder and has reported some usefulness with this kind of checklist approach.

Most of the studies that measured prevalence used validated psychiatric assessment and diagnostic tools. Some of the more common instruments used in studies referenced in this chapter are the Referral Decision Scale (Teplin & Swartz, 1989), the Composite International Diagnostic Interview (CIDI; e.g., Kessler, Andrews, Mroczek, et al., 1999; Wittchen et al., 1999; World Health Organization, 1990), the Structured Clinical Interview for DSM-IIIR, DSM-IV, or DSM-IV-TR (First, Gibbon, & Spitzer, 2001; First, Spitzer, Gibbon, & Williams 1996; Spitzer, Williams, Gibbon, & First, 1990), and the Mini-International Neuropsychiatric Interview (Sheehan et al., 1998). These tools were developed for use in other community and clinical populations and then applied to correctional settings.

How confident can we be with the estimated prevalence rates?

As with any diagnostic screen or test, there is an inherent degree of error. While there is always the potential for bias associated with self-report, the very nature and underlying purpose of the assessment tool/screen/instrument needs to be taken into account. For example, some screening tools are designed to be overly inclusive so as to catch as many of the target group as possible, thus leading to a number of false positives. While many authors have highlighted the sometimes significant limitations with the standard brief prison health screening processes (e.g., Andersen, 2004; Steadman et al., 2005; Teplin, 1990), some have also questioned the validity of using standardized diagnostic screens and tests in correctional environments (e.g., Andersen, 2004). While Heffernan and colleagues (2003) note the validity of the CIDI with respect to substance-related disorders, Falissard and colleagues (2006) point to some potential pitfalls with making valid and reliable mental health diagnoses in jails and prisons, suggesting that the standardized measures underestimate the true prevalence of mental disorders. By comparing diagnoses identified through use of the MINI with clinician assessments (using an open-ended clinical interview), Falissard and colleagues reported that the rates of all mental disorders were consistently higher with open-ended clinical interviews. This finding supports earlier research in other contexts that concluded that the administration of diagnostic measures by trained lay interviewers represented a conservative case ascertainment method compared to detailed clinical assessment (Murphy, Monson, Laird, et al., 2000). Falissard and colleagues also raised another issue: They reported good to excellent levels of interrater reliability overall between the clinicians according to the kappa coefficient, but the level of agreement varied quite a bit when individual disorders were considered. Levels of interrater agreement were lowest for manic episodes, bipolar disorder, and schizophrenia (k = 0.53, k = 0.68, and k = 0.64, respectively) and highest for drug dependence and alcohol dependence (k = 0.95 and k = 0.91, respectively). The authors suggest that the impact of the correctional environment itself on the individual (e.g., Baksheev et al., 2012b) may contribute to the lower levels of agreement found.

Summary

While a great deal of international research has been conducted on the prevalence of mental disorders in the prisons, a synthesis of this evidence demonstrates substantial heterogeneity. Due to the varying methodologies used, it is necessary to drill down beyond the headline findings to understand the basis on which the mental disorder was determined and what inclusion/exclusion criteria were used. What is apparent across many, if not all, jurisdictions, however, is that the need for mental health care is far greater than is currently being provided for; the result is that many prisoners are being held in suboptimal treatment and rehabilitation environments. The available evidence shows that substance use disorders are common (both primary and comorbid) and that there is a pressing need for more effective treatment for prisoners during and immediately after incarceration. The common comorbidity of substance use and personality disorders found in inmate populations potentially complicates standard treatment approaches and suggests that a different suite of strategies may need to be considered (see Chapters 36 and 42). Finally, the overrepresentation of more severe disorders, especially psychotic disorders, among prisoners continues to present a challenge for already overburdened and overstretched correctional health services.

To conclude, a clarion call—we need to move beyond prevalence studies; we now know all too well the overrepresentation of mental disorders in prisons. Now we must focus on improving the responsiveness and cohesion of multiagency service responses to fulfill our public health obligations. Prisons do, in fact, represent an excellent treatment opportunity and a chance to connect individuals with health and social welfare services. While we should continue to exercise caution in assigning mental health diagnoses to individuals (Taylor & Gunn, 2008), we are obliged to identify psychiatric vulnerability as early as possible and to provide timely, quality assessment and treatment where required.

References

Abram, K., Teplin, L., & McClelland, G. (2003). Comorbidity of severe psychiatric disorders and substance use disorders among women in jail. *American Journal of Psychiatry, 160*(5), 1007–1010.

Andersen, H. S. (2004). Mental health in prison populations: A review—with special emphasis on a study of Danish prisoners on remand. *Acta Psychiatrica Scandinavica, 424,* 5–59.

Baillargeon, J., Binswanger, I. A., Penn, J. V., Williams, B. A., & Murray, O. J. (2009). Psychiatric disorders and repeat incarcerations: The revolving prison door. *American Journal of Psychiatry, 166*(1), 103–109.

Baksheev, G. N., Ogloff, J., & Thomas, S. (2012a). Identification of mental illness in police cells: A comparison of police processes, the Brief Jail Mental Health Screen and the Jail Screening Assessment Tool. *Psychology, Crime and Law, 18*(6), 529–542.

Baksheev, G. N., Thomas, S. D. M., & Ogloff, J. R. P. (2012b). Psychopathology in police custody: The role of importation, deprivation and interaction models. *International Journal of Forensic Mental Health, 11*(1), 24–32.

Bennett, D. J., Ogloff, J. R., Mullen, P. E., Thomas, S. D., Wallace, C., & Short, T. (2011). Schizophrenia disorders, substance abuse and prior offending in a sequential series of 435 homicides. *Acta Psychiatrica Scandinavica, 124*(3), 226–233.

Birmingham, L. (1999). Prison officers can recognise hidden psychiatric morbidity in prisoners. *British Medical Journal, 319,* 853.

Birmingham, L., & Mullee, M. (2005). Development and evaluation of a screening tool for identifying prisoners with severe mental illness. *The Psychiatrist, 29,* 334–338.

Brinded, P. M. J., Simpson, A. I. F., Laidlaw, T. M., Fairley, N., & Malcolm, F. (2001). Prevalence of psychiatric disorders in New Zealand prisons: A national study. *Australian and New Zealand Journal of Psychiatry, 35,* 166–173.

Brooke, D., Taylor, C., Gunn, J., & Maden, A. (2002). Substance misusers remanded to prison: a treatment opportunity. *Addiction, 93*(12), 1851–1856.

Butler, T., Allnutt, S., Cain, D., Owens, D., & Muller, C. (2005). Mental disorder in the New South Wales prisoner population. *Australian and New Zealand Journal of Psychiatry, 39,* 407–413.

Butler, T., Andrews, G., Allnutt, S., Sakashita, C., Smith, N. E., & Basson, J. (2006). Mental disorders in Australian prisoners: A comparison with a community sample. *Australian and New Zealand Journal of Psychiatry, 40,* 272–276.

Côte, G., & Hodgins, S. (1990). Co-occurring mental disorders among criminal offenders. *Bulletin of the American Academy of Psychiatry and the Law, 18*(3), 271–281.

Crockford, D. N., & el-Guebaly, N. (1998). Psychiatric comorbidity in pathological gambling: A critical review. *Canadian Journal of Psychiatry, 43,* 43–50.

DiCataldo, F., Greer, A., & Profit, W. E. (1995). Screening prison inmates for mental disorder: An examination of the relationship between mental disorder and prison adjustment. *Bulletin of the American Academy of Psychiatry and the Law, 23*(4), 573–585.

Draine, J. (2002). Where is the "illness" in the criminalization of mental illness? In W. H Fisher (Ed.). *Community-based interventions for criminal offenders with severe mental illness, research in community and mental health* (pp. 9–21). Cambridge, MA: Emerald Group Publishing Limited.

Earthrowl, M., O'Grady, J., & Birmingham, L. (2003). Providing treatment to prisoners with mental disorders: Development of a policy. *British Journal of Psychiatry, 156,* 40–45.

Engel, R. S., & Silver, E. (2001). Policing mentally disordered suspects: A re-examination of the criminalization hypothesis. *Criminology, 39*(2), 225–252.

Falissard, B., Loze, J. Y., Gasquet, I., Duburc, A., de Beaurepaire, C., Fagnani, F., & Rouillon, F. (2006). Prevalence of mental disorders in French prisons for men. *BMC Psychiatry, 6,* 33.

Fazel, S., Bains, P., & Doll, H. (2006). Substance abuse and dependence in prisoners: a systematic review. *Addiction, 101,* 181–191.

Fazel, S., & Danesh, J. (2002). Serious mental disorder in 23000 prisoners: a systematic review of 62 surveys. *Lancet, 359,* 545–550.

First, M. B., Gibbon, M., & Spitzer, R. L. (2001). *Guide for the Structured Clinical Interview for DSM-IV-TR Axis I Disorders: SCID-I, Research Version.* New York: New York State Psychiatric Institute, Biometric Research Department.

First, M. B., Spitzer, R. L., Gibbon, M., & Williams, J. B. W. (1996). *Structured Clinical Interview for DSM-IV Axis I Disorders,*

Clinician Version (SCID-CV). Washington, DC: American Psychiatric Press, Inc.

Ford, J. D., Trestman, R. L., Wiesbrock, V. H., & Zhang, W. (2007). Validation of a brief screening instrument for identifying psychiatric disorders among newly incarcerated adults. *Psychiatric Services, 60,* 842–846.

Forsythe, L., & Gaffney, A. (2012). Mental disorder prevalence at the gateway to the criminal justice system. *Trends and Issues in Crime and Criminal Justice,* 438, July. Canberra, Australia: Australian Institute of Criminology.

Gunn, J., Maden, A., & Swinton, M. (1991). Treatment needs of prisoners with psychiatric disorders. *British Medical Journal, 303,* 338–341.

Heffernan, E. B., Finn, J., Saunders, J. B., & Byrne, G. (2003). Substance use disorders and psychological distress among police arrestees. *Medical Journal of Australia, 179,* 408–411.

James, D. J., & Glaze, L. E. (2006). *Mental health problems of prison and jail inmates* (NCJ 213600). Washington, DC: Department of Justice. Office of Justice Programs—Bureau of Justice and Statistics.

Kessler, R. C., Andrews, G., Mroczek, D., Ustun, T. B., & Wittchen, H-U. (1998). The World Health Organization Composite International Diagnostic Interview Short Form (CIDI-SF). *International Journal of Methods in Psychiatric Research, 7*(4), 171–185.

Martin, M. S., Colman, I., Simpson, A., & McKenzie, K. (2013). Mental health screening tools in correctional institutions: A systematic review. *BMC Psychiatry, 13,* 275.

McEvoy, A., & Spirgen, N. (2012). Gambling among prison inmates: Patterns and implications. *Journal of Gambling Studies, 28*(1), 69–76.

Murphy, J. M., Monson, R. R., Laird, N. M., Sobol, A. M., & Leighton, A. H. (2000). A comparison of diagnostic interviews for depression in the Stirling County study: Challenges for psychiatric epidemiology. *Archives of General Psychiatry, 57,* 230–236.

Nicholls, T. L., Lee, Z., Corrado, R. R., & Ogloff, J. R. (2004). Women inmates' mental health needs: Evidence of the validity of the Jail Screening Assessment Tool (JSAT). *International Journal of Forensic Mental Health, 3*(2), 167–184.

Parsons, S., Walker, L., & Grubin, D. (2001). Prevalence of mental disorder in female remand prisoners. *Journal of Forensic Psychiatry, 12,* 194–202.

Reed, J. (2003). Mental health care in prisons. *British Journal of Psychiatry, 182,* 287–288.

Senior, J., & Shaw, J. (2008). Mental healthcare in prison. In K. Soothill, P. Rogers, & M. Dolan (Eds.), *Handbook of forensic mental health* (pp. 175–195). Devon, UK: Willan Publishing.

Sheehan, D. V., Lecrubier, Y., Harnett Sheehan, K., et al. (1998). The Mini-International Neuropsychiatric Interview (M.I.N.I.): The development and validation of a structured psychiatric interview for DSM-IV and ICD-10. *Journal of Clinical Psychiatry, 59*(Suppl. 20), 22–33.

Singleton, N., Farrell, M., & Meltzer, H. (2003). Substance misuse among prisoners in England and Wales. *International Review of Psychiatry, 15,* 150–152.

Smith, N., & Trimboli, L. (2010). *Comorbid substance and non-substance mental health disorders and re-offending among NSW prisoners.*

Contemporary Issues in Crime and Justice. BOCSAR, NSW Bureau of Crime Statistics and Research.

Spitzer, R. L., Williams, J. B. W., Gibbon, M., & First, M. B. (1990). *Structured Clinician Interview for DSM-III-R Axis II Disorders, (SCID-II).* Washington, DC: American Psychiatric Press, Inc.

Spitzer, R. L., Williams, J. B. W., Gibbon, M., & First, M. B. (1992). The Structured Clinical Interview for DSM-IIIR (SCID) 1: History, rationale and description. *Archives of General Psychiatry, 49,* 624–629.

Steadman, H. J., Osher, F. C., Robbins, P. C., Case, B., & Samuels, S. (2009). Prevalence of serious mental illness among jail inmates. *Psychiatric Services, 60*(6), 761–765.

Steadman, H. J., Scott, J. E., Osher, F., Agnesa, T. K., & Robbins, P. C. (2005). Validation of the Brief Mental Health Screen. *Psychiatric Services, 56,* 816–822.

Taylor, P., & Gunn, J. (2008). Diagnosis, medical models and formulations. In K. Soothill, P. Rogers, & M. Dolan (Eds.), *Handbook of forensic mental health* (pp. 237–243). Devon, UK: Willan Publishing.

Teplin, L. A. (1984). Criminalizing mental disorder: The comparative arrest rate of the mentally ill. *American Psychologist, 39,* 794–803.

Teplin, L. (1990). Detecting disorder: The treatment of mental illness among jail detainees. *Journal of Consulting and Clinical Psychology, 58,* 233–236.

Teplin, L. A., & Swartz, J. (1989). Screening for severe mental disorder in jails: The development of the Referral Decision Scale. *Law and Human Behavior, 13*(1), 1–18.

Thomas, S., McCrone, P., & Fahy, T. (2008). How do psychiatric patients on prison healthcare centres differ from inpatient in secure psychiatric inpatient units? *Psychology, Crime and Law, 15*(8), 729–742.

Torrey, E. F., Kennard, A. D., Eslinger, D., Lamb, R., & Pavle, J. (2010). *More mentally ill persons are in jails and prisons than hospitals: A survey of the states.* Treatment Advocacy Center and National Sheriffs' Association. Retrieved from https//www.treatmentadvocacycenter. org/storage/documents/final_jails_v_hospitals

Trestman, R., Ford, J., Zhang, W. W., & Wiesbrock, V. (2007). Current and lifetime psychiatric illness among inmates not identified as acutely mentally ill at intake in Connecticut's jails. *Journal of the American Academy of Psychiatry and the Law, 35*(4), 490–500.

Tye, C. S., & Mullen, P. E. (2006). Mental disorders in female prisoners. *Australian and New Zealand Journal of Psychiatry, 40*(3), 266–271.

Walker, N., & McCabe, S. (1973). *Crime and insanity in England,* vol. 2. Edinburgh, UK: Edinburgh University Press.

Williams, R. J., Royston, J., & Hagen, B. F. (2005). Gambling and problem gambling within forensic populations. A review of the literature. *Criminal Justice and Behavior, 32*(6), 665–689.

Wittchen, H-U., Hofler, M., Gander, F., et al. (1999). Screening for mental disorders: Performance of the Composite International Diagnostic Screener (CID-S). *International Journal of Methods in Psychiatric Research, 8*(2), 59–70.

World Health Organization (1990). *Composite International Diagnostic Interview.* Geneva, Switzerland: World Health Organization.

World Health Organization International Consortium in Psychiatric Epidemiology (2000). Cross-national comparisons of the prevalence and correlates of mental disorders. *Bulletin of the World Health Organization, 78,* 413–425.

CHAPTER 33

Psychotic disorders

Johann Brink and Todd Tomita

Introduction

The presentation and management of psychotic disorders in jails and prisons present many opportunities but also confront the clinician with many challenges. In addition to schizophrenia-spectrum and substance-induced psychotic disorders, there are many disorders of unclear etiology or secondary to neurodevelopmental or neuropsychiatric disturbance. This chapter discusses the evidence basis for appropriate treatment of psychotic disorders and the range of opportunities for psychotherapy and psychopharmacology in correctional settings.

Background and context

Psychosis may present in various forms. Typically and as observed prototypically in the schizophrenia-spectrum disorders (schizophrenia, schizophreniform psychosis, delusional disorder, and schizoaffective and schizotypal personality disorder), psychosis is characterized by abnormalities in one or more of the following five domains: delusions (fixedly held false beliefs), hallucinations (perception-like experiences that occur without an external stimulus), disorganized thinking (off the point, tangential, illogical, or unintelligible statements or responses to questions), grossly abnormal behavior (e.g., childlike silliness, catatonia, stupor, or mutism), and so-called negative symptoms (e.g., diminished emotional expression and avolition; American Psychiatric Association, 2013).

The expressed behavior and symptomatology of psychotic disorders may vary in duration from a few days to weeks (e.g., in most substance-induced psychotic states and the time-limited regression into psychosis seen in persons with severe personality disorder with few coping strengths and in crisis), months, or years (schizophreniform psychosis, schizophrenia, and delusional disorder; American Psychiatric Association, 2013). Prolonged use of certain illicit substances (e.g., crystal methamphetamine) may result in prolonged and even permanent psychosis, thus rendering problematic the unambiguous distinction between substance-induced psychosis and schizophrenia (Lecomte et al., 2013; Ujike & Sato, 2004).

For individuals with severe forms of psychotic disorder, tenure in a correctional environment may provide more opportunities for stabilizing treatment than if the individual remained in the community. Also, the structure of prison itself may help diminish positive psychotic symptoms (Adams & Ferrandino, 2008; Blaauw, Roozen, & Marle, 2007). The positive outcomes that flow from incarceration might be attributable to factors such as safety, structure, reduced drug and alcohol consumption, and consistent access to medication and health care services (Blaauw et al., 2007; Hassan, Senior, Edge, & Shaw, 2011; Taylor et al., 2010).

Identification and proper diagnosis are critical issues as they often influence the management of disruptive inmates. Often, correctional officers are not in a position to differentiate volitionally produced problem behaviors from those produced by psychotic illness (e.g., undiagnosed bipolar disorder may be misidentified as behaviorally driven mischief-making, requiring segregation). Because correctional officers and operational managers have a mandate to prioritize the safe and orderly management of the institution, it makes sense that security and administrative means are primary methods used to manage disruptive inmates. However, sanctions such as administrative segregation can aggravate the condition of inmates with psychotic symptoms. Nevertheless, correctional officers are able to make important contributions to the interdisciplinary management and treatment of offenders (Appelbaum, Hickey, & Packer, 2001). Clinical presentations in prison can be complex, with comorbidity the rule rather than the exception. Limited access to intoxicating substances eliminates the contribution of this comorbidity to psychotic symptoms, allowing more clarity about diagnosis. Malingering of psychotic symptoms in order to find "easier time," particularly for individuals with previous incarceration experience, presents challenges that are not found in the community. Psychopathology can be different from that found in community settings. Experienced clinicians will identify cases of ostensibly personality-disordered inmates with a missed underlying delusional disorder who respond well to treatment once identified. Similarly, psychotic individuals who remain unidentified and untreated may deteriorate quietly and, once identified, prove to be resistant to treatment.

The differential diagnosis of psychotic disorders will vary depending on the stage of incarceration. Recently incarcerated individuals, for example, are at greater risk of substance-induced psychotic conditions than those serving long-term sentences, where confident diagnosis of primary psychotic disorder and treatment response is easier.

Psychosis has a strong effect on offending behavior in prison, with paranoia the strongest predictor of violent offenses (Felson, Silver, & Remster, 2012). Psychotropic medications relieve many of the manifestations of mental illness; therefore, disruptive behaviors are most likely to occur when individuals with psychotic disorders are not taking their medication (O'Keefe & Schnell, 2007).

Psychopharmacological interventions

Antipsychotic medications are the most commonly prescribed form of treatment for offenders with psychotic disorders.

Treatment providers need to maintain an awareness of the pressures and biases that may increase the likelihood of unnecessary antipsychotic medication use. This is particularly the case in patients who may not necessarily fit the prototypical psychotic disorder diagnostic categories. For example, self-limited psychotic symptoms may occur in patients with a personality disorder when in crisis. In these cases, off-label use of antipsychotic medication may be appropriate; care needs to be maintained in ascertaining the target symptoms being treated.

The independence of prescribers may be challenged by the desires and concerns of other staff about the potential for violent behavior in certain prisoners, as they may be encouraged to prescribe more sedating drugs for those patients considered to be a risk. The response of operational staff to disruptive behavior that looks like apparent mental disorder may create unique pressures within the health care system in a correctional network (Adams & Ferrandino, 2008). Although clinical staff may be able to differentiate volitionally disruptive behaviors in personality-disordered inmates from involuntary psychotically produced behavior, operational staff may understandably be searching for a convenient method for settling a disruptive inmate. Whether a psychiatric disorder is producing the problematic behavior becomes the core issue in determining the need for and duration of treatment with antipsychotic medication.

Treatment of psychotic disorders in correctional settings should be guided by general clinical practice standards, with modifications as needed for the correctional context. Evidence-based clinical practice guidelines offer a scientific and clinically sound basis for making treatment decisions and are consistent with the evolving community standard of care (Scott, 2010).

The adoption of any clinical practice guideline into correctional settings requires careful planning. Guidelines typically focus on specific diagnoses. In correctional settings, however, other psychotic disorders (e.g., delusional disorder) and intermittent psychotic symptoms that may accompany certain personality disorders may be the focus of treatment. For example, medication algorithms have been implemented for offenders with major psychotic disorders (Buscema, Abbasi, Barry, & Lauve, 2000; Moore et al., 2007; Rush et al., 1999) and with bipolar disorder (Kamath et al., 2010, 2013; Suppes et al., 2003). The objective of one such project (Buscema et al., 2000) was the creation of antipsychotic and mood stabilization medication, placement, and treatment needs algorithms in a correctional context. In an evaluation of one such algorithm for bipolar disorder, statistically significant improvement was reported on specific outcome measures (Kamath et al., 2010).

Choices of medications to treat psychotic disorders depend on the correctional formulary in the jurisdiction. Given the prevalence of mental disorders in inmate populations, a correctional formulary should include antipsychotic, antidepressant, and mood-stabilizing medications. It is also important that correctional policy permits access to nonformulary medications on a case-by-case basis to ensure access to appropriate treatment for serious mental illness (Scott, 2010).

A systematic literature review of psychotropic medication prescribing for Australian prisoners identified several main themes, including polypharmacy, high-dose therapy, duration of treatment, documentation and monitoring, and correctional contextual issues (Griffiths, Willis, & Spark, 2012). The authors concluded that models of good practice could be derived both from avoiding the numerous poor practices that exist and framing guidelines for improved psychopharmacological prescribing practice (Griffiths et al., 2012).

Although most guidelines discourage the simultaneous use of multiple antipsychotic medications, polypharmacy is common in correctional settings. One common example, although not unique to corrections, is the combination of an oral atypical antipsychotic with a depot injection of a typical antipsychotic (Griffiths et al., 2012). While limited data support the efficacy of this practice, several justifications typically are advanced: insufficient response to monotherapy, concerns about safety and adherence, a desire to leave medications unchanged if patients were reasonably well, and the need to avoid further deterioration (Bains & Nielssen, 2003; Haw & Stubbs, 2003).

Griffiths and colleagues (2012) found that high-dose medication therapy was common despite the ready availability of general recommendations for the therapeutic dose range of psychotropic medications. In one study cited, polypharmacy was the greatest predictor of high-dose therapy: Patients who were prescribed more than one antipsychotic medication were 41 times more likely to be on high doses than those on monotherapy (Griffiths et al., 2012).

Ongoing monitoring and regular medication reviews are critical for avoiding unnecessary psychotropic medication prescriptions. Polypharmacy may be the result of an insufficient trial of monotherapy before a second drug was prescribed, or patients may be on medications too long due to periods of high-dose antipsychotic therapy without reexamination (Griffiths et al., 2012). Griffiths and colleagues (2012) also found that documentation and patient monitoring were consistently problematic, with a lack of adherence to guidelines for monitoring. Nonadherence involved poorly documented assessment of treatment needs and "as-needed" (PRN) medications; discrepancies between clinical staff on how and when PRN medications are to be used (see Chapter 30); inconsistent monitoring and documentation of side effects and adverse drug reactions; and nonexistent documentation of consent to high-dose treatment before intervention (Griffiths et al., 2012).

Prescribing issues may be influenced by environmental and contextual factors, with a lack of consistency often noted between prescribers within a facility and between different sites (Griffiths et al., 2012). Prescribers who work solely in correctional facilities may also lack unbiased information that community practitioners have in abundance, both on best practice and on their prescribing patterns compared with national data. Limited financial resources often mean that psychotherapeutic treatment options are limited or unavailable, resulting in increased prescriber workload (see Chapters 41 and 42). The resulting high demand shortens appointment times, which may be one explanation for prisoners feeling they did not receive sufficient information about their treatment (Griffiths et al., 2012).

Psychotic disorders have an impact not only on an individual but also on effective prison functioning. Correctional mandates are generally twofold: public safety and offender rehabilitation. The resulting tension in managing and treating individuals with psychotic disorders in the correctional setting affects operational, staffing, formulary funding, and clinical decision making, with clinicians often feeling pressured to cooperate with lower-cost options (Adams & Ferrandino, 2008).

A detailed discussion of available antipsychotic and mood-stabilizing medications is beyond the scope of this chapter; details of classes of medications and recommended dosage and side-effect profiles are available from standard psychiatric and pharmacological texts. Within the correctional context, clinicians need to be attentive to the risk of prescribed medication abuse (see Chapter 31), especially quetiapine, benzodiazepines, hypnotics, and certain antidepressants (e.g., bupropion).

Psychosocial interventions

The objectives of psychotherapeutic interventions are to maximize adaptation and coping capacities, minimize vulnerability and stress, and reduce recidivism. The scientific literature indicates that psychosocial programs for offenders demonstrate the highest efficacy and clinical benefit when interventions are designed in accordance with the principles of effective correctional programs and use cognitive-behavioral therapy (CBT) components that target identified treatment needs (Andrews, Bonta, & Hoge, 1990a; Andrews, Zinger, Hoge, & Bonta, 1990b; Douglas, Nicholls, & Brink, 2008; Gendreau & Goggin, 1996; Gendreau, Little, & Goggin, 1996).

CBT is best articulated as a short-term, focused, and goal-oriented treatment that requires collaboration between the patient and therapist (Friendship, Blud, Erikson, et al., 2003). In a detailed review, Mueser and colleagues (2002) identified the treatment domains (broad-based psychoeducation; coping skills training; CBT for psychotic symptoms) deemed central to empirically informed programming, with recommendations and a comprehensive reference list that provides useful information about evidence-based models of care.

Douglas and colleagues (2008) provided a description of the Risk-Need-Responsivity (RNR) construct, which has emerged as an empirically informed treatment framework (Andrews & Bonta, 2003; Andrews et al., 1990a). The RNR principles align the results of assessment with interventions to enhance desistance from reoffending behaviors. The risk principle maintains that higher-risk individuals should be offered more intense services, and the need principle directs that services should target identified criminogenic needs—that is, dynamic risk factors that, "when changed, are associated with changes in the probability of recidivism" (Andrews & Bonta, 2003, p. 261). The responsivity principle holds that treatment should be matched to the abilities and learning styles of the offender. RNR-informed treatments adopt CBT-based approaches such as cognitive skills training (e.g., identifying and addressing maladaptive, overly simplistic, judgmental, or pro-criminal thinking styles), emotional dysregulation (e.g., anger management), problem-solving skill development (internalized prosocial conflict resolution), and realignment of dysfunctional behavioral styles with prosocial norms. Behavior modification through reinforcement, modeling, or role rehearsal is a typical component. These programs usually are offered in group-based, psychoeducational formats and may be supplemented with more specific programs that target other common criminogenic needs such as substance use (Douglas et al., 2008).

Examples of RNR-informed CBT programs for general offenders include Reasoning and Rehabilitation (Ross & Fabiano, 1985), Moral Reconation Therapy (Little, Robinson, & Burnette, 1993), Aggression Replacement Training (Goldstein, Glick, Irwin, Pask-McCartney, & Rubama, 1989), and Thinking for a Change (Bush, Glick, & Taymans, 1997). Dialectical Behavior Therapy (DBT; Linehan, 1987) has been adapted for use in complex and difficult-to-treat populations, including male and female offenders (Berzins & Trestman, 2004), with the goal of attaining a sense of personal acceptance and validation through acquisition of prosocial problem-solving skills (Robins & Chapman, 2004). In a study of DBT in a forensic sample, Evershed and colleagues (2003) reported that DBT patients showed greater reductions on measures of cognitive and dispositional aspects of hostility and anger and were significantly better than the treatment-as-usual group at managing outward expression of anger and hostility. While the frequency of violent behaviors remained unchanged, the severity of violent behaviors decreased by 53% in the DBT group compared to 22% in the treatment-as-usual group (Evershed et al., 2003).

In correctional settings, CBT has received the most systematic scientific scrutiny as a contemporary, systematic therapeutic approach (Douglas et al., 2008). Researchers have reported therapeutic benefit from a range of CBT-based interventions (Allen, MacKenzie, & Hickman, 2001; Ashford, Wong, & Sternbach, 2008; Baillargeon, Black, Contreas, et al., 2001; Berman, 2004; Bertand-Godfrey & Loewenthal, 2011; Huffman, 2006; Jew, Clanon, & Mattocks, 1972; Johnson & Zlotnick, 2008, 2012; Morgan & Flora, 2002; Morgan, Kroner, & Mills, 2006; Morgan & Winterowd, 2002; Morgan, Winterowd, & Ferrell, 1999a; Morgan, Winterowd, & Fuqua, 1999b). Metaanalytic reviews (Landenberger & Lipsey, 2005; D. B. Wilson, Bouffard, & MacKenzie, 2005; G. L. Wilson, 1990; S. Wilson, Attrill, & Nugent, 2003; S. Wilson & Forrester, 2002) provide further support for CBT-based programs as showing the greatest promise in terms of mental health recovery and lowered rates of reoffending. Chapter 42 presents a more extensive discussion on this topic.

For offenders with psychotic disorders, programs with psychoeducational components regarding the benefits and side effects of medication and teaching strategies for managing side effects generally, but not invariably, produce greater gains (Mueser et al., 2002). Effective CBT strategies include incorporating simplified medication regimens into the inmate's daily routine, motivational interviewing, and social skills training. Motivational interviewing, developed for the treatment of substance abuse (Miller & Rollnick, 1991), is effective in helping persons develop personally meaningful goals and in exploring the usefulness of medication in achieving those goals, including enhanced communication with their physician.

The Illness Management and Recovery (IMR) program (Mueser et al., 2006) incorporates the scientific evidence from 40 randomized controlled studies indicating the therapeutic benefit of psychoeducation and revised behavioral habits to improve medication adherence, relapse, and length of stay reduction through relapse prevention approaches. These CBT strategies improve coping skills and reduce the severity and distress of persistent symptoms. IMR has been modified for use in forensic settings; however, to date, there is no scientific review of this potentially valuable addition as a treatment option (K. Mueser, personal communication, May 20, 2013).

In comprehensive reviews (Bewley & Morgan, 2011; Morgan et al., 2012), researchers evaluated 26 empirical studies of psychotherapy services for male offenders with mental illness in North American correctional facilities to examine the degree to which correctional interventions adhered to the principles of effective programming as articulated by Andrews and colleagues (1990a) and Gendreau and Goggin (1996). Consistent with the principles of effective treatment for nonmentally ill offenders, the most frequently endorsed theoretical orientation was CBT-based treatment. It reduced symptoms of distress, improved offenders' ability to cope with their problems, and resulted in enhanced behavioral control (Morgan et al., 2012). Furthermore, interventions that targeted specific psychiatric and criminal justice needs produced significant reductions in psychiatric and criminal recidivism (Morgan et al., 2012). Other CBT and RNR mixed designs have been used and are described by Douglas and colleagues (2008).

Implementing evidence-based practices in correctional mental health settings

The challenges of implementing evidence-based practices are well articulated in a review of treatment services for persons with mental illness in the US criminal justice system (Brandt, 2012). Indeed, the problems posed by high prevalence rates, uneven availability and implementation of evidence-based programs, dearth of trained staff, and difficulties in establishing and sustaining a therapeutic milieu and program fidelity, as well as fiscal constraints and correctional-context related issues, present barriers to the provision of evidence-based care in many, if not most, nations.

The dearth of outcome analyses of larger-scale, controlled, multisite studies on offending populations with psychosis suggests caution when making recommendations regarding best practice treatment models. Nevertheless, the literature reviewed here, which is specifically guided by the acknowledged principles of effective correctional treatment (i.e., the RNR model) and the emergence of empirically informed CBT-based interventions, indicates that treatment approaches that are attentive to the subsequent recommendations are most likely to yield improvements in mental health, recovery, and public safety, including the following:

Psychiatric diagnoses should be assessed using standardized protocols such as the DSM-5 (2013) or *International Statistical Classification of Diseases and Related Health Problems*-10 (World Health Organization, 2008).

Psychopharmacological treatments should adhere to clinical practice guidelines while remaining cognizant of the specific challenges presented by the correctional context.

All consent, treatment-related decisions and progress evaluations should be clearly documented.

Nonpharmacological psychiatric treatments such as electroconvulsive treatment should be available for resistant psychosis, mania, and depression and administered by qualified clinicians.

Psychiatric and psychosocial treatment should focus on identified, specific (e.g., positive and negative psychotic symptoms or mood dysregulation; criminogenic risk markers; medication noncompliance; substance use disorders) and general (vocational, educational) treatment needs.

Psychosocial treatment approaches should be multifaceted and coordinated and should adhere to the principles of effective correctional treatment (e.g., RNR).

Programs should incorporate empirically informed CBT-based skills development (e.g., cognitive skills development, social learning, behavioral modification).

As far as possible, treatment should be provided in an appropriate milieu with well-trained interdisciplinary staff committed to person-centered therapeutic excellence (see Chapter 22).

Treatment fidelity should be protected through assurances of:
Support from senior management of program integrity,
Dedicated program space
Therapeutic milieu
Adequate, stable budget
Stable roster of well-trained, therapeutic program staff
Supported evaluation and research framework

While many jurisdictions offer the offender the support of parole or probation services, additional assistance may be required to ensure successful transition and continuity of care for those with mental illness (see Chapter 15). Liaison with community support services therefore is essential. Specialized team-based interventions such as Critical Time Intervention (Herman et al., 2011) and Assertive Community Treatment teams are evidence-based examples of such support (Evershed et al., 2003).

Summary

The provision of empirically informed care for incarcerated offenders with psychotic disorders presents significant clinical, security, and administrative challenges. However, strong scientific evidence exists that a configuration of CBT-informed components, designed and presented within an RNR framework and combined with appropriate pharmacological interventions, has strong empirical support as best practice in the treatment of severe mental illness in the correctional population.

References

Adams, K., & Ferrandino, J. (2008). Managing mentally ill inmates in prisons. *Criminal Justice and Behavior, 35*, 913–927.
Allen, L.C., MacKenzie, D. L., & Hickman, L. J. (2001). The effectiveness of cognitive behavioral treatment for adult offenders: A methodological, quality-based review. *International Journal of Offender Therapy and Comparative Criminology, 45*, 498–514.
American Psychiatric Association (2013). *Diagnostic and statistical manual of mental disorders* (5th ed.). Arlington, VA: American Psychiatric Association.
Andrews, D. A., & Bonta, J. (2010). *The psychology of criminal conduct* (5th ed.). Cincinnati, OH: Anderson Publishing.
Andrews, D. A., Bonta, J., & Hoge, R. D. (1990a). Classification for effective rehabilitation: Rediscovering psychology. *Criminal Justice and Behavior, 17*, 19–52.
Andrews, D. A., Zinger, I., Hoge, R. D., Bonta, J., Gendreau, P., & Cullen, F. T. (1990b). Does correctional treatment work? A clinically relevant and psychologically informed meta-analysis. *Criminology, 28*, 369–404.
Appelbaum, K. L., Hickey, J. M., & Packer, I. (2001). The role of correctional officers in multidisciplinary mental health care in prisons. *Psychiatric Services, 52*, 1343–1347.
Ashford, J. B., Wong, K. W., & Sternbach, K. O. (2008). Generic correctional programming for mentally ill offenders: A pilot study. *Criminal Justice and Behavior, 35*, 457–473.
Baillargeon, J., Black, S. A., Contreas, S., Grady, J., & Pulvino, J. (2001). Anti-depressant prescribing patterns for prison inmates with depressive disorders. *Journal of Affective Disorders, 63*, 225–231.

Bains, J. S., & Nielssen, O. B. (2003). Combining depot antipsychotic medications with novel antipsychotics in forensic patients: A practice in search of a principle. *Psychiatric Bulletin, 27,* 14–16.

Berman, A. H. (2004). The Reasoning and Rehabilitation Program: Assessing short- and long-term outcomes among male Swedish prisoners. *Journal of Offender Rehabilitation, 40,* 85–103.

Bertand-Godfrey, B., & Loewenthal, D. (2011). Delivering therapy in prison: An IPA study researching the lived experience of psychotherapists and counsellors. *European Journal of Psychotherapy and Counselling, 13,* 335–355.

Berzins, L. G., & Trestman, R. L. (2004). The development and implementation of Dialectical Behavior Therapy in forensic settings. *International Journal of Forensic Mental Health, 3,* 93–103.

Bewley, M. T., & Morgan, R. D. (2011). A national survey of mental health services available to offenders with mental illness: Who is doing what? *Law and Human Behavior, 35,* 351–363.

Blaauw, E., Roozen, H. G., & Marle, H. G. C. (2007). Saved by structure? The course of psychosis within a prison population. *International Journal of Prisoner Health, 3,* 248–256.

Brandt, A. L. S. (2012). Treatment of persons with mental illness in the criminal justice system: A literature review. *Journal of Offender Rehabilitation, 51,* 541–558.

Buscema, C. A., Abbasi, Q. A., Barry, D. J., & Lauve, T. H. (2000). An algorithm for the treatment of schizophrenia in the correctional setting: The Forensic Algorithm Project. *Journal of Clinical Psychiatry, 61,* 767–783.

Bush, J., Glick, B., & Taymans, J. (1997). *Thinking for a Change: Integrated cognitive behavior change program.* Washington, DC.

Douglas, K. S., Nicholls, T. L., & Brink, J. (2008) Psychological/behavioural treatment of the potentially violent patient. In P. Kleespies (Ed.), *Evaluating and managing behavioral emergencies: An evidence-based resource for the mental health practitioner* (p. 290). Washington, DC: American Psychiatric Association Books.

Evershed, S., Tennant, A., Boomer, D., Rees, A., Barkham, M., & Watson, A. (2003). Practice-based outcomes for dialectical behaviour therapy (DBT) targeting anger and violence, with male forensic patients: A pragmatic and non-contemporaneous comparison. *Criminal Behaviour and Mental Health, 13,* 198–213.

Felson, R. B., Silver, E., & Remster, B. (2012). Mental disorder and offending in prison. *Criminal Justice and Behavior, 39,* 125–143.

Friendship, C., Blud, L., Erikson, M., Travers, R., & Thornton, D. (2003). Cognitive-behavioural treatment for imprisoned offenders: An evaluation of HM Prison Service's cognitive skills programme. *Legal and Criminological Psychology, 8,* 103–114.

Gendreau, P., & Goggin, C. (1996a). Principles of effective programming with offenders. *Forum on Corrections Research, 8,* 38–40

Gendreau, P., Little, T., & Goggin, C. (1996b). A meta-analysis of the predictors of adult recidivism: What works! *Criminology, 34,* 401–433.

Goldstein, A. P., Glick, B., Irwin, M. J., Pask-McCartney, C., & Rubama, I. (1989). *Reducing delinquency: Intervention in the community* (1st ed.). New York: Pergamon Press.

Griffiths, E. V., Willis, J., & Spark, M. J. (2012). A systematic review of psychotropic drug prescribing for prisoners. *Australian and New Zealand Journal of Psychiatry, 46,* 407–421.

Hassan, L., Senior, J., Edge, D., & Shaw, J. (2011). Continuity of supply of psychiatric medicines for newly received prisoners. *The Psychiatrist, 35,* 244–248.

Haw, C., & Stubbs, J. (2003). Combined antipsychotics for 'difficult-to-manage' and forensic patients with schizophrenia: Reasons for prescribing and perceived benefits. *Psychiatric Bulletin, 27,* 449–452.

Herman, D., Conover, S., Gorroochurn, P., Hinterland, K., Hoepner, L., & Susser, E. (2011). Randomized trial of critical time intervention to prevent homelessness after hospital discharge. *Psychiatric Services, 62,* 713–719.

Huffman, E. G. (2006). Psychotherapy in prison: The frame imprisoned. *Clinical Social Work Journal, 34,* 319–333.

Jew, C. C., Clanon, T. L., & Mattocks, A. L. (1972). The effectiveness of group psychotherapy in a correctional institution. *American Journal of Psychiatry, 129,* 602–605.

Johnson, J. E., & Zlotnick, C. (2008). A pilot study of group interpersonal psychotherapy for depression in substance-abusing female prisoners. *Journal of Substance Abuse Treatment, 34,* 371–377.

Johnson, J. E., & Zlotnick, C. (2012). Pilot study of treatment for major depression among women prisoners with substance use disorder. *Journal of Psychiatric Research, 46,* 1174–1183.

Kamath, J., Temporini, H., Quarti, S., et al. (2010). Best practices: Disseminating best practices for bipolar disorder treatment in a correctional population. *Psychiatric Services, 61,* 865–867.

Kamath, J., Zhang, W., Kesten, K., Wakai, S., Shelton, D., & Trestman, R. L. (2013). Algorithm-driven pharmacological management of bipolar disorder in Connecticut prisons. *International Journal of Offender Therapy and Comparative Criminology, 57*(2), 251–264.

Landenberger, N. A., & Lipsey, M. W. (2005). The positive effects of cognitive-behavioral programs for offenders: A meta-analysis of factors associated with effective treatment. *Journal of Experimental Criminology, 1,* 451–476.

Lecomte, T., Mueser, K. T., MacEwan, W., et al. (2013). Predictors of persistent psychotic symptoms in persons with methamphetamine abuse receiving psychiatric treatment. *Journal of Nervous and Mental Disease, 201,* 1085–1089.

Linehan, M. M. (1987). Dialectical behavioral therapy: A cognitive behavioral approach to parasuicide. *Journal of Personality Disorders, 1,* 328–333.

Little, G. L., Robinson, K. D., & Burnette, K. D. (1993). Cognitive behavioral treatment of felony drug offenders: A five-year recidivism report. *Psychological Reports, 73,* 1089–1090.

Miller, W. R., & Rollnick, S. (1991). *Motivational interviewing: Preparing people to change addictive behavior.* New York: Guilford.

Moore, T. A., Buchanan, R. W., Buckley, P. F., et al. (2007). The Texas Medication Algorithm Project antipsychotic algorithm for schizophrenia. *Journal of Clinical Psychiatry, 68,* 1751–1762.

Morgan, R. D., & Flora, D. B. (2002). Group psychotherapy with incarcerated offenders: A research synthesis. *Group Dynamics: Theory, Research, and Practice, 6,* 203–218.

Morgan, R. D., Flora, D. B., Kroner, D. G., Mills, J., Varghese, F., & Steffan, J. S. (2012). Treating offenders with mental illness: A research synthesis. *Law and Human Behavior, 36,* 37–50.

Morgan, R. D., Kroner, D. G., & Mills, J. F. (2006). Group psychotherapy in prison: Facilitating change inside the walls. *Journal of Contemporary Psychotherapy, 36,* 137–144.

Morgan, R. D., & Winterowd, C. L. (2002). Interpersonal process-oriented group psychotherapy with offender populations. *International Journal of Offender Therapy and Comparative Criminology, 46,* 466–482.

Morgan, R. D., Winterowd, C. L., & Ferrell, S. W. (1999a). A national survey of group psychotherapy services in correctional facilities. *Professional Psychology: Research and Practice, 30,* 600–606.

Morgan, R. D., Winterowd, C. L., & Fuqua, D. R. (1999b). The efficacy of an integrated theoretical approach to group psychotherapy for male inmates. *Journal of Contemporary Psychotherapy, 29,* 203–222.

Mueser, K. T., Corrigan, P. W., Hilton, D. W., et al. (2002). Illness management and recovery: A review of the research. *Psychiatric Services, 53,* 1272–1284.

Mueser, K. T., Meyer, P., Penn, D. L., Clancy, R., Clancy, D. M., & Saleyers, M. P. (2006). The Illness Management and Recovery Program: Rationale, development, and preliminary findings. *Schizophrenia Bulletin, 32,* 532–543.

O'Keefe, M. A., & Schnell, M. J. (2007). Offenders with mental illness in the correctional system. *Journal of Offender Rehabilitation, 45,* 81–104.

Robins, C. J., & Chapman, A. L. (2004). Dialectical Behavior Therapy: Current status, recent developments, and future directions. *Journal of Personality Disorders, 18*, 73–89.

Ross, R. R., & Fabiano, E. A. (1985). *Time to Think: A cognitive model of delinquency prevention and offender rehabilitation.* Johnson City, TN: Institute of Social Sciences and Arts.

Rush, A. J., Rago, W. V., Crismon, M. L., et al. (1999). Medication treatment for the severely and persistently mentally ill: The Texas Medication Algorithm Project. *Journal of Clinical Psychiatry, 60*, 284–291.

Scott, C. L. (2010). *Handbook of correctional mental health* (2nd ed.). Arlington, VA: American Psychiatric Publishing.

Suppes, T., Rush, A. J., Dennehy, E. B., et al. (2003). Texas Medication Algorithm Project, phase 3 (TMAP-3): Clinical results for patients with a history of mania. *Journal of Clinical Psychiatry, 64*, 370–382.

Taylor, P. J., Walker, J., Dunn, E., Kissell, A., Williams, A., & Amos, T. (2010). Improving mental state in early imprisonment. *Criminal Behaviour and Mental Health, 20*, 215–231.

Ujike, H., & Sato, M. (2004). Clinical features of sensitization to methamphetamine observed in patients with methamphetamine dependence and psychosis. *Annals of the New York Academy of Sciences, 21*, 279–287.

Wilson, D. B., Bouffard, L. A., & MacKenzie, D. L. (2005). A quantitative review of structured, group-oriented, cognitive-behavioral programs for offenders. *Criminal Justice and Behavior, 32*, 172–204.

Wilson, G. L. (1990). Psychotherapy with depressed incarcerated felons: A comparative evaluation of treatments. *Psychological Reports, 67*, 1027–1041.

Wilson, S., Attrill, G., & Nugent, F. (2003). Effective interventions for acquisitive offenders: An investigation of cognitive skills programmes. *Legal and Criminological Psychology, 8*, 83–101.

Wilson, S., & Forrester, A. (2002). Too little, too late? The treatment of mentally incapacitated prisoners. *Journal of Forensic Psychiatry, 13*, 1–8.

World Health Organization (2008). *International statistical classification of diseases and related health problems* (10th rev.). New York: World Health Organization.

CHAPTER 34

Mood disorders

Jayesh Kamath and Ajay Shah

Introduction

Mood disorders have long been a part of humanity's historical narrative; more than 2,000 years ago Hippocrates wrote, "If fear or distress last for a long time it is melancholia." Mood disorders refer to a broad category that encompasses unipolar depressive disorders and bipolar disorders (BDs; American Psychiatric Association, 2013). Decades of research conducted in community and correctional settings have shown close but controversial relationships among mood disorders, aggression, and criminality. This chapter reviews some of these relationships and presents best practice and evidence-based approaches to correctional management and treatment of the mood disorders.

Epidemiology, associated disability, and recidivism

The National Commission on Correctional Health Care reported rates as high as 18.1% for major depressive disorder (MDD) and 4.3% for BD in US state prison populations (Veysey & Bichler-Robertson, 2002). A 2006 survey found that 23.5% of state prisoners met criteria for MDD within the past 12 months, three times the national 12-month prevalence (Bureau of Justice Statistics, 2006). A study conducted in the Iowa prison system using standardized assessments found that 54% of surveyed inmates met criteria for a mood disorder (Gunter et al., 2008). Several studies conducted in other countries also indicate a high prevalence of these disorders in their correctional settings (Fazel & Seewald, 2012; Pondé, Freire, & Mendonça, 2011). Studies also suggest a higher prevalence of MDD in female inmates than male inmates (Fazel & Seewald, 2012). Gunter and colleagues (2008) reported no gender-based difference for other major mood disorders (e.g., dysthymia, BDs). Elderly prisoners may have higher rates of depression than younger prisoners (Fazel et al., 2001). In the future, larger studies are needed to investigate prevalence differences by gender, race, age, and ethnicity as such knowledge may guide policy and resource decisions.

A persistent and bidirectional relationship exists between mood disorders and incarceration (Schnittker et al., 2012). The 12-month prevalence of MDD and BD was much higher in individuals with a past history of incarceration compared to those without a history of incarceration (MDD, 9.2% versus 6.4%; BD, 5.8% versus 2.5%; Schnittker et al., 2012). Conversely, incarceration was associated with a 45% increase in the odds of lifetime MDD (Schnittker et al., 2012). Incarceration also showed strong associations with other mood disorders, especially dysthymia and BD (Schnittker et al., 2012). Schnittker and colleagues (2012) also reported that incarceration was related to a higher risk of subsequent mood disorders and these disorders, in turn, were strongly related to increased disability (Fig. 34.1).

Mood disorders also play an important role in recidivism. Baillargeon and colleagues (2009a) reported that inmates with major psychiatric disorders, including MDD and BD, had a substantially increased risk of multiple incarcerations in the Texas correctional setting. The greatest increase in risk was observed among inmates with BDs, who were 3.3 times more likely to have had four or more previous incarcerations compared with inmates who had no major psychiatric disorders. A study conducted among recently paroled men in California reported high levels of depressive symptoms; predictors of these symptoms included a history of childhood abuse, nonresidential alcohol treatment, violent behavior, and low self-esteem (Nyamathi et al., 2011). Furthermore, evidence suggests that each incarceration has a negative impact on an existing mood disorder and increases the risk and severity of subsequent mood disorders (Schnittker et al., 2012).

Common comorbidities and their impact on disease burden

Substance use disorders represent the most common comorbidity in inmates with mood disorders. Results from the Epidemiologic Catchment Area Study show that comorbidity of addictive disorders with mental illness was highest in prison populations and was particularly high in inmates with BD (Regier et al., 1990). Studies have reported significantly higher rates of cooccurring addictive disorders in both male and female individuals with serious mental illness who have a history of incarceration compared with similar patients without such a history (Abram & Teplin, 1991; Abram et al., 2003; Regier et al., 1990). Studies have consistently shown higher rates of substance use disorders in inmates with BDs compared with inmates with other mood disorders or other serious mental illness. In male detainees, rates of co-occurring addictive disorders were higher among persons with BD than those with unipolar depression (Abram & Teplin, 1991). Similarly, in female detainees with BD, 50.7% met criteria for alcohol disorders, 54.9% met criteria for drug disorders, and, overall, 72% to 74% of female detainees with mood disorders met criteria for either alcohol or drug disorders (Abram et al., 2003).

Anxiety disorders and impulse control disorders are also highly comorbid with mood disorders. Lifetime prevalence of an anxiety disorder was seen in 86.7% of bipolar I patients and in 89.2% of bipolar II patients. Compared to the general population, patients with bipolar I disorder have more than a sevenfold increase in

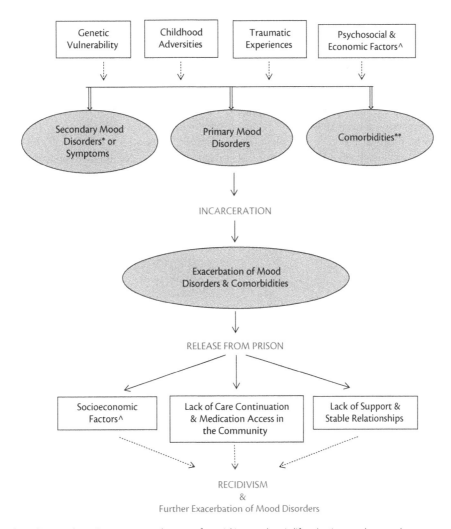

Fig. 34.1 Mood disorders and recidivism. ^, homelessness, unemployment, financial issues, chaotic lifestyles; *, secondary to substance use or PTSD; **, substance use disorders, anxiety disorders, impulse control disorders, and similar disorders.

lifetime prevalence of intermittent explosive disorder (5.2% compared to 38.1%; Kessler et al., 2005; Merikangas et al., 2007). Patients with BDs also have high rates of comorbid personality disorders, specifically antisocial and borderline personality disorder (Lenzenweger et al., 2007).

Coexistence of these disorders with mood disorders, especially BD, can present unique management challenges in the correctional setting. Inadequate symptom control combined with difficulties adapting to the correctional environment can exacerbate maladaptive behaviors. Such behaviors include aggression (toward other inmates, correctional officers, and other staff; see Chapter 48) or self-injurious behaviors, both with or without suicidal intent (see Chapters 43 and 9). As a consequence, inmates with serious mental illness are more likely than other inmates to be charged with facility rule violations or infractions and, as a result, serve longer sentences (Bureau of Justice Statistics, 2006). The relationship between mood disorders and violent behaviors is complex (Lamb & Weinberger, 2011). While it is generally accepted that the vast majority of persons with serious mental illness are no more dangerous than the general population, a subgroup of patients with certain cooccurring disorders (e.g., BD combined with recent substance use) may be at greater risk for violence. This

is especially true when symptoms are inadequately controlled in a stressful environment such as a correctional setting (Lamb & Weinberger, 2011).

Individuals with serious mental illness and an incarceration history are much more vulnerable to traumatic life experiences than the general population. Social instability and other socioeconomic issues increase the likelihood of traumatic experiences, including risk of physical abuse, violent assaults, and sexual victimization (Gunter et al., 2012; Reed et al., 2009). Studies conducted in correctional settings further suggest a close relationship between traumatic experiences and mood disorders (Gunter et al., 2012; Reed et al., 2009). Trauma is a significant predictor of suicide risk and is associated with substance use, especially in women (Gunter et al., 2012; Reed et al., 2009). Posttraumatic stress disorder (PTSD) is also highly comorbid with mood disorders in incarcerated individuals, again especially women (Binswanger et al., 2010; Gunter et al., 2012).

Incarcerated individuals with mood disorders also have frequent medical comorbidities (Binswanger et al., 2010). These comorbidities are partially the result of socioeconomic issues such as a chaotic lifestyle, social instability, and poor nutritional choices. Antipsychotics and certain mood stabilizers used in the management of mood disorders are known to cause weight gain and increase the risk of metabolic syndrome (Vancampfort et al., 2013). Chronic medical conditions can, in turn, can cause and/or contribute to exacerbation of mood disorders in inmates (Murdoch et al., 2008).

Although not a comorbidity per se, socioeconomic issues have major and direct contributions to the management and prognosis of mood disorders in the correctional setting. Homelessness and unemployment, a chaotic lifestyle due to social instability, unstable relationships, and family members with substance use disorders and/or a history of incarceration are common among offenders with serious mental illness (Fontanarosa et al., 2013). Each issue may exacerbate mood disorders, increase the risk of substance use, and subsequently present management challenges during incarceration. More importantly, addressing these socioeconomic issues can lead to improved outcomes during transition to the community (see Chapter 15).

Suicide risk

Studies conducted with both genders in the correctional setting have shown a strong association between depression and near-lethal suicide attempts (Marzano et al., 2010; Rivlin et al., 2010). Both individual and prison-related factors have shown associations with suicide attempts (Marzano et al., 2011). Individual factors include recent life events; past trauma; childhood abuse; family history of suicide; high scores on measures of depression, anxiety, aggression, impulsivity, and hostility; and low levels of self-esteem and social support (Lekka et al., 2006; Marzano et al., 2011). Prison-related factors include being on remand to custody from parole or probation, being housed alone, and negative prison experiences (Marzano et al., 2011). Baillergeon and colleagues (2009b) reported an elevated risk of completed suicide in patients with MDD and BD in the Texas prison system. Chapter 43 includes a more extensive discussion of correctional suicide risks and management.

Differential diagnosis and clinical presentation

Incarcerated individuals with mood disorders present diagnostic challenges that are similar to those in the community. Such diagnostic challenges include differentiating between unipolar and bipolar depression and between primary and secondary (e.g., substance-induced) mood disorders. Incarcerated individuals also present with special diagnostic issues not encountered in community patients. These issues are most common in the first months in prison. Use of substances prior to incarceration and detoxification following incarceration exacerbate or generate mood and anxiety symptomatology. Similarly, distress associated with incarceration, disappointments with court decisions, guilt and/or feelings of abandonment toward loved ones in the community, and adjustment to the correctional environment can cause or exacerbate mood disorders. Loss of freedom, in some cases for decades, can lead to grieving with prominent anger and despair. Such issues may result in misdiagnosis of depressive disorders rather than adjustment disorders. Withdrawal from substances can present with mood lability, leading to a misdiagnosis of BD. Substance withdrawal and adjustment issues may generate anxiety symptoms and insomnia, requiring diagnostic differentiation between primary and secondary anxiety disorders. In certain individuals, especially in women, extensive traumatic histories and PTSD may complicate mood disorder diagnosis.

These unique diagnostic challenges require correctional clinicians to adapt their assessment and management strategies (see Chapter 20). Similar to the community setting, differentiating between primary and secondary disorders is the key first step. A single cross-sectional clinical interview is frequently inadequate and can lead to misdiagnosis. Critical elements of appropriate correctional diagnostic assessments include comprehensive and longitudinal evaluation of past mood episodes; evidence of mood episodes during substance-free periods; typical symptoms experienced during substance withdrawal; prior therapeutic trials and estimates of adherence to treatment; and contribution of psychiatric and medical comorbidities to current mood symptoms, including the impact of traumatic experiences. Assessment of psychosocial factors and their contribution to presenting symptoms is crucial in any diagnostic assessment. It is frequently necessary to consider other sources such as past medical/psychiatric records; reports from community providers; and information from family, friends, and loved ones. Communication with a community pharmacy regarding recent medications and date(s) of refills can provide valuable data (see Chapter 19). Laboratory assessments such as substance screens and status of medical comorbidities (e.g., diabetes control) are also necessary parts of diagnostic assessments at the time of entry to the correctional setting. Similar to psychiatric medications, inadequate access to medications used to treat medical comorbidities (e.g., insulin, antihypertensives) and/or nonadherence with these medications are common just prior to incarceration. Furthermore, many inmates do not have primary care physicians or miss medical appointments. Exacerbation or inadequate control of multiple medical conditions may present as symptoms of mood disorders and require consideration (see Chapter 38).

Reassessment of symptomatology at every visit, especially in the first few months of incarceration, enhances accurate diagnosis. As described earlier, substance withdrawal, adjustment issues, and other comorbidities frequently confound the clinical presentation of these individuals when they enter the correctional setting. The clinical picture frequently evolves over weeks to months. The clinical presentation is complicated by diagnostic challenges but also presents an opportunity for accurate diagnoses (over time) due to the lack of confounding factors such as substances and other community factors.

Studies conducted in community settings, such as the National Institute of Mental Health–sponsored study known as the Systematic Treatment Enhancement Program for Bipolar Disorder (STEP-BD), have shown that comorbid anxiety and/or anxiety disorders can increase severity, have a negative impact on recovery from a mood episode, increase suicide risk, and significantly worsen prognosis (Simon et al., 2007). In STEP-BD, lifetime comorbid anxiety disorders were associated with a more than doubling of the odds of a past suicide attempt, while current anxiety comorbidity was associated with a more than two-fold increase in the odds of current suicidal ideation (Simon et al., 2007). The STEP-BD outcomes suggest that patients with mixed features, compared with those with classic presentations, are more difficult to manage, have worse prognoses, and are significantly more likely to have an early age of illness onset, rapid cycling in the past year, bipolar I subtype, history of suicide attempts, and more days in the preceding year with irritability or mood elevation (Goldberg et al., 2010). In this context, it is notable that inmates with BD, especially incarcerated men, frequently present in mixed states with high comorbid anxiety (Kamath et al., 2013). Similar to the mixed state in BD, irritability and agitation are commonly seen in incarcerated individuals who present with unipolar depression. Such "agitated depression" in patients with unipolar depression is frequently resistant to treatment, with higher behavioral risks, including an increased risk of suicidal behaviors (Swann, 2013).

Studies have evaluated the use of structured or semistructured interviews and validated questionnaires to diagnose mood disorders in the correctional setting. The Structured Clinical Interview for DSM (*Diagnostic and Statistical Manual of Mental Disorders*)-III-R is often considered the gold standard for diagnostic assessment. It is a useful research tool but, realistically, too time-consuming for clinical use. Several prison studies have evaluated briefer structured instruments such as the Mini-International Neuropsychiatric Interview (MINI) or the MINI-Plus (Falissard et al., 2006; Gunter et al., 2008). Use of standardized assessments in prison settings is highly recommended given the complexity of diagnostic issues. To date, such assessments are rarely used in practice due to lack of resources, funding, and time (Easton et al., 2008). Development of briefer standardized assessments designed specifically for correctional settings may address this issue.

Management and release planning

Similar to the management of mood disorders in the community (American Psychiatric Association, 2006), both pharmacotherapy and psychotherapy play critical roles in the treatment of mood disorders in correctional settings. Treatment considerations should account for psychiatric comorbidities (e.g., PTSD, substance use disorders), symptomatology driven by these comorbidities, medical issues (including the possibility of pregnancy), and other complicating factors (e.g., psychosocial). Other considerations include the individual's psychotropic medication regimen in the community (see Chapter 19), including any medications with withdrawal risks (e.g., selective serotonin reuptake inhibitors) and drug–drug interactions. Inmates who are withdrawing from substances or experiencing significant adjustment difficulties with exacerbation of symptoms might require short-term, heightened symptomatic management with anxiolytics, mood stabilizers, and, in some cases, antipsychotics. Substance withdrawal protocols should be implemented when required (see Chapter 17). However, the use of medications with addictive potential (e.g., benzodiazepines, hypnotics) should be minimized due to high substance use comorbidities and vulnerability to physiological dependence in these individuals (see Chapter 16). As discussed earlier, the symptomatology might change as the initial symptoms related to adjustment issues or substance withdrawal resolve. Continuous symptom and diagnostic reevaluation should drive optimization of medication regimens, considering both risk and benefit. In a study conducted in the Connecticut Department of Correction, algorithm-driven treatment of BD demonstrated significant

benefits, including improved clinical outcomes, improved quality of life, and reduced polypharmacy by optimizing utilization of evidence-based medications (Kamath et al., 2013). Adaptation of evidence-based treatment algorithms such as the Texas Implementation of Medication Algorithm (Rush et al., 1999) to the correctional setting can reduce inappropriate variations in clinical practice, improve outcomes, and reduce costs by eliminating ineffective practices (Ehret et al., 2013; Kamath et al., 2010). Correctional formularies are frequently restricted in order to manage costs, enhance consistency of care, and, at times, prevent the risk of abuse and diversion of prescribed medications (Tamburello et al., 2012; see Chapters 28 and 31). Correctional clinicians can have access to nonformulary medications with special approval but are generally expected to work within formulary restrictions. In some cases, this can affect management. Kamath and colleagues (2013) reported the effectiveness and benefits of algorithm-driven treatment of BD while working within formulary restrictions. During the implementation process, researchers had to accommodate certain variations to the algorithm in order to be consistent with formulary restrictions. The implementation was successful despite restrictions, partially because the algorithm included several generic medication options.

Psychotherapy, either as monotherapy or adjunctive treatment, can play a critical role in managing mood disorders in the correctional setting. Individual or group psychotherapy can be very helpful in managing the initial despair of incarceration and ongoing distress and in improving coping skills. Psychotherapies such as cognitive-behavioral therapy and Dialectical Behavioral Therapy have been adapted to treat offenders with serious mental illness (see Chapter 42). A randomized controlled study investigated the efficacy of group interpersonal therapy in the treatment of women with MDD participating in a prison substance use program (Johnson & Zlotnik, 2012). Participants reported significantly lower depressive symptoms after eight weeks of in-prison treatment compared with the control group. Dual-diagnosis treatment programs can be helpful in the management of comorbid substance use disorders in the correctional setting (Edens et al., 1997).

Finally, planning for transition to the community upon release is critical to ensure successful reentry and integration of inmates and thus to reduce recidivism (see Chapters 15 and 47). Crucial aspects of release planning include ensuring access to medications immediately after release, ensuring continuity of clinical care, and addressing socioeconomic needs in a comprehensive manner.

Summary

Inmates with mood disorders present significant diagnostic and treatment challenges to correctional clinicians due to higher severity of symptoms, frequent psychiatric and medical comorbidities, and complicated psychosocial and economic issues. Management of these individuals in the correctional setting is further complicated by their higher risk of suicidality, the challenges of the correctional environment, and repeated incarcerations. These issues demand distinct management strategies. Brief but structured diagnostic assessments and use of evidence-based treatments (pharmacotherapy and psychotherapy) can significantly improve management and outcomes of mood disorders in correctional settings.

References

Abram, K. M., & Teplin, L. A. (1991). Co-occurring disorders among mentally ill jail detainees. Implications for public policy. *American Psychologist, 46*(10), 1036–1045.

Abram, K. M., Teplin, L. A., & McClelland, G. M. (2003). Comorbidity of severe psychiatric disorders and substance use disorders among women in jail. *American Journal of Psychiatry, 160*(5), 1007–1010.

American Psychiatric Association (2013). *Diagnostic and statistical manual of mental disorders* (5th ed.). Washington, DC: American Psychiatric Publishing.

American Psychiatric Association Practice Guidelines (2006). Available at: psychiatryonline.org/guidelines.aspx

Baillargeon, J., Binswanger, I. A., Penn, J. V., Williams, B. A., & Murray, O. J. (2009a). Psychiatric disorders and repeat incarcerations: the revolving prison door. *American Journal of Psychiatry, 166*(1), 103–109.

Baillargeon, J., Penn, J. V., Thomas, C. R., Temple, J. R., Baillargeon, G., & Murray, O. J. (2009b). Psychiatric disorders and suicide in the nation's largest state prison system. *Journal of the American Academy of Psychiatry and the Law, 37*(2), 188–193.

Binswanger, I. A., Merrill, J. O., Krueger, P. M., White, M. C., Booth, R. E., & Elmore, J. G. (2010). Gender differences in chronic medical, psychiatric, and substance-dependence disorders among jail inmates. *American Journal of Public Health, 100*(3), 476–482.

Bureau of Justice Statistics (2006). *Special Report: Mental health problems of prison and jail inmates.* Washington, DC: U.S. Department of Justice. Available at: bjs.gov/content/pub/pdf/mhppji.pdf

Easton, C. J., Devine, S., Scott, M., & Wupperman, P. (2008). Commentary: implications for assessment and treatment of addictive and mentally disordered offenders entering prisons. *Journal of the American Academy of Psychiatry and the Law, 36*(1), 35–37.

Edens, J. F., Peters, R. H., & Hills, H. A. (1997). Treating prison inmates with co-occurring disorders: an integrative review of existing programs. *Behavioral Sciences and the Law, 15*(4), 439–457.

Ehret, M. J., Shelton, D., Barta, W., et al. (2013). Medication adherence among female inmates with bipolar disorder: results from a randomized controlled trial. *Psychological Services, 10*(1), 106–114.

Falissard, B., Loze, J. Y., Gasquet, I., et al. (2006). Prevalence of mental disorders in French prisons for men. *BMC Psychiatry, 6*, 33–40.

Fazel, S., Hope, T., O'Donnell, I., & Jacoby, R. (2001). Hidden psychiatric morbidity in elderly prisoners. *British Journal of Psychiatry, 179*, 535–539.

Fazel, S., & Seewald, K. (2012). Severe mental illness in 33,588 prisoners worldwide: systematic review and meta-regression analysis. *British Journal of Psychiatry, 200*(5), 364–373.

Fontanarosa, J., Uhl, S., Oyesanmi, O., & Schoelles, K. M. (2013). *Interventions for adult offenders with serious mental illness* [Internet]. Rockville, MD: Agency for Healthcare Research and Quality.

Goldberg, J. F., Perlis, R. H., Bowden, C. L., et al. (2009). Manic symptoms during depressive episodes in 1,380 patients with bipolar disorder: findings from the STEP-BD. *American Journal of Psychiatry, 166*(2), 173–181.

Gunter, T. D., Arndt, S., Wenman, G., et al. (2008). Frequency of mental and addictive disorders among 320 men and women entering the Iowa prison system: use of the MINI-Plus. *Journal of the American Academy of Psychiatry and the Law, 36*(1), 27–34.

Gunter, T. D., Chibnall, J. T., Antoniak, S. K., McCormick, B., & Black, D. W. (2012). Relative contributions of gender and traumatic life experience to the prediction of mental disorders in a sample of incarcerated offenders. *Behavioral Sciences and the Law, 30*(5), 615–630.

Johnson, J. E., & Zlotnick, C. (2012). Pilot study of treatment for major depression among women prisoners with substance use disorder. *Journal of Psychiatric Research, 46*(9), 1174–1183.

Kamath, J., Temporini, H., Quarti, S., et al. (2010). Best practices: disseminating best practices for bipolar disorder treatment in a correctional population. *Psychiatric Services, 61*(9), 865–867.

Kamath, J., Zhang, W., Kesten, K., Wakai, S., Shelton, D., & Trestman, R. (2013). Algorithm-driven pharmacological management of bipolar disorder in Connecticut prisons. *International Journal of Offender Therapy and Comparative Criminology, 57*(2), 251–264.

Kessler, R. C., Berglund, P., Demler, O., Jin, R., Merikangas, K. R., & Walters, E. E. (2005). Lifetime prevalence and age-of-onset distributions of DSM-IV disorders in the National Comorbidity Survey Replication. *Archives of General Psychiatry, 62*(6), 593–602.

Lamb, H. R., & Weinberger, L. E. (2011). Meeting the needs of those persons with serious mental illness who are most likely to become criminalized. *Journal of the American Academy of Psychiatry and the Law, 39*(4), 549–554.

Lekka, N. P., Argyriou, A. A., & Beratis, S. (2006). Suicidal ideation in prisoners: risk factors and relevance to suicidal behaviour. A prospective case-control study. *European Archives of Psychiatry and Clinical Neuroscience, 256*(2), 87–92.

Lenzenweger, M. F., Lane, M. C., Loranger, A. W., & Kessler, R. C. (2007). DSM-IV personality disorders in the National Comorbidity Survey Replication. *Biological Psychiatry, 62*(6), 553–564.

Marzano, L., Fazel, S., Rivlin, A., & Hawton, K. (2010). Psychiatric disorders in women prisoners who have engaged in near-lethal self-harm: case-control study. *British Journal of Psychiatry, 197*(3), 219–226.

Marzano, L., Hawton, K., Rivlin, A., & Fazel, S. (2011). Psychosocial influences on prisoner suicide: a case-control study of near-lethal self-harm in women prisoners. *Social Science and Medicine, 72*(6), 874–883.

Merikangas, R. C., Akiskal, H. S., Angst, J., et al. (2007). Lifetime and 12-month prevalence of bipolar spectrum disorder in the National Comorbidity Survey Replication. *Archives of General Psychiatry, 64*(5), 543–552.

Murdoch, N., Morris, P., & Holmes, C. (2008). Depression in elderly life sentence prisoners. *International Journal of Geriatric Psychiatry, 23*(9), 957–962.

Nyamathi, A., Leake, B., Albarran, C., et al. (2011). Correlates of depressive symptoms among homeless men on parole. *Issues in Mental Health Nursing, 32*(8), 501–511.

Pondé, M. P., Freire, A. C., & Mendonça, M. S. (2011). The prevalence of mental disorders in prisoners in the city of Salvador, Bahia, Brazil. *Journal of Forensic Sciences, 56*(3), 679–682.

Reed, E., Raj, A., Falbo, G., et al. (2009). The prevalence of violence and relation to depression and illicit drug use among incarcerated women in Recife, Brazil. *International Journal of Law and Psychiatry, 32*(5), 323–328.

Regier, D. A., Farmer, M. E., Rae, D. S., et al. (1990). Comorbidity of mental disorders with alcohol and other drug abuse. Results from the Epidemiologic Catchment Area (ECA) Study. *Journal of the American Medical Association, 264*(19), 2511–2518.

Rivlin, A., Hawton, K., Marzano, L., & Fazel, S. (2010). Psychiatric disorders in male prisoners who made near-lethal suicide attempts: case-control study. *British Journal of Psychiatry, 197*(4), 313–319.

Rush, A. J., Rago, W. V., Crismon, M. L., et al. (1999). Medication treatment for the severely and persistently mentally ill: the Texas Medication Algorithm Project. *Journal of Clinical Psychiatry, 60*(5), 284–291.

Schnittker, J., Massoglia, M., & Uggen, C. (2012). Out and down: incarceration and psychiatric disorders. *Journal of Health and Social Behavior, 53*(4), 448–464.

Simon, N. M., Zalta, A. K., Otto, M. W., et al. (2007). The association of comorbid anxiety disorders with suicide attempts and suicidal ideation in outpatients with bipolar disorder. *Journal of Psychiatric Research, 41*(3-4), 255–264.

Swann, A. C. (2013). Activated depression: mixed bipolar disorder or agitated unipolar depression? *Current Psychiatry Reports, 15*(8), 376.

Tamburello, A. C., Lieberman, J. A., Baum, R. M., & Reeves, R. (2012). Successful removal of quetiapine from a correctional formulary. *Journal of the American Academy of Psychiatry and the Law, 40*(4), 502–508.

Vancampfort, D., Vansteelandt, K., Correll, C. U., et al. (2013). Metabolic syndrome and metabolic abnormalities in bipolar disorder: a meta-analysis of prevalence rates and moderators. *American Journal of Psychiatry, 170*, 265–274.

Veysey, B. M., & Bichler-Robertson, G. (2002). Providing psychiatric services in correctional settings. In: *Health status of soon-to-be released inmates.* Vol. 2, Report to Congress. Chicago: National Commission on Correctional Health Care.

CHAPTER 35

Anxiety disorders including post traumatic stress disorder (PTSD)

Catherine F. Lewis

Introduction

Over the past two decades, an increasing number of studies of correctional populations have emphasized diagnosis with structured clinical instruments (Jordan, Schlenger, Fairbanks, et al., 1996; Lewis, 2006; Lynch, DeHart, Beknap, et al., 2014; Teplin, Abram, McClelland, et al., 1996, 1997; Trestman, Ford, Zhang, et al., 2007; Zlotnick, 1997). These studies have primarily focused on serious mental illness (i.e., psychotic and affective illness), substance use disorders, and personality disorders. The focus has made sense because of the need to identify the severely mentally ill who are incarcerated and to identify the most common disorders (i.e., substance use and personality pathology, particularly antisocial personality disorder [ASPD]). This emerging literature also has robustly established a high prevalence of posttraumatic stress disorder (PTSD) among incarcerated women and men (Jordan et al., 1996; Lewis, 2006; Lynch et al., 2014; Teplin et al., 1996; Trestman et al., 2007; Zlotnick, 1997). Despite the renewed focus on PTSD, little work has focused on the presence of other anxiety disorders in these populations.

This chapter first examines PTSD, a particularly prevalent anxiety disorder in correctional systems. Second, other anxiety disorders are reviewed with a focus on the difficulty caused when they are not recognized and managed. This is done using case vignettes. Emphasis is placed on existing treatment algorithms that are feasible within the correctional system.

Background

PTSD is a recognized issue and challenge within correctional populations. This recognition may be more common for populations of women, where abuse in the community has been better documented. However, recent studies support the finding that male inmates have a higher prevalence of abuse than men in the community (Fazel & Danesh, 2002; Trestman et al., 2007). In community samples observed in the National Comorbidity Study Replication, the total 12-month prevalence of all anxiety disorders (28.8 percent) exceeded that of impulse control disorders (24.8 percent), mood disorders (20.8 percent), and substance use disorders (14.6 percent; Kessler, Berglun, Demler, et al., 2005).

Not surprisingly, data from general populations are quite different from those from correctional settings. Individuals who enter the correctional system have increased exposure to victimization and are more likely to have personality pathology as well as substance abuse (Browne, Miller, & Maguin, 1999; Fazel & Danesh, 2002; Lewis, 2006; Lynch et al., 2014). PTSD is highly prevalent in both male and female populations, as are substance use disorders and mood disorders. Relatively little work has been done to identify specific anxiety disorders beyond PTSD. There are two major reasons why the identification of anxiety disorders beyond PTSD is important. First, it is well established that total disease burden, symptom counts, and diagnoses are associated with outcomes (Kessler, Borges, & Walters, 1999). Second, individuals with undiagnosed anxiety disorders are difficult to manage and often are high users of services within correctional settings. This is particularly true when the anxiety disorders are coupled with personality pathology (Teplin et al., 1997; Wright, Van Voorhis, Salisbury, & Bauman, 2012; Zlotnick, 1999).

Posttraumatic stress disorder within the correctional system

While initial studies of correctional mental health disorders justifiably focused on the seriously mentally ill (i.e., psychotic, manic, depressed), it is now recognized that PTSD is highly prevalent among incarcerated men and women. There has been more work to date on incarcerated women, likely because of their higher exposure to sexual and physical abuse in the community (Browne et al., 1999; Greenfeld & Snell, 1999; Zlotnick, 1997, 1999). In one of the few studies to compare the prevalence of male and female PTSD, jail detainees not identified as mentally ill were significantly more likely to have lifetime PTSD if they were female (41.8 percent versus 20.0 percent; Trestman et al., 2007). Of note in that study, however, is the significant elevation in prevalence for men when compared with community samples. This finding confirms that PTSD is a diagnosis important to recognize and treat in both men and women in corrections.

Incarcerated people are likely to meet the criteria for multiple diagnoses (e.g., PTSD, ASPD, multiple substance use diagnoses, and depression). It has been established that this disease burden places people at higher risk for morbidity and mortality, including death by suicide (Brodsky, Oquendo, Ellis, et al., 2001; Kessler et al., 1999). While controversial (Taylor, Asmundson, & Carleton, 2006), the concept of "complex PTSD," including symptoms of pervasive personality disturbance and somatization (Herman, 1992), appears relevant to management of these populations.

The first step in managing inmates with complex psychopathology including PTSD is to ensure that they are safe from revictimization and from harming themselves. For those with acute symptomatology, this may require placement in an observation cell, psychiatric hospital unit, or specialized housing unit. Limited treatment outcome data demonstrating reduced self-mutilation and suicidal behavior exist for women with PTSD using interventions such as Seeking Safety, dialectical behavioral therapy, and the trauma recovery and empowerment model (Fallot & Harris, 2002; Najavits, 2002; Najavits, Weiss, Shaw, et al., 1998). More work must be done with male populations to assess effectiveness. The research, even for women, is in its infancy.

The American Psychiatric Association Guidelines for PTSD (American Psychiatric Association, 2010) outline basic steps to follow when assessing and treating PTSD. The first critical step is to conduct an initial assessment. Because of the high prevalence of ASPD in the correctional system and the ease with which PTSD can be malingered (Resnick, 1997; see Chapters 23 and 36), collateral data and nonleading questions are important. Structured instruments are helpful as adjuncts to the clinical interview. It can be difficult to establish rapport with inmates with complex pathology including PTSD, but the formation of a therapeutic alliance is critical. These inmates sometimes do best in specialized structured housing units where therapy assists them in developing strategies to manage their symptoms (see Chapters 22 and 42).

An essential component of treatment is to target comorbid conditions (e.g., major depression). As comorbidity is common, it is important to develop integrated strategies that minimize therapeutic burden or polypharmacy. Psychopharmacological interventions for PTSD include selective serotonergic reuptake inhibitors (SSRIs) and selective serotonergic noradrenergic reuptake inhibitors (SNRIs) for both men and women with PTSD (American Psychiatric Association, 2010). While head-to-head trials between specific SSRIs have not been performed, the guidelines note that it is most useful to consider side effects and tolerance when selecting an agent. While some of the literature suggests efficacy of tricyclic antidepressants and monoamine oxidase inhibitors in treating PTSD, use in corrections is not optimal because of cardiac side effects, adverse medication interactions, and risk of lethal overdose if hoarded. Benzodiazepines are generally not used widely in correctional systems because of the likelihood of abuse and diversion and the relative contraindication of use for those with addiction histories. Further, the guidelines note that the efficacy of benzodiazepines in treating core symptoms of PTSD is not established (American Psychiatric Association, 2010). While some studies have suggested a role for atypical antipsychotics, the literature does not robustly support their use at this time; antipsychotics are generally expensive and have negative metabolic side effects for a population often already struggling with obesity. Atypical antipsychotics may be considered in refractory cases of PTSD or cases when psychotic symptoms are present. Finally, some studies suggest that the use of alpha$_1$ adrenergic antagonists (e.g., prazosin) and the alpha$_2$ agonist clonidine may reduce nightmares and hyperarousal, respectively. These compounds have had success in trials to treat combat veterans (American Psychiatric Association, 2010). There are practical concerns relating to the use of these medications with incarcerated patients because they can be lethal in overdose, can cause significant hypotension, and can cause significant rebound hypertension if the inmate is nonadherent for a period of time.

The various permutations of cognitive-behavioral therapies for PTSD are outlined elsewhere (see Chapters 41 and 42). A number of therapies have shown preliminary efficacy and are of substantial utility in treating incarcerated individuals with PTSD (Zlotnick, et al., 2003).

Treatment vignettes related to posttraumatic stress disorder

Posttraumatic stress disorder in an adolescent male

Background: JB is a 17-year-old male who was bound over to the adult prison after shooting his father to death. JB has no other legal history. The father had a lengthy history of sexually abusing JB. A family member noted that "ever since JB's mother died, JB became 'the woman' and endured sexual abuse for years." These facts came to light only after the homicide, when the home was thoroughly searched and police found pornographic films and pictures of JB and his father. JB has a history of learning disabilities, depression, substance use, and multiple suicide attempts. He also self-mutilates because it is "the only thing other than dying that would relax me." A screen for PTSD is strongly positive, even as he attempts to minimize symptoms.

Treatment: JB needs a risk assessment and may require a suicide watch for a period of time following incarceration. Optimally he would then be placed in a mental health housing unit that treats young adults with trauma. A major challenge will be to ensure that he is placed with young men who will not further victimize him socially or physically. JB would benefit from a specific therapist and case manager with whom he can develop trust and rapport. The focus of therapy should be on general strategies for JB to get through the day and maintain safety. Medication (e.g., an SSRI or SNRI) should be initiated to treat major depression. Finally, JB should receive psychoeducation about PTSD and be placed in programs that empower him by teaching concrete skills (i.e., educational, vocational, and substance use treatment).

Complex ptsd in an adult woman

Background: KA is a 30-year-old woman with a lengthy history of trauma. This includes rape by her father at the age of 2 (which resulted in uterine rupture), multiple rapes in adulthood (primarily when she was prostituting to support a drug habit), and severe physical abuse at the hands of multiple boyfriends. On one of these instances, she was hung naked out of a sixth-story window as a boyfriend mocked her and told her he could kill her. She has a history of multiple incarcerations dating to adolescence, including arrests for violent crime (armed robbery, attacking a person over the age of 60, accessory to rape of a minor, and assault with a weapon). She self-mutilates by cutting and burning and has made two suicide attempts by hanging while in jail. Attempts to house her in the mental health unit have been thwarted by her fighting with other inmates, assaulting staff, and openly mocking other women during group therapy. Her comments have been sadistic; she told one woman that she "deserved what she got" when she was raped at age 4. KA has also been found with contraband on the unit more than once, has been involved with other women sexually, and has openly encouraged others to self-mutilate. Staff are split about how to manage KA. One group is empathic to the horror of her childhood and committed to her, while the other wants her off the unit and ticketed for her behavior. Correctional staff advocate ticketing her for breaches of rules and holding her fully accountable for her behavior.

Treatment: KA engages in behavior that disrupts the therapeutic community and has been refractory to multiple interventions. Testing shows that she meets criteria for PTSD, major depression, and ASPD; she also has a high score on a measure of psychopathy. As her consistent behavior limits the effectiveness of treatment for anyone on the unit, KA should be ticketed for behavior that deviates from the rules of the correctional facility and the unit. She would benefit from treatment of symptoms related to depression and PTSD, but psychopathy is a bigger challenge. Her treatment must be arranged so that it does not compromise the safety of other inmates and staff. She should be assigned a counselor who will assist in developing a behavioral plan for KA (see Chapter 50). If she is able to follow it and maintain control, KA could be introduced to group settings where other women with similar pathology (including psychopathy) are being treated.

Other anxiety disorders within the correctional system

While not as extensively studied, anxiety disorders in jails and prisons are nevertheless prevalent and carry significant risk. Studies suggest that of incarcerated males with ASPD, fully one half to two thirds have a lifetime history of anxiety disorder (Hodgins, De Brito, Chhabra, & Côté, 2010) and may represent a distinct diagnostic subtype (Coid & Ullrich, 2010). In one large study, inmates with mood disorders had a comorbid anxiety disorder (including PTSD) at a rate of 73 percent for men and 82 percent for women; the co-occurrence of anxiety and psychotic disorders was 67 percent for men and 90 percent for women (Butler, Indig, Allnutt, & Mamoon, 2011). In addition to the known complexities of treating comorbid disorders, anxiety disorders appear to carry a specific additional risk during incarceration: suicide. In a study of near-lethal suicide in prison (Rivlin, Hawton, Marzano, & Fazel, 2010), the odds ratio (OR) of having a diagnosis of any anxiety disorder was 6.0 (95 percent confidence interval [CI], 2.3–15.5); for panic disorder, OR 10.0 (95 percent CI, 1.3–78); and for social anxiety, OR 9.5 (95 percent CI, 2.2–40.8). The following case vignettes provide examples of anxiety disorder diagnoses common to correctional settings and potential treatment interventions.

Treatment vignettes of other anxiety disorders

Claustrophobia

Background: AB is a 32-year-old man well known to the correctional system. His first incarceration was at age 21, with multiple incarcerations since that time. For the past five years, he has adamantly refused to get into the van that transports inmates to court.

He states he is terrified of being in an enclosed space with other inmates and fears enclosed spaces in general. He has received multiple tickets for refusing to go, and once struck a correctional officer who was trying to place him in the van. One treatment provider recommends a one-time dose of a benzodiazepine, while another says to give him a dose of diphenhydramine. The situation has now escalated to the point that advocates are demanding that he be transferred individually by car to all court hearings.

Treatment: To assess this situation, a longitudinal history of AB's behavior is required, as well as a review of any trauma that occurred in the van or elsewhere. Gathering collateral information from the unit about how he functions, particularly when in enclosed spaces, is useful. A structured and nonleading interview to assess AB for panic disorder, agoraphobia, PTSD, or another specific phobia is appropriate. He must also be assessed for malingering. Finally, any medical efforts must be coordinated with correctional staff. If they are unwilling to transfer AB in the van, that is fine. A car may be an option the correctional system chooses. Regardless, the AB should be psychiatrically treated. While a benzodiazepine may work, it sets a dangerous precedent in reinforcing similar behavior from the inmate as well as others. Additionally, a claim of being overmedicated may present issues in court or if he claims assault in the van. If AB is found to have comorbid disorders (e.g., either anxiety disorders or depression), these should be addressed both psychopharmacologically and therapeutically (i.e., cognitive-behavioral therapy). For his claustrophobic symptoms, medications (e.g., SSRIs) are of benefit, as is cognitive-behavioral therapy. Concrete steps other than transporting the inmate in a car might include allowing him to sit near the door or window of the van, working to focus his thoughts on something else (with skills gained from cognitive-behavioral therapy), or transporting him with officers he knows.

Panic disorder

Background: CD is a 49-year-old woman with chronic obstructive pulmonary disease, coronary artery disease with two prior heart attacks, and insulin-dependent diabetes mellitus. She has a history of heroin dependence and is HIV positive. Her history is significant for trauma dating to childhood, but she consistently refuses to engage mental health staff in her treatment. She complains of multiple somatic symptoms, and a number of medical emergency codes have been called as a result. During these codes, she is rushed to the infirmary complaining of shortness of breath, palpitations, sweating, and a sense of impending death. Multiple workups, including two performed at an outside hospital, were negative. The medical staff is exhausted with her multiple (up to four a week) emergent visits and want the behavior to stop. At the same time, they recognize that CD is at real risk for medical complications and cannot be ignored.

Treatment: An integrated approach is indicated. Medical and mental health staff should see CD on the same day (preferably proximate in time and even enabling two providers to speak to her at the same time). Her symptoms, while most consistent with panic attacks, are viewed by the patient as purely physical. She should ideally be treated with an SSRI that minimally interacts with her other medications. The psychiatrist, along with the primary care physician, should schedule regular nonemergent appointments with CD. In so doing, they can explain that the medication they plan to treat her with is safe despite all her comorbid conditions and will help with anxiety related to her health. She should also receive either one-on-one or group cognitive therapy to assist her in managing her stress. This therapy can be presented as a support group for women with chronic illness. Finally, any contribution of substance use disorder should be fully assessed. In this instance, CD, partially due to fear of another attack of shortness of breath, was overusing an asthma inhaler (i.e., albuterol), a short-acting beta agonist, which exacerbated her attacks.

Anxiety secondary to a medical condition and substance use

Background: EF is a 62-year-old man who is serving 10 years on his most recent sentence. He has been in and out of corrections since he was young. Most recently, he demanded a single cell because he says he is claustrophobic and cannot tolerate a double cell. Two much younger cellmates have assaulted him in the past six months. EF assaulted another inmate by punching him so that he could "go to segregation and be in peace." He describes feeling panicked and cooped up with another inmate in his cell but fine when alone. He had no history of assaults or altercations throughout his previous sentences.

Treatment: Because of his lengthy history of functioning well with a cellmate in the past, the suspicion for malingering must be high. EF should be observed in his cell when he is not aware he is being watched. In this initial phase, he should not be medicated and should be informed that the diagnostic assessment is ongoing. When observed alone, EF shows no signs of impairment but is noted to drink more than two quarts of coffee per day. He is also noted to use the toilet frequently and to stand for a lengthy period before he urinates. As EF waits to urinate, he becomes anxious and shaky. Follow-up on this case revealed that EF had developed an enlarged prostate, which made him go the bathroom repetitively during the night, thus waking his cellmate. This had angered his cellmates, who, in reality, had picked fights with him. EF had increased his coffee intake in an effort to "try to get things out easier." This increased caffeine exacerbated his worry related to his medical condition. Once the prostate issues were solved, EF did not have issues while being in a double cell.

Specific phobia of blood, injection, and blood draws

Background: BL is a 26-year-old man who has hepatitis C, which was virulent during his time in the community. He has been admitted to corrections several times and, on each occasion, refused blood work or was not present when called to get blood work. His explanation for this is that there is "no point" since his sister died of HIV. BL becomes frustrated and angry when his case manager attempts to discuss the issue; he simply states that he has the right to refuse blood work. He threatens to sue the staff if they make him get the blood test. The social worker is able to obtain from BL a release of information for his mother. The mother confirms that BL's sister died of HIV but says that has nothing to do with the refusal to have his blood drawn. She notes that he has

been "absolutely terrified of needles" since childhood and had to be held down to get shots at the pediatrician's office. She routinely accompanied him when he had mandatory blood work done in the community. She has seen BL faint when blood is drawn. His maternal uncle and brother both have the same difficulty.

Treatment: BL is exhibiting symptoms of a specific phobia. While specific phobias are common, they rarely cause significant impairment because the individual avoids the stimuli (e.g., snakes, spiders, heights). In this case, BL's phobia is jeopardizing his health and should be addressed. He should be assessed and treated for any comorbid disorders appropriately. If there were no comorbid disorders, he would ideally be managed with a cognitive-behavioral intervention; however, BL must be willing to participate.

Anxiety secondary to withdrawal from a substance

Background: AK is a 44-year-old man who was admitted to a lockup facility following a domestic charge that resulted from an incident in which he struck his wife while drinking. He is put on a suicide watch and two days later goes to his court arraignment. Following his court appearance, AK is brought to jail and begins to act agitated and anxious. He then complains that people are out to get him. He pushes away staff and tries to run from them. AK is placed in the segregation unit but does not calm with time. He becomes more agitated and begins to yell that people should get out of his cell, although he is alone in it.

Treatment: AK is exhibiting signs and symptoms of potential alcohol or benzodiazepine withdrawal. Ideally, he would have been questioned on admission about his use of these substances, and any prescribed benzodiazepine use would have been confirmed with a pharmacy. Review of his admission notes shows that he admits to drinking a pint of whiskey plus a six-pack of beer per day. His anxiety and mental status changes are most consistent with those seen in alcohol withdrawal. When staff takes his vital signs, AK is hypertensive, tachycardic, and febrile. He does not know where he is and is hallucinating and agitated. The correct intervention is to medicate him with a benzodiazepine and an antipsychotic (e.g., haloperidol) for agitation, with rapid transfer to the hospital unit. He is beginning to show signs of delirium tremens, which if not treated has a high risk of morbidity and mortality.

Summary

Anxiety disorders are common in the corrections population. One anxiety disorder that stands apart from others is PTSD, which occurs at much higher rates in both incarcerated men and women than in the community. Despite this fact, other anxiety disorders are often comorbid and add to the overall disease burden and impair the ability to function. Individuals with a greater disease burden (i.e., number of diagnoses, symptom counts) have worse outcomes than those with uncomplicated disorders. These impaired outcomes include a deteriorating trajectory of illness, increased health service use, a poor prognosis, and an increased likelihood of morbidity and mortality (Kessler et al., 1999; Wu, Kouzina, & Leaf, 1999). Thus, while anxiety disorders may not be the primary focus of the correctional system, they must be recognized as important. Unrecognized anxiety disorders can result in behavior that is disruptive and may appear to be volitional. They can also lead to overuse of health services that are already facing substantial demands. Appropriate, available, and consistent assessment, diagnosis, and treatment that are well integrated can successfully intervene in the range of anxiety disorders that present in correctional settings.

References

American Psychiatric Association (2010). *Guideline watch (March 2009): Practice guideline for the treatment of patients with acute stress disorder and posttraumatic stress disorder*. Arlington, VA: American Psychiatric Publishing, Inc.

Brodsky, B. S., Oquendo, M., Ellis, S. P., et al. (2001). The relationship of childhood abuse of impulsivity and suicidal behavior in adults with major depression. *American Journal of Psychiatry, 158*, 1871–1877.

Browne, A., Miller, B., & Maguin E. (1999). Prevalence and severity of lifetime physical and sexual victimization among incarcerated women. *International Journal of the Law and Psychiatry, 22*, 2301–2322.

Butler, T., Indig, D., Allnutt, S., & Mamoon, H. (2011). Co-occurring mental illness and substance use disorder among Australian prisoners. *Drug and Alcohol Review, 30*(2), 188–194.

Coid, J., & Ullrich, S. (2010). Antisocial personality disorder and anxiety disorder: A diagnostic variant? *Journal of Anxiety Disorders, 24*(5), 452–460.

Fallot, R. D., & Harris, M. (2002). The trauma recovery and empowerment model (TREM): conceptual and practical issues in a group intervention for women. *Community Mental Health Journal, 38*, 475–485.

Fazel, S., & Danesh, J. (2002). Serious mental disorder in 23,000 prisoners: a systemic review of 62 surveys. *The Lancet, 359*, 545–550.

Greenfeld, L. A., & Snell, T. L. (1999). *Bureau of Justice Statistics Special Report: Women offenders*. Washington, DC: Bureau of Justice Statistics.

Herman, J. L. (1992). Complex PTSD: a syndrome in survivors of prolonged and repeated trauma. *Journal of Traumatic Stress, 5*(3), 377–391.

Hodgins, S., De Brito, S. A., Chhabra, P., & Côté, G. (2010). Anxiety disorders among offenders with antisocial personality disorders: A distinct subtype? *Canadian Journal of Psychiatry, 55*(12), 784–791.

Jordan, B. K., Schlenger, W. E., Fairbanks, J. A., et al. (1996). Prevalence of psychiatric disorders among incarcerated women, II: Convicted felons entering prison. *Archives of General Psychiatry, 55*, 513–519.

Kessler, R. C., Berglund, P., Demler, O., et al. (2005). Lifetime prevalence and age-of-onset distributions of DSM-IV disorders in the National Comorbidity Survey Replication. *Archives of General Psychiatry, 62*(6), 593–602.

Kessler, R. C., Borges, G., & Walters, E. E. (1999). Prevalence of and risk factors for lifetime suicide attempts in the National Comorbidity Survey. *Archives of General Psychiatry, 56*, 617–626.

Lewis, C. F. (2006). Treating incarcerated women: gender matters. *Psychiatric Clinics of North America, 29*, 773–789.

Lynch, S. M., DeHart, D. D., Beknap, J. E. et al. (2014). A multisite study of the prevalence of serious mental illness, PTSD, and substance use disorders of women in jail. *Psychiatric Services In Advance*, February 3, 1–5.

Najavits, L. M. (2002). "Seeking Safety": therapy for trauma and substance abuse. *Corrections Today, 64*, 136–141.

Najavits, L. M., Weiss, R. D., Shaw, S. R., et al. (1998). "Seeking Safety": outcome of a new cognitive-behavioral psychotherapy for women with PTSD and substance use disorder. *Journal of Trauma and Stress, 11*, 437–456.

Resnick, P. J. (1997). Malingering of posttraumatic disorders. In Richard Rogers (Ed.), *Clinical assessment of malingering and deception* (pp. 130–152). New York: The Guilford Press.

Rivlin, A., Hawton, K., Marzano, L., & Fazel, S. (2010). Psychiatric disorders in male prisoners who made near-lethal suicide attempts: case–control study. *British Journal of Psychiatry, 197*(4), 313–319.

Taylor, S., Asmundson, G. J., & Carleton, R. N. (2006). Simple versus complex PTSD: A cluster analytic investigation. *Journal of Anxiety Disorders, 20*(4), 459–472.

Teplin, L. A., Abram, K. M., & McClelland, G. M. (1996). Prevalence of psychiatric disorders among incarcerated women, 1: Pre-trial jail detainees. *Archives of General Psychiatry, 53*, 505–512.

Teplin, L. A., Abram, K. M., & McClelland, G. M. (1997). Mentally disordered women in jail, who receives services? *American Journal of Public Health, 87*, 604–609.

Trestman, R. L., Ford, J., Zhang, W. Z., et al. (2007). Current and lifetime psychiatric illness among inmates not identified as mentally ill at intake in Connecticut's jails. *Journal of the American Academy of Psychiatry and the Law, 35*, 490–500.

Wright, E., Van Voorhis, P., Salisbury, E. J., & Bauman, A. (2012). Gender-responsive lessons learned and policy implications for women in prison: a review. *Criminal Justice and Behavior, 39*, 1612–1632.

Wu, L. T., Kouzina, A. C., & Leaf, P. J. (1999). Influence of co-morbid alcohol and psychiatric disorders on utilization of mental health services in the National Comorbidity Survey. *American Journal of Psychiatry, 156*(8), 1230–1236.

Zlotnick, C. (1997). PTSD comorbidity and childhood abuse among incarcerated women. *Journal of Nervous and Mental Disorders, 185*, 761–763.

Zlotnick, C. (1999). Antisocial personality disorder, affective dysregulation and childhood abuse among incarcerated women. *Journal of Personality Disorders, 13*, 90–95.

Zlotnick, C., Najavits, L. M., Rohsenow, D. J., et al. (2003). A cognitive-behavioral treatment for incarcerated women with substance abuse disorder and posttraumatic stress disorder: findings from a pilot study. *Journal of Substance Abuse Treatment, 25*, 99–105.

CHAPTER 36

Personality disorders

Sundeep Virdi and Robert L. Trestman

Introduction

Personality disorders, by definition, are associated with significant functional impairment of affected individuals and may also have negative impacts on those around them. That impairment results from the way these individuals think and feel about themselves and others (American Psychiatric Association, 2013, pp. 645–684). Patients with personality disorders are challenging to manage; the difficulties associated with their care are accentuated in correctional settings. Inmates with personality disorders often require a disproportionate level of attention from correctional staff (Barrett & Byford, 2012), and their behavior can contribute to a dangerous environment inside a facility (Coid, 2002). Compared to offenders with other psychiatric disorders or nonmentally disordered offenders, offenders with personality disorders have higher rates of violence, criminality, and recidivism (Rigonatti et al., 2006; Yu et al., 2012).

DSM-5 (*Diagnostic and Statistical Manual of Mental Disorders*) personality disorders are divided into three clusters (American Psychiatric Association, 2013). Cluster A consists of paranoid, schizoid, and schizotypal personality disorders; Cluster B comprises antisocial, histrionic, borderline, and narcissistic; and Cluster C is made up of avoidant, dependent, and obsessive–compulsive personality disorders. Forensic implications of the DSM-5 personality disorder update are reviewed elsewhere (Trestman, 2014).

The following four personality disorders are particularly relevant to the correctional psychiatry setting: borderline personality disorder (BPD), antisocial personality disorder (ASPD), narcissistic personality disorder (NPD), and paranoid personality disorder (PPD). Research reflects that these four have the highest correctional prevalence rates among the personality disorders (Black et al., 2010; Coid et al., 2013; Fazel et al., 2002; Trestman et al., 2007). For each of these four disorders, this chapter presents a description and some management challenges, data on correctional prevalence, appropriate psychotherapy, and potential psychopharmacological interventions.

Borderline personality disorder
Description and management challenges

DB is a 29-year-old woman awaiting trial for reckless endangerment of her 3-year-old child. She was incarcerated two months ago with diagnoses of BPD and cocaine abuse. Her community medications, which she acknowledges taking inconsistently, included divalproex, escitalopram, and quetiapine. Since her incarceration, she has self-injured (cutting with bits of metal,
removed stiches to a deeper laceration), threatened suicide, received four disciplinary infractions, and attempted suicide. Custody staff is frustrated with her and wants the mental health team to deal with her.

According to DSM-5, the criteria for diagnosing BPD are "significant impairments in personality functioning manifest by impairment in self-functioning and impairment in interpersonal functioning." These patients have many characteristics that prove to be problematic in a corrections setting, such as impulsivity, emotional lability, aggression, difficulty controlling anger, distress intolerance, and self-harming behavior (Black et al., 2007; Trestman, 2000). These same qualities contribute to criminal behavior and also place patients at a higher risk of recidivism than the general population (Black et al., 2007).

In a corrections setting, the mindset of patients with BPD leads to several management concerns. Their behavior often provokes strong responses in prison personnel that range from irritation to frustration and anger (Trestman, 2000). The tension that these patients cause among fellow inmates often leads to violence and endangers prison staff and inmates. Patients with BPD also place themselves in danger with self-mutilating and self-harming behavior (see Chapter 49); these patients are at high risk for suicide (Trestman, 2000). Also, forensic patients with BPD have been shown to engage in behaviors such as fire-setting, property damage, and assaults; evidence suggests that these behaviors provide borderline patients with relief from the tension and dysphoria they may be experiencing (Coid, 2002).

Correctional prevalence

The prevalence of BPD in the corrections populations is significantly higher than in the general community or even in clinical psychiatric settings (Trestman et al., 2007). Studies indicate that the community prevalence of BPD is between 1.6% and 5.9%, depending on sample and methodology (Grant et al., 2008; Zanarini et al., 2011). Historically, about 75% of diagnosed cases are female, but newer data suggest that, while the clinical presentation may differ, the actual gender ratio is closer to 1:1 (Grant et al., 2008). In correctional settings, the prevalence for men has been reported to be between 12.9% and 26.8% and for women between 20% and 54.5% (Black et al., 2007; Trestman et al., 2007; Tye & Mullen, 2006).

Psychotherapy

Psychotherapy is the treatment of choice for patients with BPD (National Institute for Health and Clinical Excellence, 2009). Treatment is important to enhance function in correctional settings and subsequently in society upon release from incarceration (Berzins & Trestman, 2004). One extensive review (Stoffers et al., 2012) found community-based clinical trials of a half-dozen psychotherapies for treating BPD; the strongest data exist for Dialectical Behavioral Therapy (DBT). DBT is a cognitive-behavioral treatment that combines the basic strategies of behavior therapy with the practice of mindfulness. DBT has been implemented in correctional settings (Berzins & Trestman, 2004), with evidence of benefit in terms of reduced aggression and management problems (Sampl et al., 2010; Shelton et al., 2009, 2011). When adapted to the forensic setting, the goal of DBT is to help patients with severe behavioral dyscontrol who engage in life-threatening and unit-destructive behavior to learn to control their behavior (Berzins & Trestman, 2004). The costs of training, staff turnover, and maintenance of an appropriate milieu are some of the pragmatic challenges of implementing and sustaining DBT in correctional environments.

Other psychotherapies have been implemented in correctional settings to treat this population, with varying degrees of research support. These include Reasoning and Rehabilitation (R&R; Ross & Fabiano, 1985), Systems Training for Emotional Predictability and Problem Solving (STEPPS; Black et al., 2008), and START NOW (Shelton, 2011); also see Chapter 42.

Psychopharmacology

Psychopharmacological treatment focuses on the symptoms associated with BPD—emotional lability, impulsivity, perceptual distortions, anxiety—and not the disorder itself (Trestman, 2000). Very little data support the effectiveness of medications in patients with BPD. One extensive, structured review concluded that mood stabilizers and antipsychotics may provide modest benefit and may be helpful in the presence of comorbid conditions. Total BPD severity was not significantly influenced by any drug. No promising results are available for the core BPD symptoms of chronic feelings of emptiness, identity disturbance, and abandonment (Stoffers et al., 2010). Of the available data, the greatest amount exists for anticonvulsant use for impulsivity and emotional instability. Lithium may be of benefit as well (see Chapter 48). One challenge is effective patient engagement for adherence with these medications; without adherence, more harm than good may be the result. Antidepressants are best reserved for treating comorbid depression; while antipsychotics are frequently used, their benefit in this population is modest at best and the side-effect burden is significant (Stoffers et al., 2010). At this time, there are no randomized clinical trials demonstrating that the use of two or more medications in this population results in a better outcome than a single medication.

Antisocial personality disorder
Description and management challenges

> RL is a 22-year-old man sentenced to eight years for manslaughter. This is his fifth incarceration. He was admitted while on methadone, which he supplemented with street heroin. He has received multiple disciplinary reports for flagrant disregard of direct orders and for fighting. He often presents to mental health with requests for treatment and then refuses to participate in therapy or to take the medications prescribed.

ASPD is characterized by a pervasive pattern of socially irresponsible, exploitative, and guiltless behavior, long seen as a significant risk factor for criminality and imprisonment (Anton et al., 2012). Individuals with ASPD have difficulty dealing with authority and living in a structured setting such as prison (Trestman, 2000). Traits that make these individuals difficult to manage include their disregard for the rights of others and their lack of empathy and remorse (Black et al., 2010). They are also more likely to be gang members than those without an ASPD diagnosis (Coid et al., 2013). These qualities lend themselves to violence in a correctional setting, given that such settings are typically extremely regimented and have many authority figures, and the congregate living environment generates many interpersonal interactions due to proximity.

These individuals often require a high level of mental health services because of the frequent comorbidities associated with ASPD, which include mood, anxiety, and substance use disorders and attention-deficit/hyperactivity disorder (Black et al., 2010). Patients with ASPD have high rates of comorbid psychiatric illnesses (Black et al., 2010) and medical conditions (Goldstein et al., 2008).

Correctional prevalence

It has been said that ASPD is "endemic to correctional settings" (Trestman, 2000). While estimates vary, studies have demonstrated rates of ASPD in the prison population to be as high as 75% (Zeier et al., 2012). While ASPD is often seen as a diagnosis of men, it is important not to overlook the diagnosis in women. An extensive review of international studies available prior to 2000 found the average prevalence of ASPD in correctional settings to be 47% in men and 21% in women, with little variation in sentenced and unsentenced samples (Fazel & Danesh, 2002). One study of a US prison system found a 35% prevalence of ASPD, with no gender difference (Black et al., 2010). In a study of 2,196 individuals conducted in Connecticut jails, ASPD was present in 39.5% of men and 27% of women (Trestman et al., 2007). This study also demonstrated racial disparities in the diagnosis of ASPD, with 53.7% of Hispanic males meeting criteria for ASPD versus 35.5 of black males and 35.7 of white males (Trestman et al., 2007). Despite the prevalence of ASPD, it is important to keep in mind that not everyone with ASPD breaks the law and not everyone who engages in criminal behavior has ASPD (National Institute for Health and Clinical Excellence, 2009).

Psychotherapy

Patients with ASPD generally deny responsibility for any problem and thus can be quite difficult to engage when asked to change their behaviors. The motivation to seek mental health assistance, when it happens, is typically related to ultimatums by family, friends, or law enforcement. ASPD patients often work to discontinue therapy once an obligation no longer exists. They routinely incite and test the limits of those trying to work with them. Staff working with and treating patients with ASPD must maintain both therapeutic boundaries and therapeutic optimism; individuals with ASPD may still respond well to crisis interventions and treatment of comorbid disorders (Trestman & Lazrove, 2010).

The National Institute for Health and Clinical Excellence (NICE; 2013) in Great Britain has published guidelines on the treatment of ASPD. These guidelines discuss possible pharmacological and psychological interventions to be used in ASPD and indicate that due to the limited number of randomized clinical trials assessing therapeutic interventions in ASPD, further research is necessary to determine the benefits of various therapies, including pharmacotherapy and group-based therapy. Similar results were found in another structured review that used rigorous standards (Gibbon et al., 2010).

Despite these caveats, several studies have been conducted with ASPD patients in correctional settings using primarily manualized cognitive-behavioral therapies such as Moral Reconation Therapy (Little & Robinson, 1988) and R&R (Ross & Fabiano, 1985). The best-studied ones are variants of R&R. While benefits were found in terms of improved attitudes and behavior at R&R program completion (Clarke et al., 2010) and at 12-month follow-up (Cullen et al., 2011), dropout rates were as high as 76%. Shorter variants of R&R have been tested with improved retention rates but more modest impact (Young et al., 2013).

Going beyond the studies, the basics of psychotherapy still apply. Maintaining a respectful attitude; being direct, clear, and honest; and following through with any commitments (e.g., "I will be back later today to listen to your concerns") will help to establish an effective therapeutic alliance.

Psychopharmacology

Much like BPD, pharmacological treatment for ASPD centers on treating symptoms. The NICE guidelines (2009) suggest that "pharmacological interventions should not be routinely used for the treatment of ASPD or associated behaviors of aggression, anger and impulsivity." One structured review found no randomized clinical trial demonstrating evidence of benefit from using medication in the treatment of ASPD (typically frequency or intensity of aggression; Khalifa et al., 2010). However, some data indicate that pharmacological intervention may be of some utility in the corrections environment (Trestman, 2000). For instance, impulsive aggression in these patients may potentially be managed with anticonvulsants, selective serotonergic reuptake inhibitors (SSRIs), or beta blockers (see Chapter 48). It is also important to treat any comorbid disorders that may be present with appropriate psychotherapy or pharmacological therapy.

Narcissistic personality disorder
Description and management challenges

Convicted for fraud, AS is a 32-year-old man diagnosed with depression. Since his incarceration, he devotes his time to challenging the custody and health care staff by asking difficult questions in an attempt to prove their incompetence and embarrass them. He has submitted multiple grievances about alleged failures of the health care staff and has received multiple disciplinary infractions for disrespectful behavior. He describes himself as superior and disdains people who he feels have lower standards and different values than his own. He describes himself as intellectually unique. He has few close friends, a general anhedonia, and a sense of detachment. His weight is stable; appetite and sleep are fine.

NPD is characterized by a "pervasive pattern of grandiosity, lack of empathy, and hyper-sensitivity to evaluation of others, together with the over-inflated self-image considered the source of the narcissistic personality style" (Coid, 2002).

The grandiosity associated with NPD leads these inmates to create difficult situations for themselves (Trestman, 2000). Their behavior and inflated sense of self-worth can antagonize corrections staff

and fellow inmates (Coid, 2002). The highly structured corrections environment becomes difficult for them because they feel that they are better than those around them, and this often leads to violence (Trestman, 2000). Their expectations of how they should be managed differ significantly from the harsh reality of prison, and this also contributes to behavioral problems in these inmates (Coid, 2002).

In addition to grandiosity, NPD is associated with other qualities that make it challenging to manage in a corrections population. Inmates with NPD have increased anger and aggression, which can lead to threatening behavior and an inability to follow rules (Warren & South, 2009). They often see no solution to problems other than violence. Behavior can include violence against corrections staff, which may be related to pride in their fighting skills (Coid, 2002). One study of women demonstrated that violent and homicidal behavior was significantly increased among women diagnosed with NPD (Warren & South, 2009).

Correctional prevalence

The community prevalence of NPD is estimated to be approximately 1% (Dhawan et al., 2010). Very limited data on correctional NPD prevalence are available. One prison study in New Zealand found a 12% female prevalence rate (Tye & Mullen, 2006). A study of the UK prison system found a mixed-gender NPD prevalence of 7% (Ullrich et al., 2008).

Psychotherapy

To date, only sporadic theoretical approaches and case studies, and no randomized controlled studies, of psychotherapy with NPD patients are available, whether in the community or in correctional settings (Dhawan et al., 2010). Current recommendations focus on targeted clinical engagement that emphasizes interpersonal functioning, emotion regulation, and frustration tolerance (Ronningstam & Weinberg, 2013).

Psychopharmacology

Symptomatic control of NPD typically targets control of impulsive aggression (Trestman, 2000). The aggression these patients often demonstrate may be managed with SSRIs, beta blockers, antipsychotics, and anticonvulsants (see Chapter 48).

Paranoid personality disorder
Description and management challenges

EJ is a 41-year-old woman with no prior history of psychiatric care who was convicted of multiple assault charges. Since incarceration, she has made no friends and shares virtually no information about herself. She often interprets innocent remarks as intentional insults or as veiled threats. Following one such remark from a cellmate, she nursed a grudge and developed a fear that her cellmate intended to attack her. One evening, she viciously attacked her cellmate without apparent provocation. When questioned, she acknowledged that she did so to prevent an anticipated attack.

PPD is important in the corrections population because these inmates tend to be suspicious of those around them and exhibit "hypersensitivity, distrust and jealousy" (Birkeland, 2013). There is an association between PPD and criminal behavior (Kellett & Hardy, 2013). PPD is associated with an increased risk of violent behavior in the community (Pulay et al., 2008); women incarcerated for a violent crime have an elevated likelihood of a PPD diagnosis (Warren et al., 2002).

These qualities make such inmates see the environment around them through a lens of paranoia, and they tend to perceive aggression where none may exist (Trestman, 2000). In this context, these patients will lash out and respond to perceived slights or aggression with violence; in doing so, they create an unsafe environment for themselves, other inmates, and staff (Trestman, 2000). PPD is associated with violence toward other inmates and the hoarding of weapons and may be motivated by "a belief that violence is the only solution to interpersonal difficulties" or a "blow to self-esteem" (Coid, 2002). These individuals can feel such humiliation that they will exert considerable energy plotting retaliation (Coid, 2002). The violent nature of some of these patients makes management in a corrections setting extremely challenging.

Correctional prevalence

The community prevalence of PPD is approximately 4.4%, with men at slightly greater risk than women (Grant et al., 2004). The study of Connecticut jails discussed previously found no gender difference in the prevalence of PPD, with approximately 10% of men and women in the sample meeting criteria (Trestman et al., 2007). In other studies, 33% of women in New Zealand prisons (Tye & Mullen, 2006), 44.5% of men in a London intake prison (Slade & Forrester, 2013), and 23% in a mixed-gender national prison survey in the United Kingdom (Ullrich et al., 2008) met diagnostic criteria for PPD.

Psychotherapy

Few data on psychotherapy for patients with PPD exist. Treatment would target specific behaviors, addressable issues, and any comorbid diagnoses. Specific challenges of transference are significant with this population. At times, very detailed behavior management plans that target specific problematic behaviors (e.g., public masturbation) may be used; these are addressed in more detail in Chapter 50. Where available, individual psychotherapy that focuses on the creation of a therapeutic alliance may be appropriate (see Chapter 41). More commonly, group therapy with co-facilitation may be used to minimize likely transference issues (see Chapter 42).

Psychopharmacology

As with NPD, few data exist on pharmacological treatment of PPD. The few data that do exist suggest the potential use of antipsychotics. Typical of the few reports available, one small community-based case series did note functional improvement and symptom reduction with the use of antipsychotics (Birkeland, 2013). Once a therapeutic relationship is established between clinician and patient, thoughtful discussion and clarification of issues and concerns may help define specific and objective targets for treatment.

Summary

Inmates with personality disorders present many challenges to operational and clinical management in correctional settings. Prevalence, morbidity, and consumption of resources can be disproportionately high. Evolving knowledge, evidence-based protocols, and the development of situation-specific skills are improving our ability to assist personality-disordered individuals to function much more effectively and safely while incarcerated and to reintegrate into the community more effectively.

References

American Psychiatric Association (2013). *Diagnostic and statistical manual of mental disorders* (5th ed.). Arlington, VA: American Psychiatric Association.

Anton, M. E., Baskin-Sommers, A. R., Vitale, J. E., Curtin, J. J., & Newman, J. P. (2012). Differential effects of psychopathy and antisocial personality disorder symptoms on cognitive and fear processing in female offenders. *Cognitive, Affective and Behavioral Neuroscience*, 12, 761.

Barrett, B., & Byford, S. (2012). Costs and outcomes of an intervention program for offenders with personality disorders. *British Journal of Psychiatry*, 200, 336.

Berzins, L. G., & Trestman, R. L. (2004). The development and implementation of Dialectical Behavior Therapy in forensic settings. *International Journal of Forensic Mental Health*, 3(1), 94–95.

Birkeland, S. F. (2013). Psychopharmacological treatment and course in paranoid personality disorder: a case series. *International Clinical Psychopharmacology*, 28, 283–285.

Black, D. W., Gunter, T., Allen, J., et al. (2007). Borderline personality disorder in male and female offenders newly committed to prison. *Comprehensive Psychiatry*, 48, 400–403.

Black, D. W., Blum, N., Eichinger, L., McCormick, B., Allen, J., & Sieleni, B. (2008). STEPPS: Systems Training for Emotional Predictability and Problem Solving in women offenders with borderline personality disorder in prison: a pilot study. *CNS Spectrum*, 13(10), 881–886.

Black, D. W., Gunter, T., Loveless, P., et al. (2010). Antisocial personality disorder in incarcerated offenders: Psychiatric comorbidity and quality of life. *Annals of Clinical Psychiatry*, 22, 113–120.

Clarke, A. Y., Cullen, A. E., Walwyn, R., & Fahy, T. (2010). A quasi-experimental pilot study of the reasoning and rehabilitation program with mentally disordered offenders. *Journal of Forensic Psychiatry & Psychology*, 21, 490–500.

Coid, J. W. (2002). Personality disorders in prisoners and their motivation for dangerous and disruptive behavior. *Criminal Behavior and Mental Health*, 12, 213–218, 220–223.

Coid, J. W., Ullrich, S., Keers, R., et al. (2013). Gang membership, violence, and psychiatric morbidity. *American Journal of Psychiatry*, 170(9), 985–993.

Cullen, A. E., Clarke, A. Y., Kuipers, E., Hodgins, S., Dean, K., & Fahy, T. (2011). A multi-site randomized controlled trial of a cognitive skills program for male mentally disordered offenders: Social-cognitive outcomes. *Psychological Medicine*, 1–13.

Dhawan, N., Kunik, M. E., Oldham, J., & Coverdale, J. (2010). Prevalence and treatment of narcissistic personality disorder in the community: a systematic review. *Comprehensive Psychiatry*, 51(4), 333–339.

Fazel, S., & Danesh, J. (2002). Serious mental disorder in 23,000 prisoners: A systematic review of 62 surveys. *Lancet*, 359, 545–550.

Gibbon, S., Duggan, C., Stoffers, J., et al. (2010). Psychological interventions for antisocial personality disorder. *Cochrane Database Systematic Review*, (6):CD007668.

Goldstein, R. B., Dawson, D. A., Chou, S. P., et al. (2008). Antisocial behavioral syndromes and past-year physical health among adults in the United States: Results from the National Epidemiologic Survey on Alcohol and Related Conditions. *Journal of Clinical Psychiatry*, 69(3), 368–380.

Grant, B. F., Chou, S. P., Goldstein, R. B., et al. (2008). Prevalence, correlates, disability, and comorbidity of DSM-IV borderline personality disorder: results from the Wave 2 National Epidemiologic Survey on Alcohol and Related Conditions. *Journal of Clinical Psychiatry*, 69(4), 533–545.

Grant, B. F., Hasin, D. S., Stinson, F. S., et. al. (2004). Prevalence, correlates, and disability of personality disorders in the United

States: results from the National Epidemiologic Survey on Alcohol and Related Conditions. *Journal of Clinical Psychiatry, 65*(7), 948–958.

Kellett, S., & Hardy, G. (2013). Treatment of paranoid personality disorder with cognitive analytic therapy: A mixed-methods single-case experimental design. *Clinical Psychology and Psychotherapy,* DOI:10.1002/cpp.1845

Khalifa, N., Duggan, C., Stoffers, J., et al. (2010). Pharmacological interventions for antisocial personality disorder. *Cochrane Database Systematic Review,* DOI:10.1002/14651858.CD007667.pub2

Little, G. L., & Robinson, K. D. (1988). Moral Reconation Therapy: a systematic step-by-step treatment system for treatment-resistant clients. *Psychological Reports, 62*(1), 135–151.

National Institute for Health and Clinical Excellence (2009). *Borderline personality disorder: treatment, management and prevention.* NICE Clinical Guideline 78. Accessed December 28, 2013, at: http://www.nice.org.uk/nicemedia/live/12125/43045/43045.pdf

National Institute for Health and Clinical Excellence (2013). *Antisocial personality disorder: treatment, management and prevention.* NICE Clinical Guideline 77. Accessed December 28, 2013, at: http://www.nice.org.uk/nicemedia/live/11765/42993/42993.pdf

Pulay, A. J., Dawson, D. A., Hasin, D. S., et al. (2008). Violent behavior and DSM-IV psychiatric disorders: results from the national epidemiologic survey on alcohol and related conditions. *Journal of Clinical Psychiatry, 69*(1), 12–22.

Rigonatti, S. P., Serafim, A., Caires, M. A., Filho, A. H., & Arboleda-Florez, J. (2006). Personality disorders in rapists and murderers from a maximum security prison in Brazil. *International Journal of Law and Psychiatry, 29,* 361.

Ronningstam, E., & Weinberg, I. (2013). Narcissistic personality disorder: Progress in recognition and treatment. *FOCUS: The Journal of Lifelong Learning in Psychiatry, 11*(2), 167–177.

Ross, R. R., & Fabiano, E. A. (1985). *Time to Think: A cognitive model of delinquency prevention and offender rehabilitation.* Johnson City, TN: Institute of Social Sciences and Arts.

Shelton, D., Sampl, S., Kesten, K., Zhang, W., & Trestman, R. L. (2009). Treatment of impulsive aggression in correctional settings. *Behavioral Sciences and the Law, 27,* 787–800.

Sampl, S., Wakai, S., & Trestman, R. L. (2010). Translating evidence-based practices from community to corrections: An example of implementing DBT-CM. *Journal of Behavioral Analysis of Offender and Victim Treatment and Prevention, 2*(2), 114–123.

Shelton, D., Kesten, K., Zhang, W., & Trestman, R. L. (2011). Impact of a Dialectic Behavior Therapy Corrections modified upon behaviorally challenged incarcerated male adolescents. *Journal of Child and Adolescent Psychiatric Nursing, 24,* 105–113.

Shelton, D., & Wakai, S. (2011). A process evaluation of START NOW skills training for inmates with impulsive and aggressive behaviors. *Journal of the American Psychiatric Nurses Association, 17*(2), 148–157.

Slade, K., & Forrester, A. (2013). Measuring IPDE-SQ personality disorder prevalence in pre-sentence and early-stage prison populations, with

sub-type estimates. *International Journal of Law and Psychiatry, 36,* 207–212.

Stoffers, J., Völlm, B. A., Rücker, G., Timmer, A., Huband, N., & Lieb, K. (2010). Pharmacological interventions for borderline personality disorder. *Cochrane Systematic Reviews,* DOI:10.1002/14651858.CD005653.pub2

Stoffers, J. M., Völlm, B. A., Rücker, G., Timmer, A., Huband, N., & Lieb, K. (2012). Psychological therapies for people with borderline personality disorder. *Cochrane Database Systematic Review, 8.* DOI: 10.1002/14651858.CD005652.pub2

Trestman, R. L. (2000). Behind bars: personality disorders. *Journal of the American Academy of Psychiatry and the Law, 28,* 2–6.

Trestman, R. L., Ford, J., Zhang, W., & Wiesbrock, V. (2007). Current and lifetime psychiatric illness among inmates not identified as acutely mentally ill at intake in Connecticut's jails. *Journal of the American Academy of Psychiatry and Law, 35,* 492–496.

Trestman, R. L., & Lazrove, S. (2010). On the coming of age of antisocial personality disorder: A commentary on the NICE treatment guidelines for antisocial personality disorder. *Personality and Mental Health, 4,* 12–15.

Trestman, R. L. (2014). Forensic implications of changes in DSM-5 on personality disorders. *Journal of the American Academy of Psychiatry and Law, 42*(2), 173–181.

Tye, C. S., & Mullen, P. E. (2006), Mental disorders in female prisoners. *Australian and New Zealand Journal of Psychiatry, 40,* 266–271.

Ullrich, S., Deasy, D., Smith, J., et al. (2008). Detecting personality disorders in the prison population of England and Wales: comparing case identification using the SCID-II screen and the SCID-II clinical interview. *Journal of Forensic Psychiatry & Psychology, 19*(3), 301–322.

Warren, J. I., Burnette, M., South, S. C., Chauhan, P., Bale, R., & Friend, R. (2002). Personality disorders and violence among female prison inmates. *Journal of the American Academy of Psychiatry and the Law Online, 30*(4), 502–509.

Warren, J. I., & South, S. C. (2009). A symptom-level examination of the relationship between Cluster B personality disorders and patterns of criminality and violence in women. *International Journal of Law and Psychiatry, 32*(1), 10–17.

Young, S., Hopkin, G., Perkins, D., Farr, C., Doidge, A., & Gudjonsson, G. (2013). A controlled trial of a cognitive skills program for personality-disordered offenders. *Journal of Attention Disorders, 17*(7), 598–607.

Yu, R., Gedder, J. R., & Fazel, S. (2012). Personality disorders, violence, and antisocial behavior: a systematic review and meta-regression analysis. *Journal of Personality Disorders, 26*(5), 784–786.

Zanarini, M. C., Horwood, J., Wolke, D., Waylen, A., Fitzmaurice, G., & Grant, B. F. (2011). Prevalence of DSM-IV borderline personality disorder in two community samples: 6,330 English 11-year-olds and 34,653 American adults. *Journal of Personality Disorders, 25*(5), 607–619.

Zeier, J. D., Baskin-Sommers, A. R., Newman, J. P., & Racer, K. H. (2012). Cognitive control deficits associated with antisocial personality disorder and psychopathy. *Journal of Personality Disorders, 3*(3), 284.

CHAPTER 37

Attention deficit disorders

Kenneth L. Appelbaum and Kevin R. Murphy

Introduction

Few disorders in correctional settings present the degree of diagnostic and treatment controversy as does attention-deficit/ hyperactivity disorder (ADHD). The nature of the condition, its assessment, and its management combine to create a perfect storm of potentially vexing challenges for the prison psychiatrist. This chapter reviews those diagnostic and treatment challenges, including the risk of diversion and misuse of controlled substances among inmates. An assessment and treatment model is also presented that minimizes risk while ensuring access to care in appropriately selected cases.

Adult prevalence

Some research findings suggest that ADHD occurs at far greater prevalence rates among criminal justice populations than in the population at large. Prevalence estimates among inmates range from 9% to 50% (Curran & Fitzgerald, 1999; Daderman et al., 2004; Dalteg et al., 1998; Eyestone & Howell, 1994; Lindgren, 2002; Rasmussen et al., 2001; Rosler et al., 2004; Ziegler et al., 2003; Ginsberg et al., 2010; Moore et al., 2013; Westmoreland et al., 2010; Young et al., 2009). Although this broad range may accurately reflect diverse settings, significant methodological shortcomings exist in these prevalence studies: nonrepresentative inmate samples, use of adolescent rather than adult populations, reliance on single sources of information, exclusive use of self-reports, use of community-based screening tools not validated in correctional settings, and overreliance on simplistic symptom counts on self-administered ADHD rating scales or screening instruments. Inmates often present with complex psychiatric histories and multiple comorbidities that make it challenging for even seasoned diagnosticians to reliably identify ADHD in such patients, especially without a more comprehensive diagnostic evaluation. One screening tool, for example, consists of six questions including, "How often are you distracted by activity or noise around you?" Given the typically crowded, cacophonous, and often hazardous environment in jails and prisons, a positive response to this question has little discriminatory value. Concluding that an inmate has ADHD based solely on self-report, symptom counts, use of nonspecific screening instruments, or other insufficient sources or information compromises the reliability of most of the correctional prevalence literature.

Moreover, population prevalence studies estimate that 2.5% to 4% of adults worldwide meet diagnostic criteria for ADHD (Fayyad et al., 2007; Kessler et al., 2006; Simon et al., 2009). Based on US Census Bureau statistics, the population of adult males 18 years and older was approximately 115 million in 2010. At a prevalence rate of between 2.5% and 4%, approximately 3 to 4.5 million of them had ADHD. At the start of 2010, approximately 6 million adult males were under state or federal criminal justice supervision or incarceration according to US Department of Justice statistics (Glaze, 2010). That translates into 150,000 adult male offenders with ADHD at a 2.5% prevalence rate. If 50% of them had ADHD, however, this would represent nearly all adult males with ADHD in the United States.

Accurate diagnosis generally requires obtaining a thorough clinical history; reliably establishing a childhood onset of symptoms; gaining input from collateral informants who know the patient well; inspecting objective records such as school report cards, teacher comments, prior evaluation reports, and special education records for evidence of chronic ADHD-like symptoms and impairments; using *Diagnostic and Statistical Manual of Mental Disorders* (DSM)–based symptom rating scales; and having a qualified professional perform a diagnostic interview to rule out other possible diagnoses and alternative explanations for the symptoms before concluding that ADHD is present (Murphy & Gordon, 2006). Most prison systems do not have the time and resources to conduct such rigorous assessments. This also compromises the reliability of making accurate ADHD diagnoses in prison settings.

Diagnostic considerations

Although commonly thought of as a disorder of childhood, in most individuals with ADHD the symptoms persist into adulthood, especially inattention, restlessness, poor planning, and impulsivity (Turgay et al., 2012). Regardless of age, however, ADHD remains difficult to diagnose for several reasons (Murphy & Gordon, 2006). Inattention and impulsivity, the hallmark symptoms of ADHD, are part of the universal human experience, which leads to diagnostic dimensional uncertainty. These symptoms also occur with many other mental disorders and thus lack categorical specificity. On top of these basic challenges, other factors increase diagnostic difficulties among adults. Inaccurate or poor recall of childhood symptoms and impairment, lack of available collateral informants who know the inmate well, and inability to obtain corroborating data or historical records complicate the validation of childhood onset of dysfunction required to qualify for an ADHD diagnosis as an adult. Moreover, ADHD-like symptoms are commonly found in many adult psychiatric diagnoses, medical disorders, or even stressful life events that have an onset during adulthood. All of this further underscores the diagnostic complexities inherent in making accurate ADHD diagnoses in adults.

Psychiatric disorders that share symptoms with ADHD include affective disorders, some personality disorders, generalized anxiety disorder, obsessive–compulsive disorder, intermittent explosive disorder, substance abuse, sleep disorders, cognitive impairments due to head injury or dementia, and psychotic disorders. Some of these conditions also can arise as comorbid complications from ADHD, further complicating the differential diagnosis. Endocrine, nutritional, metabolic, cardiac, and other medical conditions, along with the effects of some medications, can also mimic symptoms of ADHD, as can adverse interpersonal, vocational, financial, or other significant life events or stressors. Accurate diagnosis relies on a well-documented, life-long history of problems, ideally with third-party corroboration. It can be especially difficult to identify *bona fide* ADHD among inmates as these patients routinely present with complex histories that may include multiple comorbidities, personality disorders, trauma, longstanding substance use, poverty, head injuries, or major mental illness.

The first and most important step in an evaluation for ADHD focuses on the degree and chronicity of impairment. The diagnosis among children and adolescents requires at least six symptoms of inattention and/or hyperactivity–impulsivity that result in clinically significant impairment in social, academic, or occupational functioning (American Psychiatric Association, 2013). These maladaptive features typically begin relatively early in childhood and persist until late adolescence or early adulthood, if not beyond. Although DSM-IV criteria included the presence of some disabling symptoms before age 7, DSM-5 sets symptom onset to prior to age 12 in recognition of the difficulties in precise retrospective determinations (Kieling et al., 2010). The new criteria also establish a lower threshold of five, as opposed to six, symptoms to diagnose the disorder among adults. Individuals with fewer symptoms, brief or episodic symptoms, or symptoms that do not result in significantly maladaptive impairment do not qualify for a DSM-5 diagnosis. These represent important dimensional and categorical diagnostic restrictions. Few, if any, individuals go through life without experiencing moments of inattention to details, poor organization of tasks and activities, restlessness, or impulsive decisions. With ADHD, however, symptoms have readily apparent persistence and severity, resulting in significant disruption and underachievement in major life activities including social, academic, and vocational areas (Barkley et al., 2008). A reliable diagnosis requires objective evidence of major dysfunction, not merely self-perceptions of underachievement.

Along with a complete psychosocial history, rating scales can aid in the diagnosis. Some standardized self-report measures for ADHD include Conners' Adult ADHD Rating Scale, the Brown Attention Deficit Disorder Scale, the Barkley Symptom Rating Scale, and the Adult ADHD Self-Report Scale v1.1 Symptom Checklist (ASRS-V1.1). A shorter version of the ASRS-V1.1, the Adult ADHD Self-Report Scales v1.1 Screener, consists of only six items and can be used as a starting point to determine whether a more thorough assessment for ADHD is warranted. Murphy and Adler (2004) have described these rating scales in more detail. As noted, however, interpreting community instruments not standardized for correctional settings requires caution.

Treatment

In addition to medications, interventions for adults with ADHD include education about the disorder, organizational strategies, cognitive-behavioral therapy, and psychotherapy. The most effective approach to treatment combines these modalities with medication (Murphy, 2005; Safren et al., 2005).

Although not as well studied as medications for children, medications for adults can help reduce symptoms and improve functioning. The US Food and Drug Administration (FDA) has approved four stimulants, all long-acting, for adults with ADHD: dextroamphetamine/amphetamine, an osmotic-controlled release form of methylphenidate, extended-release dexmethylphenidate, and lisdexamfetamine dimesylate. Methylphenidate and amphetamine formulations each block dopamine and norepinephrine reuptake and differ slightly in their mechanism of action; response and tolerance vary among individuals. Treatment sometimes results in hypertension, and common, usually mild side effects include decreased appetite, abdominal symptoms, nervousness, difficulty sleeping, and mood disturbance. Special cautions apply to patients with cardiovascular disease, and the risk of adverse events increases with concurrent use of caffeine or sympathomimetic agents.

The nonstimulant norepinephrine reuptake inhibitor atomoxetine also has FDA approval for treatment of adults with ADHD, with response rates somewhat lower than with stimulants. Although less well studied than other agents, bupropion, tricyclic antidepressants, modafinil, guanfacine, and alpha-adrenergic agonists have been used off-label to treat ADHD.

The logic and potential strategies for the use of psychotropic treatment of ADHD in correctional settings are discussed in more detail below in the section "Recommendations."

Special considerations for the correctional setting

Several problems can arise with the prescription of stimulants in correctional facilities. These medications have substantial economic value among inmates, which may lead to diversion, both voluntary and involuntary through threats or extortion. Falsified or exaggerated symptom presentations in an effort to obtain medication can consume precious psychiatric time. Inmates may file grievances, board of licensure or registration complaints, or legal actions against psychiatrists who fail to provide a desired prescription. Disparate prescribing thresholds increase the likelihood of complaints against more conservative psychiatrists, especially when the psychiatrist decides to discontinue a medication started by an inmate's provider in the community or elsewhere in the correctional system. Such time-wasting or adversarial encounters make for an unpleasant experience that many practitioners would rather avoid.

Nursing staff often face equally vexing challenges. The special handling, monitoring, and documentation required for controlled substances demands substantial time, potentially overwhelming an institution's capacity as the number of inmates on these medications mounts. Custody staff also have valid concerns about the consequences of substance availability and misuse within correctional facilities.

The high prevalence of substance-related disorders among inmates leads many clinical and custody staff to question the wisdom of introducing prescribed stimulants, or other controlled substances, into the environment. These concerns have merit. In the month prior to their offense, 12% of state prisoners reported using stimulants and 56% reported using any drug (Mumola & Karberg, 2006).

Given these potential problems, should correctional systems simply make stimulants unavailable, or do the benefits of their use outweigh the risks? A decision to restrict access to current standards of care requires compelling reasons. A task force report of the American Psychiatric Association states, "The fundamental policy goal for correctional mental health care is to provide the same level of mental health services to each patient in the criminal justice process that should be available in the community" (2000, p. 6). The report goes on to state that "[a] full range of psychotropic medications . . . must be available" and represents an "essential service" (2000, p. 45).

Ensuring that inmates have access to common and beneficial treatments for their disorders might alone provide sufficient reason to keep stimulants available for appropriate cases, but other considerations also support this. If inadequate treatment of ADHD interferes with the ability of inmates to function, this, too, can have adverse security implications. An inmate's participation in work assignments, educational activities, and other programs has benefits for correctional facilities and for society in general, as well as for the inmate.

Medication for adults with ADHD also might affect the risk of further criminality. Although confounding variables could account for the results, a large-scale pharmacoepidemiologic study in Sweden found that current treatment with ADHD medication was associated with reduced criminal convictions (Lichtenstein et al., 2012). If this represents a true medication effect, a similar reduction in disciplinary infractions might occur for inmates who are treated during their incarcerations. At least one program has noted such benefits (McCallon, 2000), with other studies reporting an association between ADHD symptoms and both violent and nonviolent breaches of prison discipline (Gordon et al., 2012; Young et al., 2009). As with the literature on ADHD prevalence among inmates, however, interpreting studies on the relationship between ADHD and criminality requires caution. A conclusion that ADHD accounts for a significant proportion of crime or that most individuals with the disorder engage in criminal activity lacks an adequate evidence base and does a disservice to this population. Another recent prospective study, for example, found no relationship between ADHD and criminal recidivism (Grieger & Hosser, 2012).

Finally, misuse and diversion of medications occurs in community as well as correctional settings. However, for inmates, at least one component of this risk does not apply: The correctional psychiatrist can confidently know that the patient does not have access to stimulant prescriptions from multiple prescribers.

Unfortunately, the same confidence does not exist regarding illicitly obtained medications or other substances, which few facilities can eliminate.

Recommendations

In the absence of a complete ban on access to stimulant medications—an option we do not recommend or consider necessary—facilities need an approach that mitigates adverse effects on staffing resources, security, and litigation. In the experience of one author of this chapter (K.L.A.), as director of correctional mental health for a state prison system, a carefully implemented protocol for stimulant prescriptions can go a long way toward achieving this goal (Appelbaum, 2009). This approach enhances diagnostic consistency in a multiprovider environment and helps support psychiatrists when they make treatment decisions that are consistent with a system's established criteria and approval process. The recommended protocol has several key provisions, which are described later.

Before describing this protocol, however, some important considerations warrant attention. Custody employees and mental health professionals can have different perspectives on the goal or purpose of treating inmates with stimulant medication. Mental health professionals (or researchers who conduct prevalence studies) may try to identify and treat all inmates who meet diagnostic criteria for ADHD. Custody personnel might not share this goal; instead, they may have more pragmatic and utilitarian goals. Their primary interests may include reducing disruptive behavior and conflict, minimizing functional impairments in programming and activities, and generally having facility operations run as smoothly as possible. In this sense, efforts targeted toward providing ADHD assessments and treatment only to obviously impaired inmates with persistent difficulties in their daily activities might prove more fruitful for all. If these impaired inmates have *bona fide* ADHD and respond positively to treatment by exhibiting fewer functional problems, everybody wins. Although this strategy would result in the treatment of far fewer inmates with stimulant medications, it has the advantage of ensuring treatment for the inmates who need it most, minimizing administrative and monitoring responsibilities, reducing risks of diversion and misuse, and diminishing disability for some individuals.

Whether to use stimulants for an inmate whose only significant problem involves disruptive activities presents a dilemma. As previously noted, impulsivity and other ADHD symptoms could contribute to disciplinary infractions, and these behaviors might improve with effective treatment. If this is the sole basis for treatment, however, some inmates might intentionally misbehave to gain access to stimulants. This can become an especially dangerous situation if it encourages self-injury, assaults, or other harmful acts. For this reason, prudence would suggest that the functional justification for treatment with stimulants requires more than just transient serious misbehavior. Legitimate ADHD results in a chronic and pervasive pattern of impairment rather than a sudden onset in a circumscribed situation associated with secondary gain.

Other than making an accurate diagnosis, the single most important consideration when deciding whether to treat an inmate with stimulant medications concerns current functioning and activities. Unless ADHD symptoms significantly interfere with an inmate's active engagement, or attempts to engage, in work assignments, educational activities, or other programming, the benefits of stimulants do not warrant the cost in resources or risks. We recommend making such dysfunction a prerequisite for stimulant treatment. Difficulties with leisure or recreational activities by themselves would not meet this functional threshold. The importance of active and observable impairment before initiating treatment makes sense for anyone, not just inmates. A diagnosis of ADHD requires the presence of symptoms in two or more settings and "clear evidence that the symptoms interfere with, or reduce the quality of . . . functioning" (American Psychiatric Association, 2013). Impairment could be measured by a combination of methods, including observations by custody staff, documented behavioral problems, input from family members or significant others when possible, and use of brief, easily administered rating scales that survey the presence of ADHD symptoms and associated functional impairments (Barkley & Murphy, 2006). These rating scales include self-report versions and versions that would allow others (e.g., correctional officers, work supervisors, family members, treatment providers) to rate an inmate's symptoms and impairments. Murphy and Barkley (2006) also provide scales to assist psychiatrists in rating side effects and measuring medication efficacy, a sample diagnostic interview, and questionnaires regarding developmental, social, vocational, and health histories.

Whenever possible, third-party sources can provide an important confirmation of an inmate's dysfunction in meaningful activities. These sources include work assignment supervisors, programming staff, continuing education teachers, and health care providers. The richest source of third-party information, however, may come from correctional officers who have regular contact with inmates during these activities and on their housing units. All of these observers have valuable information relevant to assessing ADHD, making the initial treatment decision, and performing ongoing assessments of treatment response. Use of observer and self-report rating scales can aid in both diagnosis and monitoring. Although not central to the diagnosis of ADHD, neuropsychological testing may help assess deficits in cognition, attention, learning, and executive functioning (American Academy of Child and Adolescent Psychiatry, 2007).

The special risks and challenges associated with the prescription of controlled substances in correctional facilities support an initial preference for nonstimulants, absent contraindications or previously adequate but unsuccessful trials. When stimulants prove necessary, the shorter-acting agents, although not FDA approved for adults, have the benefit of being crushable and thus not as susceptible to diversion and misuse. The disadvantage of more frequent administration lessens if dosing occurs only when needed for important activities.

Continuing prescriptions for inmates who misuse or divert their medications makes little sense and undermines the credibility of the psychiatrist among nursing and custody staff. The same concerns apply to the possession or distribution of any substances, including other prescription medications. We recommend warning inmates of the consequences of such behavior, which include immediate discontinuation of their ADHD medication.

Access to medications should also require engagement in appropriate nonpharmacological interventions. An inmate who does not meaningfully participate in recommended ADHD educational and therapeutic activities has not shown full investment in managing the disorder.

This approach to assessment and treatment in correctional settings appropriately limits the number of inmates who receive stimulant medications. Those who truly need these medications will receive them, and those who do not, won't. Some may view this practice as unjustifiably restrictive and others may see it as injudiciously permissive (Appelbaum, 2009; Burns, 2009), but we believe that it strikes a reasonable balance. The implementation of this protocol in a relatively well-staffed and -resourced correctional mental health system resulted in a stimulant treatment prevalence of about 1% of all state inmates over a two-year time span (Appelbaum, 2011). Although below the ADHD prevalence estimates reported in the literature, these inmates represented an entire state prison population and had verified current impairment in areas of important functioning, rather than simply screening positive on self-report or other rating scales. Thus, the implementation experience of one system may provide a more realistic estimate of the number of inmates likely to qualify for stimulant medications under a similar protocol.

Summary

The existing literature gives widely disparate estimates of ADHD prevalence among inmates. Regardless of the actual numbers, some inmates have a compelling need for treatment, including stimulant medications. Neither unbridled use nor complete elimination of stimulants makes good clinical or administrative sense for correctional systems. An approach that relies on current impairment in significant functional areas, meaningful involvement in treatment, and absence of active misuse of substances will allow access to medication for those with verifiable need while lessening the risks associated with the prescription of controlled substances in jails and prisons.

References

American Academy of Child and Adolescent Psychiatry (2007). Practice parameter for the assessment and treatment of children and adolescents with attention-deficit/hyperactivity disorder. *Journal of the American Academy of Child and Adolescent Psychiatry, 46*(7), 894–921.

American Psychiatric Association (2000). *Psychiatric services in jails and prisons: Task Force to Revise the APA Guidelines on Psychiatric Services in Jails and Prisons* (Rep. No. 2). Washington, DC: American Psychiatric Association.

American Psychiatric Association (2013). *Diagnostic and Statistical Manual of Mental Disorders* (5th ed.). Arlington, VA: American Psychiatric Publishing.

Appelbaum, K. L. (2009). Attention deficit hyperactivity disorder in prison: a treatment protocol. *Journal of the American Academy of Psychiatry & the Law, 37,* 45–49.

Appelbaum, K. L. (2011). Stimulant use under a prison treatment protocol for attention-deficit/hyperactivity disorder. *Journal of Correctional Health Care, 17,* 218–225.

Barkley, R. A., & Murphy, K. R. (2006). *Attention-deficit hyperactivity disorder: A clinical workbook.* New York: Guilford Press.

Barkley, R. A., Murphy. K. R., & Fischer, M. (2008). *ADHD in adults: What the science says.* New York: Guilford Press.

Burns, K. A. (2009) The top ten reasons to limit prescription of controlled substances in prisons. *Journal of the American Academy of Psychiatry & the Law, 37,* 50–52.

Curran, S., & Fitzgerald, M. (1999) Attention deficit hyperactivity disorder in the prison population. *American Journal of Psychiatry, 156,* 1664–1665.

Daderman, A. M., Lindgren, M., & Lidberg, L. (2004) The prevalence of dyslexia and AD/HD in a sample of forensic psychiatric rapists. *Nordic Journal of Psychiatry, 58,* 371–381.

Dalteg, A., Gustafsson, P., & Levander, S. (1998). [Hyperactivity syndrome is common among prisoners. ADHD not only a pediatric psychiatric diagnosis]. *Lakartidningen, 95,* 3078–3080.

Eyestone, L. L., & Howell, R. J. (1994). An epidemiological study of attention-deficit hyperactivity disorder and major depression in a male prison population. *Bulletin of the American Academy of Psychiatry & the Law, 22,* 181–193.

Fayyad, J., De Graaf, R., Kessler, R., et al. (2007). Cross-national prevalence and correlates of adult attention-deficit hyperactivity disorder. *British Journal of Psychiatry, 190,* 402–409.

Ginsberg, Y., Hirvikoski, T., & Lindefors, N. (2010). Attention deficit hyperactivity disorder (ADHD) among longer-term prison inmates is a prevalent, persistent and disabling disorder. *BMC Psychiatry, 10,* 112.

Glaze, L. E. (2010). Correctional populations in the United States, 2009. *Bureau of Justice Statistics Bulletin,* December, 2010, NCJ 231681. Washington, DC, U.S. Department of Justice. Available at http://www.bjs.gov/index.cfm?ty=pbdetail&iid=2316

Gordon, V., Williams, D. J., & Donnelly, P. D. (2012). Exploring the relationship between ADHD symptoms and prison breaches of discipline amongst youths in four Scottish prisons. *Public Health, 126,* 343–348.

Grieger, L., & Hosser, D. (2012). Attention deficit hyperactivity disorder does not predict criminal recidivism in young adult offenders: Results from a prospective study. *International Journal of Law and Psychiatry, 35,* 27–34.

Kessler, R. C., Adler, L., Barkley, R., et al. (2006). The prevalence and correlates of adult ADHD in the United States: results from the National Comorbidity Survey Replication. *American Journal of Psychiatry, 163,* 716–723.

Kieling, C., Kieling, R. R., Rohde, L. A., et al. (2010). The age at onset of attention deficit hyperactivity disorder. *American Journal of Psychiatry, 167,* 14–16.

Lichtenstein, P., Halldner, L., Zetterqvist, J., et al. (2012) Medication for attention deficit-hyperactivity disorder and criminality. *New England Journal of Medicine, 367,* 2006–2014.

Lindgren, M., Jensen, J., Dalteg, A., Meurling, A. W., Ingvar, A. H., & Levandar, S. (2002). Dyslexia and AD/HD among Swedish prison inmates. *Journal of Scandinavian Studies in Criminology and Crime Prevention, 3,* 84–95.

McCallon, D. (2000). Diagnosing and treating ADHD in a men's prison. In D. Fishbein (Ed.), *The science, treatment, and prevention of antisocial behaviors: application to the criminal justice system* (pp. 1–21). Kingston, NJ: Civic Research Institute.

Moore, E., Sunjic, S., Kaye, S., et al. (2013). Adult ADHD among NSW prisoners: Prevalence and psychiatric comorbidity. *Journal of Attention Disorders* (Epub Oct 17).

Mumola, C., & Karberg, J. (2006). *Drug use and dependence, state and federal prisoners, 2004.* US Department of Justice, Bureau of Justice Statistics.

Murphy, K. (2005). Psychosocial treatments for ADHD in teens and adults: a practice-friendly review. *Journal of Clinical Psychology, 61,* 607–619.

Murphy, K. R., & Adler, L. A. (2004). Assessing attention-deficit/hyperactivity disorder in adults: focus on rating scales. *Journal of Clinical Psychiatry, 65*(Suppl 3), 12–17.

Murphy, K. R., & Gordon, M. (2006). Assessment of adults with ADHD. In R. A. Barkley (Ed.), *Attention–deficit hyperactivity disorder: a handbook for diagnosis and treatment* (3rd ed.). New York: The Guilford Press.

Rasmussen, K., Almvik, R., & Levander, S. (2001) Attention deficit hyperactivity disorder, reading disability, and personality disorders in a prison population. *Journal of the American Academy of Psychiatry & the Law, 29,* 186–193.

Rosler, M., Retz, W., Retz-Junginger, P., et al. (2004). Prevalence of attention-deficit/hyperactivity disorder (ADHD) and comorbid disorders in young male prison inmates. *European Archives of Psychiatry and Clinical Neuroscience, 254,* 365–371.

Safren, S. A., Otto, M. W., Sprich, S., et al. (2005). Cognitive-behavioral therapy for ADHD in medication-treated adults with continued symptoms. *Behavioral Research and Therapy, 43,* 831–842.

Simon, V., Czobor, P., Balint, S., et al. (2009). Prevalence and correlates of adult attention-deficit hyperactivity disorder: meta-analysis. *British Journal of Psychiatry, 194,* 204–211.

Turgay, A., Goodman, D. W., Asherson, P., et al. (2012). Lifespan persistence of ADHD: the life transition model and its application. *Journal of Clinical Psychiatry, 73,* 192–201.

Westmoreland, P., Gunter, T., Loveless, P., et al. (2010). Attention deficit hyperactivity disorder in men and women newly committed to prison: clinical characteristics, psychiatric comorbidity, and quality of life. *International Journal of Offender Therapy and Comparative Criminology, 54,* 361–377.

Young, S., Gudjonsson, G. H., Wells, J., et al. (2009). Attention deficit hyperactivity disorder and critical incidents in a Scottish prison population. *Personality and Individual Differences, 46,* 265–269.

Ziegler, P., Blocher, D., Gross, J., et al. (2003). Erfassung von Symptomen aus dem Spektrum des Hyperkinetischen Syndroms bei Haftlingen einer Justizvollzugsanstalt [Assessment of attention deficit hyperactivity disorder (ADHD) in prison inmates]. *Recht & Psychiatrie, 21,* 17–21.

CHAPTER 38

General medical disorders with psychiatric implications

Erik J. Garcia and Warren J. Ferguson

Introduction

Medical conditions that have psychiatric symptoms represent a significant diagnostic dilemma, particularly in the correctional health setting. More than half of the inmates in the United States have symptoms of a major mental illness (James & Glaze, 2006). However, the pervasiveness of substance use disorders, the increasing prevalence of elderly inmates (Carson & Sabol, 2012), and limited access to a patient's past medical and psychiatric records all contribute to the challenge of discerning when a psychiatric presentation results from an underlying medical condition. One early study underscored this challenge, noting that 46% of the patients admitted to community psychiatric wards had an unrecognized medical illness that either caused or exacerbated their psychiatric illness (Hall et al., 1981). A more recent study observed that 55 of 1,340 admissions (2.8%) to inpatient psychiatry were due to unrecognized medical conditions (Reeves et al., 2010). Emergency room medical clearance of patients who present for psychiatric admission has revealed an increased risk for such underlying medical conditions among patients with any of the following five characteristics: advanced age, a history of substance abuse, no prior history of mental illness, lower socioeconomic status (SES), or significant preexisting medical illnesses (Gregory et al., 2004).

This chapter examines several of these risk groups and focuses on the presenting symptoms of delirium, mood disorders, and psychosis and the underlying medical conditions that can mimic or exacerbate them.

High-risk association

Inmates share many risk factors, especially substance abuse and low SES, associated with higher incidence of psychiatric presentation of medical illnesses. Patients recently incarcerated may experience withdrawal from prescribed or abused substances for up to two weeks following admission (Kosten & O'Connor, 2003), with symptoms ranging from depression and anxiety to frank psychosis (see Chapter 17). Traumatic brain injury (TBI), seen in 48% to 72% of inmates (McKinlay et al., 2013), is closely associated with substance abuse and low SES and may present with delirium and dementia, depression, mood lability, and impulsivity (see Chapter 53). Finally, elderly patients, particularly those with multiple significant medical conditions, have higher risk for a psychiatric presentation of medical issues. With almost 10% of

inmates aged >55 years and that % on the rise (Carson & Sabol, 2012), this scenario will become more prevalent (see Chapter 57). Past medical and mental health evaluations should be obtained whenever possible to help assess the etiology of current psychiatric symptoms. Lack of prior mental health diagnoses should prompt a particularly thorough evaluation.

Delirium and dementia

Delirium is an acute state of confusion or disturbance of consciousness caused by an underlying medical condition and characterized by rapid onset and fluctuating severity (Lipowski, 1989; Sood & McStay, 2009). Features include inability to sustain attention, global disruption of cognition, and disruption of the sleep–wake cycle, with symptoms often worse at night. The most common causes of delirium are substance use and withdrawal in younger patients and medication side effects in older patients. Anticholinergic medications are most commonly associated with delirium in the elderly, but nonsteroidal antiinflammatory drugs, diuretics, antihypertensives, and cimetidine have also been implicated (Lipowski, 1989). Infections, especially urinary tract and pulmonary, also commonly cause delirium in the elderly, while central nervous system (CNS) infection (encephalitis) can cause delirium in all age groups. Patients with HIV have a significant risk for delirium because of HIV CNS infection, CNS encephalitis (often due to cytomegalovirus or herpes simplex virus), and mass lesions (commonly lymphoma or toxoplasmosis). Other conditions associated with delirium include metabolic derangements such as hepatic failure and uremia, hyponatremia, hypokalemia, hypocalcemia, and hypoglycemia. Hyperosmolar states, as seen in severe hyperglycemia, can also present with delirium. Vitamin B12 deficiency caused by malabsorption, proton pump inhibitor use, or bariatric surgery (also a risk for thiamine [vitamin B1] deficiency) can present with acute delirium or dementia (Kibirige et al., 2013).

In the *Diagnostic and Statistical Manual of Mental Disorders*–5, dementia has been grouped among neurocognitive disorders (NCDs), which include cognitive changes from TBI or HIV (American Psychiatric Association, 2013, pp. 591–643). Dementia more commonly describes cognitive decline in the elderly. As with delirium, dementia can present with global cognitive impairment, affecting memory, thought process, and orientation. Unlike delirium, however, dementia has a slow and insidious onset; stable, instead of fluctuating, symptoms; and no alteration of consciousness or attention. Language skills are often minimally affected, which may delay early recognition of the disorder.

In younger patients, NCD most commonly occurs with TBI, a condition suffered by more than half of the current prison population (McKinlay et al., 2013). Prolonged alcohol abuse, particularly in patients with poor nutritional intake, is associated with Korsakoff dementia. Although less frequent now that highly active antiretroviral therapy is available, HIV-associated CNS diseases remain common. HIV encephalopathy, progressive multifocal leukoencephalopathy (PML), and toxoplasmosis may all present as dementia (Garvey et al., 2011). Other infections such as Lyme disease and neurosyphilis should also be considered in the evaluation (Miklossy, 2008). In older patients, Alzheimer's dementia and multi-infarct (vascular) dementia remain the most common causes of NCD, but the differential includes mass-occupying lesion (particularly with focal neurological findings), Parkinson's disease, frontotemporal neurocognitive disorder, Lewy body dementia, and prion-associated disease (Manning & Ducharme, 2010).

Medical conditions presenting as mood disorders

A strong association exists between many medical conditions and major depressive disorder (MDD). Between 10% and 15% of patients with a recent myocardial infarction or stroke, especially a left middle carotid artery, have symptoms of MDD (Gadalla, 2008); MDD occurs at a rate 1.2 to 2 times higher in adults with type 2 diabetes (Anderson et al., 2001; Markowitz et al., 2011). Depression is the most common comorbidity found in patients who have one or more chronic diseases (Sinnige et al., 2013). While the causality of debilitating medical illness and major depression is complex and multifactorial, several medical conditions present with symptoms of MDD, which often resolve with treatment.

Endocrine disorders, which are frequently unrecognized, often present with symptoms of depression. These disorders include hypothyroidism, hyperadrenalism (Cushing syndrome), adrenal insufficiency (Addison's disease), hyperparathyroidism, and hypoparathyroidism. Other presenting symptoms can include slowed mental processing and impaired memory with hypothyroidism, irritability and mental slowing with hyperparathyroidism (resulting in hypercalcemia), and hypoparathyroidism (Levenson, 2006; O'Brien et al., 2006). Each condition has associated physical and laboratory hallmarks that can aid in recognition, but they are often detected in routine lab tests (see "Patient Evaluation"). Finally, with the growing prevalence of obesity, obstructive sleep apnea is an important consideration. A clear link has been established between obstructive sleep apnea and major depression (Schroder & O'Hara, 2005).

Between 38% and 45% of patients with HIV have depression (Rabkin, 2008). Inmates infected through intravenous drug use may have an even higher prevalence given the independent association between intravenous drug use and depression (Mackesy-Amiti et al., 2012). Of particular concern, depression in patients with HIV may indicate an underlying opportunistic infection (e.g., toxoplasmosis), a mass-occupying lesion (e.g., CNS lymphoma), or HIV-related cognitive decline (e.g., HIV

encephalopathy, PML; Cohen et al., 1999). Even some treatment regimens, specifically those containing efavirenz, have severe depression as a common side effect.

Anxiety and panic attacks can be associated with many medical conditions, presenting a diagnostic challenge. The new or sudden onset of anxiety or panic should prompt a rapid evaluation for several serious physiological causes such as hypoxemia and hypoglycemia. Hypoglycemia is nearly always iatrogenic. Atrial fibrillation, congestive heart failure, myocardial infarction, asthma, and use of beta-agonist inhalers (the mainstay of treatment for bronchospasm) may present with symptoms of anxiety. Anxiety can also occur with endocrine disorders such as hypothyroidism, hyperthyroidism, and pheochromocytoma; the latter two are associated with tremor and tachycardia. As with depression, anxiety may accompany chronic medical conditions, most notably TBI, Parkinson's disease, and chronic obstructive pulmonary disease (Lavery & White, 2009).

Medical conditions presenting with psychosis or mania

Delusions or hallucinations caused by medical illness are most frequently a component of delirium and dementia seen in patients aged ≥65 years (Patkar et al., 2004; Rabins et al., 1982). Up to 40% of patients with Alzheimer's disease have auditory or visual hallucinations (Paulsen et al., 2001). Hallucinations and paranoia commonly occur with Parkinson's disease and its treatment with dopamine agonists and in conjunction with the characteristic rigidity and ataxia; psychosis with Huntington's disease often precedes the characteristic choreiform movements (Shiwach, 1994). Psychotic symptoms may occur with systemic lupus erythematous (SLE; Rogers, 1996) and multiple sclerosis, but depression is more common. Refractory epilepsy has been associated with an increased prevalence of schizophrenia (Fruchter et al., 2014), and some seizures can cause hallucinations. For example, nondominant hemisphere temporal lobe seizures happen with mania and psychoses, while isolated auditory hallucinations occur with dominant temporal lobe seizures (Mula, 2014).

Metabolic and endocrine abnormalities such as thyrotoxicosis and rarely hypothyroidism (Prasad's syndrome) can present with mania and psychosis (Mula, 2014). Adrenal insufficiency (Addison's disease) and, more commonly, Cushing syndrome can also present with depression, mania, and psychosis (Kelly, 1996; Leigh & Kramer, 1984). In addition, treatment with high doses of corticosteroids may produce psychotic symptoms such as hallucinations or behavior that may be confused with mania.

Olfactory or gustatory hallucinations suggest underlying seizures, while tactile hallucinations suggest substance intoxication or withdrawal. Auditory hallucinations, while more commonly seen in schizophrenia, may be a feature of medically related psychosis.

Patient evaluation

Some features should raise the suspicion that a psychiatric presentation is the result of an underlying medical condition. As noted previously, the elderly inmate, those with multiple medical conditions, and patients with HIV and substance use disorders are at particular risk.

Patients with a well-established history of major mental illness and documented response to appropriate treatment are unlikely to have a causative medical illness, though accurate records are rarely available in the correctional setting. Conversely, the new or abrupt onset of psychiatric symptoms should prompt further evaluation, especially when accompanied by somatic complaints or physical findings such as tachycardia, tremor, or alteration in cognitive function.

Clinical evaluation should include vital signs with oxymetry and finger-stick blood sugar, if available. In addition to a mental status evaluation, physical exam should include thyroid palpation, vascular exam (carotid bruits and pulse), cardiac and respiratory exam, and a thorough neurological exam. If there is suspicion of dementia, the Montreal Cognitive Test is particularly useful for diverse populations, as it has been validated in many languages (see http://www.mocatest.org/). Preliminary lab testing should include renal and hepatic functions, thyroid-stimulating hormone and free T4, vitamin B12, electrolytes, glucose, and serum calcium. Urinalysis or dipstick analysis is especially important for elderly patients with delirium. HIV and syphilis tests and toxicology screens should be obtained. Further lab evaluation might include testing for SLE.

Focal neurologic changes, evidence of a CNS infection such as meningeal signs, fever, and headache, or the new onset of psychosis or delirium all merit prompt referral for further evaluation and care.

Summary

Inmates have a high prevalence of mental illness, substance abuse, and chronic medical conditions that are often untreated prior to incarceration. The aging of incarcerated populations, frequent histories of TBI, and attention-seeking behavior further complicate systematic evaluation of behavioral health symptoms. Priority should be given to assessing patients for treatable, serious medical conditions that can mimic mental illness. Chief among these are metabolic derangements, conditions that lead to hypoxemia, acute substance withdrawal, CNS infections or space-occupying lesions, and iatrogenic side effects of prescribed medications.

References

American Psychiatric Association. (2013). *The Diagnostic and Statistical Manual of Mental Disorders, Fifth Edition.* Arlington, VA: American Psychiatric Association.

Anderson, R. J., Freedland, K. E., Clouse, R. E. & Lustman, P. J. (2001). The prevalence of comorbid depression in adults with diabetes: a meta-analysis. *Diabetes Care, 24,* 1069–1078.

Carson, E. A., & Sabol, W. J. (2012). *Prisoners in 2011.* (NCJ 239808). Washington, DC: Bureau of Justice Statistics, US Department of Justice.

Cohen, P. T., Sande, M. A., & Volberding, P. (1999). *The AIDS knowledge base: A textbook on HIV disease from the University of California* (Third Edition). Philadelphia: Lippincott-Raven.

Fruchter, E., Kapara, O., Reichenberg, A., Yoffe, R., Fono-Yativ, O., Kreiss, Y., et al. (2014). Longitudinal association between epilepsy and schizophrenia: A population-based study. *Epilepsy and Behavior, 31,* 291–294.

Gadalla, T. (2008). Association of comorbid mood disorders and chronic illness with disability and quality of life in Ontario, Canada. *Chronic Diseases and Injuries in Canada, 28,* 148–154.

Garvey, L., Winston, A., Walsh, J., et al. (2011). HIV-associated central nervous system diseases in the recent combination antiretroviral therapy era. *European Journal of Neurology, 18,* 527–534.

Gregory, R. J., Nihalani, N. D., & Rodriguez, E. (2004). Medical screening in the emergency department for psychiatric admissions: a procedural analysis. *General Hospital Psychiatry, 26,* 405–410.

Hall, R. C., Gardner, E. R., Popkin, M. K., Lecann, A. F., & Stickney, S. K. (1981). Unrecognized physical illness prompting psychiatric admission: A prospective study. *American Journal of Psychiatry, 138,* 629–635.

James, D., & Glaze, L. (2006). *Mental health problems of prison and jail inmates.* (NCR 213600). Washington, DC: US Department of Justice, Office of Justice Programs, Bureau of Justice Statistics.

Kelly, W. F. (1996). Psychiatric aspects of Cushing's syndrome. *QJM, 89,* 543–551.

Kibirige, D., Wekesa, C., Kaddu-Mukasa, M. & Waiswa, M. (2013). Vitamin B12 deficiency presenting as an acute confusional state: a case report and review of literature. *African Health Sciences, 13,* 850–852.

Lavery, L. L., & White, E. M. (2009). Other cognitive and mental disorders due to a general medical condition. In B. J. Sadock, V. A. Sadock, & P. Ruiz (Eds.), *Kaplan & Sadock's comprehensive textbook of psychiatry* (9th ed., p. 1226). New York: Lippincott, Williams & Wilkins.

Leigh, H., & Kramer, S. I. (1984). The psychiatric manifestations of endocrine disease. *Advances in Internal Medicine, 29,* 413–445.

Levenson, J. L. (2006). Psychiatric issues in endocrinology. *Primary Psychiatry, 13,* 27–30.

Lipowski, Z. J. (1989). Delirium in the elderly patient. *New England Journal of Medicine, 320,* 578–582.

Mackesy-Amiti, M. E., Donenberg, G. R., & Ouellet, L. J. (2012). Prevalence of psychiatric disorders among young injection drug users. *Drug and Alcohol Dependence, 124,* 70–78.

Manning, C. A., & Ducharme, J. K. (2010). Dementia syndromes in the older adult. In P. A. Lichtenberg (Ed.), *Handbook of Assessment in Clinical Gerontology* (2nd ed., pp. 155–178). San Diego, CA: Academic Press. DOI:10.1016/B978-0-12-374961-1.10006-5

Markowitz, S. M., Gonzalez, J. S., Wilkinson, J. L., & Safren, S. A. (2011). A review of treating depression in diabetes: emerging findings. *Psychosomatics, 52,* 1–18.

McKinlay, A., Corrigan, J., Horwood, L. J., & Fergusson, D. M. (2013). Substance abuse and criminal activities following traumatic brain injury in childhood, adolescence, and early adulthood. *Journal of Head Trauma Rehabilitation* [Epub ahead of print]. doi:10.1097/HTR.0000000000000001

Miklossy, J. (2008). Biology and neuropathology of dementia in syphilis and Lyme disease. *Handbook of Clinical Neurology, 89,* 825–844.

Mula, M. (2014). Epilepsy-induced behavioral changes during the ictal phase. *Epilepsy and Behavior, 30,* 14–16.

O'Brien, R. F., Kifuji, K., & Summergrad, P. (2006). Medical conditions with psychiatric manifestations. *Adolescent Medicine Clinics, 17,* 49–77.

Patkar, A. A., Mago, R., & Masand, P. S. (2004). Psychotic symptoms in patients with medical disorders. *Current Psychiatry Reports, 6,* 216–224.

Paulsen, J. S., Ready, R. E., Hamilton, J. M., Mega, M. S. & Cummings, J. L. (2001). Neuropsychiatric aspects of Huntington's disease. *Journal of Neurology, Neurosurgery and Psychiatry, 71,* 310–314.

Rabins, P. V., Mace, N. L., & Lucas, M. J. (1982). The impact of dementia on the family. *Journal of the American Medical Assocaiton, 248,* 333–335.

Rabkin, J. G. (2008). HIV and depression: 2008 review and update. *Current HIV/AIDS Reports, 5,* 163–171.

Rogers, M. (1996). Psychiatric aspects. In P. H. Schur (Ed.), *The clinical management of systemic lupus erythymatosus* (2nd ed.). Philadelphia, PA: Lippincott-Raven.

Schroder, C. M., & O'Hara, R. (2005). Depression and obstructive sleep apnea (OSA). *Annals of General Psychiatry, 4,* 13.

Shiwach, R. (1994). Psychopathology in Huntington's disease patients. *Acta Psychiatrica Scandinavica, 90,* 241–246.

Sinnige, J., Braspenning, J., Schellevis, F., Stirbu-Wagner, I., Westert, G., & Korevaar, J. (2013). The prevalence of disease clusters in older adults with multiple chronic diseases—a systematic literature review. *PLoS One, 8,* e79641.

Sood, T. R., & McStay, C. M. (2009). Evaluation of the psychiatric patient. *Emergency Medical Clinics of North America, 27,* 669–683, ix.

CHAPTER 39

Psychiatric aspects of pain management

Psychiatric assessment and management of chronic pain in correctional settings

Robert L. Trestman

Introduction

Chronic pain differs from acute pain in many ways. First, by definition, the pain has become enduring and goes beyond the expected period of healing, whether post-trauma, post-surgery, or as part of a degenerative or progressive disease. The typical time frame used for defining chronic pain is longer than six months (Turk & Okifuji, 2001). Another characteristic that distinguishes chronic from acute pain is the emotional element of perceived suffering (Turk & Okifuji, 2001). In this context, suffering is the experiential component distinct from nociceptive activity that typically defines the experience of acute pain (Turk & Okifuji, 2001). This component of chronic pain becomes important in the assessment and subsequent treatment of chronic pain.

Chronic pain management in a correctional setting is very challenging due to a host of factors. First, the majority of people being treated have a history of substance abuse disorders (Fazel et al., 2006). Further, as a whole, the population of incarcerated adults has a disproportionate prevalence of significant chronic medical and psychiatric conditions (Rich et al., 2011). Finally, access to illicit drugs is limited, if not completely eliminated, in correctional settings, shifting the environmental demand characteristics to prescription medication misuse.

This chapter addresses issues of the psychiatric assessment and management of chronic pain in correctional settings. Apropos of the assessment, information is provided regarding the factors to be elicited in a chronic pain interview, the methods used to assess chronic pain, and the assessment factors appropriate to integrate into a management plan. Subsequently, the methods used to manage chronic pain from a psychiatric perspective in the correctional setting are discussed. The need for consistent communication and interdisciplinary coordination, which are key elements of successful pain management, is reviewed. The factors involved in a management plan and various methods for tracking the outcomes of treatment, some unique to correctional settings, are also described.

Assessment of chronic pain

Biological factors

As with any appropriate assessment of chronic pain, a comprehensive history, physical examination, and review of any available prior records should be conducted. General health status, relevant laboratory data, and current and past medications should be documented, as well as the character of current pain and other physiological symptoms. Any recent changes, such as precipitating events that elicited the referral (e.g., increased pain, decreased function, contemplation of surgery) should be noted. Specific characteristics of the pain problem that should be recorded include the nature, location, and frequency of symptoms. Any needed diagnostic tests should be ordered and conducted to rule in or out treatable underlying conditions.

Psychiatric diagnoses to consider

Multiple psychiatric conditions may present with complaints of pain, may co-occur with the disorder causing the pain, or may exacerbate the pain. These psychiatric illnesses include mood disorders, anxiety disorders, personality disorders, somatoform disorders, factitious disorders, and malingering. Treatment for primary disorders of mood, anxiety, and personality would proceed as per standard practice and are addressed elsewhere in this text (Chapters 33, 34, and 35). Complaints of pain associated with or exacerbated by these disorders would be expected to be alleviated as the disorders are treated. In one study of chronic pain patients in a community setting, fully 70% had a cooccurring psychiatric disorder (Workman et al., 2002). More than 90% of those patients without a psychiatric illness responded well to therapy for chronic pain, but fewer than 40% of those with a *Diagnostic and Statistical Manual of Mental Disorders* (DSM)–IV psychiatric condition on Axis I or II improved in response to treatment (Workman et al., 2002).

Psychiatric disorders that relate directly to the presentation of pain include somatic symptom disorder, factitious disorder, and malingering. These syndromes are discussed here.

Somatic symptom disorder

As outlined in DSM-5, a focused pain complaint that cannot be entirely attributed to a specific medical disorder, and yet is causing genuine suffering and distress, is the core characteristic of somatic symptom disorder with predominant pain (American Psychiatric Association, 2013, pp. 311–315). Specific symptoms of somatic symptom disorder with predominant pain include the following: (A) pain in one or more anatomical sites that produces a predominant clinical focus and that is distressing or impairs daily activity; (B) psychological factors (excessive thoughts, feelings, or behaviors associated with the pain) that are disproportionate to the symptoms, are associated with persistent high levels of anxiety, and/or involve excessive devotion of time or energy; and (C) pain symptom(s) that persist for more than six months (American Psychiatric Association, 2013, p. 311). The disorder is classified as mild if only one of the criterion B symptoms are present, moderate if two or more are present, and severe if two or more are present and there are multiple somatic complaints. The prevalence rate of DSM-IV pain somatoform disorders (a more restrictive diagnosis than DSM-5 somatic symptom disorder with predominant pain) is 5.4%; 25% of diagnosed cases are positively assigned to psychological factors (Grabe et al., 2003). The sex ratio has been reported to be 2:1 female to male (Grabe et al., 2003). While the exact prevalence of somatic symptom disorder with predominant pain has not yet been determined, it is anticipated to be slightly higher than pain somatoform disorder (American Psychiatric Association, 2013, p. 312).

Factitious disorder

Factitious disorder involves physical or psychological symptoms that are intentionally produced or feigned to assume the sick role (American Psychiatric Association, 2013, pp. 324–326). The three key criteria for this disorder are falsification of symptoms or signs or intentional induction of illness or injury; presentation by the patient as being impaired or injured; and the occurrence of the behavior in the absence of obvious external rewards (American Psychiatric Association, 2013, p. 324). Typically, there are subjective symptoms such as complaints of acute abdominal pain in the absence of objective evidence of such pain. There may be self-inflicted conditions, which might include the production of abscesses by injection of saliva or feces into the skin. There may also be exaggeration or exacerbation of preexisting general medical conditions. This situation might present as, for example, feigning of a grand mal seizure by an individual with a previous history of seizure disorder. A defining characteristic of a factitious disorder is that external incentives for the behaviors, such as economic gain or avoiding legal responsibility, are absent. Factitious disorder with mostly physical symptoms is commonly referred to as Munchausen syndrome, named for an eighteenth-century German officer known to embellish his life story.

Malingering

Malingering is defined as the "intentional production of false or grossly exaggerated physical or psychological symptoms, motivated by external incentives such as avoiding military duty, avoiding work, obtaining financial compensation, evading criminal prosecution, or obtaining drugs" (American Psychiatric Association, 2013, p. 726). Generally speaking, there are four core criteria, two or more of which must be met for the diagnosis. The criteria are financial or legal benefit—there is no reason to malinger without an incentive; marked discrepancy between claimed disability and objective findings—potential malingering exists when the behavior is conscious and purposeful; lack of cooperation with testing or treatment; and a confirmed diagnosis of antisocial personality disorder (American Psychiatric Association, 2013, p. 727).

Correctional settings clearly set the stage for malingering behavior, since opportunities to manage and control the environment by the offender are typically otherwise very limited. However, real caution must be exercised in making a diagnosis of malingering. The risk of inappropriately withholding appropriate treatment is a major concern. Also, once someone is labeled as a malingerer, his or her concerns or threats (e.g., of suicide) may be ignored, with potentially serious consequences.

Case example

A patient with low back pain in a medium-security facility was repeatedly observed ambulating with a walker by program personnel. On one occasion, when he was unaware that he was being observed, he was seen casually carrying his walker over his shoulder while ambulating with appropriate body posture and gait. Staff subsequently conducted a thorough assessment to determine the motive: Was the patient keeping the walker to use as a weapon, as a method to conceal contraband, or perhaps as evidence of continued need for pain medication?

First, there is no simple test for malingering. Formal assessments do exist (McDermott & Feldman, 2007). One example is the Structured Interview of Reported Symptoms–2, which takes about 60 minutes to administer and score (Rogers et al., 2010, 1990). Beyond formal assessment, the clinician must look for supporting data and for a compelling pattern. Such data would include a self-reported history that is discrepant with the documented history. The reported complaints might be inconsistent with physiology—for example, a midline split of sensation (Stone, Carson & Sharpe, 2005). Self-reported symptoms that are inconsistent with observations by clinical or correctional staff are another important observation when available. Malingering is possible when the symptoms do not improve with appropriate treatment or when test results dispute information provided by the patient (Aronoff et al., 2007). Additional patient behaviors that are consistent with malingering include accurately predicting physical deteriorations; providing inconsistent, selective, or misleading information; refusing to sign appropriate releases of information for community providers; and focusing on "victimization" by medical personnel (McDermott & Feldman, 2007).

Differential diagnosis

In contrast to factitious disorders and malingering, somatic symptom disorders are not under voluntary (conscious) control. Somatic symptom disorders are conceptualized as having a predominantly psychological etiology (American Psychiatric Association, 2013, p. 314).

The clinical interview

The individual methods used are not as important as the comprehensive nature of the assessment. Any psychological testing results, mental status examination, or other data must be interpreted within the context of the chronic pain problem and symptoms. Elements of a comprehensive psychiatric assessment of chronic pain include a clinical interview, medical history, substance abuse history, pain history, relevant psychosocial histories (family, work, educational), legal history in the context of civil litigation, and specific assessment of pain-coping skills.

The initial history should include a focus on how the pain is interfering with the patient's daily life rather than subjective reports of how strong the pain is. In addition to the standard information to be gathered, specific elements are important to address. How well does the patient understand the pain problem and the expected course of treatment? What is the patient's attitude toward health, illness, and health care providers? How substantial is the perceived threat of illness to the patient's life and functional level? What perceived control over the symptoms does the patient have? What are the patient's expectations about the future? What are the patient's religious beliefs that could affect his or her engagement in treatment? History of childhood sexual abuse may be a contributing risk factor to the development of chronic pain (Paras et al., 2009).

The extent and prominence of substance abuse are key in the assessment. The degree to which the patient turns to medication or drugs as a solution to problems (as opposed to self-motivation, effort, and active participation in treatment) may inform the expected complexity and prognosis of therapy. For example, while a history of opiate abuse does not absolutely rule out opiate pain management, it does complicate treatment because the patient probably has opiate tolerance levels that will require high-dose treatment.

What is the pain history? While the primary care physician, internist, or specialist may have already established this, it is important to hear from the patient the characteristics and variability of the pain. Key elements here include circadian variability and activities that may increase or diminish the experience of pain. Use of a structured tool to assess coping strategies may also prove valuable (Harland & Georgieff, 2003).

Observation serves as a critical basis for the assessment. Is the behavior consistent with the experience of pain? Does the patient talk about or complain about the pain during the day among staff or other inmates? Is there grimacing, moaning, limping, or retarded movement consistent with the expressed pain? Does the patient rub the painful area, use assistive devices such as a cane or brace, or avoid certain activities? Beyond the complaints of symptoms, assessment of functional impairment is important. Are there limitations to activities of daily living such as self-care, exercise, or interpersonal skills?

The correctional environment offers something that outpatient evaluation in the community does not: round-the-clock observation by custody staff. It is very useful to ask custody staff on the inmate's unit about the inmate's activities when he or she is not conscious of being observed. Is there a difference in behavior?

The pattern of general health care use is also an area to explore. What are the nature, frequency, and pattern of past contacts with the health care team? Is there evidence in the chart of current and past history of adherence to recommended treatment? Is there documentation that medication has been taken as prescribed? Did the patient generally keep scheduled appointments? Did the patient tend to follow through on previous recommendations? This information can help give context to the likely ability and motivation of the patient to engage in treatment of chronic pain.

Given the correctional environment, careful examination of potential secondary gains must be conducted. The typical concerns include addiction-related behavior, secondary market issues, and environmental issues. Substance use disorders are pandemic in correctional settings; enforced abstinence, which is the general rule in correctional settings, may complicate assessment but may clarify the disorders as well. Using DSM-5 criteria for substance use disorders (American Psychiatric Association, 2013, pp. 483–485), careful documentation in the medical record of the integrated assessment is important to guide treatment decisions. Specific factors associated with an increased risk of misuse of prescribed opiate medications for chronic pain include a prior history of opiate misuse, sedative-hypnotic abuse, family history of substance misuse, history of heavy tobacco use, and age <50 years (Sehgal et al., 2012).

Simply because a person with drug addiction is incarcerated does not mean that he or she no longer engages in drug-seeking behavior. The clinical challenge is to tease apart the relative contributions of genuine pain and motivation for treatment from an addict's desire for a high. A separate concern is the existence of secondary markets in many correctional settings. A patient may cheek, or even regurgitate, medication for resale. Extortion is also possible; other offenders may threaten an inmate with harm unless they are provided with the prescribed opiate. Environment is a challenge in correctional settings. The use of illness to manipulate the environment happens with some regularity. Inmates may complain of chronic pain and impaired mobility in an effort to be moved to a more comfortable housing unit or a bottom bunk.

Case example

Mr. Smith had been disabled for one year after a low-back work injury during his arrest. The patient had undergone a variety of diagnostic tests that did not identify likely pain generators. Although he complained of extreme pain, the physical findings simply did not explain his level of suffering and disability. During incarceration, Mr. Smith was placed in a lower bunk in a preferred housing unit with accommodations for those with disabilities.

Informed with a differential diagnosis and a detailed understanding of the extent and nature of the pain, the clinician can formulate an effective treatment plan to address the issues of chronic pain management, which is the topic of the following section.

Psychiatric management of chronic pain in a correctional setting

Psychiatric management of chronic pain is not done in isolation; to succeed it must be a coordinated team effort. Close collaboration with the treatment team, which should include primary or specialty care physicians, nurses, clinical therapists, and, where appropriate, custody staff, begins with a review of the treatment plan, a definition of everyone's roles, and the sequence of interventions. Clinical therapists, including both physical and occupational therapists, are often not available in a correctional setting.

Existing medical conditions must be identified and treated. Psychiatric conditions such as depression or anxiety should be treated aggressively. Existing substance abuse disorder should also be treated, even in the situation of enforced abstinence. If not, the underlying pathology, both physiological craving as well as psychological dependence, will continue to complicate the treatment of chronic pain (Garland et al., 2013).

Psychiatric disorders

Any co-occurring psychiatric disorder should be treated aggressively to improve the response to chronic pain management. Depression and anxiety are the most common co-occurring psychiatric conditions. While major advances are being made in the treatment of these disorders (Kupfer et al., 2012), realistic treatment options in correctional settings are often limited primarily to psychotropic medications and, to a facility-specific degree, appropriate cognitive-behavioral psychotherapy (CBT).

The treatment of somatic symptom disorder with predominant pain is often complicated, and there is little consensus in the field. There is conflicting evidence that CBT alone (Kroenke et al., 2007), CBT in combination with an antidepressant such as a selective serotonin reuptake inhibitor (SSRI; Kroenke, 2007), or an SSRI alone (Fishbain et al., 1997; Luo et al., 2009) may each prove effective in reducing the severity of the complaints and enhancing daily function. None of these studies was conducted in correctional settings, so the clinician and patient will likely be best served by an individually adapted approach that takes into account local resources and patient acceptance. This chapter does not address interventional therapies, which range from site-specific steroid injections to corrective surgeries.

Initiating treatment

Following the assessment, an important first step is to engage the patient in a review of findings and recommendations. A clearly written informed consent should be drafted and reviewed carefully with the patient. The informed consent should specify the nature of treatment and the responsibilities of the patient for adherence. If opiates are to be used, directly observed therapy is a near-universal requirement in correctional settings. Consequences for violations should be specified. Diversion of medication, failure of random urine drug testing (if indicated), falsification of continued disability, and similar actions should have clearly staged consequences, up to and including immediate tapering off of opiate medication.

Pain medication

Although it is beyond the scope of this chapter, it is important to recognize the limitations of medications in the management of chronic pain, particularly opiate medications (Chou et al., 2009; van Tulder & Koes, 2012). Their lack of clearly demonstrated effectiveness in chronic noncancer pain and their adverse side effects (Manchikanti et al., 2010), coupled with the risks of use in correctional settings (as noted previously), should make their use the exception rather than the rule. Sequential approaches to medication selection, starting with nonsteroidal antiinflammatories and progressing through opiates of increasing potency, should be followed (e.g., see Chou et al., 2009), with attention being paid to decreasing benefit over time and increasing side-effect burden (van Tulder & Koes, 2012). Adjuvant medications,

including anticonvulsants (gabapentin, pregabalin, topiramate) and antidepressants (amitriptyline, nortriptyline, duloxetine, venlafaxine), may also play an important role (Chou et al., 2009). In general, it is important to avoid the use of benzodiazepines whenever possible, as abuse potential in this context is substantial (Hojsted et al., 2013). Careful monitoring and documentation of ongoing benefit, potential dose escalation, and treatment adherence are critical to effective management of chronic pain with medications in the correctional setting.

Motivational interviewing

Miller and Rollnick (1991) developed a approach called Motivational Interviewing for use with drug-abusing patients. It has found extensive use over the intervening decades and is very relevant in the treatment of chronic pain (Kerns & Rosenberg, 2000). The concepts of rolling with resistance, change talk, self-efficacy, and ambivalence bring flexibility and often enhance engagement in the treatment process (Miller & Rollnick, 1991).

Cognitive–behavioral therapy

As noted previously, chronic pain incorporates substantial psychological components beyond pure physiological nociceptive stimulation. These psychological elements have generally been most successfully addressed with variants of CBT to target coping skills, self-regulation, and perceived functional limitations (Morley, 2011; Turk et al., 2002, 2008). One study that used CBT for patients with chronic pain and co-occurring substance abuse disorders found that 50% of patients were functioning well and were opiate-free at 12 months following the intervention. Components of this study included opiate medication reduction and CBT with resultant decease in perceived pain, improved functioning, and reduced distress (Currie et al., 2003). CBT is well suited to the correctional environment, as its various manualized versions allow for ease of learning, use, and monitoring and can generally be adapted to the specific facility requirements. While typically group-based, it can be delivered to an individual patient. It is highly structured and has integrated defined exercises to reinforce learning and generalizability to the specific problems being addressed. In CBT, people are seen as active processors of information rather than passive receivers. Thoughts are seen to affect affective and physiological arousal, both of which may serve to change behavior. Individuals are expected to take an active role. As outlined later, treatment includes targeted improvement in cognitive, emotional, physiological, and behavioral dysfunction.

Coping strategies

Basic psychotherapeutic coping strategies include avoiding negatives, focusing on the present tense, using first person, and keeping ideas realistic (Peres & Lucchetti, 2010). Examples include teaching patients to think in terms of "I will be confident and calm" in contrast to "I can't be nervous about the pain increasing" (avoiding negatives). Another example might be "I will work to recover fully after the surgery" versus the unrealistic thought that "the surgery will make my pain go away." Defining the strategies can be operationalized with a standardized assessment (Harland & Georgieff, 2003).

Functional analysis

A core component of many forms of CBT is functional analysis, wherein the patient is taught to deconstruct an event and then restructure it to allow for a positive outcome when a similar situation arises in the future (Rummel et al., 2012). The basic outline follows an easily remembered ABC format: (1) describe clearly the Activating event (e.g., back pain), (2) recognize the Belief associated with that event ("I can't cope with this"), and (3) describe the Consequent emotion(s) (hopelessness, fear, anger). The intervention consists of guided development of alternative, positive beliefs and consequent emotions to minimize distress (Rummel et al., 2012).

Relaxation therapy

Modern relaxation therapy techniques have been in use for more than 70 years (Jacobson, 1938). They have evolved substantially and include a variety of breathing techniques, progressive muscle relaxation, visualization exercises, meditation, and various forms of guided imagery (Chen & Francis, 2010). Practiced twice daily at times of relative quiet while in a comfortable position, relaxation techniques have been demonstrated to be a useful element in the psychotherapy of chronic pain management (Chen & Francis, 2010).

Monitoring progress

Individualized objective measures of progress provide a structured way to assess progress in these often-difficult cases. Multiple approaches that are used in concert will likely provide the best assessment. Typical assessments include pain questionnaires that target both symptoms and function (Haanpaa, 2011); daily diaries and scales maintained by the patient to record pain severity and functional activity (Haanpaa, 2011); and, in the correctional setting, perhaps most valuably, observation by clinical and custodial staff. Taken as a whole, these assessments can serve the clinician and patient as a valuable guide to treatment progress.

Summary

Chronic pain management is among the more challenging conditions to address in community settings. In correctional settings, with circumscribed boundaries, limited access to drugs of abuse, and careful monitoring, coherent treatment still requires close coordination by the treatment team and effective engagement by the patient. It does, nevertheless, offer significant opportunities to deliver effective treatment with significant functional improvement and symptom reduction beyond what may be possible in the community for patients with chronic pain and complex comorbidities, including substance abuse.

References

Aronoff, G. M., Mandel, S., Genovese, E., et al. (2007). Evaluating malingering in contested injury or illness. *Pain Practice, 7*(2), 178–204.

Chen, Y. L., & Francis, A. J. (2010). Relaxation and imagery for chronic, nonmalignant pain: Effects on pain symptoms, quality of life, and mental health. *Pain Management Nursing, 11*, 159–168.

Chou, R., Fanciullo, G. J., Fine, P. G., Adler, J. A., Ballantyne, J. C., Davies, P., . . . & Miaskowski, C. (2009). Clinical guidelines for the use of chronic opioid therapy in chronic noncancer pain. *The Journal of Pain, 10*(2), 113–130.

Currie, S. R., Hodgins, D. C., Crabtree, A., Jacobi, J., & Armstrong, S. (2003). Outcome from integrated pain management treatment for recovering substance abusers. *Journal of Pain, 4*(2), 91–100.

Fazel, S., Bains, P., & Doll, H. (2006). Substance abuse and dependence in prisoners: a systematic review. *Addiction, 101*(2), 181–191. DOI:10.1111/j.1360-0443.2006.01316.x

Fishbain, D. A., Cutler, R. B., Rosomoff, H. L., & Rosomoff, R. S. (1998). Do antidepressants have an analgesic effect in psychogenic pain and somatoform pain disorder? A meta-analysis. *Psychosomatic Medicine, 60*, 503–509.

Garland, E. L., Froeliger, B., Zeidan, F., Suveg, K., & Howard, M. O. (2013). The downward spiral of chronic pain, prescription opioid misuse, and addiction: Cognitive, affective, and neuropsychopharmacologic pathways. *Neuroscience and Biobehavioral Reviews.* doi:pii: S0149-7634(13)00196-6 10.1016/j.neubiorev.2013.08.006

Grabe, H. J., Meyer, C., Hapke, U., Rumpf, H. J., Freyberger, H. J., Dilling, H., & John, U. (2003). Somatoform pain disorder in the general population. *Psychotherapy and Psychosomatics, 72*(2), 88–94. DOI:10.1159/000068681

Harland, N. J., & Georgieff, K. (2003). Development of the Coping Strategies Questionnaire 24, a clinically utilitarian version of the coping strategies questionnaire. *Rehabilitation Psychology, 48*(3) 296–230.

Hojsted, J., Ekholm, O., Kurita, G. P., Juel, K., & Sjogren, P. (2013). Addictive behaviors related to opioid use for chronic pain: A population-based study. *Pain,* Accessed Sept. 1, 2013 at http://www.sciencedirect.com/science/article/pii/S0304395913004144

Institute for Clinical Systems Improvement (2011). *Assessment and management of chronic pain* (5th ed.). Bloomington, MN: Institute for Clinical Systems Improvement.

Jacobson, E. (1938). *Progressive relaxation.* Chicago: University of Chicago Press.

Kerns, R. D., & Rosenberg, R. (2000). Predicting responses to self-management treatments for chronic pain: application of the pain stages of change model. *Pain, 84*(1), 49–55.

Kroenke, K. (2007). Efficacy of treatment for somatoform disorders: A review of randomized controlled trials. *Psychosomatic Medicine, 69*, 881–888.

Kupfer, D. J., Frank, E., & Phillips, M. L. (2012). Major depressive disorder: New clinical, neurobiological, and treatment perspectives. *Lancet, 379*(9820), 1045–1055.

Luo, Y. L., Zhang, M. Y., Wu, W. Y., Li, C. B., Lu, Z., & Li, Q. W. (2009). A randomized double-blind clinical trial on analgesic efficacy of fluoxetine for persistent somatoform pain disorder. *Progress in Neuro-Psychopharmacology and Biological Psychiatry. 33*(8), 1522–1525.

Manchikanti, L., Benyamin, R., Datta, S., Vallejo, R., & Smith, H. (2010). Opioids in chronic noncancer pain. *Expert Review of Neurotherapeutics, 10*(5), 775–789. DOI:10.1586/ern.10.37

McDermott, B. E., & Feldman, M. D. (2007). Malingering in the medical setting. *Psychiatric Clinics of North America, 30*(4), 645–662.

Miller, W. R., & Rollnick, S. (1991). *Motivational Interviewing: Preparing people to change addictive behavior.* New York: Guilford Press.

Morley, S. (2011). Efficacy and effectiveness of cognitive behaviour therapy for chronic pain: Progress and some challenges. *Pain, 152*(3), S99–S106.

Haanpaa, M. (2011). NeuPSIG guidelines on neuropathic pain assessment. *Pain, 152*(1), 14–27.

Paras, M. L., Murad, M. H., Chen, L. P., et al. (2009). Sexual abuse and lifetime diagnosis of somatic disorders: a systematic review and meta-analysis. *Journal of the American Medical Association, 302*(5), 550–561. DOI:10.1001/jama.2009.1091

Peres, M. F., & Lucchetti, G. (2010). Coping strategies in chronic pain. *Current Pain and Headache Reports, 14*, 331–228.

Rich, J. D., Wakeman, S. E., & Dickman, S. L. (2011). Medicine and the epidemic of incarceration in the United States. *New England Journal of Medicine, 364*(22), 2081–2083. DOI:10.1056/NEJMp1102385

Rogers, R., Gillis, J. R., & Bagby, R. M. (1990). The SIRS as a measure of malingering: A validation study with a correctional sample. *Behavioral Sciences & the Law, 8*, 85–92. DOI:10.1002/bsl.2370080

Rogers, R., Sewell, K. W., & Gillard, N. D. (2010*). Structured Interview of Reported Symptoms (SIRS), 2nd edition, professional manual*. Lutz, FL: Psychological Assessment Resources, Inc.

Rummel, C., Garrison-Diehn, C., Catlin, C., & Fisher, J. E. (2012). Clinical functional analysis: Understanding the contingencies of reinforcement. In W. O'Donahue & J. S. Fisher (Eds.), *Cognitive behavior therapy: core principles for practice* (pp. 13–36). J. Wiley & Sons, DOI:10.1002/9781118470886

Sehgal, N., Manchikanti, L., & Smith, H. S. (2012). Prescription opioid abuse in chronic pain: A review of opioid abuse predictors and strategies to curb opioid abuse. *Pain Physician, 15*, ES67–ES92.

Stone, J., Carson, A., & Sharpe, M. (2005). Functional symptoms in neurology: management. *Journal of Neurology, Neurosurgery & Psychiatry, 76*(suppl 1), i13–i21.

Turk, D. C., & Okifuji, A. (2001). Pain terms and taxonomies. In D. Loeser, S. H. Butler, J. J. Chapman, et al. (Eds.), *Bonica's management of pain* (3rd ed., pp. 18–25). Philadelphia: Lippincott Williams & Wilkins.

Turk, D. C., & Okifuji, A. (2002). Psychological factors in chronic pain: Evolution and revolution. *Journal of Consulting and Clinical Psychology, 70*(3), 678–690. DOI:10.1037//0022-006X.70.3.678

Turk, D. C., Swanson, K. S., & Tunks, E. R. (2008). Psychological approaches in the treatment of chronic pain patients—when pills, scalpels, and needles are not enough. *Canadian Journal of Psychiatry, 53*(4), 213–223.

van Tulder, M., & Koes, B. (2012). International guidelines for the diagnostics and treatment of acute, subacute, and chronic back pain. In M. I. Hasenbring, A. C. Rusu, & D. C. Turk (Eds.), *From acute to chronic back pain: risk factors, mechanisms, and clinical implications* (pp. 419–432). New York: Oxford University Press.

Workman, E. A., Hubbard, J. R., & Felker, B. L. (2002). Comorbid psychiatric disorders and predictors of pain management program success in patients with chronic pain. *Primary Care Companion to the Journal of Clinical Psychiatry, 4*(4), 137–140.

SECTION VIII

Psychotherapeutic options

CHAPTER 40

Applicability of the recovery model in corrections

Debra A. Pinals and Joel T. Andrade

Introduction

Mental health professionals and substance use treatment providers have worked with "recovery" concepts for many years (Onken et al., 2007). President George W. Bush's New Freedom Commission on Mental Health (2002) spoke to important aspects of mental health care systems that were challenged, recognizing that "care must focus on increasing consumers' ability to successfully cope with life's challenges, on facilitating recovery, and on building resilience, [and] not just on managing symptoms." The report went on to state that "recovery will be the common, recognized outcome of mental health services." These words related to general mental health services, and yet correctional settings have become a place where mental health services are increasingly needed. Prisons and jails, however, are built around confinement and the general principles of sentencing that include retribution, deterrence, incapacitation, and rehabilitation (Appelbaum & Zaitchik, 1995). Thus, it might seem that there is such a fundamental distinction between a prison or jail and a place of treatment that a "recovery" orientation seems inappropriate or unrealistic.

In this chapter, we address recovery, describing ways of defining this construct. We also review considerations related to recovery-oriented services that may be feasible and even helpful in correctional environments and describe some of the tensions between recovery and responsibility when working with an offender population. Finally, we present recommendations for combining evidence-based treatments for incarcerated individuals with a recovery-based model for inmates with mental health needs.

Correctional departments and mental health

The past 30 years has seen a significant and dramatic increase in the number of incarcerated individuals with mental health conditions (Pew, 2008). This has fundamentally and rapidly changed the landscape of correctional mental health. The prevalence of serious mental illness in state correctional settings is between 8% and 19% (Metzner & Fellner, 2010). The prevalence of incarcerated individuals with any history of mental health issues is significantly higher, approximately 50% to 60% (Bureau of Justice Statistics, 2006).

The basic, fundamental obligation of a place of detention is to maintain the life and health of those incarcerated. Custody in a correctional institution is sufficiently restrictive that those incarcerated must depend on their keepers for the basics of survival, which include food, water, clothing, and medical care. In the United States, a detainee's or prisoner's right to mental health care comes from the Due Process Clause of the Fourteenth Amendment and the prohibition of cruel and unusual punishment in the Eighth Amendment of the US Constitution. All incarcerated individuals are entitled to the minimal conditions necessary to sustain life and to avoid needless suffering. Courts understand that prisons and jails are not likely to be models of comfort and free from stress and conflict. However, there is a legal duty to identify and treat inmates with serious illness, including serious mental illness (see Chapter 3). Therefore, the role of correctional mental health professionals has historically been to identify and treat serious mental illness, often in the form of voluntary and involuntary psychopharmacological treatment. The changing landscape in correctional psychiatry, with significant numbers of individuals with serious mental illness and high levels of acuity, as well as individuals with significant mental health needs that do not meet criteria for a serious mental illness, requires that we continue to improve upon previous treatment models. In this vein, recovery concepts offer correctional settings the opportunity to improve outcomes for incarcerated individuals with mental illness, decrease recidivism for this population, and increase facility safety and security as long as the limits of recovery structures are recognized and priority given to safety considerations when needed. The following sections provide an overview of the underpinnings of the recovery framework and conceptualization.

Recovery: shared definitions

According to the US Substance Abuse and Mental Health Services Administration (SAMHSA, 2014), recovery from mental disorders and/or substance use disorders can be defined as "a process of change through which individuals improve their health and wellness, live a self-directed life, and strive to reach their full potential." The historical conceptualization of recovery in the treatment of substance use disorders has followed a different trajectory from recovery from mental disorders, although these are increasingly becoming integrated concepts. Regarding substance use, for example, the framework of engaging in a 12-step model with a "sponsor" stems from the origins of Alcoholics Anonymous in the 1930s (Alcoholics Anonymous, 2014), with a goal of abstinence defining recovery. There is a robust literature on the benefits of engaging in these 12-step models to assist in achieving abstinence from substance use (Alcoholics Anonymous, 2014; Chappel & Dupont, 1999). Recovery from mental disorders is a more recent concept. In the 1990s, conceptualizations of psychiatric rehabilitation and recovery, and how these relate to the treatment of mental disorders, were refined and expanded. This resulted in a shift in thinking from mental disorders as lifetime conditions to disorders from which individuals can recover and for which services can be brought to assist individuals to live productive, meaningful lives even if some symptoms persist.

Ideas behind recovery in psychiatric services have been viewed as a vision, a process, and a potential outcome (Onken et al., 2007). Recovery involves individuals, but equally and necessarily has affected systems of services that have become "recovery-oriented." Although symptom reduction can be a critical element of a recovery story, societal challenges (e.g., discrimination, access to entitlements and rehabilitative services) also may become part of a recovery journey and can affect the process of recovery. Onken and colleagues (2007) further delineated elements of recovery to include personal narratives that encompass stories of coping, healing, wellness, and thriving. SAMHSA has established 10 principles of recovery:

◆ Hope

◆ Person-driven

◆ Many pathways

◆ Holistic

◆ Peer support

◆ Relational

◆ Culture

◆ Addresses trauma

◆ Strengths/responsibility

◆ Respect

These guideposts, taken in turn, can help managers of behavioral health services in a correctional setting identify what might and might not be suitable for system care delivery.

Criminogenic focus of treatment

Correctional mental health populations present with unique characteristics, including higher rates of personality disorder (see Chapter 36), psychopathy (Hare, 1991/2003), violence, and substance use. Based on the criminogenic aspects of this population, research in offender treatment finds that treatment interventions that address the Risk-Need-Responsivity (RNR) principles are more effective in reducing criminal recidivism than treatments that do not (Andrews et al., 1990; Andrews & Bonta, 2010). How do recovery tenets fit into a system that is geared to treat individuals with mental illness who may have propensities toward criminal conduct? It is first important to understand basic elements of RNR treatment to see where it can all fit together.

The three areas—risk, need, and responsivity—are each made up of certain principles. The Risk principle calls for matching an individual's risk level with the intensity of intervention: High-risk offenders should receive the most intense treatment interventions, followed by their medium-risk and low-risk counterparts. The Need principle calls for specific interventions aimed at addressing these criminogenic needs (Andrews et al., 2006). The Responsivity principle calls for the specific characteristics of an individual's ability to engage in treatment, such as cognitive ability and motivation for treatment, to be addressed and can also include the treatment provider's ability to address the individual's needs. Research on responsivity finds that the most effective treatments for addressing criminal recidivism are based on cognitive-behavioral, behavioral, and social learning techniques (Smith et al., 2009). Metaanalyses have found a 28% reduction in recidivism when programs adhere to RNR principles (Andrews & Bonta, 2010). A study that compared inmates with versus without serious mental illness found that antisocial attitudes and criminal thinking patterns were similar between these two groups (Morgan et al., 2010). Such findings support adherence to RNR principles in the treatment of inmates with mental illness to decrease recidivism and problematic behavior while incarcerated.

Rehabilitation

Correctional environments have historically been thought of as places where an individual could be rehabilitated from criminal behavioral patterns (Bosworth, 2010). In some ways, current RNR-framed treatment programs are a developmental next step toward this type of criminal rehabilitation and, as noted, are geared toward identifying and confronting antisocial attitudes and behaviors as a focus of treatment (Osher et al., 2012).

According to Anthony (1993), the rehabilitation model for severe mental illness includes a recognition that psychiatric illness includes impairments, such as those seen with active symptoms; dysfunction, which may mean that as a result of such symptoms the person cannot perform certain functions or tasks otherwise considered "normal"; disability, which reflects that because of dysfunction and impairment a person may not be able to perform in a certain role; and disadvantage, which reflects that opportunities for individuals with serious mental illness may be limited. Psychiatric rehabilitation is an important concept that helps clinicians approach individuals with these challenges separate from their antisocial cognitions and behaviors.

In mental health services, rehabilitation and recovery become intermingled concepts. Deegan (1988) noted important distinctions between them. Specifically, rehabilitation refers to "services and technologies made available to persons with disabilities so that they might learn to adapt to their world" (Deegan, 1988, p. 11). Recovery relates more to the person's individualized process of change as he or she overcomes his or her disabilities. As Deegan (1988) notes, rehabilitation services that do not take into account the individual's personal motivations, abilities, and readiness, as well as symptoms, may be of no use. Thus, recovery processes become the frame of reference for rehabilitation efforts.

Attention to the rehabilitation needs of inmates with mental illness may be more or less robust depending on correctional facilities. That said, one might conceptualize rehabilitative work done in a correctional environment as one step toward recovery.

Traditional reentry services focus on inmates as a whole. However, linkages with community mental health agencies prior to release may help identify rehabilitative options after release and potential barriers that inmates often need to overcome before and after release (McCoy et al., 2004).

Systems and recovery "readiness"

Individual recovery can affect systems and services, and these can affect recovery. As such, increased attention has been paid to elements in a system that make it "recovery-oriented." Anthony (2000) outlined initial standards one might consider in examining whether a system is recovery-oriented. Key themes include using language that supports recovery, integrating consumers of services into all levels of service planning and feedback, identifying where recovery can be incorporated into policy, and recognizing that one of the missions of the service system is to improve role functioning, quality of life, and empowerment and satisfaction with services.

There may be significant barriers for a correctional system as it adopts some of these elements, and the need for institutional security cannot be overlooked. That said, programming for inmates with substance use and mental health disorders could be supported by recovery principles. This requires a careful understanding of how, given the value of self-determination and personal choice in the recovery construct, recovery principles must be balanced by important safety considerations and the legal realities of an individual's situation. These matters may need to be continually revisited for both individuals and the correctional system. There should not be confusion about recovery from symptoms, or improved functioning and social integration even with residual symptoms, and recovery from all of life's complexities and problems.

Recovery versus safety in a correctional setting

Individuals in correctional environments have either been charged with criminal conduct (pretrial detainees) or adjudicated guilty of a criminal offense (sentenced inmates). Unique clinical aspects of this population require special attention. For example, among incarcerated offenders, the base rate of antisocial personality disorder has been found to be between 60% (Côté & Hodgins, 1990) and 80% (Hare, 1991/2003). The construct of psychopathy is much more discriminant, and findings indicate that 15% to 25% of incarcerated individuals meet criteria for psychopathy (Hare, 1991/2003). Psychopathic individuals engage in significantly more institutional violence than their nonpsychopathic peers. This has been shown in incarcerated samples (Hill et al., 1996) and civil psychiatric samples (Heilbrun et al., 1998). Instrumental/calculated self-injurious behavior, which can be challenging with this population, can also compromise institutional safety. Therefore, recovery orientation may need to be more circumspect with some individuals by helping to motivate positive behavioral choices (rather than verbal attestations that they are willing and ready to change) that may move them toward improved outcomes.

Complicated questions have been raised about recovery and personal responsibility for individuals whose criminal behavior may be related to mental illness (Pouncey & Lukens, 2010). Mental health, administration, and security personnel have important obligations to maintain institutional safety and to provide care and treatment for inmates. Recovery does not give permission for individuals to do whatever they want to support their independence. Autonomy and personal choice cannot override the social contract that requires public safety. Correctional mental health services may have administrative and clinical obligations to lessen the risk of harm to self or others that an individual with mental illness (or substance use issues) might pose.

Thus, although a recovery framework emphasizes shared decision making, with the patient at the center, there may also be a need to balance competing institutional needs and general public safety concerns. Provisions to override treatment refusal, for example, have been considered permissible under the US Constitution when institutional safety is at risk (*Washington v. Harper*, 1990). However, the laws or constitutions of some states do not allow such overrides for inmates in nonemergencies. Safety and security may subjugate an individual's wishes and self-determination in some situations and jurisdictions. Correctional providers are typically familiar and comfortable with these constructs in service delivery, more so than treatment providers in the community. That said, even when coercion in care is needed, how one perceives services vis-a-vis coercion can affect outcomes. For example, increased perceptions of coercion were negatively correlated with perceptions of recovery and predictive of subsequent criminal involvement in one criminal justice sample (Pratt et al., 2013). Research continues to emerge; over time, we may learn more about how conversations with inmates can foster a sense of autonomy, even when providers have legal and/or institutional mandates to act in ways that contradict inmates' wishes. When dialogue and person-centered care occur in a correctional environment, individuals may have more prominent voices in their behavioral and other treatment interventions that could lead to improved outcomes.

Examples of institutional efforts to support recovery goals

Trauma-informed services

Trauma histories among incarcerated individuals are known to be common (Miller & Najavits, 2012), and this includes witnessing prior violence and experiencing physical and sexual abuse. These histories can contribute to aggressive behavior (Sarchiapone et al., 2009) and behavioral health treatment needs. For example, justice-involved men and women showed high rates of childhood trauma (Wolff & Shi, 2012), which contributed to more significant behavioral health challenges and needs, especially in cases of early sexual trauma.

Correctional systems can be traumatizing. The Prison Rape Elimination Act of 2003 (2003) reflects this, as it was recognized that the prevalence of sexual assault among prisoners needed further study and attention and mandated protections for the inmate population. Miller and Najavits (2012) point out several elements in the correctional environment that can be traumatizing or can serve as a trigger for individuals with trauma histories, such as shackling, overcrowding, lighting, lack of privacy, security personnel operating to maintain order, pat-downs, strip searches, restricted movement, and disciplinary actions (see also Owens et al., 2008). Institutions with a trauma-informed perspective recognize the practices that may inadvertently create additional challenges for individuals who have trauma histories.

As part of a focus on recovery, correctional departments need to consider their level of trauma awareness and whether trauma-informed services are available. The department will also need to determine whether it is ready to become more trauma-informed. Trauma-informed strategies are strongly recommended. In addition, trauma-specific interventions such as Seeking Safety (Najavits, 2002) and Trauma Recovery and Empowerment (Harris, 2014) have been used effectively (Fallot & Harris, 2002; Lynch et al., 2012; Najavits, 2006). Other models also exist and can be found at the National Center on Trauma Informed Care website of SAMHSA (NCTIC, 2014). See Chapter 35 for further discussion of trauma and correctional settings.

Peer support and consumer-guided services

In recent years, there has been growing awareness of the importance of having someone who has lived experience with mental illness support another individual in his or her recovery. Even in correctional settings, programs have been designed to demonstrate the impact of inmates helping inmates. For example, Loeb and colleagues (2013) described how inmates can assist other inmates who are facing terminal illness by providing support and companionship to the dying. In the mental health context, peer support helps individuals move through their illness and inspires hope and meaning for their lives, while giving the individuals a sense of social connectedness. Similarly, forensic peers, which include individuals with a history of criminal justice involvement and behavioral health challenges, are increasingly recognized as an important source of support for persons with co-occurring disorders in the justice system (Davidson & Rowe, 2008). These peers become part of the workforce. When peer supporters are hired to come into correctional institutions, there may be challenges to overcome, including appropriate screening and vetting of criminal backgrounds prior to hire (Miller & Massaro, 2008).

As noted previously, it is important to obtain consumer viewpoints about service delivery in a recovery-oriented system (Clossey & Rheinheimer, 2013). Correctional institutions may do this through special meetings between inmates and the leadership of the institution, allowing inmates to have a regular process and forum where their voices can be heard to help improve services. General inmate surveys and reviews of medical and mental health services can be informative in identifying shortfalls or even abuses. There may be the risk of unfounded inmate complaints; however, routine reviews of inmates' perspectives of treatment services, especially those delivered in segregation and specialized treatment units, can provide helpful data to inform system improvements.

Hope in the context of a prison environment

Hope in a correctional setting may seem elusive, especially for individuals serving lengthy or life sentences. However challenging, finding hope while incarcerated will foster positive outcomes and lead to reduced institutional infractions and lower rates of recidivism (Dekhtyar et al., 2012). Working with inmates to help support their ability to find meaning can be an important contribution to making the institution more recovery-oriented. This support can, in turn, help individuals "give back" as appropriate, where there may be opportunities for personal narrative or sharing of recovery journeys to help others find similar hope and meaning.

Training

For correctional departments to fully benefit from recovery-model concepts, the leadership throughout the department must embrace the basic tenets of this model. Initial training must be provided to all leaders in the institution to gain initial buy-in and long-term adherence to recovery-based principles. After such training, the leadership group, composed of correctional and mental health professionals, can work collaboratively to implement the aspects of the model that seem to fit best, while considering all safety and security concerns. The next section provides some "hands-on" recommendations for application.

Initial steps for implementing a recovery-based model in a correctional setting

Planning

Without a well-defined and structured approach supported by all key stakeholders, recovery-focused programming will not succeed. A small preplanning committee should include key stakeholders from the correctional department and mental health administration (including high-ranking individuals with decision-making power). This group will identify how the recovery-based model can be supported and implemented in their system. This group should hold regular meetings to review the literature on recovery, attend training, and visit recovery-based programs. Individuals with experience designing mental health units in correctional settings will be particularly helpful in leadership roles, especially if additional mental health units are contemplated.

Implementation

Once the vision for the systemic implementation has been determined, an oversight committee should be established to work out the details. The participants may include general planning committee members and a larger group of professionals with experience providing mental health services to incarcerated individuals. It would be helpful, when feasible in the correctional environment, to include "consumers" in the planning process. A group of inmates with mental health needs should be recruited from the general population for membership in the workgroup. To maintain the integrity and security of the department, the process for selecting this group of inmates must be thorough. Also, the inmate participants should not be privy to information that would pose a security risk (e.g., detailed plans, descriptions of facility design, schedules for transferring inmates between facilities). Inmate members provide consumer-based input into the planning of the treatment program (e.g., identify needs and incentives for active participation).

Leadership and infrastructure with services to focus on recovery

Use of a system where officers and treatment staff are trained to deliver services respectfully can help make an institution more recovery-centered. Programs and services that focus on an individual's strengths, instead of on barriers to success, comport with a recovery orientation and can help individuals take responsibility for their actions.

This might require major institutional adjustments. However, in the authors' experience, this can best occur when the leadership embraces these approaches and demonstrates them through role modeling, while training and supporting staff with this new way of thinking. This is best done when leadership emphasizes how these approaches will improve safety and security. The leaders should emphasize that these philosophical shifts do not equate to ignoring the critical need for caution and vigilance and that policies and protocols on safety and security will be enforced.

The availability and development of specialized mental health units in a correctional department can set the stage for programs that support rehabilitation and recovery. The number of facilities and units will depend on the size of the department. This model allows mental health professionals to select participants based on preestablished clinical criteria and to make placement decisions more rapidly based on clinical need and acuity. This also allows inmates with mental health issues to more fully engage in the recovery process in a safe setting. To ensure that security is not compromised by transferring offenders to programs not consistent with their security classification level, treatment units should be available across security levels (e.g., maximum security and medium security). This should include access for inmates in segregation and protective custody.

Summary

The recovery model provides correctional systems with unique opportunities to more fully engage individuals with serious mental illness and other mental health needs. Moreover, this model is being embraced in community settings, making it an important framework to use where feasible in any behavioral health setting. Application in correctional settings requires adjustments and flexibility related to recovery frameworks used in the community, but the underlying philosophy can still be used. To provide a comprehensive program, the basic tenets of recovery should be combined with evidence-based practice in correctional settings. This will benefit the entire inmate population and correctional staff by increasing safety and security. This is also in the interest of public safety, as at least 95% of incarcerated individuals will be released to the community. By providing programs based on evidence, including criminogenic risk factors, coupled with individual-focused recovery-based initiatives for inmates with mental illness, the chance of successful reintegration into society improves.

References

Alcoholics Anonymous (2014). *Historical data: the birth of A.A. and its growth in U.S./Canada.* Available at http://www.aa.org/lang/en/subpage.cfm?page=288 (accessed January 12, 2014).

Andrews, D. A., & Bonta, J. (2010). *The psychology of criminal conduct.* New Providence, NJ: Matthew Bender & Company, Inc., a member of the LexisNexis Group.

Andrews, D. A., Bonta, J., & Wormith, S. J. (2006). The recent past and near future of risk and/or need assessment. *Crime and Delinquency, 52,* 7–27.

Andrews, D. A., Zinger, I., Hoge, R. D., Bonta, J., Gendreau, P., & Cullen, F. T. (1990). Does correctional treatment work? A psychologically informed meta-analysis. *Criminology, 28,* 369–404.

Anthony, W. A. (1993). Recovery from mental illness: the guiding vision of the mental health service system in the 1990s. *Psychosocial Rehabilitation Journal, 16*(4), 11–23.

Anthony, W. A. (2000). A recovery-oriented system: setting some system level standards. *Psychiatric Rehabilitation Journal, 24* (2), 159–168.

Appelbaum, K. L., & Zaitchik, M. C. (1995) Mental health professionals play critical role in presentencing evaluations. *Mental & Physical Disability Law Reporter, 19*(5), 677–684.

Bosworth, M. (2010). *Explaining U.S. imprisonment.* Thousand Oaks, CA: SAGE Publications, Inc.

Bureau of Justice Statistics (2006). *Mental health problems of prison and jail inmates.* Special Report. Washington, DC: U.S. Department of Justice.

Chappel, J. N., & DuPont, R. L. (1999). Twelve-step and mutual-help programs for addictive disorders. *Psychiatric Clinics of North America, 22*(2), 425–446.

Clossey, L., & Rheinheimer, D. (2013). Exploring the effect of organizational culture on consumer perceptions of agency support for mental health recovery. *Community Mental Health Journal* [Epub ahead of print].

Côté, G., & Hodgnis, S. (1990). Co-occurring mental disorders among criminal offenders. *Bulletin of the American Academy of Psychiatry & the Law, 18*(3), 271–281.

Davidson, L., & Rowe, M. (2008). *Peer support within criminal justice settings: The role of forensic peer specialists.* Delmar, NY: CMHS National GAINS Center.

Deegan, P. E. (1988) Recovery: The lived experience of rehabilitation. *Psychosocial Rehabilitation Journal, 11*(4), 11–19.

Dekhtyar, M., Beasley, C. R., Jason, L. A., & Ferrari, J. R. (2012). Hope as a predictor of reincarceration among mutual-help recovery residents. *Journal of Offender Rehabilitation. 51,* 474–483.

Fallot, R. D., & Harris, M. (2002). The Trauma Recovery and Empowerment Model (TREM): Conceptual and practical issues in a group intervention for women. *Community Mental Health Journal, 38,* 475–485.

Hare, R. D. (1991/2003). *The Hare Psychopathy Checklist-Revised, 2nd ed.* Toronto, Canada: Multi-Health Systems.

Harris, M. (2014). *Trauma Recovery and Empowerment (TREM) and Men's Trauma Recovery and Empowerment (M-TREM).* Available at http://www.communityconnectionsdc.org/web/page/657/interior.html (accessed January 13, 2014).

Hill, C. D., Rogers, R., & Bickford, M. E. (1996). Predicting aggressive and socially disruptive behavior in a maximum security forensic psychiatric hospital. *Journal of Forensic Sciences, 41*(1), 56–59.

Heilbrun, K., Hart, S. D., Hare, R. D., Gustafson, D., Nunez, C., & White, A. (1998). Inpatient and post-discharge aggression in mentally disordered offenders: The role of psychopathy. *Journal of Interpersonal Violence, 13,* 514–527.

Loeb, S. J., Hollenbeak, C. S., Penrod, J., Smith, C. A., Kitt-Lewis, E., & Crouse, S. B. (2013). Care and companionship in an isolating environment: inmates attending to dying peers. *Journal of Forensic Nursing, 9*(1), 35–44.

Lynch, S. M., Health, N. M., Mathews, K. C., & Cepeda, G. J. (2012). Seeking Safety: an intervention for trauma-exposed incarcerated women? *Journal of Trauma and Dissociation, 13*(1), 88–101.

McCoy, M. L., Roberts, D. L., Hanrahan, P., Clay, R., & Luchins, D. J. (2004). Jail linkage assertive community treatment services for individuals with mental illness. *Psychiatric Rehabilitation Journal, 27*(3), 243–250.

Metzner, J. L., &Fellner, J. (2010). Solitary confinement and mental illness in U.S. prisons: A challenge for medical ethics. *Journal of the American Academy of Psychiatry and Law, 38,* 104–108.

Miller, L. D., & Massaro, J. (2008). *Overcoming legal impediments to hiring forensic peer specialists.* Delmar, NY: CMHS National GAINS Center.

Miller, N. A., & Najavits, L. M. (2012). Creating trauma-informed correctional care: a balance of goals and environment. *European Journal of Psychotraumatology, 3,* 17246. DOI:10.3402/ejpt.v.20.17246

Morgan, R. D., Fisher, W. H., Duan, N., Mandracchia, J. T., & Murray, D. (2010). Prevalence of criminal thinking among state prison inmates with serious mental illness. *Law and Human Behavior, 34,* 324–336.

Najavits, L. M. (2002). *Seeking Safety: A treatment manual for PTSD and substance abuse.* New York: Guilford Press.

Najavits, L. M. (2006). Managing trauma reactions in intensive addiction treatment environments. *Journal of Chemical Dependency Treatment, 8,* 153–161.

National Center for Trauma-Informed Care, Substance Abuse and Mental Health Services Administration (2014). Available at http://www.samhsa.gov/nctic/ (accessed January 13, 2014).

Onken, S. J., Craig, C. M., Ridgway, P., Ralph, R. O. & Cook, J. A. (2007). An analysis of the definitions of recovery: a review of the literature. *Psychiatric Rehabilitation Journal, 31,* 9–22.

Osher, F. D'Amora, D. A., Plotkin, M., et al. (2012). *Adults with behavioral health needs under correctional supervision: a shared framework for reducing recidivism and promoting recovery.* Council of State Governments Justice Center, Criminal Justice/Mental Health Consensus Project.

Owens, B., Wells, J., Pollock, Muscat, B., & Torres, S. (2008). *Gendered violence and safety: a contextual approach to improving security in women's facilities.* Washington, DC: U.S. Department of Justice, Office of Justice Programs, National Institute of Justice.

Pew Charitable Trusts (2008). *One in 100: Behind bars in America 2008.* Washington, DC: Pew Charitable Trusts.

Pouncy, C. L., & Lukens, J. M. (2010). Madness versus badness: the ethical tension between the recovery movement and forensic psychiatry. *Theoretical Medicine and Bioethics, 31,* 93–105.

Pratt, C., Yanos, P. T., Kopelovich, S. L., Koerner, J., & Alexander, M. J. (2013). Predictors of criminal justice outcomes among mental health courts participants: The role of perceived coercion and subjective mental health recovery. *International Journal of Forensic Mental Health, 12*(2), 116–125.

President's New Freedom Commission on Mental Health. *Transforming mental health care in America.* Available at http://govinfo.library.unt.edu/mentalhealthcommission/reports/FinalReport/FullReport-1.htm (accessed January 9, 2014).

Prison Rape Elimination Act of 2003, P.L. 108–179.

Substance Abuse and Mental Health Services Administration (2014). *SAMHSA announces a working definition of "recovery" from mental disorders and substance use disorders.* Available at http://www.samhsa.gov/newsroom/advisories/1112223420.aspx (accessed January 12, 2014).

Sarchiapone, M., Carli, V., Cuomo, C., Marchetti, M., & Roy, A. (2009). Association between childhood trauma and aggression in male prisoners. *Psychiatry Research, 165,* 1–2, 187–192.

Smith, P., Gendreau, P., & Swartz, K. (2009). Validating the principles of effective intervention: A systematic review of the contributions of meta-analysis in the field of corrections. *Victims and Offenders, 4,* 148–169.

Washington v. Harper, 494 U.S. 2010, 1990.

Wolff, N., & Shi, J. (2012). Childhood and adult trauma experiences of incarcerated persons and their relationship to adult behavioral health problems and treatment. *International Journal of Environmental Research and Public Health, 9,* 1908–1926.

CHAPTER 41

Individual psychotherapy

James L. Knoll, IV

Introduction

The abandonment of the medical model in corrections almost half a century ago left a scorched-earth policy for rehabilitation and, in turn, for psychotherapeutic efforts with inmates (Martinson, 1974). Fortunately, the promise of new progress is returning (Simon, 2013). Along with the imperative of improving psychiatric treatment in corrections, mental health professionals have brought the science of psychotherapeutic intervention back into corrections, this time reinforced by a social science evidence base (Ameen, Loeffler-Cobia, Clawon, & Guevara, 2010; Andrews, Bonta, & Wormith, 2011).

This chapter includes a discussion of the practical and fundamental aspects of individual psychotherapy with inmate patients, followed by an overview of evidence-based paradigms for psychotherapy in corrections. While much of the evidence base supports cognitive-behavioral approaches, the importance of maintaining competence in psychodynamically informed therapy is also discussed.

Practical considerations

It is important to have a sense of one's motives, both manifest and latent, for choosing what many in society would consider unusual work. The clearer one is on one's own motivations, the less likely they will impair one's judgment and effectiveness as a therapist. Achieving insight into such dynamics will be beneficial to clinical judgment and help prevent inappropriate identification with inmate patients. Regardless of one's motivations, being clear about them is a prerequisite to doing correctional psychotherapy. Other practical considerations include therapeutic style, setting, informed consent, and confidentiality.

Style

Therapeutic style is cultivated over time. In correctional therapy, a worthwhile style is genuine and humanistic while also firm and realistic. A useful rule to keep in mind is "when in doubt, be human" (Gabbard, 2010). Inmates often come from harsh and traumatic backgrounds and respond better to a genuine as opposed to a distant therapist. Genuine does not here refer to relaxing one's style. Instead, it refers to a willingness to respond in a relatively undefended way and without making value judgments. It also involves treating the inmate patient with dignity and respect, as noted in the American Psychiatric Association's *Principles of Medical Ethics with Annotations Especially Applicable to Psychiatry* (American Psychiatric Association, 2001). Inmates' struggles are often intense and occur in a crucible that tests the human will.

Common themes

Correctional psychotherapy brings the therapist in contact with the harsh realities of inmate patients' difficult and traumatic life circumstances. Salient themes can be expected to arise repetitively. The two major themes used as examples here are nihilism and the need to find meaning. Clinical observations suggest that a significant portion of inmate patients struggle with a persecutory mindset (Hyatt-Williams, 1998) and develop a nihilistic attitude toward treatment and life (Knoll, 2009). Such cognitions reduce an inmate's ability to participate in and benefit from treatment efforts. Regardless of the type of individual therapy used, therapists will likely encounter inmate patients' sense of hopelessness and need to find meaning in their personal struggles.

Psychiatrist Victor Frankl's experience as a Nazi concentration camp prisoner led him to conclude that a primary motivation is a drive to find meaning and purpose in life (Frankl, 1963). In contrast, a failure to find meaning may result in hopelessness, suicidality, and self-defeating actions (Edwards & Holden, 2001). Trauma literature and research suggest that "meaning making" can be a "central process in healing from trauma or loss" (Lemaire, 2011). The path to reconstructing meaning will depend on the individual's background, culture, and spiritual beliefs. A common central theme to meaning making involves intolerable conditions, causing one to reach one's limit—followed by acceptance, dissolution of defenses, and finally positive transformation (Andresen, 1991; Chodron, 2008).

Setting

The therapy setting depends on the security level of the inmate, the security level of the facility, and overall institutional resources. In most cases, the therapist should strive to see the inmate patient in a private room. When this is not possible, other arrangements can sometimes suffice. For example, a group room that allows a correctional officer to see both therapist and patient, yet not hear them, may be adequate. Convenience or other factors do not justify "cell-side" therapy or similarly nonconfidential arrangements. The setting should be chosen for both confidentiality and safety. Ultimately, correctional administrators have the responsibility to ensure that clinical staff have adequate and appropriate space for treatment. Given the significant amount of psychiatric treatment rendered in corrections, it is appropriate for correctional mental health leaders to diplomatically advocate for confidential therapy space when it is lacking.

There is currently controversy over the use of so-called therapy cells. These are phone booth–like structures used for both group and individual therapy. Arguments against their use include possible dehumanizing effects and the distraction of the inmate patient remaining in a caged structure. Security rules may result in therapy cells being the only option allowed for those on high-security levels or with histories of severe violence. There is limited research evidence on their effects on individual psychotherapy.

Informed consent

The patient's right to consent to treatment is a basic ethical principle in medicine (Appelbaum, 2007). To give legally and ethically appropriate consent, the patient must be competent, have adequate information about the proposed treatment, and be in a position to voluntarily choose the treatment. However, the requirement that a patient be provided adequate information to make rational treatment decisions regarding psychotherapy is unclear (Beahrs & Gutheil, 2001; Simon, 1992). This is despite the American Psychiatric Association's position statement that notes: "Whether or not required by the law, it seems reasonable to encourage psychiatrists to discuss with their patients the nature of psychotherapy, likely benefits and risks (where applicable), and alternative approaches (both psychotherapeutic and non-psychotherapeutic) to their problems" (American Psychiatric Association, 1997). It is recommended that the correctional therapist obtain and document the inmate patient's informed consent for therapy at the initial meeting (Appelbaum, 1997).

Confidentiality

The therapist should explain the limits of confidentiality and, in particular, the limits that apply in the correctional setting. No clear consensus exists among correctional and forensic mental health staff about how to approach explaining limits to confidentiality (Bruggen, Eytan, Gravier, & Elger, 2013). However, standards of inmate patient confidentiality should generally be the same as those in the community (Pinta, 2009). Thus, the usual exceptions to confidentiality apply, such as risk of harm to self or others (Slovenko, 1975). Ideally, in the first session, the inmate patient should be informed about circumstances that may require the therapist to breach confidentiality (Mossman, 2006; Pinta, 2010). When a potential duty to protect a third party arises, correctional therapists should carefully consider the relevant options. Options may include hospitalization, warning third parties, or increasing the frequency of outpatient therapy appointments.

There are some important exceptions to confidentiality specific to the correctional setting. These include when an inmate patient informs the therapist that he is an escape risk or is involved in a prison riot or some activity that would cause "disorder within the facility" (American Psychiatric Association, 2000). The correctional therapist should be clear on any other exceptions to confidentiality that may be specified in the facility's policies and procedures.

Psychotherapy approaches

Engaging, cost-effective, and evidence-based approaches are preferred in today's budget-restricted, overpopulated prisons. The number of therapeutic programming options delivered in group and manualized form has grown faster than evidence-based individual therapies. However, many of the newer evidence-based programs incorporate individual sessions within their overall paradigm. Evidence-based psychotherapy approaches for inmate patients have not made strong gender distinctions. This may change in the future, given research findings on differences between male and female offenders. For example, women with antisocial personality disorder (ASPD) are more likely than men with ASPD to report childhood neglect, sexual abuse, and victimization during adulthood (Alegria, Blanco, Petry, et al., 2013). It is not uncommon for female inmate patients to have comorbid post-traumatic stress disorder and substance use disorders that require special trauma-focused treatment.

Dialectical behavior therapy (DBT) has been shown to be an effective approach for both men and women inmate patients. DBT has been modified for a correctional setting (DBT–Corrections Modified) and used to help reduce impulsive–aggressive behaviors, particularly those that result in disciplinary tickets (Shelton, Kesten, Zhang, & Trestman, 2011; Shelton, Sampl, Kesten, et al., 2009). This approach is often used in conjunction with group sessions and manuals. The Connecticut correctional system has had success with a psychotherapy program that integrates cognitive-behavioral therapy (CBT) and motivational interviewing (MI), designed for impulsive–aggressive behavior in high-security settings (Shelton & Wakai, 2011). The program, called START NOW, is a manualized program (Trestman, 2013) that consists of skills training group sessions; it may be combined with individual therapy using MI and/or CBT. CBT and MI have been combined and used to treat dually diagnosed inmate patients (Weldon & Ritchie, 2010).

MI is an evidence-based therapy used to facilitate behavior change (Triana & Olson, 2013). It has been effective in treating substance use disorders in nonincarcerated populations. In the correctional setting, MI is used to engage and build motivation for treatment. Additionally, MI can be modified for use with intellectually disabled inmate patients (Frielink & Embregts, 2013). There are four main strategies in MI, which are easily taught to multidisciplinary therapists (Miller & Moyers, 2006; Miller & Rollnick, 2002). The first principle involves engaging inmate patients by appropriately expressing empathy and acceptance of their unique issues. The second principle is to elicit dialogue about change. This is done by developing important areas of discrepancy. For example, therapists would assist patients in describing differences in current personal efficacy versus how they would like things to be in the future. The third MI principle is called "rolling with resistance." This requires therapists to pay attention to defensiveness and recognize it as a signal that a modified approach to the issue is needed. This involves a series of reflective, reframing comments by the therapist in order to emphasize the role of personal choice. The fourth MI principle is to support self-efficacy by reinforcing expressions of willingness to understand therapist input, acknowledge problems, and take steps toward positive change.

Preliminary evidence suggests that mentalization-based therapy (MBT) may be effective for individuals with ASPD (Bateman, Bolton, & Fonagy, 2013). MBT was initially designed for individuals with borderline personality disorder (Fonagy & Bateman, 2006) but has been expanded for use in other populations. MBT is a type of psychodynamically oriented psychotherapy. However, it does not focus on developing insight. Rather, its focus is on the present and on enhancing mentalization, which refers to the capacity to understand emotions and behaviors in self and others. Mentalization also involves the implicit and explicit interpretation of actions of oneself and others as intentional (Bateman et al., 2013). It is theorized that persons with ASPD are biased toward external mentalizing, with difficulty understanding the internal mentalizing of others. MBT is typically conducted twice per week, with sessions alternating between group and individual therapy. The overarching goal of MBT is to enhance the patient's appreciation of the emotions, behaviors, and intentions of self and others.

The mindfulness movement

The New York State Department of Corrections and Community Supervision, in collaboration with the New York State Office of Mental Health, has developed an intervention for inmate patients with serious mental illness and/or severe personality disorders who are difficult to engage, behaviorally challenging, and frequently sentenced to punitive isolation. The program is held in a facility called the residential mental health unit (RMHU) with a capacity for approximately 100 inmate patients. The RMHU places heavy emphasis on programming, psychotherapy, and behavioral analysis.

Both group and individual psychotherapy use a CBT–DBT approach, focusing on skills training, insight development, and medication management. The RMHU helps engage inmate patients by expunging their punitive isolation time after successful program participation. The program uses daily multidisciplinary ratings for behavioral analysis, symptom checklists, and measures of improvement. The psychotherapy approach of mindfulness is strongly emphasized, as outlined in Linehan's DBT manual (Linehan, 1993). Mindfulness training helps inmate patients learn to focus their attention on moment-by-moment experience and has become popular as a complementary therapeutic strategy for medical and psychiatric conditions (Marchand, 2012; Robins, Keng, Ekblad, & Brantley, 2012). It has been used as part of stress-reduction programs and mindfulness-based cognitive therapy. Evidence suggests a role as an adjunct treatment for depression, anxiety, pain management, and general psychological health.

Mindfulness training relies on principles taught in meditation; one advantage of this method is that meditation-based programs are low-cost, effective treatments. Mindfulness and meditation training in corrections is in the relatively early stages of psychotherapy research; however, there is growing evidence in favor of meditation-based programs as rehabilitative for incarcerated populations (Himelstein, 2011). Meditation-based programs can assist inmate patients in enhancing psychological well-being and decreasing substance use. The advantage of mindfulness training is that it can be done with minimal resources and in either a group or individual setting (Bateman & Krawitz, 2013). Its practical, easily grasped application appeals to a broad population of inmate patients; its principles can be either divorced from spiritual traditions or related to them. Core objectives include control of attention, improved emotional regulation, and effective problem solving.

Psychodynamic knowledge in correctional psychotherapy

There are many reasons to maintain a broad psychodynamic viewpoint of inmate patients, even when psychodynamic psychotherapy is not used. Psychodynamically oriented therapists have begun to subject their approach to the scientific method (Gabbard, 2010; Gerber, Kocsis, Milrod, et al., 2011; Perry &

Bond, 2012), and important lessons have been learned. For example, nonpsychodynamic therapies may be effective, in part, because more skilled practitioners use techniques that have long been central to psychodynamic theory and practice (Shedler, 2010). Further, inmate patients will commonly bring more than one illness or problem to therapy. Therapists find themselves using a mix of evidence-based treatments with other empirically supported approaches and a good measure of creativity (Douglas, 2011; Vaillant, 2012).

An understanding of the inmate patient's childhood development is critical to the therapeutic relationship, approach, and goal setting. In addition to its instructive focus on the therapeutic relationship and countertransference, psychodynamic theory involves other distinctive features that are of particular concern to correctional therapists. These features include identification of recurring behavior or thought patterns, understanding of interpersonal relations, and recognizing style of emotional expression (Gabbard, 2010). Regardless of psychotherapy approach, there remains a need to understand inmate patients' use of defense mechanisms, as well as important transference and countertransference themes. Countertransference to an inmate patient may provide valuable data about the emotions and cognitions induced in others, which will inform future therapy directions. Specific personality disorders and styles are associated with fairly consistent emotional responses in therapists, allowing the therapist to make diagnostic and therapeutic use of these responses (Colli, Tanzilli, Dimaggio, & Lingiardi, 2014). For example, therapist countertransference involving feelings of being devalued, criticized, or mistreated has been associated with patient diagnoses of ASPD, paranoid personality disorder, and narcissistic personality disorder (Perry, Presniak, & Olson, 2013). Borderline personality disorder is associated with countertransference feelings of helplessness and being overwhelmed and overinvolved.

In the United Kingdom, "forensic psychotherapists" place importance on understanding "the meaning of a violent act for the offender" and believe that a "psychodynamic approach can inform effective therapeutic interventions in hard-to-treat patients" (Yakeley & Adshead, 2013). Forensic psychotherapists are particularly interested in how an individual's offending behavior may represent a repetition of early experience. For example, it has been observed that for some, shame and humiliation resulted in violent acting out (Gilligan, 2002). Thus, future inability to tolerate such emotions results in violence toward others.

The use of psychodynamic thinking helps in the individual therapy setting and in managing multidisciplinary staff's responses to inmates. Unexplored countertransference in staff may result in a host of adverse outcomes such as staff division, boundary violations, breaches of security, and a toxic team milieu. Finally, knowledge of psychodynamic theory assists in developing a psychodynamic formulation that informs future therapy. A psychodynamic formulation remains valuable because it provides a biopsychosocial summary of personal strengths, vulnerabilities, and core conflicts.

Offender development

Inmate patients often share similar developmental histories that profoundly affect and challenge psychotherapeutic efforts. It helps to have a good understanding of a patient's developmental history prior to treatment. Histories of neglect and trauma are common and forewarn of difficulties with treatment readiness, trust in the therapeutic alliance, and realistic treatment goal setting.

Childhood abuse and neglect are associated with an increased risk of personality disorders (Johnson, Cohen, Brown, Smailes, & Bernstein, 1999). Poor or abusive parenting is believed to play a major role in the development of adult criminality (Lykken, 1998). Object relations theory suggests that children who experience developmentally adverse events develop distorted internal models of interpersonal relationships and self-regulation (Craissati, 2006). Early maltreatment and adverse conditions are theorized to play a role in creating structural changes in the brain, as evidenced by preliminary neuroimaging findings (McCollum, 2006). Childhood exposure to violence and abuse may adversely affect infant neurocircuitry, leading to underdevelopment in the frontal and prefrontal cortex (Keeshin, Cronholm, & Strawn, 2012). Childhood abuse and stress can result in chronically increased cortisol levels, leading to hippocampal volume loss and associated learning problems (Bair-Merritt, Zuckerman, Augustyn, & Cronholm, 2013). Such neuropsychiatric deficits may produce problems in behavioral self-regulation, emotional regulation, and executive function that may significantly affect the inmate patient's treatment readiness (Fishbein, Sheppard, Hyde, et al., 2009).

Common countertransference themes in correctional psychotherapy

The capacity to "hold, and examine anti-social thoughts and feelings is not just a requirement for psychiatrists and their patients. It is a need for everyone" (Simon, 1996). Recognizing and making use of countertransference with inmate patients, particularly those with antisocial traits, is critical to therapy success, cohesive staff functioning, and safety. The term "countertransference" is used here in its broadest sense to mean the emotional reaction of the therapist to the patient (Ursano, Sonnenberg, & Lazar, 1991). Regardless of style, therapists working with inmate patients invariably come to realize that treatment cannot be a "dispassionate technical endeavour" (Friedrich & Leiper, 2006). The therapist must recognize, tolerate, and "hold" the inmate patient's feelings in a safe way that helps the patient (Slochower, 1991). Lack of attention to countertransference may cause the therapist to reflexively avoid internal discomfort by responding in an attacking or rejecting manner. Inmate patients with strong psychopathic traits may engender particularly corrosive countertransference emotions, causing the therapist to feel controlled or deceived.

Friedrich and Leiper (2006) found that countertransference themes reported by clinicians treating sex offenders fell into three main domains: negative and problematic reactions, the clinicians' experience of having something done to them, and struggles to create a therapeutic relationship. The reactions discussed here fall primarily into the first and second domains. Correctional therapists may find themselves using isolation of affect to deal with unpleasant or difficult emotional reactions to some patients. An absence or lack of feelings about the patient will be the hallmark of this reaction. For example, therapists working with psychopathic offenders have described a process of engaging in detached, ritualistic task performance to avoid unpleasant countertransference feelings (Grounds et al., 1987). This type of reaction can create

excessive distance from the inmate patient or cause the therapist to overlook important clinical warning signs.

Therapeutic nihilism is a countertransference reaction experienced with difficult-to-treat or help-rejecting inmate patients and patients with strong psychopathic traits (Meloy, 1988). Many therapists assume that all such individuals are similar in their lack of response, and therefore treatment is pointless. This reaction should be tempered by the fact that inmate patients are a heterogeneous group with unique personal characteristics; there is no evidence that all are immune to treatment efforts (Barbaree, 2005; Salekin, 2002). It is critical to have realistic expectations; however, therapeutic nihilism is often the result of "oral tradition," passed down in the absence of objective data (Meloy, 1988). The therapist must carefully navigate between the Scylla and Charybdis of therapeutic nihilism and therapeutic naiveté. This is a challenge that requires efforts to prohibit moral judgment from impinging on an objective, professional approach.

Malignant pseudoidentification is a potentially hazardous reaction described in the treatment of highly antisocial inmate patients (Meloy, 1988). It involves the process by which the inmate patient consciously imitates (or unconsciously simulates) the narcissistic characteristics of the therapist. This results in a strengthening of the therapist's identification with the offender, which may cause the therapist to become vulnerable to manipulation. The process may involve the inmate patient simulating values, beliefs, or even mannerisms of the therapist. The pseudo-flattery may be taken as a positive sign of improvement by the therapist, who then assumes a therapeutic alliance and "healthy" identification.

Some inmate patients may realistically carry a poor long-term prognosis. Such cases have the potential to induce subtle feelings of worthlessness and self-devaluation in the therapist. Similar self-devaluing reactions include excessive questioning of one's abilities or feeling that one's work is insignificant. Some inmate patients may demonstrate attitudes that the therapist will find disgusting or off-putting. Feelings of hatred may be acted on by the therapist in the form of inappropriate criticisms, hostile remarks, or premature withdrawal of care. In all such cases, supervision and/or case consultation is highly recommended. The therapist must be particularly thoughtful if an inmate patient's crime "touches on a specific area of sensitivity for the therapist" (Hyatt-Williams, 1998). Countertransference hatred is less likely to be acted on when the therapist is conscious of it and can reevaluate clinical decisions more objectively. A reflective processing of such countertransference may be required on a treatment team level. This is especially important when other staff also have conscious or unconscious wishes to destroy or punish the inmate patient.

Meloy and Meloy (2002) hypothesized that clinicians' fearful responses to psychopathic individuals are merely a natural biological reaction of prey to a predator. In contrast, some therapists may respond in the opposite manner, with a counterphobic denial of actual danger. A thorough clinical risk assessment will enable the therapist, in collaboration with a treatment team, to make more objective estimates of the precautions necessary for the psychotherapy setting. Ultimately, when a therapist finds, after consultation and/or supervision, that a particular inmate patient engenders intractable, destructive countertransference, it may be necessary to transfer the patient to another therapist.

Summary

Individual psychotherapy with inmate patients can be as gratifying as it is challenging. The evidence base for correctional psychotherapy approaches is advancing, with an emphasis on cognitive-behavioral methods and mindfulness training. However, there remains an important place for psychodynamic competence, particularly in the areas of biopsychosocial formulations and effective management of countertransference. Finally, the correctional therapist's effectiveness will be enhanced by liberal use of consultation and supervision.

References

Alegria, A. A., Blanco, C., Petry, N. M., et al. (2013). Sex differences in antisocial personality disorder: Results from the National Epidemiological Survey on Alcohol and Related Conditions. *Personality Disorders, 4*(3), 214–222.

Ameen, C. A., Loeffler-Cobia, J., Clawon, E., & Guevara, M. (2010). *Evidence-based practice skills assessment for criminal justice organizations.* Crime and Justice Institute at Community Resources for Justice, Version 1.0. Washington, DC: National Institute of Corrections.

American Psychiatric Association (1997). American Psychiatric Association resource document on principles of informed consent in psychiatry. *Journal of American Academy of Psychiatry Law, 25*(1), 121.

American Psychiatric Association (2000). *Psychiatric services in jails and prisons* (2nd ed.). Washington, DC: American Psychiatric Publishing.

American Psychiatric Association (2001). *The principles of medical ethics with annotations especially applicable to psychiatry.* Washington, DC: American Psychiatric Association.

Andresen, J. J. (1991). Biblical job: Changing the helper's mind. *Contemporary Psychoanalysis, 27*(3), 454–481.

Andrews, D. A., Bonta, J., & Wormith, J. S. (2011). The risk-need-responsivity (RNR) model: Does adding the good lives model contribute to effective crime prevention? *Criminal Justice and Behavior, 38*(7), 735–755.

Appelbaum, P. (1997). Informed consent to psychotherapy: Recent developments. *Psychiatric Services, 48*(4), 445.

Appelbaum, P. (2007). Assessment of patients' competence to consent to treatment. *New England Journal of Medicine, 357,* 1834–1840.

Bair-Merritt, M., Zuckerman, B., Augustyn, M., & Cronholm, P. F. (2013). Silent victims: an epidemic of childhood exposure to domestic violence. *New England Journal of Medicine, 369*(18), 1673–1675.

Barbaree, H. (2005). Psychopathy, treatment behavior, and recidivism: An extended follow-up of Seto and Barbaree. *Journal of Interpersonal Violence, 20*(9), 1115–1131.

Bateman, A., Bolton, R., & Fonagy, P. (2013). Antisocial personality disorder: A mentalizing framework. *FOCUS: The Journal of Lifelong Learning in Psychiatry, 11*(2), 178–186.

Bateman, A. W., & Krawitz, R. (2013). *Borderline personality disorder: An evidence-based guide for generalist mental health professionals.* New York: Oxford University Press.

Beahrs, J. O., & Gutheil, T. G. (2001). Informed consent in psychotherapy. *American Journal of Psychiatry, 158*(1), 4–10.

Bruggen, M. C., Eytan, A., Gravier, B., & Elger, B. S. (2013). Medical and legal professionals' attitudes towards confidentiality and disclosure of clinical information in forensic settings: A survey using case vignettes. *Medical Science Law, 53*(3), 132.

Chodron, P. (2008). *Comfortable with uncertainty: 108 teachings on cultivating fearlessness and compassion.* Boston, MA: Shambhala Publications.

Colli, A., Tanzilli, A., Dimaggio, G., & Lingiardi, V. (2014). Patient personality and therapist response: An empirical investigation. *American Journal of Psychiatry, 171,* 102–108. doi:10.1176/appi. ajp.2013.13020224

Craissati, J. (2006). Attachment problems and sex offending, In A. R. Beech, L. A. Craig, & K. D. Browne (Eds.), *Assessment and Treatment of Sex Offenders: A Handbook,* Chapter 2, Malden, MA: John Wiley & Sons.

Douglas, C. (2011). Studying the efficacy of psychodynamic psychotherapy. [Letter to the editor.] *American Journal of Psychiatry, 168,* 649.

Edwards, M., & Holden, R. (2001). Coping, meaning in life, and suicidal manifestations: Examining gender differences. *Journal of Clinical Psychology, 57*(12), 1517–1534.

Fishbein, D., Sheppard, M., Hyde, C., et al. (2009). Deficits in behavioral inhibition predict treatment engagement in prison inmates. *Law and Human Behavior, 33*(5), 419–435.

Fonagy, P., & Bateman, A. W. (2006). Mechanisms of change in mentalization based treatment of BPD. *Journal of Clinical Psychology, 62*(4), 411–430.

Frankl, V. E. (1963). *Man's search for meaning.* (Originally published in 1959.)

Friedrich, M., & Leiper, R. (2006). Countertransference reactions in therapeutic work with incestuous sexual abusers. *Journal of Child Sexual Abuse, 15*(1), 51–68.

Frielink, N., & Embregts, P. (2013). Modification of motivational interviewing for use with people with mild intellectual disability and challenging behaviour. *Journal of Intellectual and Developmental Disability, 38*(4), 279–291.

Gabbard, G. (2010). *Long-term psychodynamic psychotherapy: A basic text.* Washington, DC: American Psychiatric Publishing.

Gerber, A. J., Kocsis, J. H., Milrod, B. L., et al. (2011). A quality-based review of randomized controlled trials of psychodynamic psychotherapy. *American Journal of Psychiatry, 168*(1), 19–28.

Gilligan, J. (2002). *Violence: Reflections on our deadliest epidemic.* London: Jessica Kingsley Publishers.

Grounds, A. T., Quayle, M. T., France, J., Brett, T., Cox, M., & Hamilton, J. R. (1987). A unit for 'psychopathic disorder'patients in Broadmoor Hospital. *Medicine, Science and the Law, 27*(1), 21–31.

Himelstein, S. (2011). Meditation research: The state of the art in correctional settings. *International Journal of Offender Therapy and Comparative Criminology, 55*(4), 646–661.

Hyatt-Williams, A. (1998). *Cruelty, violence and murder: Understanding the criminal mind.* Northvale, NJ: Jason Aronson, Inc.

Johnson, J., Cohen, P., Brown, J., Smailes, E., & Bernstein, D.. (1999). Childhood maltreatment increases risk for personality disorders during early adulthood. *Archives of General Psychiatry, 56*(7), 600–606.

Keeshin, B. R., Cronholm, P. F., & Strawn, J. R. (2012). Physiologic changes associated with violence and abuse exposure an examination of related medical conditions. *Trauma, Violence, & Abuse, 13*(1), 41–56.

Knoll J. (2009). Treating the morally objectionable. In J. Andrade (Ed.), *Handbook of violence risk assessment and treatment: New approaches for mental health professionals* (pp. 311–345). New York: Springer Publishing Company.

Lemaire, C. (2011). Grief and resilience. In F. Stoddard, A. Pandya, & C. Katz (Eds.), *Disaster psychiatry: Readiness, evaluation, and treatment* (Chapter 11). Washington, DC: American Psychiatric Publishing, Inc.

Linehan, M. (1993). *Cognitive-behavioral treatment of borderline personality disorder.* New York, NY: Guilford Press.

Lykken, D. T. (1998). The case for parental licensure. In T. Millon, E. Simonsen, M. Birket-Smith, & R. D. Davis (Eds.), *Psychopathy: Antisocial, criminal, and violent behavior* (Chapter 8). New York, NY: Guilford Press.

Marchand, W. R. (2012). Mindfulness-based stress reduction, mindfulness-based cognitive therapy, and Zen meditation for depression, anxiety, pain, and psychological distress. *Journal of Psychiatric Practice®, 18*(4), 233–252.

Martinson, R. (1974). What works? Questions and answers about prison reform. *The Public Interest, 35,* 22.

McCollum, D. (2006). Child maltreatment and brain development. *Minnesota Medicine, 89*(3), 48–50.

Meloy, J. (1988). *The psychopathic mind: Origins, dynamics, and treatment.* Lanham, MD: Jason Aronson, Inc.

Meloy, J., & Meloy, M. (2002). Autonomic arousal in the presence of psychopathy: A survey of mental health and criminal justice professionals. *Journal of Threat Assessment, 2*(2), 21–33.

Miller, W. R., & Moyers, T. B. (2006). Eight stages in learning motivational interviewing. *Journal of Teaching in the Addictions, 5*(1), 3–17.

Miller, W. R., & Rollnick, S. (2002). *Motivational interviewing: Preparing people for change.* New York: Guilford Press.

Mossman, D. (2006). Critique of pure risk assessment or, Kant meets *Tarasoff. University of Cincinnati Law Review, 75,* 523.

Perry, J. C., & Bond, M. (2012). Change in defense mechanisms during long-term dynamic psychotherapy and five-year outcome. *American Journal of Psychiatry, 169*(9), 916–925.

Perry, J. C., Presniak, M. D., & Olson, T. R. (2013). Defense mechanisms in schizotypal, borderline, antisocial, and narcissistic personality disorders. *Psychiatry: Interpersonal & Biological Processes, 76*(1), 32–52.

Pinta, E. R. (2009). Decisions to breach confidentiality when prisoners report violations of institutional rules. *Journal of the American Academy of Psychiatry and the Law Online, 37*(2), 150–154.

Pinta, E. R. (2010). *Tarasoff* duties in prisons: Community standards with certain twists. *Psychiatric Quarterly, 81*(2), 177–182.

Robins, C. J., Keng, S., Ekblad, A. G., & Brantley, J. G. (2012). Effects of mindfulness-based stress reduction on emotional experience and expression: A randomized controlled trial. *Journal of Clinical Psychology, 68*(1), 117–131.

Salekin, R. (2002). Psychopathy and therapeutic pessimism: Clinical lore or clinical reality? *Clinical Psychology Review, 22,* 79–112.

Shedler, J. (2010). The efficacy of psychodynamic psychotherapy. *American Psychologist, 65*(2), 98.

Shelton, D., Kesten, K., Zhang, W., & Trestman, R. (2011). Impact of a dialectic behavior therapy—Corrections Modified (DBT-CM) upon behaviorally challenged incarcerated male adolescents. *Journal of Child and Adolescent Psychiatric Nursing, 24*(2), 105–113.

Shelton, D., Sampl, S., Kesten, K. L., Zhang, W., & Trestman, R. L. (2009). Treatment of impulsive aggression in correctional settings. *Behavioral Sciences & the Law, 27*(5), 787–800.

Shelton, D., & Wakai, S. (2011). A process evaluation of START NOW Skills Training for inmates with impulsive and aggressive behaviors. *Journal of the American Psychiatric Nurses Association, 17*(2), 148–157.

Simon, J. (2013). The return of the medical model: Disease and the meaning of imprisonment from John Howard to *Brown v. Plata. Harvard Civil Rights-Civil Liberties Law Review, 48,* 217–325.

Simon, R. (1992). Informed consent: Maintaining a clinical perspective. *Clinical psychiatry and the law* (2nd ed., pp. 121–153). Washington, DC: American Psychiatric Press.

Simon, R. (1996). *Bad men do what good men dream* (p. 17). Washington, DC: APA Press, Inc.

Slovenko, R. (1975). Psychotherapy and confidentiality, *Cleveland State Law Review, 24,* 375–395.

Slochower, J. (1991). Variations in the analytic holding environment. *The International Journal of Psychoanalysis, 72*(4), 709–718.

Trestman, R. (2013). *Motivational interviewing and mental health: START NOW.* Central New York Psychiatry Center Statewide Medical Staff Meeting, Marcy, NY.

Triana, A. C., & Olson, M. (2013). Motivational interviewing as a pedagogical approach in behavioral science education: 'Walking the talk'. *International Journal of Psychiatry Medicine, 45*(4), 389.

Ursano, R., Sonnenberg, S., & Lazar, S. (1991). *Concise guide to psychodynamic psychotherapy.* Washington, DC: American Psychiatric Press.

Vaillant, G. (2012). Lifting the field's "repression" of defenses. *American Journal of Psychiatry, 169*(9), 885–887.

Weldon, S., & Ritchie, G. (2010). Treatment of dual diagnosis in mentally disordered offenders: Application of evidence from the mainstream. *Advances in Dual Diagnosis, 3*(2), 18.

Yakeley, J., & Adshead, G. (2013). Locks, keys, and security of mind: Psychodynamic approaches to forensic psychiatry. *Journal of the American Academy of Psychiatry and the Law Online, 41*(1), 38–45.

CHAPTER 42

Group psychotherapy

Shama Chaiken and Brittany Brizendine

Introduction

This chapter provides an overview of literature related to the use of group therapy with offender populations. Group therapy outcomes and factors related to efficacy of group therapy are reviewed. Information is included regarding selection of participants, therapist core competencies, and management of issues unique to the correctional population. Structured approaches for treatment of specific correctional populations and nationally recognized evidence-based programs and practices (Substance Abuse and Mental Health Services Administration, 2013) are described.

Overview

Research indicates that group psychotherapy can be an effective form of treatment for a variety of disorders, and many studies indicate that it is as effective as individual therapy (DeLucia-Waack, 2004; Fuhriman & Burlingame, 1994; McEvoy, 2007; McRoberts et al., 1998; Tasca & Bone, 2007). Yalom (2005) defines the following 11 therapeutic factors of group therapy:

◆ Installation of hope

◆ Universality

◆ Imparting information

◆ Altruism

◆ Corrective recapitulation of the primary family group

◆ Development of socializing techniques

◆ Imitative behavior

◆ Interpersonal learning

◆ Group cohesiveness

◆ Catharsis

◆ Existential factors

A variety of outcomes have been used to evaluate the effectiveness of group psychotherapy with offender populations, including behaviors such as recidivism, disciplinary behavior, and substance abuse (Allen et al., 2001; Little et al., 2000; Sandahl et al., 1998).

There is considerable clinical consensus that patients are extremely poor candidates for a heterogeneous outpatient therapy group if they are brain-damaged, paranoid, hypochondriacal, addicted to drugs or alcohol, acutely psychotic, or sociopathic (Yalom, 2005; Yalom & Leszcz, 1995). However, Yalom (2005) indicates that specialized group therapy with a more homogeneous population may be the most effective type of treatment for individuals who cannot benefit from standard group therapy.

Group therapy has been found to be more effective than individual therapy for treatment of specific conditions. Although some studies find no impact of group therapy on measured outcomes, only a few studies have found deleterious effects for specific treatment populations (e.g., Kanas et al., 1980). The group treatment modality can be particularly helpful in improving social support and interpersonal relationships (Kanas, 1996; Yalom, 2005) and for treatment of individuals who engage in harmful secretive behaviors, including sex offenders (Salter, 1988). Outcomes of group therapy are most positive when participants are appropriately selected, goals of treatment are carefully defined, and the group facilitator is adequately trained and skilled (Barlow, 2004). According to Andrews and colleagues (1990), nondirective therapies are less effective than directive approaches that target criminogenic needs such as cognitive-behavioral therapies (CBTs) that are matched to the participants' learning styles. Gendreau (1996) went so far as to assert that effective offender rehabilitation programs must include CBT. Most empirically supported interventions for offender populations use a CBT framework (Andrews et al., 1990). Group-based therapy, using a cognitive-behavioral model, is a primary forum for sex offender treatment (McGrath et al., 2003) and is discussed in Chapter 59.

Therapy groups may be "closed," where the same participants attend the group over time, or "open," where new participants may join the group. There are four broad categories of group therapy used with correctional populations: self-help, psychoeducational, recreational, and psychotherapy. Regardless of the type of group, the group facilitator's main job is to help participants to interact without aggressive, violent, destructive, or other inappropriate behavior during the session (Chaiken et al., 2005).

The correctional treatment literature has primarily focused on interventions that target criminal behavior with offenders who do not have serious mental illness (Andrews et al., 2006; Gendreau, 1996). This body of literature supports the risk-need-responsivity approach, which is likely the most commonly used model of offender assessment and treatment (Ward et al., 2007). This approach matches the level of services to the offender's level of risk for reoffending so that offenders with greater levels of risk receive more intensive services. The literature supports the principle of responsivity, which includes providing treatments tailored to the specific needs of the offender, such as the offender's learning style, motivation, personality functioning, and cognitive functioning.

Logistics and supporting quality group therapy

Pregroup interviews

Appropriate patient selection is an important factor in treatment success, and one recommended method is pregroup interviews with the offender. The terms of treatment or patient agreements should be reviewed with the offender during this pregroup session. Therapy readiness should be evaluated prior to acceptance; this should include an agreement to engage in the treatment for the specified period of time, with the possibility of the treatment being renewed. The agreement also informs the offender about what to expect from the facilitator.

Group therapy facilitator skills

Group therapy services commonly provided for offenders often are implemented by clinicians without substantial resources and who have not received standardized training. Treatment of offenders may be affected by staff turnover, staff burnout, poor fidelity monitoring, and other institutional priorities that divert from a focus on meaningful and effective group therapy (Gendreau et al., 1999; Hamm & Schrink, 1989; Hollin, 1995; Smith, 2006).

To provide effective group therapy for correctional populations, facilitators must have adequate training, a passion for providing group therapy, and support systems to prevent burnout and compassion fatigue due to trauma exposure. Strategies to prevent burnout and foster a psychologically healthy workplace for facilitators providing group therapy include the following:

◆ Circumscribed time frames for groups with clear start and stop dates,

◆ Time to reflect on and renew group syllabi,

◆ Clinical supervision,

◆ Autonomy with patient selection and discretion in use of standardized materials,

◆ Positive and collaborative custody and clinical relationships, and

◆ Inclusion in treatment planning and treatment team decisions.

Supervisors should meet regularly with facilitators to provide supervision and consultation. These meetings should have clear goals and objectives, including review of group syllabi, countertransference and transference, and decisions about self-disclosure. Effective facilitation of group therapy requires an artful balance of empathic support and confrontation (Kominars & Dornheim, 2004).

Language

Little information is available about offenders who speak English as a second language and are included in English-speaking groups. Use of language interpreters for group therapy without assistive technology is cumbersome. Assigning individuals to groups with a facilitator and participants who speak their preferred language is clearly best but not always logistically possible. Where interventions are not designed to account for cultural factors, facilitators should acknowledge the differences between people in the group and stimulate discussion to overcome any cultural barriers to full participation and benefit.

Learning and intellectual disabilities

Modification of group therapy for offenders with learning disabilities is a challenge in many settings. Offenders who have neurological disorders and/or cognitive-developmental disabilities pose unique treatment challenges. Individuals who have deficits in memory processing or difficulty in learning new information may not be appropriate for inclusion in psychoeducational or psychotherapy groups with offenders who have higher cognitive functioning. Offenders with developmental disabilities may need structured activities to fulfill the human need for basic social interaction. Group therapies recommended for this population include sex education, substance abuse education/treatment, anger management, vocational training, and recreation therapy. A requirement for success using these therapies with this population is concrete, repetitious training using simple terms (Shively, 2004). Accommodation and adaptation of materials for individuals with cognitive disabilities is critical to efficacy of treatment.

Severe mental illness

While the correctional literature is limited, a substantial body of research supports the efficacy of group therapy as a treatment for people with severe mental illness. Group therapy for this population may focus on symptom reduction, skills training, substance abuse prevention, and/or behavioral goals such as reducing recidivism. Group therapy can be as effective as, or more effective than, individual therapy for treatment of psychotic disorders (Kanas, 2005; Kanas et al., 2006). Empirical studies have demonstrated that group therapy is a useful adjunct to antipsychotic medication for psychotic patients and, in many cases, is superior to individual therapy. Group therapy can be used to provide education about psychotropic medication, including the risks and benefits of specific medications, with the goal of improving medication adherence (Kanas, 1996).

Security and group therapy in lockup units

Secured housing units such as administrative segregation and security housing require the offender to be segregated from other offenders for safety and security of the institution. Due to the segregated status of a lockup unit, providing group therapy to these offenders typically requires a physical barrier between each offender and the staff to ensure safety and security. Chapter 14 provides a summary that is pertinent to such arrangements.

Length and duration of treatment

The length of treatment may depend on its purpose and on the composition of the offenders and the milieu. For inpatient programs, it is common for group therapy to occur daily or multiple times a week for a short time. For outpatient programs, group treatment typically occurs weekly or twice a month for 8 to 16 weeks. Some longer-term programs may last up to a year or longer. It is not uncommon for group treatment in corrections to end abruptly; reasons include unanticipated offender transfer to another facility. Regardless of treatment duration, active planning and discussion of termination should begin in the first session (Linehan, 1993) and continue throughout the span of treatment to prepare the offender and to allow for appropriate emotional closure.

Reinforcing participation

Inconsistent attendance has been identified as one of the most common problems in therapy groups. There is often increased reluctance to disclose private information when attendance among group members is unstable (MacNair-Semands, 2002). Poor attendance by some group participants can disrupt group solidarity and may hinder meaningful work for the rest of the group (MacNair & Corazzini, 1994).

Incentives for participation in group therapy may include avoidance of incarceration, reduced incarceration time, or release to a less restrictive environment from settings such as inpatient hospitalization or segregation units. In some state prisons and jails, behavioral reinforcers such as television and radio access are used to encourage disciplinary-free behavior accompanied by group therapy participation.

When the reason for inconsistent participation is ambivalence to change, motivational interviewing (Miller & Rollnick, 2002) may be used. Motivational interviewing supports change in a way that is congruent with an individual's own values and beliefs. In the corrections population, research has supported motivational interviewing as a way to enhance motivation to change and reduce offending behaviors (McMurran, 2009).

Confidentiality issues in correctional group therapy

Providers who treat offenders often are required to make decisions about disclosure of information, especially when patients reveal violent thoughts. Exceptions to confidentiality in group therapy need to be disclosed as part of the informed consent process prior to treatment. While the group facilitator remains bound to ethical requirements of confidentiality in the group therapy setting, other group participants are not (Rapin, 2004). Informed consent requires that participants understand that the facilitator does not have the ability to protect the confidentiality of information disclosed during group therapy (Chaiken et al., 2005). Participants may not understand that disclosure of their personal history could lead to danger from other offenders; systems should be in place to evaluate such safety issues. At a minimum, custody and clinical staff should be aware of offenders who have a history of violence against others with specific characteristics (e.g., sex crimes or specific gang affiliation) and consider these factors in group therapy participant selection. To maximize group therapy effectiveness, leaders should facilitate ongoing discussion of the importance of confidentiality and the impact of disclosure outside the group on the therapeutic process (Koocher & Keith-Spiegel, 2008).

Cultural competence and gang culture

Heterogeneity of group participants can either facilitate group process or hinder communication and trust (Yalom, 2005). One important job of the group leader in any setting is to help participants identify and discuss differences in values and beliefs that are based on group affiliation, including gender, ethnicity, race, socioeconomic status, education level, sexual orientation, and religion. Facilitators need to work within their scope of training and seek additional information when working with individuals from a cultural group with which they are less familiar.

Another job of the facilitator is to match the group therapy techniques to the treatment population because some types of group therapy are more effective with specific cultural groups. For example, group therapy using a direct confrontational approach to treat stimulant abuse led to a higher dropout rate for Asian and female participants and was more effective with African-American males (Pérez-Arce et al., 1993).

Group facilitators who work with offenders need to be aware of issues related to inmate gang affiliation, type of offense, and length of commitment. In settings where differences can spark violence, such as high-security jails and prisons, facilitators may need to direct the conversation to areas of common interest and agreement instead of expecting cultural differences to be resolved during group sessions. In some cases, combining specific offenders together in a group can be dangerous and counterproductive. The underlying differences may lead to extreme emotions such as fear, hatred, anger, and mistrust that are unlikely to be resolved in the group therapy setting.

Certain gang cultures discourage mental health treatment. In that context, it is recommended that the facilitator work with the local gang investigation unit to better understand these "politics" relative to the institution. Group facilitators should be astute to cultural competency related to prison politics and the gang culture in conjunction with general cultural and diversity-related issues. Chapter 58 discusses gang-related concerns in more detail.

Research indicates that certain populations have more positive outcomes despite cultural differences within a group setting. These include groups treating bulimia nervosa, obsessive–compulsive disorder, social phobia, and panic disorder. Group therapy is hypothesized to be more effective for such groups because the similarity and intensity of the disorder tend to outweigh cultural differences (Yalom, 2005).

Women: trauma-informed care

Compared to men, incarcerated women have higher rates of poverty, substance abuse, and mental illness, and a history of physical, psychological, and sexual abuse is more common (see Chapter 51). Researchers suggest that group therapy with women avoid confrontational techniques and incorporate affective, spiritual, and trauma-informed curriculum (Spiropoulos, Spruance, van Voorhis, & Schmitt, 2005). Trauma-informed care is an approach to engaging people with histories of trauma that recognizes the presence of trauma symptoms and acknowledges the role that trauma has played in their lives (Substance Abuse and Mental Health Services Administration, 2013). Gender-responsive group therapy has been demonstrated to be more effective than standard therapeutic community group therapy in reducing drug use and recidivism (Messina et al., 2010). Helping Women Recover and Beyond Trauma are examples of manual-driven group therapy treatment programs that, when combined, serve women in criminal justice or correctional settings who have substance use disorders and are likely to have co-occurring trauma histories such as sexual or physical abuse (Substance Abuse and Mental Health Services Administration, 2013).

Structured approaches
Cognitive-behavior therapies

One of the most replicated and studied forms of CBT used with forensic populations is Moral Reconation Therapy (MRT; Little & Robinson, 1988). According to the Substance Abuse and

Mental Health Services Administration National Registry of Evidence-Based Programs and Practices (SAMHSA NREPP; 2013), MRT is a systematic treatment strategy that seeks to decrease recidivism among juvenile and adult criminal offenders by increasing moral reasoning. MRT includes specific group exercises and prescribed homework assignments. Participants meet in groups once or twice weekly and can complete all steps of the MRT program in three to six months. Studies have demonstrated the efficacy of this treatment with a range of felony offenders (Allen et al., 2001; Little et al., 2010).

A program called Reasoning and Rehabilitation (R&R) was designed by Ross and Fabian (1988) to combine successful elements of cognitive training programs focused on reducing recidivism. This 36-session manualized program, delivered by probation officers to groups of high-risk probationers, was successful in reducing rates of re-arrest and incarceration. A revised version of R&R was shortened to 16 sessions and adapted to be responsive to the needs of mentally disordered offenders. This revised program, R&R2–MHP, was effective in reducing violent attitudes and improving problem-solving abilities (Rees-Jones et al., 2012).

Several other manualized treatments are being developed for treating mental illness in correctional settings. These include STEPPS, which targets patients with borderline personality disorder (Black et al., 2008), and START NOW, which grew out of prison-based research and is gender-specific, is written at a fifth-grade reading level, and incorporates elements of CBT, motivational interviewing, neurocognitive rehabilitation, and trauma-informed care (Shelton & Wakai, 2011).

Dialectical behavior therapy

Dialectical Behavior Therapy is a cognitive-behavioral treatment that incorporates mindfulness-based interventions and was developed by Marsha M. Linehan (Linehan, 1993). DBT comprises four modules: mindfulness, distress tolerance, emotion regulation, and interpersonal effectiveness. The treatment is delivered in two components: individual and group therapy. DBT was initially validated as an evidence-based approach for patients diagnosed with borderline personality disorder but has since shown promising outcomes for other disorders, including substance abuse, eating disorders, and bipolar disorder. DBT has been found to be effective in the setting of substance abuse, anger, interpersonal difficulties, treatment dropout, and inpatient hospitalizations; it has been shown to reduce suicidal behavior (Behavioral Tech, LLC, 2013). DBT has been adapted for use with incarcerated populations; however, there are no published standardized manuals for DBT generalizable to correctional settings (Berzins & Trestman, 2004). Nee and Farman (2005) used DBT with female prisoners and found an overall reduction in self-harm behavior.

Recovery model

The recovery model is a treatment philosophy that focuses on treating individuals with mental illness by focusing on life satisfaction, hope and optimism, knowledge about mental illness and services, and empowerment (see Chapter 40). The New York State Office of Mental Health piloted a program called Illness Management and Recovery (IMR), a curriculum-based treatment that uses research-informed psychosocial approaches that help adults to manage serious mental health problems and make progress toward specific goals. The research led to adaptation of the IMR curriculum and creation of the Wellness Self-Management (WSM) curriculum, which is organized into a workbook that belongs to the participants and includes self-directed action steps. The process for WSM groups is organized around a specific group facilitation format, and online training is available for facilitators. Research indicates that 75% of participants demonstrated significant progress with respect to their identified goal areas over the course of the program (Salerno et al., 2011).

Substance abuse

Group therapy has been shown to be an effective treatment for alcohol dependence and other substance abuse disorders (Sandahl et al., 1998), as well as substance abuse co-occurring with other mental disorders such as social anxiety (Courbasson & Nishikawa, 2010). Empirical studies demonstrate that approaches such as motivational interviewing and CBT, in conjunction with 12-step programs, are effective in treating substance abuse (Sobell & Sobell, 2011). The SAMHSA NREPP (2013) includes three programs designed to treat substance abuse, Living in Balance, Forever Free, and Helping Woman Recover/Beyond Trauma.

In corrections settings, treatment of substance abuse may be complicated by institutional rules related to disclosure of substance use or trafficking. The group therapist should regularly remind participants of limits of confidentiality and consequences of disclosure of substance abuse during incarceration.

Community reentry

Many corrections settings provide group therapy with a focus on preparation for community reentry; however, there are few empirical studies that measure the impact of these groups on recidivism. One study of a structured intervention demonstrated significant reduction in recidivism for a population with serious mental illness (Kesten et al., 2012). A widely used curriculum (Shrum, 2012) includes information about specific community resources, including support service programs, education and training opportunities, employment supports for ex-offenders, budgeting/finance management, and strategies for homeless living.

Process groups

Process groups focus on the "here and now" of interactions between group members to create a social microcosm that allows experiential learning and insight development (Yalom, 2005). The goal of the process group is to reduce dysfunctional interactions between group participants in order to increase self-awareness and facilitate behavioral change that generalizes to life outside the group. Doctoral-level providers typically facilitate psychotherapy groups because extensive clinical training and experience are required to appropriately use the group process as a catalyst for emotional growth and behavioral change.

Recreation therapy

Recreation therapy is an evidence-based treatment used to improve a person's overall functioning in physical, cognition, emotion, and psychosocial areas; this, in turn, helps support health and wellness by improving daily living skills (American Therapeutic Recreation Association, 2013; Booth, 1981). Activities such as sports, games, art, music, drama, and reading are used to encourage improvement in social skills, exploration of relationships, and reduction of the impact of isolation. In the corrections setting, recreation groups may include opportunities to watch television or movies as a behavioral reinforcement or to stimulate discussion and interactions between group members.

Summary

Evidence-based group therapy is a cost-effective way to treat mental illness and substance abuse and to reduce criminal behavior. Administrators and legislators who are responsible for developing treatment plans for correctional populations should ensure that the goals of group therapy are carefully defined and that resources are allocated appropriately for training, implementation, and fidelity monitoring.

References

Allen, L. C., MacKenzie, D. L., & Hickman, L. J. (2001). The effectiveness of cognitive behavioral treatment for adult offenders: A methodological, quality-based review. *International Journal of Offender Therapy and Comparative Criminology, 45*, 498–514.

American Therapeutic Recreation Association (2013). *Frequently asked questions about recreational therapy.* Available at: http://www.atra-online.com/associations/10488/files/TR_FAQ.pdf (accessed November 24, 2013).

Andrews, D. A., Bonta, J., & Wormith, J. S. (2006). The recent past and near future of risk and/or need assessment. *Crime and Delinquency, 52,* 7–27.

Andrews, D. A., Zinger, I., Hoge, R. D., Bonta, J., Gendreau, P., & Cullen, F. T. (1990). Does correctional treatment work? A clinically relevant and psychologically informed meta-analysis. *Criminology, 28,* 369–404.

Barlow, S. (2004). A strategic three-year plan to teach group competencies. *Journal of the Specialists in Group Work, 29,* 113–126.

Behavioral Tech, LLC (n.d.). *DBT Resources: What is DBT?* Available at: http://www.behavioraltech.com/resources/whatisdbt.cfm (accessed August 17, 2013).

Berzins, L. G., & Trestman, R. L. (2004). The development and implementation of dialectical behavior therapy in forensic settings. *International Journal of Forensic Mental Health, 3,* 93–103.

Black, D. W., Blum, N., Eichinger, L., McCormick, B., Allen, J., & Sieleni, B. (2008). STEPPS: Systems Training for Emotional Predictability and Problem Solving in women offenders with borderline personality disorder in prison—a pilot study. *CNS Spectrums, 13,* 881–886.

Booth, M. A. (1981). *Recreation and leisure time activities in the correctional setting: A selected bibliography.* Washington, DC: U.S. Dept. of Justice, National Institute of Justice.

Chaiken, S., Thompson, C., & Shoemaker, W. (2005). Mental health interventions in correctional settings. In C. L. Scott & J. B. Gerbasi (Eds.), *Handbook of correctional mental health* (pp. 345–376). Washington, DC: American Psychiatric Publishing, Inc.

Courbasson, C. M., & Nishikawa, Y. (2010). Cognitive behavioral group therapy for patients with co-existing social anxiety disorder and substance use disorders: A pilot study. *Cognitive Therapy and Research, 34,* 82–91.

DeLucia-Waack, J. L. (2004). *Handbook of group counseling and psychotherapy.* Thousand Oaks, CA: Sage Publications.

Fuhriman, A., & Burlingame, G. M. (1994). Group psychotherapy: Research and practice. In A. Fuhriman & G. M. Burlingame (Eds.), *Handbook of group psychotherapy: An empirical and clinical synthesis* (pp. 3–40). New York: Wiley.

Gendreau, P. (1996). Offender rehabilitation: What we know and what needs to be done. *Criminal Justice and Behavior, 23,* 144–161.

Gendreau, P., Goggin, C., & Smith, P. (1999). The forgotten issue in effective correctional treatment: Program implementation. *International Journal of Offender Therapy and Comparative Criminology, 43,* 180–187.

Hamm, M. S., & Schrink, J. L. (1989). The conditions of effective implementation: A guide to accomplishing rehabilitative objectives in corrections. *Criminal Justice and Behavior, 16,* 166.

Hollin, C. R. (1995). The meaning and implications of "programme integrity." In J. McGuire (Ed.), *What works: Effective methods to reduce reoffending* (pp. 269–287). Chichester: Wiley.

Kanas, N., Rogers, M., Kreth, E., Patterson, L., & Campbell, R. (1980). The effectiveness of group psychotherapy during the first three weeks of hospitalization: A controlled study. *Journal of Nervous and Mental Disease, 168,* 487–492.

Kanas, N. (1996). *Group therapy for schizophrenic patients.* Washington, DC: American Psychiatric Press.

Kanas, N. (2005). Group therapy for patients with chronic trauma-related stress disorders. *International Journal of Group Psychotherapy, 55,* 161–165.

Kanas, N., Penn, D. L., Waldheter, E. J., Perkins, D. O., et al. (2006). Group therapy with schizophrenia patients/Dr. Penn and colleagues reply. *American Journal of Psychiatry, 163,* 937–938.

Kesten, K. L., Leavitt-Smith, E., Rau, D. R., Shelton, D., Zhang, W., Wagner, J., & Trestman, R. L. (2012). Recidivism rates among mentally ill inmates impact of the Connecticut Offender Reentry Program. *Journal of Correctional Health Care, 18,* 20–28.

Kominars, K., & Dornheim, L. (2004) Group approaches in substance abuse treatment. In J. L. DeLucia-Waack, D. A. Gerrity, C. R. Kalodner, & M. T. Riva (Eds.), *Handbook of group counseling and psychotherapy* (pp. 563–575). Thousand Oaks, CA: Sage Publications.

Koocher, G. P., & Keith-Spiegel, P. (2008). *Ethics in psychology and the mental health professions: Standards and cases.* Oxford: Oxford University Press.

Kominars, K., & Dornheim, L. (2004). *Group approaches in substance abuse treatment.* Thousand Oaks, CA: Sage Publications Ltd.

Linehan, M. M. (1993). *Cognitive behavioral treatment of borderline personality disorder.* New York: The Guilford Press.

Little, G. L., & Robinson, K. D. (1988). Moral reconation therapy: A systematic step-by-step treatment system for treatment resistant clients. *Psychological Reports, 62,* 135–151.

Little, G., Robinson, K. D., Burnette, K. D., & Swan, S. (2000). Ten-year outcome data MRT-treated DWI offenders. *Alternatives to Incarceration, 6,* 16–18.

Little, G. L., Robinson, K. D., Burnette, K. D., & Swan, E. S. (2010). Twenty-year recidivism results for MRT-treated offenders. *Cognitive Behavioral Treatment Review, 19,* 1–5.

MacNair, R. R., & Corazzini, J. G. (1994). Client factors influencing group therapy dropout. *Psychotherapy: Theory, Research, Practice, Training, 31,* 352–362.

MacNair-Semands, R. (2002). Predicting attendance and expectations for group therapy. *Group Dynamics: Theory, Research, and Practice, 6,* 219–228.

McGrath, R. J., Cumming, G. F., & Burchard, B. L. (2003). *Current practices and trends in sexual abuser management: The Safer Society 2002 nationwide survey.* Brandon, VT: Safer Society.

McEvoy, P. M. (2007). Effectiveness of cognitive behavioural group therapy for social phobia in a community clinic: A benchmarking study. *Behaviour Research and Therapy, 45,* 3030–3040.

McMurran, M. (2009). Motivational interviewing with offenders: A systematic review. *Legal and Criminological Psychology, 14,* 83–100.

McRoberts, C., Burlingame, G. M., & Hoag, M. J. (1998). Comparative efficacy of individual and group psychotherapy: A meta-analytic perspective. *Group Dynamics: Theory, Research, and Practice, 2,* 101–117.

Messina, N., Grella, C. E., Cartier, J., & Torres, S. (2010). A randomized experimental study of gender-responsive substance abuse treatment for women in prison. *Journal of Substance Abuse Treatment, 38,* 97–107.

Miller, W. R. & Rollnick, S. (2002). *Motivational interviewing: Preparing people for change.* New York: Guilford Press.

Nee, C., & Farman, S. (2005). Female prisoners with borderline personality disorder: Some promising treatment developments. *Criminal Behaviour and Mental Health, 15,* 2–16.

Pérez-Arce, P., Carr, K. D., & Sorensen, J. L. (1993). Cultural issues in an outpatient program for stimulant abusers. *Journal of Psychoactive Drugs, 25,* 35–44.

Rapin, L. S. (2004). *Guidelines for ethical and legal practice in counseling and psychotherapy groups.* Thousand Oaks, CA: Sage Publications Ltd.

Rees-Jones, A., Gudjonsson, G., & Young, S. (2012). A multi-site controlled trial of a cognitive skills program for mentally disordered offenders. *BMC Psychiatry, 12,* 44.

Salerno, A., Margolies, P., Cleek, A., Pollock, M., Gopalan, G., & Jackson, C. (2011). Best practices: Wellness Self-Management: An adaptation of the illness management and recovery program in New York state. *Psychiatric Services, 62,* 456–458.

Salter, A. C. (1988). *Treating child sex offenders and victims: A practical guide.* Thousand Oaks, CA: Sage Publications, Inc.

Sandahl, C., Herlitz, K., Ahlin, G., & Ronnberg, S. (1998). Time-limited group psychotherapy for moderately alcohol dependent patients: A randomized controlled clinical trial. *Psychotherapy Research, 8,* 361.

Shelton, D., & Wakai, S. (2011). A process evaluation of START NOW skills training for inmates with impulsive and aggressive behaviors. *Journal of the American Psychiatric Nurses Association, 17*(2), 148–157.

Shively, R. (2004). Treating offenders with mental retardation and developmental disabilities. *Corrections Today, 66,* 84–86, 141

Shrum, H. E. (2012). *The ex-offender's guide to a responsible life: A national directory of re-entry tips and resources.* Manassas Park, VA: Impact Publications.

Smith, P. (2006). *The effects of incarceration on recidivism: A longitudinal examination of program participation and institutional adjustment in federally sentenced adult male offenders.* Order No. NR41222, University of New Brunswick, Canada.

Sobell, L. C., & Sobell, M. B. (2011). *Group Therapy for Substance Use Disorders: A Motivational Cognitive-Behavioral Approach.* New York, NY: Guilford Press.

Spiropoulos, G. V., Spruance, L., van Voorhis, P., & Schmitt, M. M. (2005). Pathfinders and problem solving: Comparative effects of two cognitive-behavioral programs among men and women offenders in community and prison. *Journal of Offender Rehabilitation, 42*(2), 69–94. doi:10.1300/J076v42n0205

Substance Abuse and Mental Health Services Administration (n.d.). *NREPP home.* Available at: http://www.nrepp.samhsa.gov/ (accessed September 29, 2013).

Tasca, G. A., & Bone, M. (2007). Individual versus group psychotherapy for eating disorders. *International Journal of Group Psychotherapy, 57,* 399–403.

Ward, T., Melser, J., & Yates, P. M. (2007). Reconstructing the risk-need-responsivity model: A theoretical elaboration and evaluation. *Aggression and Violent Behavior, 12,* 208–228.

Yalom, I. D. (2005). *The theory and practice of group psychotherapy* (5th ed.). New York: Basic Books.

Yalom, I. D., & Leszcz, M. (1995). *The theory and practice of group psychotherapy.* New York: Basic Books.

SECTION IX

Suicide risk management

CHAPTER 43

Suicide risk management

Kerry C. Hughes and Jeffrey L. Metzner

Introduction

The risk of suicide is a significant concern for incarcerated individuals. This chapter reviews issues relevant to prevalence, demographics, trends, screening, and assessment of suicide risk, as well as identification of key factors associated with increased risk and managing that risk safely and appropriately in correctional facilities. Suicide risk factors that are often more specific to prisons, such as restrictive housing, facility transfers, and loss of community social support systems, which often require proactive interventions, are highlighted.

Suicide in jails and prisons

Prevalence of suicide in prisons and jails

Suicide was the leading cause of death for jail inmates in 2009 and 2010. Available data indicate that the rate of suicide in jails showed an initial decline over the past decades, with some recent increase in the rate. Information from the Bureau of Justice Statistics indicates that jail suicide rates have declined steadily from 129 per 100,000 inmates in 1983 to 47 per 100,000 in 2002 (Mumola, 2005). A subsequent review noted that the local jail suicide rate declined from 49 per 100,000 inmates in 2001 to 36 per 100,000 in 2007. The rate increased slightly in 2010 to 42 per 100,000 (Noonan, 2012).

In contrast, suicide was the fifth most common cause of death in prisons during 2010 (Noonan, 2012). The suicide rate in state prisons decreased from 34 per 100,000 in 1980 to 14 per 100,000 in 2002 (Mumola, 2005). State prison suicide rates remained essentially unchanged after 2002; the rate was 16 per 100,000 in 2004, 17 per 100,000 in 2006, 15 per 100,000 in 2009, and 16 per 100,000 in 2010 (Noonan, 2012).

Several factors have been cited to explain the decrease over time in the suicide rate for incarcerated individuals. Increased awareness of the issue due to national studies of correctional suicide, improved training curricula that incorporate research about suicide prevention, evolving national correctional standards, and inmate suicide litigation have been identified as factors that have influenced the overall decrease in suicide rates (Hayes, 2013). While such improvements are critical, they are not permanent. Continuing and consistent efforts on the part of both clinicians and administrators are required to maintain and advance suicide risk reduction. This chapter details some of the many elements involved in this process.

Demographics of suicide in jails and prisons

Incarcerated individuals are at a higher risk for suicide than the general population for several reasons. Higher rates of mental illness and substance abuse, lack of social supports, conditions of confinement, access to medical and mental health services, and psychosocial stressors of incarceration play significant roles in the increased suicide risk for incarcerated individuals.

Several studies have examined demographic factors related to suicide in jails and prisons. In one study that examined jail suicides in 2005 and 2006, the following factors were identified: 67 percent of the individuals were white; 93 percent were male; the average age was 35; 42 percent were single; 43 percent were held on a personal and/or violent charge (e.g., assault, armed robbery); and they had histories of substance abuse (47 percent), medical problems (28 percent), mental illness (38 percent), treatment with psychotropic medications (20 percent), and suicidal behavior (34 percent; Hayes, 2010). Additionally, the Bureau of Justice Statistics reported that white jail inmates were six times more likely to commit suicide than black inmates and three times more likely than Hispanic inmates. Violent offenders committed suicide at nearly triple the rate of nonviolent offenders in jails (Mumola, 2005). Jail inmates aged ≥55 years had the highest suicide rate and committed suicide at twice the rate of jail inmates aged 18–24 years, who had the lowest suicide rate (Noonan, 2012). Based on these factors, the typical individual who may present with increased suicide risk in jails is an older white male arrested for a violent offense with a history of substance abuse, concomitant medical and mental health problems, and a history of suicidal behavior.

Other factors that have been noted regarding jail suicides include the method and timing of suicides. Hayes (2010) reported that 93 percent of jail suicide victims used hanging as the method, with 30 percent using a bed or bunk as the anchoring device and 66 percent using bedding as the ligature. The deaths were evenly distributed throughout the year, 32 percent occurred between 3 PM and 9 PM, 23 percent occurred within the first 24 hours of incarceration, 27 percent between 2 and 14 days of incarceration, and 20 percent between 1 and 4 months of incarceration. Twenty percent of the victims were intoxicated at the time of death (Hayes, 2010). These data indicate that hanging remains the most common method for suicide in jails, and approximately half of suicides occurred within the first 2 weeks of jail incarceration.

Other significant factors that may assist in improved assessment and intervention include the following: 31 percent of the victims were found dead more than 1 hour after the last observation; cardiopulmonary resuscitation was administered in only 63 percent of the incidents; 38 percent of the victims were held in isolation; 8 percent were on suicide watch at the time of death; no-harm contracts were used in 13 percent of the cases; 35 percent of the deaths occurred close to the date of a court hearing, with 80 percent occurring within 2 days; 47 percent of the victims were assessed by a clinician within 3 days of death; and 22 percent occurred close to the date of a telephone call or visit, with most of them occurring within the first 24 hours (Hayes, 2010). These data are informative in that they illustrate critical factors for increased scrutiny due to higher risk for suicide, including individuals housed in isolation and those who may have received unfavorable news in court, by telephone, or during a visit. Many of the individuals who committed suicide had been seen recently by a clinician, highlighting the need for adequate suicide risk assessment. This information also demonstrates that no-harm contracts were ineffective in preventing suicide.

Suicide in state prison systems from 2001 to 2010 shares many characteristics with suicide in jails, with some important distinctions. On average, age appeared to have little effect on the suicide rate; prisoners committed suicide at nearly equal rates across all age groups (Noonan, 2012). White state prisoners had the highest suicide rates; their rate was 22 percent higher than the Hispanic suicide rate. Black inmates had the lowest rate of suicide and were one-third as likely as whites to commit suicide and less than half as likely as Hispanics (Mumola, 2005). In contrast to local jails, the suicide rate for violent offenders in state prison was much lower (19 suicides per 100,000 versus 92 per 100,000). Nevertheless, violent offenders were still more likely to commit suicide than nonviolent offenders (Mumola, 2005).

Suicides in prisons were less concentrated during the admission/intake period than in jails. Only 7 percent of prison suicides occurred during the first month, and most prison suicides occurred after the first year of confinement (65 percent), with 33 percent occurring after the inmate had served at least 5 years in prison (Mumola, 2005). Some common elements between jail and prison suicides included the lack of relationship to the time of day and place of occurrence (inmate's cell or room).

Studies have also examined suicide in the nation's largest state prison systems. One study of the Texas Department of Criminal Justice noted that, consistent with national data, the prevalence of suicide was reduced among blacks compared to whites and elevated among males compared to females (Baillargeon et al., 2009). The study indicated that Texas prison inmates had rates of psychiatric disorders that were higher than those in the general US population but comparable to other prison populations. It also revealed that inmates with one of four severe psychiatric disorders (major depressive disorder, 61 per 100,000; bipolar disorder, 49 per 100,000; schizophrenia, 91 per 100,000; nonschizophrenic psychotic disorder, 144 per 100,000) had a strikingly elevated risk of suicide during incarceration (Baillargeon et al., 2009).

Another study examined completed suicides that occurred in the California Department of Corrections and Rehabilitation between 1999 and 2004 (Patterson & Hughes, 2008). This study noted that several factors were likely present among individuals who committed suicide during that period. Prisoners with a history of serious mental illness or suicide attempts and those housed in a single cell (particularly in administrative segregation or a secure housing unit) were at elevated risk. Inmates who expressed safety concerns with associated anxiety and agitation, those with serious medical conditions, and those with a co-occurring mood or psychotic disorder and a severe personality disorder were also at elevated risk of suicide. Inmates whose legal status had undergone a significant change such as additional charges or prison time were at elevated risk. Consistent with other studies, white prisoners were at increased risk of suicide, although there was also a rapid increase observed in this 5-year period in suicides by Hispanic prisoners (Patterson & Hughes, 2008).

Incarcerated veterans may not receive the necessary scrutiny regarding suicide prevention. Although there is a lack of data on suicide rates among incarcerated veterans, this group may face high suicide risk due to the presence of many of the risk factors for suicide noted previously (Wortzel et al., 2009). This is an area of needed research and investigation.

Screening and assessment of suicide risk in jails and prisons

The risk of suicide differs in jail and prison settings based on differences in demographics and conditions of confinement. Early research indicated that more than 50 percent of jail suicides occurred within the first 24 hours of incarceration (Hayes, 1989). This contrasts with more recent studies that show that less than a quarter of inmates who committed suicide did so within the first 24 hours of confinement. Half committed suicide between 2 days and 4 months of confinement, highlighting the important but limited value of early screening in suicide prevention (Hayes, 2012). Screening at the time of intake to the correctional facility and ongoing suicide risk assessment at critical times during incarceration are therefore essential in decreasing the risk of suicide (Cox & Morschauser, 1997).

Suicide risk should initially be assessed at the intake into the facility. A confidential setting for the evaluation is vital to the assessment process. Although visual confidentiality may not be possible or advisable in many correctional settings, auditory confidentiality is critical during the intake assessment. Because many of the issues related to suicide risk may be sensitive and difficult to discuss, the assessment must occur in a safe setting that will prevent others from hearing. Omission of this important factor may result in the individual's reluctance to convey important information and an inaccurate assessment of suicide risk.

A trained and qualified mental health professional usually performs the suicide risk assessment; however, a trained correctional or nonmental health staff member (e.g., a nurse) may perform the initial suicide risk assessment. See Chapters 11 and 12 for more detailed information about screening, assessment, and interviewing in correctional settings. Relevant information can be obtained from the arresting or transporting officer regarding observations, reports of suicide, and other information that will help to inform the assessment. Additionally, information on prior incarcerations and placement on suicide monitoring during past incarcerations is vital to obtain (Hayes, 2013).

An adequate suicide risk screening tool or checklist is an important part of a comprehensive suicide prevention program because it

- Provides intake staff with structured questions on areas of concern to cover;

- Functions as a memory aid for busy intake staff when there is little time available to conduct an in-depth evaluation;

- Facilitates communication between officers, health care staff, and mental health staff; and

- Provides legal documentation that an inmate was screened for suicidal risk upon entrance into the facility and again as conditions changed (World Health Organization, 2007).

Screening for suicide risk may be contained in the medical screening form or a separate form and include inquiry regarding the following risk factors:

◆ Past suicidal ideation or attempts;

◆ Current suicidal ideation;

◆ Suicidal threat;

◆ Suicide plan;

◆ Prior mental health treatment and hospitalization;

◆ Recent significant loss (e.g., job, relationship, death of family member/close other, loss of status in the community due to legal concerns);

◆ History of suicidal behavior by family member/close other;

· Suicide risk during prior confinement; and

◆ Arresting/transporting officer's belief that inmate is currently at risk (Metzner & Hayes, 2006).

A positive suicide risk screening assessment may initiate referral to mental health staff for an evaluation and, when clinically appropriate, a more extensive suicide risk assessment.

There are other critical times during incarceration when a suicide risk assessment is indicated. Assessment should obviously occur at the time of report of suicidal ideation, threat, or attempt. Additionally, an assessment may also be indicated whenever a mental health referral is submitted from facility staff, other inmates, or the inmates themselves due to concerns regarding depression or possible suicidal ideation. This is particularly important when staff referrals originate from noted changes in behavior with signs and symptoms of depression and anxiety, such as giving away belongings or expressions of hopelessness and/or helplessness. Assessment is also indicated after inmates receive bad news, recent court proceedings, or contact with family members/significant others that may lead to changes in behavior. Lastly, suicide risk assessment is indicated when contemplating discontinuation of suicide monitoring. The risk assessment may be useful in helping to evaluate current stressors, whether continued monitoring is recommended, as well as the frequency of post-observation follow-up.

In comparison to jails, prisons present a unique challenge due to the generally longer term of incarceration and more residential nature of this setting. Longer-term incarceration may result in feelings of hopelessness and helplessness, which can be a risk factor for suicide. Another consequence of longer incarceration may be the deterioration or loss of social supports such as those provided by family, friends, significant others, occupation, and standing in the community. A factor unique to prisons is the transfer of individuals to other facilities within the prison system due to classification changes, the need for more specialized services, or population management concerns. This change in location and environment may be stressful for some individuals, with the attendant changes in the treatment team, friends, the proximity to family, and concerns regarding a new setting. As these individuals are new to the receiving facility, the assessment for potential suicide risk is of particular importance.

The assessment of suicide risk is a comprehensive evaluation that requires cooperation and communication among mental health, custody, and medical staff. Additionally, it may be necessary to obtain supplementary information such as outside medical records and collateral interviews from family and friends.

Placement into segregated or restrictive housing may also prompt the completion of the suicide risk screening protocol as housing in these settings has been noted to pose higher risk for suicide. The completion of such screening in an out-of-cell setting is important, unless the inmate refuses to leave the cell. Placement into restrictive or segregated housing may occur for several reasons including disciplinary, administrative, and safety concerns. Due to the isolative nature of these units and the customary practice of removal of personal items such as televisions and radios, placement into these housing units may increase the risk of suicide for those individuals (Patterson & Hughes, 2008). Access to materials to make a mental health referral (e.g., a request form) may also be limited in restrictive housing compared to a traditional housing unit.

A study in the New York State Prison system noted that most suicides in a special disciplinary housing unit occurred within 8 weeks of placement (Way et al., 2007). The previously referenced screening prior to placement into restrictive housing is essential to prevent placement of suicidal individuals into this type of housing. Additionally, enhanced clinical and custody rounds, monitoring for suicidal behavior, and access to mental health staff are necessary as described in the next section.

Restricted housing units

Clinical rounds and monitoring should occur for all individuals in restrictive housing units, not solely for those previously identified as needing mental health services. The frequency of these rounds will be determined by factors that include the usual length of stay, size of the housing unit, and demographics of the inmate population (e.g., are inmates with a serious mental illness excluded from such a housing placement?). These rounds are often unfairly criticized due to their potentially brief and superficial quality. However, these rounds are not designed to provide a formal mental health assessment of each inmate. These rounds are performed to

◆ Ensure that mental health staff have a presence in the housing unit. Prior to mental health rounds becoming a routine practice, it was common for mental health staff to avoid high-security housing units for reasons such as security regulations or personal discomfort.

◆ Screen all inmates for signs or symptoms of mental health problems that require clinical intervention and/or removal from the restrictive housing unit. This screening is an important component of a facility's suicide prevention plan.

◆ Improve access to mental health care services by supplementing the "sick call" process, which often does not work well in a restricted housing setting for reasons such as poor access to health care request forms.

By establishing a consistent presence on the unit, the mental health clinician has an opportunity to develop a good working relationship with custody staff who will aid in the previously referenced screening objectives and improve access to the unit for the clinician and access to mental health care services for the inmate.

It is not uncommon for a good correctional mental health clinician to lack the interpersonal skills needed to adequately perform mental health rounds. Many nonmentally ill inmates will initially and, at times continuously, verbally assault the clinician during rounds in a manner that is quite unpleasant. Other inmates will make requests of the clinician that are not within the scope of duties for a mental health clinician. A needed clinical skill, which is acquired under supervision and with practice, is appropriate limit-setting and the ability to say "no" in a manner that the inmate can accept and respect.

Due to the very limited property and social interactions in many restricted housing units, it is helpful if the clinician can offer inmates regular access to crossword puzzles or something equivalent to help the inmate deal with the inherent monotony of the housing unit. Reading the sports page prior to starting rounds in order to provide scores of sporting events will be appreciated by many inmates and can facilitate a working relationship with them. Rounds provide the inmate with an opportunity to speak with the clinician at the cell front. An out-of-cell interview can then be scheduled as clinically appropriate based on this triage screening.

Monitoring of inmates who are on the mental health caseload is best accomplished by out-of-cell clinical interviews that ensure adequate sound privacy. The frequency of such clinical contacts will be determined by the level of mental health care required as per the inmate's treatment plan, although the mental health rounding process often results in additional out-of-cell contacts as circumstances arise. Monitoring of nonmental health caseload inmates is accomplished by performing mental health rounds and by mental health staff attendance at custody committee meetings that review the inmates' status (e.g., a classification committee review).

Managing the risk of suicide in jails and prisons

Correctional facilities can implement other proactive measures to reduce suicides. All correctional facilities need a suicide prevention program that includes written policies and procedures and meaningful staff training regarding these plans (US Department of Health and Human Services, Substance Abuse and Mental Health Services Administration, 2011). Because correctional officers have the most contact with incarcerated individuals and can routinely intervene in a timely way to prevent suicides, they must receive training in suicide prevention. All correctional staff and health care and mental health personnel need to receive initial suicide prevention training, followed by refresher training each year. In addition, all staff who have routine contact with inmates need training in standard first aid, cardiopulmonary resuscitation, and the use of emergency equipment located in each housing unit, with incorporation of mock drills into initial and refresher training (Metzner & Hayes, 2006).

It is important that the suicide prevention plan include a suicide prevention committee (SPC) that meets regularly (monthly to quarterly depending on the size of the facility and other variables). Membership may include high-ranking staff from the custody, mental health, nursing, medical, and pharmacy departments in addition to select line staff. This committee is often cochaired by the director of mental health and the deputy warden for health care (or equivalent position). In large prisons, the SPC generally reports to the mental health subcommittee of the health care quality improvement committee. The reporting

structure in jails and smaller prisons will be determined by the local organization.

The SPC generally oversees implementation of the suicide prevention plan, policies, and procedures. It reviews, on an ongoing basis, statistics and details on suicide attempts (especially serious attempts) and training relevant to the suicide prevention plan. Corrective actions recommended by psychological autopsies (which follow any completed suicide and are described in detail later) and pertinent reports from the morbidity and mortality committee may be developed, implemented, and monitored by the SPC.

It is also important that correctional facilities provide an adequate and effective mental health care delivery system that ensures timely response to referrals to mental health for assessment and treatment and that there is a system for follow-up for ongoing mental health concerns. See Chapter 22 for more details. This system must be in place to have an effective suicide prevention program.

Another proactive measure that may be effective in decreasing the feelings of hopelessness and despondency that may occur for incarcerated individuals is the implementation of rehabilitation programs in correctional settings (Cullen & Gilbert, 2012). Education, work, and substance abuse treatment programs have been decreased and eliminated in some facilities due to budgetary concerns. The absence of these programs has resulted in a dearth of opportunities for individuals to address the issues that led to their incarceration. Additionally, these programs provide a mechanism of structure and purpose for individuals who have little opportunity for meaningful advancement due to their incarceration. Correctional facilities might consider the expansion or implementation of rehabilitation programs to assist individuals in self-improvement and possibly to decrease some of the factors that may lead to suicide.

Housing for the suicidal inmate

There is a word of caution to convey regarding the active management of an inmate with a high or imminent suicide risk. Such inmates are frequently placed in "strip cells," which often do not even include a mattress. A "suicide smock" without underwear is the only clothing usually allowed. In many correctional facilities, inmates experience suicide monitoring as punitive and unpleasant due to the harsh nature of such observation. Measures such as an uncomfortable temperature; the routine removal of clothing, assistive devices, and reading materials; and placement into harsh environments such as padded or rubberized cells without toilets may, in fact, be counterproductive. Such measures may inhibit and discourage, rather than encourage, the report of suicidal ideation, plan, or intent (Metzner & Hayes, 2006). It is important that suicide monitoring and treatment planning be individualized and that the conditions of observation provide a safe environment to prevent self-harm while also maintaining the dignity of individuals who are monitored.

The housing location of suicidal inmates is an important consideration. National correctional standards stress the need for housing in the general population, mental health unit, or medical infirmary located close to staff rather than the tendency, in many settings, to isolate suicidal individuals (Metzner & Hayes, 2006). Such housing should rarely exist in a restricted housing unit. An important consideration is the composition of the room in which an individual is monitored. These spaces may need to be modified to reduce potential means of self-harm. This includes modifying potential tie-off points such as smoke detectors, light fixtures, hooks, bars, and ventilation grates. Toilets and sinks made of metal or a nonbreakable material can prevent the use of shards as potential items for self-harm. The interior of the cell should be visible from the outside to prevent blind areas.

Facilities may also consider double-celling for appropriate suicidal individuals. Qualified mental health professionals must make individualized determinations of allowable property for inmates on suicide monitoring. Unless contraindicated, inmates receive tear-resistant mattresses and blankets.

The National Commission on Correctional Health Care (NCCHC) provides recommendations for suicide monitoring that ranges from constant observation to less frequent, staggered checks every 10 to 15 minutes (National Commission on Correctional Health Care, 2008). Acuity determines the level of suicide monitoring, with constant observation reserved for actively suicidal inmates who either threaten or engage in suicidal behavior. Inmates not actively suicidal but with suicidal ideation or recent incidents of self-injurious behavior receive less frequent monitoring (Hayes, 1995). Further, it is important that suicide prevention assessment be performed daily by a qualified mental health professional.

Correctional facilities have used several means to monitor individuals at high risk for suicide. One means has been the use of closed-circuit televisions, which should supplement and not replace constant observation for high-risk individuals, as they record but do not prevent the completion of suicide. Some systems have used inmate companions for suicide monitoring for high-risk individuals to supplement adequate suicide monitoring by facility staff. We strongly discourage the use of inmates for such purposes, for reasons that include an added burden on the nursing staff, who now must monitor not only the suicidal inmate but also the inmate companion (who is often disruptive to the unit despite training and screening for the role). There is also the risk of inappropriate use of inmate observers in lieu of staff. Contracts with inmates for "safety" have been shown to be ineffective in preventing suicides, and the use of such contracts is not recommended (Hayes, 2013).

Placement on a suicide monitoring program too often involves minimal clinical intervention and/or out-of-cell clinical contacts. The underlying dynamics for this dearth of clinical interventions is often the unspoken belief that the inmate is manipulating the system by reporting suicidality (i.e., has used the "s" word) to avoid some issue (e.g., a debt to another inmate) in the inmate's prior housing placement. Thus, some correctional staff believe that the manipulation will cease and the inmate will no longer report being suicidal if conditions of confinement are sufficiently unpleasant. Such a formulation bypasses the responsibility of the clinician to perform a competent suicide risk assessment that may be the basis for subsequent interventions.

The use of a suicide risk assessment instrument is also important at the time of consideration of discontinuing suicide monitoring and for subsequent follow-up. Clinical follow-up is essential soon after discontinuation of suicide monitoring and then based on clinical need.

Suicide risk-reduction training

The framework for a comprehensive correctional suicide prevention program includes substantial staff training. Because correctional staff are frequently the first responders after a suicide attempt or completed suicide, their training is critical.

The American Correctional Association (ACA) and the NCCHC provide guidance regarding the need for training as an integral part of an adequate suicide prevention program. ACA standard 3-4081 requires that all new correctional staff receive training in the "signs of suicide risk" and "suicide precautions"; standard 3-4364 requires staff training in the implementation of the suicide prevention program (American Correctional Association, 2003). The NCCHC standard P-54 also addresses the need for suicide training, stating that "all staff members who work with inmates should be trained to recognize verbal and behavioral curs that indicate potential suicide" (National Commission on Correctional Health Care, 2003).

The most effective approach to training correctional staff is through preservice training in state, regional, or local academies. It is important that retraining be conducted periodically, preferably at least every 2 years on an in-service basis (Rowan & Hayes, 1995). It is recommended that all correctional, medical, and mental health personnel and other staff who have regular contact with inmates receive 8 hours of initial suicide prevention training and a minimum of 2 hours of refresher training each year. This initial training includes instruction regarding administrator and staff attitudes about suicide and how negative attitudes impede suicide prevention efforts, why correctional environments are conducive to suicidal behavior, potential predisposing factors to suicide, high-risk suicide periods, warning signs and symptoms, how to identify suicidal inmates despite a denial of risk, components of the facility's suicide prevention policy, and liability. The 2-hour refresher training reviews the topics discussed during the initial training and also describes any changes to the facility's suicide prevention plan. The annual training also includes a general discussion of recent suicides and/or suicide attempts in the facility (Hayes, 2012).

In addition, it is important that all staff in contact with inmates be trained in standard first aid and cardiopulmonary resuscitation procedures and learn how to use the emergency equipment located in each housing unit. To ensure an efficient emergency response to suicide attempts, mock drills should be incorporated into both the initial and refresher training for all staff (Hayes, 2012). Staff who arrive at the scene must not presume that the inmate is dead; using emergency response equipment that is monitored and maintained in working order, staff should initiate and continue appropriate life-saving measures until relieved by medical personnel (Metzner & Hayes, 2006).

Psychological autopsy

Following a completed suicide, a formal protocol may be beneficial in assisting staff in understanding the events that led to the suicide, specifically intervening to address staff feelings that follow such a trauma and performing a psychological autopsy for quality improvement purposes. This section describes best-practice approaches to postmortem review.

What happens after a completed suicide?

The correctional suicide prevention program should include procedures regarding official documentation and report of the incident and provide the constructive feedback necessary to improve suicide prevention activities (Konrad & Daigle, 2007). Reporting requirements include notification to the appropriate facility staff, the inmate's family, and the necessary outside authorities. The medical record must be secured, and staff involved in the incident are required to write statements about their involvement.

Staff and inmates involved in the incident or with knowledge of the victim may experience a range of feelings from anger and resentment to guilt and sadness; these individuals may benefit from more detailed debriefing and/or grief counseling (World Health Organization, 2007). Vulnerable inmates who may have viewed the incident, who were housed near the victim, or who may be at higher risk for suicide may require particular attention. These individuals should be identified, screened, and monitored to prevent additional suicides. Discussions in therapeutic community-like meetings, individual sessions, and group therapy may serve as vehicles to assist identified inmates in dealing with the completed suicide of a peer. One form of assistance is critical incident stress debriefing (CISD). A CISD team is typically composed of professionals trained in crisis intervention and traumatic stress awareness (e.g., police officers, paramedics, firefighters, clergy, and mental health personnel). Use of a CISD team allows staff and inmates to process their feelings about the incident, develop an understanding of critical stress symptoms, and seek ways of dealing with those symptoms. For maximum effectiveness, the CISD process or other appropriate support services should occur within 24 to 72 hours of the critical incident (Hayes, 2012).

Postmortem review and psychological autopsy

The development and implementation of a systematic quality management process with review of all completed suicides is an important component of an effective suicide prevention program (Patterson & Hughes, 2008). To fully understand why an inmate committed suicide and whether the agency was in the best possible position to prevent the incident, every suicide and serious suicide attempt (i.e., those requiring hospitalization) must be examined through a comprehensive morbidity and mortality review process, which is separate from other formal investigations that may be required to determine the cause of death (e.g., autopsy, state police inquiry, coroner's inquest; Hayes, 1999). The morbidity and mortality review process should include the following:

* A critical inquiry of the circumstances surrounding the incident;

* Facility procedures relevant to the incident;

* Relevant training that involved staff received;

* Pertinent medical and mental health services or reports involving the victim;

* Possible precipitating factors that led to the suicide or serious suicide attempt; and

* Recommendations, if any, for changes in policy, training, physical plant, medical or mental health services, and operational procedures (Hayes, 1999).

The timely completion of a psychological autopsy may also assist in gaining an understanding of why an inmate committed suicide. The psychological autopsy is a retrospective reconstruction of a decedent's life initiated to gain better understanding of his or her death (Shneidman, 1981). This report includes a review of pertinent information, including incident reports,

health care records, prison custody records, medical autopsy and toxicology findings, an inspection of the death scene, and interviews with inmates and staff (and possibly family and friends). The reviewer may then provide an assessment of precipitating events; the motive for suicide; and recommendations on mental health and medical standards of care, suicide prevention policy and procedures, or changes in environmental design or training (Sanchez, 1999).

Summary

Correctional facilities must develop and implement effective suicide prevention programs. These programs can be successful only if they are part of a larger mental health delivery system. As suicide risk fluctuates based on changes in environment and circumstances, the assessment of suicide risk must not be seen as static; rather, it is an ongoing process throughout the individual's incarceration. In light of a changing correctional environment that includes more compromised individuals and fewer inpatient beds, there is a need for greater attention to proactive measures that will reduce the risk of suicide in jails and prisons.

Training of mental health, medical, and correctional staff is an integral part of a successful suicide prevention program, and this training may help to address many of the negative attitudes on assessment and treatment of an incarcerated suicidal individual. Finally, critical review should occur after a serious suicide attempt or completed suicide to evaluate the circumstances that led to the incident and address potential corrective actions needed to prevent future suicidal events.

References

American Correctional Association (2003). *Standards for adult correctional institutions*, 4th ed. Lanham, MD.

American Correctional Association (2004). *Performance-based standards for adult local detention facilities*, 4th ed. Lanham, MD.

American Heart Association, Emergency Cardiac Care Committee and Subcommittees (1992). Guidelines for cardiopulmonary resuscitation and emergency cardiac care. *Journal of the American Medical Association*, 268, 2172–2183.

American Psychiatric Association (2000). *Psychiatric services in jails and prisons*, 2nd ed. Washington, DC: American Psychiatric Association.

Anno, B. (1985). Patterns of suicide in the Texas Department of Corrections, 1980–1985. *Journal of Prisons and Jail Health*, 5(2), 82–93.

Appelbaum, K., Dvoskin, J., Geller, J., & Grisso, T. (1997). *Report on the psychiatric management of John Salvi in Massachusetts Department of Corrections Facilities: 1995–1996*. Worcester, MA: University of Massachusetts Medical Center.

Atlas, R. (1989). Reducing the opportunity for inmate suicide: A design guide. *Psychiatric Quarterly*, 60, 161–171.

Aufderheide, D. (2000). Conducting the psychological autopsy in correctional settings. *Journal of Correctional Health Care*, 7(1), 5–36.

Baillargeon, J., Penn, J., Thomas, C. R., Temple, J. R., Baillargeon, G., & Murray, J. (2009). Psychiatric disorders and suicide in the nation's largest state prison system. *Journal of American Academy of Psychiatry and the Law*, 37, 188–193.

Beck, A. J. (1993). *Survey of state prison inmates, 1991* (pp. 1–34). US Department of Justice, Office of Justice Programs, Bureau of Justice Statistics.

Bonner, R. (1992). Isolation, seclusion, and psychological vulnerability as risk factors for suicide behind bars. In R. Maris, A. Berman, J. Maltsberger, & R. Yufit (eds.), *Assessment and prediction of suicide* (pp. 398–419). New York: Guilford Press.

Bonner, R. (2000). Correctional suicide prevention in the year 2000 and beyond. *Suicide and Life-Threatening Behavior, 30*(4), 370–376.

Clark, D., & Horton-Deutsch, S. (1992). Assessment in absentia: The value of the psychological autopsy method for studying antecedents of suicide and predicting future suicides. In A. Maris, J. Maltsberger, & R. Yufit (eds.), *Assessment and prediction of suicide* (pp. 144–182). New York: Guilford Press.

Copeland, A. R. (1989). Fatal suicidal hangings among prisoners in jail. *Medicine, Science and the Law, 29,* 341–345.

Cox, J. F., & Lawrence, J. E. (2010). Planning services for elderly inmates with mental illness. *Corrections Today, 72,* 52–57.

Cox, J. F., & Morschauser, P. C. (1997). A solution to the problem of jail suicide. *Journal of Crisis Intervention and Suicide Prevention, 18*(4), 178–184.

Cullen, F. T., & Gilbert, K. E. (2012). *Reaffirming rehabilitation.* Waltham, MA: Anderson Publishing.

Ditton, P. M. (1999). *Mental health and treatment of inmates and probationers* (pp. 1–12). U.S. Department of Justice, Bureau of Justice Statistics Special Report, NCJ 174463.

DuRand, C. J., Burtka, G. J., Federman, E. J., & Haycox, J. A. (1995). A quarter century of suicide in a major urban jail: Implications for community psychiatry. *American Journal of Psychiatry, 152,* 1077–1080.

Felthous, A. (1994). Preventing jailhouse suicides. *Bulletin of the American Academy of Psychiatry and the Law, 22,* 477–488.

Freeman, A., & Alaimo, C. (2001). Prevention of suicide in a large urban jail. *Psychiatric Annals, 31,* 447–452.

Frost, R., & Hanzlick, R. (1988). Deaths in custody: Atlanta city jail, and Fulton county jail, 1974–1985. *American Journal of Forensic Medicine and Pathology, 9,* 207–211.

Goss, J. R., Peterson, K., Smith, L. W., Kalb, K., & Brodey, B. B. (2002). Characteristics of suicide attempts in a large urban jail system with an established suicide prevention program. *Psychiatric Services, 53*(5), 574–579.

Grattet, R., & Hayes, J. (2013). *California's changing prison population* (pp. 1–2). Public Policy Institute of California.

Harrison, P. M., & Karlberg, J. C. (2004). *Prison and jail inmates at midyear 2003* (pp. 1–14). Bureau of Justice Statistics Bulletin, NCJ 203947. Available at http://www.ojp.usdoj.gov/bjs/pub/pdf/pjm03.pdf (accessed December 3, 2004).

Hayes, L. M. (1983). And darkness closes in . . . a national study of jail suicides. *Criminal Justice and Behavior 10*(4), 461–484.

Hayes, L. M. (1989). National study of jail suicide: Seven years later. *Psychiatric Quarterly, 60,* 7–29.

Hayes, L. M. (1995). Prison suicide: an overview and guide to prevention. *Prison Journal, 75,* 431–456.

Hayes, L. M. (1996). Jail standards and suicide prevention: Another look. *Jail Suicide/Mental Health Update, 6*(4), 9–11.

Hayes, L. M. (2003). Suicide prevention and protrusion-free design of correctional facilities. *Jail Suicide/Mental Health Update, 12*(3), 1–5.

Hayes, L. M. (1999). Was it preventable? The comprehensive review of inmate suicide. *Crisis: The Journal of Crisis Intervention and Suicide Prevention, 20*(4), 147–149.

Hayes, L. M. (2010). *National study of jail suicide: 20 years later.* U.S. Department of Justice National Institute of Corrections, NIC Accession Number 024308.

Hayes, L. M. (2012). National study of jail suicide: 20 years later. *Journal of Correctional Health Care, 18,* 233–245.

Hayes, L. M. (2013). Suicide prevention in correctional facilities; Reflections and next steps. *International Journal of Law and Psychiatry, 36,* 188–194.

He, X. Y., Felthous, A. R., Holzer, C. E., Nathan, P., & Veasey, S. (2001). Factors in prison suicide: one-year study in Texas. *Journal of Forensic Sciences, 46*(4), 896.

Hughes, D. (1995). Can the clinician predict suicide? *Psychiatric Services, 46,* 449–451.

Jutzi-Johnson v. United States, 263 F.3rd 753 (7th Cir. 2001).

Konrad, N., Daigle, M. S., Daniel, A. E., et al. (2007). Preventing suicide in prisons, part 1. Recommendations from the International Association for Suicide Prevention Task Force on Suicide in Prisons. *Crisis, 28,* 113–121.

Kovasznay, B., Miraglia, R., Beer, R., & Way, B. (2004). Reducing suicides in New York State facilities. *Psychiatric Quarterly, 75,* 61–70.

Marcus, P., & Alcabes, P. (1993). Characteristics of suicides by inmates in an urban jail. *Hospital and Community Psychiatry, 44,* 256–261.

Maris, R. (1992). Overview of the study of suicide assessment and prediction. In R. Maris, A. Berman, J. Maltsberger, & R. Yufit (eds.), *Assessment and prediction of suicide* (pp. 3–22). New York: Guilford Press.

Maruschak, L. M. (2001). *HIV in prisons and jails, 1999* (pp. 1–12). U.S. Department of Justice, Bureau of Justice Statistics Bulletin, NCJ 187456.

Meehan, B. (1997). Critical incident stress debriefing within the jail environment. *Jail Suicide/Mental Health Update, 7*(1), 1–5.

Metzner, J. L. (1993). Guidelines for psychiatric services in prisons. *Criminal Behavior and Mental Health, 3,* 252–267.

Metzner, J. L. (1997). An introduction to correctional psychiatry, part I. *Journal of the American Academy of Psychiatry and Law, 25,* 375–381.

Metzner, J. L. (2002). Class action litigation in correctional psychiatry. *Journal of the American Academy of Psychiatry and the Law, 30,* 19–29.

Metzner, J., & Hayes, L. M. (2006). Suicide prevention in jails and prisons. In R. Simon & R. Hales (eds.), *Textbook of suicide Assessment and management* (pp. 139–155). Washington, DC: American Psychiatric Publishing.

Mitchell, J., & Everly, G. (1996). *Critical incident stress debriefing: An operations manual for the prevention of traumatic stress among emergency services and disaster workers,* 2nd ed. Ellicott City, MD: Chevron Publishing.

Morrissey, J. P., Swanson, J. W., Goldstrom, I., Rudolph, L., & Manderscheid, R. W. (1993). *Overview of mental health services provided by state adult correctional facilities: United States, 1988* (pp. 1–13). Department of Health & Human Services, DHHS Publication No. (SMA) 93-1993.

Mumola, C. J. (2005). *Suicide and homicide in state prisons and local jails.* Bureau of Justice Statistics Special Report. Washington, DC: US Department of Justice.

National Commission on Correctional Health Care (1999). *Correctional mental health care: Standards and guidelines for delivering services.* Chicago, IL.

National Commission on Correctional Health Care (2003). *Standards for health services in jails.* Chicago, IL.

National Commission on Correctional Health Care (2008). *Standards for health services in jails.* Chicago, IL.

Noonan, M. (2012). *Mortality in local jails and state prisons, 2000–2010— statistical tables.* Bureau of Justice Statistics. Washington, DC: US Department of Justice.

Patterson, R., & Hughes, K. (2008). Review of completed suicides in the California Department of Corrections and Rehabilitation, 1999 to 2004. *Psychiatric Services, 59,* 676–682.

Regier, D. A., Farmer, M. E., Rae, D. S., Lock, E. B. Z., Keith. S. J., Judd, L. L., & Goodwin, F. K. (1990). Comorbidity of mental disorders with alcohol and other drug abuse: results from the epidemiologic catchment area (ECA) study. *Journal of the American Medical Association, 264,* 2511–2518.

Rowan, J. R., & Hayes, L. M. (1995). *Training curriculum on suicide detection and prevention in jails and lockups.* Mansfield, MA: National Center on Institutions and Alternatives.

Ruiz v. Estelle, 503 F. Supp. 1265 (S.D. Texas 1980).

Sanchez, H. G. (1999). Inmate suicide and the psychological autopsy process. *Jail Suicide/Mental Health Update, 8*(3), 3–9.

Severson, M. (1993). Security and mental health professionals: A (too) silent partnership? *Jail Suicide Update, 5*(3), 1–6.

Shneidman, E. S. (1981). The psychological autopsy. *Suicide and Life-Threatening Behavior, 11*, 325–340.

U.S. Department of Health and Human Services, Substance Abuse and Mental Health Services Administration (2011). *The role of correctional professionals in preventing suicide.* Accessed September 28, 2014 at: http://www.sprc.org/sites/sprc.org/files/CorrectionOfficers.pdf.

Way, B., Sawyer, D. A., Barboza, S., & Nash, R. (2007). Inmate suicide and time spent in special disciplinary housing in New York State Prison. *Psychiatric Services, 58*, 558–560.

White, T. W., Schimmel, D. J., & Frickey, R. (2002). A comprehensive analysis of suicide in federal prisons: A fifteen-year review. *Journal of Correctional Health Care, 9*, 321–343.

White, T. W., & Schimmel, D. J. (1995). Suicide prevention in federal prisons: A successful five-step program. In L. Hayes (ed.), *Prison suicide: An overview and guide to prevention* (pp. 46–57). Washington, DC: National Institute of Corrections, US Department of Justice.

World Health Organization (2007). *Preventing suicide in jails and prisons.* Geneva: World Health Organization, Department of Mental Health and Substance Abuse.

Wortzel, H. S., Binswanger, I. A., Anderson, C. A., & Adler, L. E. (2009). Suicide among incarcerated veterans. *Journal of the American Academy of Psychiatry and the Law, 37*, 82–91.

Treatment of addictions

CHAPTER 44

Programming

Patrece Hairston and Ingrid A. Binswanger

Introduction

The nexus of substance use disorders and criminal justice involvement is considerable. This is particularly the case in the United States, where 48% of individuals in federal prisons were incarcerated for drug-related convictions in 2011 (Carson & Sabol, 2012). In the last year for which national data are available (2004), approximately half of the individuals incarcerated in state and federal prisons met criteria for drug abuse or dependence. These estimates were based on inmate surveys that used questions derived from the *Diagnostic and Statistical Manual of Mental Disorders*, fourth edition (DSM-IV; Mumola & Karberg, 2006) diagnostic codes, which were recently updated in DSM-5. Tobacco and alcohol use are also more common in correctional populations than in the general, noninstitutionalized population (Binswanger, Krueger, & Steiner, 2009). Thus, criminal justice populations have a significant need for evidence-based treatment of addiction and interventions to reduce the medical complications of drug use.

This chapter describes the evolution of addiction programming within correctional settings from the late 1700s to contemporary practices. Beginning with a discussion of mutual aid societies as one of the earliest providers of "treatment," this chapter outlines important aspects of early treatment. Additionally, current levels of care and specialized modalities for individuals involved in the criminal justice system, such as cognitive-behavioral interventions, drug courts, therapeutic communities, pharmacologically supported therapy, and harm-reduction approaches, are discussed.

Diagnosis and assessment considerations

Changes to our understanding of addiction, often operationalized in diagnostic criteria, affect estimates of the burden of substance use disorders in correctional populations. Released in 2013, DSM-5 included several changes to the psychiatric diagnostic system. Most notably, it combined substance dependence and abuse into a single diagnostic category of substance use disorder. Historically, the distinction between substance abuse and dependence was based on the concept that abuse represented a milder form of behavior, with dependence as the more severe manifestation (American Psychiatric Association, 2013, pp. 481–485). Previously, individuals who met criteria for substance abuse could present with severe symptomatology but no symptoms of dependence. To account for symptom severity and need for clinical intervention, a unitary diagnostic category was created; individuals are assessed on a continuum from mild to severe. Two or three symptoms are needed for a diagnosis of mild substance use

disorder compared with only one symptom for a diagnosis of substance abuse in DSM-IV.

In DSM-5, each substance is addressed as a separate use disorder (e.g., alcohol use disorder). Drug craving has been added to the list of 11 potential criteria. Additionally, the "problems with law enforcement" criterion has been eliminated (American Psychiatric Association, 2013, p. 815); this makes the diagnosis internationally more applicable, given that national policies regarding illicit substance use vary.

Gambling disorder was added to DSM-5 in a section on behavioral addictions. "Pathological gambling" was listed in DSM-IV in a different section. However, over time, brain studies have illustrated the biochemical, behavioral, and neurological similarities between gambling disorder and other substance use disorders (American Psychiatric Association, 2013). Among the criminal justice population, approximately one third could be identified as "problem" or "pathological" gamblers (Williams, Royston, & Hagen, 2005). Problem gamblers have also reported higher rates of childhood conduct disorder and antisocial personality disorder, as well as high levels of alcohol consumption—all factors correlated with violent offending (Abbott, McKenna, & Giles, 2005). Despite high prevalence rates and the impact on the criminal justice system, assessment and treatment within correctional settings remain scarce. This diagnostic change may promote the incorporation of gambling disorder into comprehensive treatment programs.

The diagnostic changes in DSM-5 have several implications for the assessment of substance use by correctional providers. First, diagnostic changes may affect the prevalence of substance use disorders. For instance, the deletion of the "problems with law enforcement" criterion may reduce prevalence estimates in the correctional and general population. These changes may subsequently affect programming access and treatment recommendations that require a substance use disorder diagnosis. Substance use assessment tools for criminal justice settings will need modification and validation to reflect the diagnostic changes. Since diagnoses drive treatment recommendations and, subsequently, outcomes, providers will require training in the new diagnostic systems to identify and assess inmates.

For correctional populations, correct classification of substance use disorder severity may have an impact on treatment outcomes. For example, in research on the effectiveness of substance abuse interventions with criminal justice populations, the most effective programs were those that targeted inmates who had substance use disorders and who tended to be moderate to high risk in terms of criminal justice failure (Bahr, Masters, & Taylor,

2012). Treatment and recidivism outcomes were not as robust for lower-risk inmates, which is expected since these inmates tend not to have substance use disorders. As such, individuals need treatment recommendations matched to their identified level of usage and current functioning (National Institute on Drug Abuse, 2012; Taxman, Perdoni, & Caudy, 2013). If not, treatment outcomes may be negatively affected since the person will not benefit from the treatment programming. Accurate assessment and diagnosis should guide tailored treatment recommendations.

Treatment evolution: early modalities

In the late 1700s, the physician Benjamin Rush began an educational campaign to warn against the potential dangers of consuming distilled alcoholic beverages. Regarded as the "father of American psychiatry," Rush advocated for the understanding of alcoholism as a medical disease in need of ongoing treatment. Based primarily on physical observation, Rush described medical conditions that he believed were caused by consuming large amounts of distilled alcoholic spirits (Katcher, 1993; White, 1998). He identified symptoms such as stomach discomfort, vomiting, liver damage, "madness," and tremors (after abstaining). Although he was astute in his clinical observations, treatment recommendations included severe whippings, sticking a feather down the throat to force vomiting, dunking patients in cold water, and inducing sweats. Despite the promotion of these early punitive remedies, Rush also advocated for "sober houses," medical communities that focused on treating individuals with alcohol problems (White, 1998). Decades later, this idea would establish Benjamin Rush as an innovator within the treatment community and lay the foundation for inpatient treatment modalities.

Throughout the 1800s, the temperance movement gained momentum; abstinence from alcoholic beverages was permeating the broader culture. During this century, the idea of developing "inebriate asylums" was born and propagated by Samuel Woodward, a physician who championed the ideal of "moral therapy" and supported a warm, compassionate approach to care (Blocker, Fahey, & Tyrell, 2003). Prior to the establishment of these institutions, many individuals with substance use disorders were housed primarily in prisons and housing facilities for the poor (Dadoly, Levin, & Palmer, 2005). Using a "patient-centered" approach to care, Woodward recommended occupational therapy, games, and spiritual treatments. He advocated against the use of physical violence and rarely used restraints. In addition to the creation of early inpatient psychiatric facilities for individuals with substance use disorders and with mental illnesses, he focused on treatment as opposed to punishment. The late 1800s spawned the continued development of alcohol-focused mutual aid societies and a new treatment for alcohol addiction and other illicit substances such as cocaine (White, 1998).

In the early 1900s, most inebriate asylums and private addiction facilities closed for a brief period (White, 1998). State laws in the United States called for mandatory sterilization of "defective" citizens, including individuals with addiction (Blocker et al., 2003). In 1935, chemical aversive conditioning was introduced in inpatient settings for alcohol abuse (Lemere & Voegtlin, 1950; White, 1998; Wilson, 1987). Individuals were given nausea-inducing drugs as a means of conditioning an aversion to the smell and taste of alcoholic beverages. Early research studies touted success but were later criticized for being uncontrolled and methodologically flawed (Wilson, 1987). This form of treatment, also called taste aversion learning, remains controversial but continues in sporadic use (Elkins, Dandala, & Whitford, 2009).

During the mid-1900s, Alcoholics Anonymous (AA) was born when the founders realized that the company and encouragement of peers could be an effective intervention. Consistent with mutual aid societies, AA furthered the message of abstinence as key to treatment success (Kurtz, 1979). The self-identified "fellowship" began with visits to hospital wards to encourage individuals to abstain from alcohol. This eventually developed into the 12-step model and spread across the globe in a few decades (Kurtz, 1979; White, 1998). A protocol has been developed specifically for correctional settings (AA document for jails and prisons, 1966). Narcotics Anonymous was founded in 1953 to address the use of other substances. AA and similar models remain heavily used in correctional settings, despite mixed findings of outcome research on their long-term effectiveness (Bahr et al., 2012).

Throughout the evolution of addiction treatment, the management of incarcerated individuals presented challenges and opportunities for medical and behavioral providers. Individuals were held in correctional facilities due to a lack of understanding of the biological underpinnings of substance use disorders. Throughout the 1700s and 1800s, treatment options were scarce and dependent on citizen-led social organizations. In the 1900s, there was a greater availability of treatment, including inpatient facilities or inebriate asylums, outpatient options, and peer-led services such as AA. The medical and psychiatric community began to understand substance use disorders as brain and behavioral disorders. The concept of levels of care emerged. Researchers studied specific populations and formulated treatment recommendations for specialized needs. This process led to multiple types of evidence-based programming at various levels of care. Evidence-based addiction treatment is now available to some criminal justice populations through inpatient, outpatient, correctional, and community-based settings.

Contemporary evidence-based programming

Treatment of criminal justice populations provides an opportunity to improve long-term outcomes in a high-need and significantly underserved population. Correctional programming for substance use disorders has evolved to account for some empirical research and cultural, sociopolitical shifts in attitudes toward substance use disorders; however, the extent of clinical intervention is limited. Whereas 56% of state prisoners met criteria for substance use disorders in the United States in the early 2000s, only 40% of them reported participating in treatment in state prison, and most of that programming is focused on alcohol and drug abuse education and self-help groups instead of clinical programming (Taxman, Perdoni, & Harrison, 2007). Of those inmates who receive treatment, most are placed in programming that is not appropriate given their needs. Less than 1% received drug maintenance treatment (Mumola & Karberg, 2006). In another study, only 10% of individuals who met criteria for substance use disorders received medically based treatment such as psychotherapeutic intervention or residential treatment while incarcerated (Belenko, 2002).

By its nature, incarceration involves enforced relative abstinence; access to illicit substances is generally curtailed, although not eliminated, through enforcement mechanisms. Among people entering correctional settings, access to detoxification units may be limited (Mumola & Karberg 2006; see Chapter 17) and withdrawal may be associated with significant discomfort. There may be risks associated with the fluctuating levels of tolerance experienced by individuals with substance use disorders moving through the criminal justice system, as demonstrated by the increased risk of drug-related death (i.e., overdose) after release from prison (Binswanger, Stern, Deyo, et al., 2007; Binswanger et al., 2013). Former inmates have a high risk of relapse and face considerable challenges when they reintegrate into community settings, in part, due to ubiquitous triggers to return to drug and alcohol use (Binswanger et al., 2011). Thus, there is an ongoing need for the widespread implementation of evidence-based programming in correctional facilities and during the transition back into the community.

Evidence-based behavioral treatment options for correctional populations

Treatment has evolved from early mutual aid societies to medically and psychologically oriented inpatient and outpatient treatment models. Behavioral and cognitive-behavioral therapeutic models are the most common approaches in correctional settings. This is largely due to the effectiveness of these modalities in treating a wide range of behavioral and substance use disorders (Hofmann, Asnaani, Vonk, et al., 2012; O'Connor & Stewart, 2010). Cognitive-behavioral therapies (CBTs) for substance use disorders have also been studied in correctional populations and have shown effectiveness as compared to drug and alcohol education or no treatment at all (Landenberger & Lipsey, 2005; Pearson, Lipton, Cleland, & Yee, 2002; Wilson, Bouffard, & MacKenzie, 2005).

Cognitive-behavioral therapy programs

The underlying tenets of CBT include identifying maladaptive thinking patterns, modifying distorted beliefs and attitudes, and changing problematic behaviors (Beck, 1995, 1970; Ellis, 1962). As a therapeutic approach, CBT is grounded in empirical research and is effective for a range of addictive, behavioral, and psychiatric conditions. For criminal justice populations, six programs have been adapted to the needs of this specialized population (Table 44.1), but few of them

Table 44.1 Common cognitive-behavioral treatment modalities

Name	Reference
Aggression Replacement Training (ART)	Goldstein, Glick, & Gibbs (1998)
Criminal Conduct and Substance Abuse Treatment:	Wanberg & Milkman (2008)
Strategies for Self-Improvement and Change	
Moral Reconation Therapy	Little & Robinson (1988)
Reasoning and Rehabilitation; Reasoning and Rehabilitation–2	Ross & Fabiano (1985); Ross & Ross (1997)
Thinking for a Change	Bush, Glick, & Taymans (1997)
Relapse Prevention Therapy	Marlatt, Parks, & Witkiewitz (2002)

have been tested extensively. Most use a cognitive-behavioral framework with added features based on the target issues and behaviors. Further, much of the evaluation effort in terms of curriculum effectiveness addresses adherence to the curriculum components. Poor adherence is a major issue in the delivery of treatment services.

Aggression replacement training

Based on a model originally developed for juvenile corrections, Aggression Replacement Therapy (ART) is a CBT intervention that addresses social skills, anger control, and moral reasoning skills (Glick, 2006; Goldstein, Glick, & Gibbs, 1998). Each skill set corresponds with a specific aspect of the cognitive triangle—behavioral, affective, and cognitive. Representing the behavioral component, the social skills training module teaches interpersonal skills to deal with anger- or fear-inducing events. Individuals learn 10 social skills that include dealing with someone else's anger, helping others, expressing affection, and responding to failure (Goldstein et al., 1998; Goldstein, Sherman, Gershaw, et al., 1978). The affective component helps individuals learn to identify triggers and cues for their anger and to develop self-control techniques to diffuse their own anger. Participants focus on self-evaluation and planning for future scenarios (Goldstein et al., 1998). The last component of this 10-week intervention is the development of moral reasoning skills, which corresponds to the cognitive component (Kohlberg, 1969). This component is intended to assist participants gain a broader understanding of relevant, but abstract, concepts related to interacting in an "unjust" world. These include activities to enhance understanding of fairness, justice, and the needs and rights of others (Goldstein et al., 1998). This program can be implemented at various levels of care (e.g., inpatient, outpatient) and in both jails and prisons, although studies have not been conducted to demonstrate that the program is effective in these various settings. In addition to being used to decrease substance abuse, ART has shown effectiveness in reducing aggression and rates of recidivism among the criminal justice population; however, studies have not clearly shown the type of patients who would benefit the most from participating in this treatment program (Barnoski & Aos, 2004; Greenberg & Lippold, 2013; Gundersen & Frode, 2006).

Criminal conduct and substance abuse treatment: strategies for self-improvement and change

Strategies for Self-improvement and Change (SSC) is a long-term, multiphasic cognitive-behavioral intervention developed for adults in the criminal justice system. This intervention was intended to develop skills and understanding of the internal (thought, emotions, beliefs, attitudes) processes and external events or circumstances that lead to substance use and involvement in the justice system (Wanberg & Milkman, 2008). The curriculum consists of 12 treatment modules with three phases. Phase I is focused on relationships, self-disclosure, self-awareness, and a relapse/recidivism prevention plan. Phase II involves active practice and change implementation (Wanberg & Milkman, 2008). This phase also includes managing cravings, regulating emotions, and developing more effective interpersonal relationships. Finally, this approach incorporates social responsibility therapy, which is designed to promote prosocial behaviors (Yokley, 2010). This curriculum has not been formally evaluated, and therefore it is unknown how well it addresses substance use disorders.

Moral reconation therapy

Originally developed for prison-based therapeutic communities, Moral Reconation Therapy (MRT) is focused on moral reasoning (CCI, 2010; Little & Robinson, 1988). Within a cognitive-behaviorist framework, MRT was influenced by Lawrence Kohlberg's theory of moral development, which asserts that moral development progresses through six stages, with few adults reaching the highest stage (Kohlberg, 1976). Advocates of MRT assert that character and personality traits are a significant reason for recidivism after release (Milkman & Wanberg, 2007). This model uses nine hierarchical personality stages of anticipated growth and recovery, each with specific personality characteristics that are amenable to change (CCI, 2010). More advanced personality stages are thought to reflect higher levels of moral reasoning ability and understanding. Participants progress through MRT's 16 steps, focused on setting goals and building skills. This curriculum is conducted in open groups and has been adapted for correctional facilities and community-based settings. A meta-analysis of MRT indicated success in reducing rates of recidivism (Ferguson & Wormith, 2012). However, a major concern is that the original study was mainly conducted by the author and the company that delivers MRT. Also, evaluations of this curriculum have primarily been conducted with populations that have been convicted of driving while intoxicated, generally white males, and generally relatively older populations (in their 40s). Probation or parole officers commonly deliver this curriculum; little is known about the clinical efficacy of these service providers.

Reasoning and rehabilitation

Reasoning and Rehabilitation (R&R) is a 35-session CBT program that focuses on the development of prosocial attitudes and perspectives, emotion regulation and self-control, and interpersonal problem solving (Ross & Fabiano, 1985). Developed for institutional, community corrections, and reentry programs, participants learn problem-solving skills, how to cope with provoking situations, empathy, and assertive communication. Focused on participant engagement, R&R includes many activities, games, role-playing, and modeling to encourage skill development. This program was developed to be run by health professionals with various levels of education (Milkman & Wanberg, 2007). However, certain skills among facilitators are deemed necessary for successful implementation of R&R, including above-average verbal skills, empathy with the criminal justice population, ability to manage group dynamics, enthusiasm, and sophisticated understanding of the cognitive model (Ross & Fabiano, 1985; Ross, Fabiano, & Ross, 1986). Developed in 1996, R&R2 is a shorter form of R&R that offers specialized versions tailored to specific subpopulations of inmates (Ross & Hilborn, 2008). R&R has shown effectiveness across cultural contexts with high- and low-level inmates, reducing rates of recidivism and criminal behavior (Joy Tong & Farrington, 2006). The limitations of the curriculum are that it is unclear what type of patients benefit from this curriculum and what type of facilitator produces the most positive results.

Thinking for a change

Developed by the National Institute of Corrections, Thinking for a Change (T4C) is a 22-session intervention that integrates cognitive restructuring, social skills, and problem solving in a CBT framework (Bush, Glick, & Taymans, 1997). This program has been implemented in state prisons, county jails, community corrections, and probation and parole departments for both juveniles and adults. The curriculum examines intrapsychic processes (feelings, beliefs, attitudes), develops social and interpersonal relationship skills, and engages in problem solving (Bush et al., 1997). The program accommodates facilitators at various educational levels, but they must have a desire to teach, experience working with criminal justice populations, training in the model, and the ability to exhibit empathy. There has only been one quasi-experimental study of T4C in a reentry facility, where it was shown to reduce recidivism (Golden, Gatchel, & Cahill, 2006; Lowenkamp, Hubbard, Makarios, & Latessa, 2009). The degree to which the curriculum was implemented and the types of patients who participated in the program are unclear.

Relapse prevention training

Developed primarily to prevent relapse following addiction treatment, Relapse Prevention Training (RPT) conceptualizes addictive behaviors as habits from a biopsychosocial perspective (Marlatt, Parks, & Witkiewitz, 2002). RPT includes five therapeutic strategies: coping skills training, "relapse roadmaps," identifying and reframing cognitive distortions, implementing health promotion activities, and anticipating and preparing for relapses. RPT emphasizes the importance of a balanced lifestyle and health promotion as key aspects in maintaining recovery (Marlatt et al., 2002). A metaanalysis of these programs in criminal justice settings suggests that they have efficacy at reducing recidivism (Dowden et al., 2003); however, there was variation in the quality of implementation in the primary studies.

Drug courts

Drug courts are becoming a widespread system-level intervention for use with the criminal justice population. The most effective drug courts serve populations with less severe problems, provide high-intensity programming, emphasize rehabilitation and recovery, use rewards and sanctions to motivate behavior, and predictably apply rewards and sanctions (Longshore, Turner, Morral, et al., 2001; Mitchell, Wilson, Eggers, & MacKenzie, 2012). The primary focus of drug courts is to divert individuals with substance use disorders to treatment rather than jail or prison. Drug courts have been implemented across the United States to increase treatment use and decrease drug-related crime (National Association of Drug Court Professionals, 1997; National Drug Court Institute, 2008). The implementation of drug courts has been shown to decrease recidivism among adults, although it is unclear whether drug treatment courts can benefit those with severe substance use disorders (Mitchell et al., 2012).

Therapeutic communities

Therapeutic communities (TCs) are among the most intensive facility-based residential treatment models for criminal justice populations. They are supported by a block grant that each state receives to offer these programs, known as residential substance abuse treatment grants. Participants generally participate in treatment for six to twelve months (Kooyman, 1993; Mitchell, Wilson, & MacKenzie, 2007). TCs vary in terms of specific programming, but most share some elements. In correctional facilities, individuals in TCs should be separated from the general population and inundated with recovery-related interventions. The TC builds a social climate to support change and involves the residents/ peers in the delivery of services (Kooyman, 1993). A metaanalysis suggests that participation in TCs increases treatment success; however, the analyses found that in-prison TCs followed by aftercare in the community are more effective (Mitchell et al., 2007). TCs can help control prison management costs and provide significant rehabilitative effects among inmates (Zhang, Roberts, & McCollister, 2009).

Pharmacologically supported treatment and harm-reduction approaches

Traditionally, evidence-based pharmacological adjuncts to behavioral treatment were largely absent from the treatment of inmates in prisons or jails (Mumola & Karberg, 2006; Rich, Boutwell, Shield, et al., 2005). Despite being shown to be highly effective in noncorrectional settings, methadone and buprenorphine for opioid dependence are largely unavailable to nonpregnant adults in jails and prisons (Rich et al., 2005). However, mounting evidence suggests that pharmacological treatment can be effectively provided in correctional settings (Dolan, Shearer, MacDonald, et al., 2003; Gordon, Kinlock, Schwartz, & O'Grady, 2008). Other emerging trends include approaches to reduce fatal overdose with substance use, such as the provision of naloxone (an opioid antidote that reverses respiratory depression in opioid overdose) for inmates leaving prison (National Services Scotland, 2013). Given the high risk of overdose death during the transitional period (Binswanger et al., 2013; Wakeman, 2009), these harm-reduction approaches have been tested in some international prison settings and appear to be gaining wider acceptance. Similar to addiction treatment in community settings, the management of addiction in corrections for many individuals will require a combination of pharmacotherapy and psychosocial interventions. Additionally, harm-reduction approaches that are designed to reduce the complications and adverse outcomes associated with alcohol and drug use may gain wider acceptance by correctional agencies in many international contexts.

Summary

Correctional facilities face challenges and opportunities in the treatment of substance use disorders. Changes in the diagnosis and assessment of substance use disorders will have implications for programming and treatment planning for criminal justice populations. The history of treatment of substance use disorders in corrections was influenced by mutual aid societies, the temperance movement, and AA. Current behavioral approaches are highly influenced by CBT and infrequently integrate pharmacological or harm-reduction approaches. While many programs to address substance use disorder among correctional populations exist, many individuals fail to receive adequate care and continue to experience complications of substance use disorders. Thus, correctional clinicians and staff, researchers, and patients need to continue to advocate for improved and enhanced dissemination of integrated, evidence-based behavioral and pharmacological treatment for substance use disorders across the continuum of criminal justice involvement.

References

Abbott, M. W., McKenna, B. G., & Giles, L. C. (2005). Gambling and problem gambling among recently sentenced male prisoners in New Zealand. *Journal of Gambling Studies, 21*(4), 537–558.

Alcoholics Anonymous World Services, Inc. (1966). *AA document for jails and prisons.* Available at: http://www.aa.org/pdf/products/p-26_AAinCF.pdf

American Psychiatric Association (2013). *Diagnostic and statistical manual of mental disorders* (5th ed.). Arlington, VA: American Psychiatric Association.

Bahr, S., Masters, A., & Taylor, B. (2012). What works in substance abuse treatment programs for offenders? *The Prison Journal, 92*(2), 155–174.

Barnoski, R., & Aos, S. (2004). *Outcome evaluation of Washington State's research-based programs for juvenile offenders.* Olympia, WA: Washington State Institute for Public Policy.

Beck, J. (1995). *Cognitive therapy: Basics and beyond.* New York: Guilford Publications, Inc.

Beck, A. T. (1970). Cognitive therapy: Nature and relation to behavior therapy. *Behavior Therapy, 1,* 184–200.

Belenko, S. (2002). *Trends in substance abuse and treatment needs among inmates: Final report.* Report to National Institute of Justice by National Center on Addiction and Substance Abuse at Columbia University, Department of Justice.

Binswanger, I., Stern M., Deyo, R., Heagerty, P., Cheadle A., & Elmore, J. (2007). Release from prison: a high risk of death for former inmates. *New England Journal of Medicine, 356*(2), 157–165.

Binswanger, I. A., Blatchford, P. J., Mueller, S. R., & Stern, M. F. (2013). Mortality after prison release: opioid overdose and other causes of death, risk factors, and time trends from 1999 to 2009. *Annals of internal medicine, 159*(9), 592–600.

Binswanger, I. A., Krueger, P. M., & Steiner, J. F. (2009). Prevalence of chronic medical conditions among jail and prison inmates in the USA compared with the general population. *Journal of Epidemiology and Community Health, 63*(11), 912–919.

Binswanger, I. A., Nowels, C., Corsi, K. F., Long, J., Booth, R. E., Kutner, J., & Steiner, J. F. (2011). Return to Drug Use and Overdose After Release from Prison: A Qualitative Study. *Substance Abuse, 32*(1), 57–58.

Blocker, J., Fahey, D., & Tyrell, I. (2003). *Alcohol and temperance in modern history: An international encyclopedia.* Santa Barbara, CA: ABC-CLIO.

Bush, J., Glick, B., & Taymans, J. (1997). *Thinking for a change.* Longmont, CO: National Institute of Corrections, United States Department of Justice.

Carson, E., & Sabol, W. (2012). *Prisoners in 2011.* Washington, DC: U.S. Department of Justice, Office of Justice Programs.

Dadoly, J., Levin, L., & Palmer, L. (2005). *Dr. Samuel B. Woodward: A 19th-century pioneer in American psychiatric care.* Presented at Medical Library Association Annual Meeting. San Antonio, TX.

Dolan, K., Shearer, J., MacDonald, M., Mattick, R., Hall, W., & Wodak, A. (2003). A randomised controlled trial of methadone maintenance treatment versus wait list control in an Australian prison system. *Drug and Alcohol Dependence, 72*(1), 59–65.

Dowden, C., Antonowicz, D., & Andrews, D. A. (2003). The effectiveness of Relapse Prevention with offenders: A meta-analysis. *International Journal of Offender Therapy and Comparative Criminology, 47*(5), 516–528.

Elkins, R., Dandala, K., & Whitford, J. (2009). *Patient and provider acceptance of chemical aversion substance dependence treatments.* Available at: http://schickshadel.com/wp-content/uploads/2013/06/Chemical-Aversion-Substance-Dependence-Treatments.pdf

Ellis, A. (1962). *Reason and emotion in psychotherapy.* New York: Lyle Stuart.

Ferguson, L. M., & Wormith, J. S. (2012). Meta-analysis of Moral Reconation Therapy. *International Journal of Offender Therapy and Comparative Criminology, 57*(9), 1076–1106.

Glick, B. (2006). *Cognitive behavioral interventions for at risk youth.* Kingston, NJ: Civic Research Institute.

Greenberg, M. T., & Lippold, M. A. (2013). Promoting healthy outcomes among youth with multiple risks: Innovative approaches. *Annual Review of Public Health, 34,* 253–270.

Golden, L. S., Gatchel, R. J., & Cahill, M. A. (2006). Evaluating the effectiveness of the National Institute of Corrections' "Thinking for a Change" program among probationers. *Journal of Offender Rehabilitation, 43*(1), 55–73.

Goldstein, A., Glick, B., & Gibbs, J. (1998). *Aggression Replacement Training* (Rev. ed.). Champaign, IL: Research Press.

Goldstein, A., Sherman, M., Gershaw, N., Sprafkin, R., & Glick, B. (1978). Training aggressive adolescents in prosocial behavior. *Journal of Youth and Adolescence, 7*(1), 72–93.

Gordon, M., Kinlock, T., Schwartz, R., & O'Grady, K. (2008). A randomized clinical trial of methadone maintenance for prisoners: findings at 6 months post-release. *Addiction, 103*(8), 1333–1342.

Gundersen, K. K., & Frode, S. (2006). Aggression Replacement Training in Norway: outcome evaluation of 11 Norwegian student projects. *Scandinavian Journal of Education Research, 50*(1), 63–81.

Hofmann, S. G., Asnaani, A., Vonk, I. J., Sawyer, A. T., & Fang, A. (2012). The efficacy of cognitive behavioral therapy: A review of meta-analyses. *Cognitive Therapy and Research, 36,* 427–440.

Joy Tong, L. S., & Farrington, D. P. (2006). How effective is the "Reasoning and Rehabilitation" programme in reducing reoffending? A meta-analysis of evaluations in four countries. *Psychology, Crime & Law, 12*(1), 3–24.

Katcher, B. (1993) Benjamin Rush's educational campaign against hard drinking. *American Journal of Public Health, 83*(2), 273–281.

Kohlberg, L. (1969) Stage and sequence: The cognitive-development approach to socialization. In D. Goslin (Ed.), *Handbook of socialization theory and research.* Chicago, IL: Rand McNally.

Kooyman, M. (1993) *The therapeutic community for addicts: intimacy, parent involvement, and treatment success.* Lisse, Netherlands: Swets and Zeitlinger Publishers.

Kurtz, E. (1979). *Not God: A history of Alcoholics Anonymous.* San Francisco: Harper and Row Publishers, Inc.

Landenberger, N. A., & Lipsey, M. W. (2005). The positive effects of cognitive–behavioral programs for offenders: A meta-analysis of factors associated with effective treatment. *Journal of Experimental Criminology, 1*(4), 451–476.

Lemere, F., & Voegtlin, W. (1950). An evaluation of aversion treatment. *Quarterly Journal of Studies on Alcohol, 11,* 199–204.

Little, G., & Robinson, K. (1988). Moral Reconation Therapy: A systematic, step-by-step treatment system for treatment resistant clients. *Psychological Reports, 62,* 135–151.

Longshore, D., Turner, S., Morral, A., Harrell, A., McBride, D., Deschenes, E., et al. (2001). Drug courts: A conceptual framework. *Journal of Drug Issues, 31,* 7–26.

Lowenkamp, C. T., Hubbard, D., Makarios, M. D., & Latessa, E. J. (2009). A quasi-experimental evaluation of Thinking for a Change: A "real world" application. *Criminal Justice and Behavior, 36*(2), 137–146.

Marlatt, G., Parks, G., & Witkiewitz, K. (2002). *Clinical guidelines for implementing Relapse Prevention Therapy: A guideline developed for the Behavioral Recovery Management Project.* Available at: http://www.bhrm.org/guidelines/RPT%20guideline.pdf

Milkman, H., & Wanberg, K. (2007). *Cognitive-behavioral treatment: A review and discussion for corrections professionals.* NIC Accession Number 021657, U.S. Department of Justice, National Institute of Corrections.

Mitchell, O., Wilson, D., & MacKenzie, D. (2007). Does incarceration-based drug treatment reduce recidivism? A meta-analytic synthesis of research. *Journal of Experimental Criminology, 3,* 353–375.

Mitchell, O., Wilson, D., Eggers, A., & MacKenzie, D. (2012) Assessing the effectiveness of drug courts on recidivism: A meta-analytic review of traditional and non-traditional drug courts. *Journal of Criminal Justice, 40,* 60–71.

Mumola, C., & Karberg J. (2006). *Drug use and dependence, state and federal prisoners, 2004.* Bureau of Justice Statistics Special Report, NCJ 213530. Washington, DC: U.S. Department of Justice, Office of Justice Programs.

National Association of Drug Court Professionals (1997). *Defining drug courts: The key components.* Washington, DC: Bureau of Justice Assistance.

National Drug Court Institute (2008). *Quality improvement for drug courts: Evidence-based practices.* Available at: http://www.ndcrc.org/sites/default/files/mono9.qualityimprovement_0.pdf

National Institute on Drug Abuse (2012). *Principles of drug abuse treatment for criminal justice populations: A research-based guide.* Available at: http://www.drugabuse.gov/sites/default/files/podat_cj_2012.pdf

National Services Scotland (2013). *National Naloxone Programme Scotland—naloxone kits issued in 2012/13.* Information Services Division. Available at: http://www.isdscotland.org/Health-Topics/Drugs-and-Alcohol-Misuse/Publications/2013-07-30/2013-07-30-naloxone-report.pdf

O'Connor, R. M., & Stewart, S. H. (2010). Substance use disorders. In D. McKay, J. Abramowitz, & S. Taylor (Eds.), *Cognitive-behavioral therapy for refractory cases: Turning failure into success* (pp. 211–229). Washington, DC: American Psychological Association.

Pearson, F. S., Lipton, D. S., Cleland, C. M., & Yee, D. S. (2002). The effects of behavioral/cognitive-behavioral programs on recidivism. *Crime and Delinquency, 48*(3), 476–496.

Rich, J. D., Boutwell, A. E., Shield, D. C., et al. (2005). Attitudes and practices regarding the use of methadone in US state and federal prisons. *Journal of Urban Health, 82,* 411–419.

Ross, R. R., & Ross, R. D. (1995). *Thinking straight: The Reasoning and Rehabilitation program for delinquency prevention and offender rehabilitation.* Ottawa: AIR Training and Publications.

Ross, R., & Fabiano, E. (1985). *Time to Think: A cognitive model of delinquency prevention and offender rehabilitation.* Johnson City, TN: Institute of Social Sciences and Arts, Inc.

Ross, R., Fabiano, E., & Ross, R. (1986). *Reasoning and Rehabilitation: A handbook for teaching cognitive skills.* Ottawa, Ontario: T3 Associates.

Ross, R., & Hilborn, J. (2008). *Rehabilitating rehabilitation: Neurocriminology for treatment of antisocial behavior.* Ottawa, Ontario: Cognitive Centre of Canada.

Substance Abuse and Mental Health Services Administration (2008). *Assertive Community Treatment: Building your program.* DHHS Pub. No. SMA-08-4344. Rockville, MD: Center for Mental Health Services, SAMHSA.

Taxman, F. S., Perdoni, M., & Caudy, M. (2013). The plight of providing appropriate substance abuse treatment services to offenders: Modeling the gaps in service delivery. *Victims & Offenders, 8*(1), 70–93.

Taxman, F. S., Perdoni, M., & Harrison, L. (2007). Drug treatment services for adult offenders: The state of the state. *Journal of Substance Abuse Treatment, 32*(3), 239–254. PMID: 17383549. PMCID: PMC2266078

Wakeman, S. E., Bowman, S. E., McKenzie, M., Jeronimo, A., & Rich, J. D. (2009) Preventing death among the recently incarcerated: an argument for naloxone prescription before release. *Journal of Addictive Diseases, 28,* 124–129.

Wanberg, K., & Milkman, H. (2008). *Criminal Conduct and Substance Abuse Treatment: Strategies for Self-Improvement and Change, Pathways to Responsible Living, providers' guide.* Thousand Oaks, CA: Sage Publications.

White, W. (1998). *Slaying the dragon: The history of addiction treatment and recovery in America.* Bloomington, IL: Chestnut Health Systems.

Williams, R. J., Royston, J., & Hagen, B. F. (2005). Gambling and problem gambling within forensic populations: A review of the literature. *Criminal Justice and Behavior, 32*(6), 665–689.

Wilson, D. B., Bouffard, L. A., & MacKenzie, D. L. (2005). A quantitative review of structured, group-oriented, cognitive-behavioral programs for offenders. *Journal of Criminal Justice and Behavior, 32*(2), 172–204.

Wilson, G. (1987). Chemical aversion conditioning as a treatment for alcoholism: A re-analysis. *Behaviour Research and Therapy, 25*(6), 503–516.

Yokley, J. (2010). Social Responsibility Therapy for harmful, abusive behavior. *Journal of Contemporary Psychotherapy, 40*, 105–113,

Zhang, S. X., Roberts, R. E., & McCollister, K. E. (2009). An economic analysis of the in-prison therapeutic community model on prison management costs. *Journal of Criminal Justice, 37*, 388–395.

CHAPTER 45

Dual diagnosis
Interventions designed to address substance abuse, mental health, and criminal offending

Faye S. Taxman

Introduction

Substance abuse and mental illness are concentrated in correctional populations. Further, nearly half of female inmates and one third of male inmates with substance use disorders have a diagnosable mental illness. Even with the higher rates of comorbid disorders of substance use and mental health, studies find that justice-involved individuals with mental illness tend to subscribe to a criminal lifestyle, criminal identity, and criminal values (Lamb & Weinberger, 2013; Morgan, Fisher, Duan, et al., 2010; Skeem, Winter, Kennealy, et al., 2013; Wilson, Farkas, Ishler, et al., 2014). Treatment for this population needs to address the syndemic of criminal lifestyle, mental illness, and substance abuse to reduce recidivism and symptoms.

The substance abuse population in most correctional settings is not homogeneous in terms of the type of drug abuse, age and gender, criminal justice history, criminal lifestyle and value system, and mental health needs. In the justice system, there is a temptation to provide generic types of drug treatment, but treatment services need to be tailored to the individual to reduce symptoms and improve overall justice outcomes. For dually diagnosed patients, the need to provide treatment for both substance abuse and mental illness along with criminal lifestyle and thinking is widely recognized (Epperson, Wolff, Morgan, et al., 2011).

This chapter reviews current knowledge about treatments for dually diagnosed patients. Included is a discussion of the factors that are unknown or unclear in the literature. Best practices and implementation issues regarding treatment for dual diagnosis patients are then discussed. An important part of these implementation issues involves the system factors required to support treatment in correctional settings. The chapter concludes with a research agenda for the future of dual diagnosis treatment in corrections.

Effective treatments

To a large extent, the recommended treatments for dual diagnosis patients are the same as for those with substance use disorders; the main distinction is that treatment for dual diagnosis should combine medication and psychosocial interventions. Appropriate medications assist the patient both to stabilize mental illness and to address the substance use disorder (see Chapter 46). Psychosocial interventions, commonly including cognitive-behavioral therapy (CBT) for dual diagnosis, need to be adapted to meet the patient's level of functioning, incorporate criminal lifestyle issues, and address relapse.

The major challenge in providing integrated treatment for both substance abuse and mental illness is whether the disorders are managed sequentially, in parallel, or in an integrated manner (Mueser, Noordsy, Drake, et al., 2003). Sequential models treat comorbid disorders one at a time. Parallel models treat co-occurring conditions concurrently, often with different providers, who may work for different agencies. In integrated treatment, both disorders (substance abuse and mental illness) are addressed concurrently by the same provider or team, ensuring coordination and communication. In this model the providers are trained in both substance abuse treatment and mental illness and are comfortable using therapies that draw on both disciplines. Sequential models generally suffer from a lack of evidence to guide the order or timing of the interventions to achieve optimal care. For example, at what point do you transition from a primary focus on the substance abuse treatment to a focus on the mental illness? Which disorder is treated first? How are relapses managed? All too often, parallel models suffer from a lack of communication or coordination between providers, the distraction of having competing providers, and potentially different therapeutic messages.

From a research perspective, three psychotherapeutic approaches are recommended for substance abusers overall (National Institute on Drug Abuse, 2012), with components that address mental health disorders: motivational interviewing (MI), CBT, and Therapeutic Communities (TCs). Another well-respected treatment in the substance abuse field is contingency management (CM), which uses structured incentives as a motivator for behavioral change (see Chapter 44). Most of the work in dual diagnosis treatment is emerging. Another intervention is self-help groups to augment treatment and provide continued support in the community.

Motivational interviewing

MI is considered a best-practice approach to providing patient-centered care. MI makes use of a special set of techniques to engage the patient in the change process and is used in stand-alone sessions, as part of cognitive-behavioral programming, and in individual therapy sessions. Frequently, MI is used before formal treatment begins to address the patient's readiness to engage in treatment. Overall, MI is regarded as an evidence-based treatment; however, few studies have explored how best to use MI for the criminal justice patient (McMurran, 2009). Both treatment providers and justice staff such as correctional officers, correctional case managers, and probation and/or parole officers use MI techniques. A few studies have assessed the varied uses of MI with offenders and the impact on patient-level outcomes (McMurran, 2009); other studies have examined how correctional staff use MI (Robinson, Lowenkamp, Holsinger, et al., 2012; Robinson, VanBenschoten, Alexander, & Lowenkamp, 2011). Overall, correctional and probation staff have a difficult time "sharing the power" over the components of a case plan and integrating patient preferences into the criminal justice system priorities (Taxman & Belenko, 2012). MI is an important advance since it focuses on empowering patients to be engaged in their own care. Its flexibility, as stand-alone sessions or intermingled with other psychosocial interventions, is noteworthy.

Martino and colleagues (2002) adapted MI for patients with dual diagnosis by creating Dual Diagnosis Motivational Interviewing (DDMI). This model is an adaptation of one-session MI for dual diagnosis patients and demonstrated lower substance abuse indicators than a group who did not receive MI (Martino et al., 2002). DDMI includes four considerations for assisting those with dual diagnosis: adopting an integrated approach that equally emphasizes substance abuse and mental illness; accommodating the cognitive impairments that patients with psychotic disorders present; modifying the core skills of MI (i.e., asking open-ended questions, active listening, reflecting and affirming) to accommodate the challenges of dual disorder patients; and modifying MI strategies to integrate personalized and engaged feedback, use of decisional balance matrices, and other clinical tools. These modifications accommodate the interplay between substance use disorders and psychotic functioning. Most of the adaptations use MI and other clinical tools to address ambivalence toward treatment for a psychiatric disorder and medication adherence. DDMI has not been tested with a justice-involved population, but its emphasis on incorporating psychiatric conditions and its functionality make it potentially useful for this population.

Cognitive-behavioral therapy

CBT uses a structured set of therapeutic tools to address maladaptive thoughts and behaviors through a series of active problem-solving approaches. The therapy instructs participants on new skills to increase awareness of problematic thinking patterns and behaviors, to assess the plausibility of alternative strategies, to consider optional approaches, and to apply the new strategies. The CBT model is one of the most effective psychotherapies for substance abusers (National Institute on Drug Abuse, 2012) as well as for those in the criminal justice system (Andrews & Bonta, 2010; Landenberger & Lipsey, 2006). As of yet, few studies have documented how best to modify CBT to meet the needs of a dual diagnosis correctional population. Clinical practice suggests the following guidelines for modifying CBT: using a slower pace when going through therapy and group sessions;

adding practice sessions; focusing attention on both symptoms of mental illness and relapse for substances; emphasizing medication adherence strategies; and integrating behavioral therapy with skills to advance stability in the community regarding housing, social supports, and transition across justice settings. In correctional settings, CBT sessions should also be adapted to address prevalent concerns such as power and control issues, anger management, criminal thinking, antisocial peer networks, and social supports. Another accommodation that may need to occur in jails is to have fewer treatment sessions, given the shorter time frame of incarceration.

As noted in Chapter 44, a number of curricula exist for CBT. Many use the CBT framework but integrate aspects of criminal thinking or antisocial cognitions such as Aggression Replacement Training, Criminal Conduct and Substance Abuse Treatment: Strategies for Self-improvement and Change, Moral Reconation Therapy, Thinking for a Change, and Reasoning and Rehabilitation. Inclusion of criminal lifestyle and offending behavior is important in these curricula because it focuses attention on antisocial values and behaviors. However, these curricula do not encompass substance abuse behaviors or relapse prevention. While readily available to the field, there is a lack of research to confirm CBT's effectiveness in reducing criminal behavior, mental illness severity, and substance use symptoms among justice-involved, dually diagnosed patients.

For patients with dual diagnosis, there is no specific evidence-based CBT curriculum that has emerged (McGovern, personal communication, 2014). Instead, there is recognition that there are a variety of psychiatric illnesses and that CBT curricula should be developed to meet the mental health needs of the individual patient. One such approach is the Unified Protocol that addresses emotional disorders as part of a unified transdiagnostic treatment (Barlow, Farchione, Fairholme, et al., 2011). Further, a number of CBT trials targeting specific pairings of mental illness and addiction are ongoing. These include, for example, social phobias and alcohol problems, anxiety disorders and alcohol problems, and depression and drug use. As noted by McGovern (personal communication, 2014), a major challenge is to translate the efficacy studies of CBT conducted with homogeneous disorders to address the various diagnostic pairings.

For example, one available curriculum that seems to cater to the needs of dual diagnosis patients, both in and out of the justice system, is Seeking Safety (Najavitis, 2002), a 25-session CBT-based curriculum delivered in either individual or group therapy format. Research findings are mixed, and it is not considered an evidence-based curriculum as of yet due to the failure to demonstrate impact on multiple outcomes. Seeking Safety is a "present-focused" CBT since it focuses attention on the person planning for today's life events; many of the other CBT criminal thinking curricula discussed previously focus on prior behaviors to help the person learn from past patterns. A recent study on incarcerated women found that the Seeking Safety curriculum specifically addresses issues present in the incarcerated population, including impulsiveness, social maladjustment, and emotional dysregulation (Wolff, Frueh, Shi, & Schumann, 2012). Overall, studies of women offenders have found mixed results of Seeking Safety on substance use outcomes, with some studies reporting positive outcomes and others reporting negative outcomes. No study has examined its impact on recidivism.

Modified therapeutic community

The Therapeutic Community (TC) model is recognized as evidence-based practice (Mitchell, Wilson, & MacKenzie, 2007). The TC model varies considerably in practice from a therapeutic residential setting to an intervention that uses the community and social setting as part of the treatment. The TC approach includes a focus on the whole individual, including a daily regimen that is structured to resocialize the individual, to develop personal responsibility, to engage in self-help in managing life difficulties, to use peer social networks as a healing agent, and to pursue change as a gradual developmental process. The model emphasizes work, self-reliance, and prosocial values that are developed through vocational and independent living skills. The TC approach typically requires no less than 12 months in a specialized living unit. Continuing aftercare following participation in a TC prolongs the impact and allows patients to practice and improve their prosocial skills. The modified TC for dual diagnosis patients addresses psychiatric symptoms, cognitive impairments, and functionality. The treatment schedule is less intense (i.e., proceeds at a slower pace) than the schedule for substance abusers and individualizes the intervention (Sacks et al., 2008). Many TC clinical programs use CBT that involves less confrontation and more focus on behavioral and social skills. A modified TC approach often addresses criminal thinking and behavior by providing psychosocial education to help patients understand the linkage among substance abuse, mental illness, and criminality; it also encourages healthy prosocial networks. This approach, in a clinical trial at one site, was found to reduce reincarceration rates. Another modified version was used as the transition from prison to the community (reentry) with similar positive impact on reincarceration and criminal activity (Sacks, Chapel, Sacks, et al., 2012).

Contingency management

CM is a well-recognized intervention for substance abusers designed to encourage patients to engage in treatment and to remain abstinent (Drake, O'Neal, & Wallach, 2008). The typical protocol involves earning points for desired behaviors (e.g., attending treatment sessions, remaining abstinent) or earning the opportunity to draw a prize from a fishbowl to reward desired behaviors. The literature on CM is strong, but again the research is primarily on substance abusers, with few involved in the justice system. A recent CM study found that many components of the model are not transportable to a justice setting (problem-solving courts) because rewarding patients for positive behaviors is not part of the cultural norm and due to difficulty disentangling a discrete set of desirable behaviors (e.g., abstinence) from general functionality (Portillo, Rudes, & Taxman, 2014).

Conclusion about treatment for this population

To date, there is very little research to support the ability of MI, CBT, or TC to effect improvements in substance use and mental health functioning (Hunt et al., 2013). Even less research is available on treatments that affect offending behaviors. Three critical treatment issues need to be answered: What are the desired outcomes? What are the required dosage units to achieve effectiveness? What is the best way to provide effective therapies for this population?

Existing research addresses some of the critical treatment issues in serving the dual diagnosis population in correctional settings. One challenge in dealing with the syndemic of disorders (offending, substance abuse, and mental illness) is which specific outcomes are considered most desirable. In the criminal justice literature, treatment effectiveness is generally based on justice-related outcomes such as arrest, conviction, or reincarceration. These outcomes serve to define the treatments and practices that are defined as "evidence-based." Reduction in psychiatric symptoms or drug use is considered secondary and generally is not part of the determination of evidence-based practices. In fact, few studies actually measure drug use and mental health outcomes simultaneously with criminal justice outcomes (Skeem et al., 2013). One challenge in developing and defining evidence-based treatments for dually diagnosed correctional populations is the recognition that some treatments may have other desirable outcomes such as medication adherence, symptom reduction, and increased abstinence; these signals of progress may, in turn, mediate or moderate criminal justice outcomes. While possible, confirmatory research has not been conducted.

Another unanswered question is the effect of intervention dosage. Dosage of psychotherapy refers to treatment duration, frequency, or intensity. Regardless of the definition, insufficient research links therapeutic dosage to optimal outcome. The original TC model was 18 months long, but many of the new TC models are shorter. The modified TC in one reentry facility was six months long (see Sacks et al., 2012). The length of time for some CBT group therapies is four months, but other CBT groups last six months. Some CBT groups meet weekly, others more often. MI can be offered as a stand-alone two-session program or integrated with other therapies of varying duration. Overall, while there are therapeutic orientations that appear to be more effective than others, we are unsure which specific characteristics lead to desired outcomes.

While clinicians generally support the use of integrated treatment, research has not addressed whether sequential, parallel, or integrated models of care are more effective. A major challenge is the array of skills required to handle criminal thinking, substance use, and mental illness. Each domain has been discipline-specific; integrated models require clinical staff competence in all three areas.

Another uncertainty relates to the complexity of the integrated material of criminal conduct, substance abuse, and mental illness. It is still unclear whether the complexity of the material is overwhelming for patients or whether simultaneous attention to all three conditions facilitates treatment engagement.

Implementation issues regarding treatments for dual diagnosis

Within a correctional setting, safety and security come first. A clear vision for how dual diagnosis treatment benefits safety and advances inmate change is important to effective implementation. In addition to having properly trained staff, treatment needs to be aligned with correctional processes, with clearly stated outcomes that incorporate security and treatment goals. Similarly, treatment agencies must see a benefit from working with corrections to support integrated programs for dual diagnosis patients within the facility and then to refer patients to appropriate aftercare following release. Without the support of the external agencies, many treatment programs for inmates "wilt" over time and lose support. Implementation must therefore attend to program quality issues as well as the complex system issues that affect sustainability (Taxman & Belenko, 2012).

Program quality

A good-quality treatment program incorporates five main elements: staff training in the program materials, patients who meet defined eligibility criteria, well-articulated program materials that identify the therapeutic goals and skills, sufficient time devoted to the mental health and substance abuse issues in the program, and well-specified outcomes that determine whether the patient is making solid progress in the program. Each element is critical to a well-administered program for complex dual diagnosis patients. The Dual Diagnosis Capability in Addiction Treatment Services Index (McGovern, Matzkin, & Giard, 2007) was developed for substance abuse and mental health systems to assess the quality of programming. The index generally revealed that community-based programs do not have the capacity to provide quality programming. While this tool has not been used in correctional settings, a review of the literature would suggest similar results.

Staffing is an important and often difficult issue for treatment programs. Dealing with psychologically and medically complex patients requires clinical skills in multiple areas. An additional challenge is staff turnover, as it creates program instability. Together, these issues can be addressed through good training of staff to build their skills in using CBT coupled with quality assurance procedures to ensure program fidelity.

Another key issue regarding program quality is to have clear eligibility guidelines regarding the type of individual best served by this program. Generally, programs have rather broad admission criteria. Studies have found that too much heterogeneity in problem behaviors is correlated with poorer treatment outcomes. It is useful to determine the type of substance abuse (e.g. opioid, cocaine, marijuana), type of mental illness (e.g. internalizing, externalizing), and criminal risk behaviors for purposes of program placement.

Treatment should be defined by a curriculum or a well-defined set of goals and approaches (National Institute on Drug Abuse, 2012). The goal of a treatment curriculum is to provide structure, goals, and key activities. Research supports the use of curricula in therapy to provide a framework for clinical goals, to ensure that the program is using standard methods across treatment groups, and to enhance staff training.

Another quality issue refers to the balance between clinical sessions devoted to problem behaviors. While the goal of a dual diagnosis program is to address both disorders, many programs provide more attention to substance abuse, leading to concerns of sufficient dosage to address mental health issues.

Finally, an effective dual diagnosis program should have clearly defined outcomes that define patient progress. Such behavioral goals might include reductions in the frequency of drug use, enhanced adherence to medications, reduction in criminal behavior or thinking, or reduction in symptoms of mental illness. With behavioral goals, the markers of progress and success are clear to the patient, the clinician, and administrators who are monitoring the program.

Internal management issues

Providing treatment in justice settings requires the cooperation and collaboration of the justice organizations, regardless of whether the treatment program is offered on site or the patients are referred to a program in a treatment facility. A key element is the degree to which the facility administrator (i.e., warden, chief, officer) supports the treatment programming. A few lessons from implementing treatment programs in correctional settings are that senior management must explicitly support the program and its goals; line correctional staff must see value in providing treatment for inmates and should be aware of the program's components; the treatment program must be aligned with existing policies and procedures; and treatment program staff, even if they are from another agency, must be aware of the security needs, which should be integrated into the treatment program's structure.

It is often necessary to adjust or refine the existing work process to offer dual diagnosis treatment. For example, attention must be given to the assessment process to ensure that sufficient information is collected on substance use and mental illness. Standard criminal justice risk-and-needs assessment tools are generally inadequate for this since they do not provide sufficient information to make a clinical diagnosis. Another workflow issue is treatment timing and location. In a jail or prison, these programs are generally on site; however, it is important that the program does not interfere with recreation time, education classes, or religious groups.

A major internal issue is preparing the correctional staff to work successfully with this population. To effectively supervise and manage individuals with dual diagnoses, correctional staff need to understand the disorders and the techniques for working with this population (e.g., use of MI, components of cognitive restructuring, social milieu, contingency management). A major goal of staff development efforts is to help staff learn to destigmatize the disease for the individual to improve treatment engagement and outcomes. While research on correctional staff remains to be done, researchers have found that probation and parole staff who understand the illness have a positive impact on outcomes (Manchak, Skeem, Kennealy, & Eno Louden, 2014). Nevertheless, integration of the correctional and treatment services is important in proper handling and management of dual diagnosis individuals.

External stakeholders

Stakeholder support is important for both initiating (capacity building) and maintaining (building resilience) a dual diagnosis program. During capacity building, justice, health, and citizen and community groups partner to develop knowledge about the issues related to substance abuse and mental illness and how they relate to justice and health issues in the community. A shared knowledge base is important because it galvanizes collective energy. Knowledge dissemination is then used to build a foundation and identify the clinical, case management, and procedural skills necessary to handle the needs of the population. A third aspect of capacity building is to reach consensus about goals and expectations; this will provide the framework for all organizations to commit to certain goals and outcomes.

The next step after a program is designed and implemented is to build resiliency, with the goal of long-term sustainability of the program and efforts to improve the outcomes of the dual diagnosis population. Building resilience requires alignment of the policies, procedures, and program(s) with all involved correctional, justice, and health agencies. This requires a commitment to review existing practice and refine it based on the expectations established. The collective efforts focus on resource distribution, continuous building of staff skills, program refinement based on outcome data, creation of a common goal and mission, development of public media messages (as appropriate), and creation and management of performance measures. Performance measures provide monitoring of progress at individual, program, and system levels. Attention to these details creates a hospitable environment for the programs and services for the dual diagnosis patients and ensures that the treatment programs can be sustained if they improve the safety and health outcomes.

Future research agenda

To a large extent, our knowledge about effective dual diagnosis programs comes from the general treatment literature (Chandler, Peters, Field, & Juliano-Bult, 2004). Borrowing from the general treatment literature is useful but does not address transportability of the treatment models or approaches for the incarcerated population of substance abusers with mental illness (Taxman & Belenko, 2012). Exploring transportability allows for closer attention to the following issues: the settings where the programs can best operate (e.g., in a prison, jail, probation office, or treatment center); the target populations that are better suited for CBT, TC, MI, CM, or other interventions; the adherence and fidelity to the treatment program and to the model of correctional oversight that best aligns with the treatment program; the alignment and fit with the organization; the assessment tool kit that can be administered; the treatment manuals that can be implemented in correctional settings; the dosage needed to improve mental health functionality and reduce substance abuse; the processes that generate better patient-level outcomes; the social media messages that obtain buy-in and support from the justice, health, and general community; and the treatment models that generate better outcomes.

Summary

While epidemiological studies clearly identify the prevalence of comorbid substance abuse and mental illness, dual diagnosis patients in the correctional system have the added morbidity of antisocial values, attitudes, and behaviors. This syndemic of conditions requires treatment that can address all three disorders. While clinical preference is for integrated care, research is needed to identify effective treatments that address all three disorders. Currently few studies have examined the impacts of various MI, CBT, and/or TC curricula on substance abuse, mental health, and criminal outcomes. More research is needed to define factors that improve the treatment provided to this population, including attention to implementation issues. This critically important (and relatively large) population deserves more attention by clinicians and researchers to develop the evidence base for treatment and services to advance clinical outcomes.

References

Andrews, D. A., & Bonta, J. (2010). *The psychology of criminal conduct* (5th ed.). Cincinnati, OH: Anderson Publishing Co.

Barlow, D. H., Farchione, T. J., Fairholme, C. P., et al. (2011). *The Unified Protocol for Transdiagnostic Treatment of Emotional Disorders: Client workbook*. New York: Oxford University Press. Accessed on April 24, 2014 at: http://bostonanxietytreatment.com/the-unified-protocol/

Chandler, R. K., Peters, R. H., Field, G., & Juliano-Bult, D. (2004). Challenges in implementing evidence-based treatment practices for co-occurring disorders in the criminal justice system. *Behavioral Sciences & the Law, 22*(4), 431–448.

Drake, R. E., O'Neal, E. L., & Wallach, M. (2008). A systematic review of psychosocial research on psychosocial interventions for people with co-occurring disorders. *Journal of Substance Abuse Treatment, 34*, 123–138.

Epperson, M. W., Wolff, N., Morgan, R., Fisher, W. H., Frueh, B. C., & Huening, J. (2011). *The next generation of behavioral health and criminal justice interventions: Improving outcomes by improving interventions*. New Brunswick, NJ: Rutgers University, Center for Behavioral Health Services & Criminal Justice Research.

Hunt, G. E., Siegfried, N., Morley, K., Sitharthan, T., & Cleary, M. (2013). Psychosocial interventions for people with both severe mental illness and substance misuse. *Cochrane Database of Systematic Reviews*, Issue 10. Art. No.: CD001088. DOI:10.1002/14651858.CD001088.pub3

Lamb, H. R., & Weinberger, L. E. (2013). Some perspectives on criminalization. *Journal of the American Academy of Psychiatry and the Law, 41*, 287–293.

Landenberger, N. A., & Lipsey, M. W. (2005). The positive effects of cognitive-behavioral programs for offenders: A meta-analysis of factors associated with effective treatment. *Journal of Experimental Criminology, 1*, 451–476.

Manchak, S. M., Skeem, J. L., Kennealy, P. J., & Eno Louden, J. (2014, April 21). High-fidelity specialty mental health probation improves officer practices, treatment access, and rule compliance. *Law and Human Behavior*, advance online publication. http://dx.doi.org/10.1037/lhb0000076

Martino, S., Carroll, K., Kostas, D., Perkins, J., & Rounsaville, B. (2002). Dual Diagnosis Motivation Interviewing: a modification of Motivational Interviewing for substance-abusing patients with psychotic disorders. *Journal of Substance Abuse Treatment, 23*(40), 297–308.

McGovern, M. P., Matzkin, A. L., & Giard, J. L. (2007). Assessing the dual diagnosis capability of addiction treatment services: The Dual Diagnosis Capability in Addiction Treatment Services (DDCAT) Index. *Journal of Dual Diagnosis, 3*(2), 111–123.

McMurran, M. (2009). Motivational Interviewing with offenders: a systematic review. *Legal and Criminological Psychology, 14*(1), 83–100.

Mitchell, O. J., Wilson, D. B., & MacKenzie, D. L. (2007). Does incarceration-based treatment reduce recidivism? A meta-analytic synthesis of the research. *Journal of Experimental Criminology, 3*(4), 353–375.

Morgan, R. D., Fisher, W. H., Duan, N., Mandracchia, J. T., & Murray, D. (2010). Prevalence of criminal thinking among state prison inmates with serious mental illness. *Law and Human Behavior, 34*, 324–336. doi:10.1007/s10979-009-9182-z

Mueser, K. T., Noordsy, D. L., Drake, R. E., et al. (2003). *Integrated treatment for dual disorders: a guide to effective practice.* New York: Guilford Press.

Najavits, L. M. (2002). Seeking Safety: A new psychotherapy for posttraumatic stress disorder and substance use disorder. In P. Ouimette & P. Brown (Eds.), *Trauma and substance abuse: Causes, consequences, and treatment of comorbid disorders* (pp. 147–170). Washington, DC: American Psychological Association.

National Institute on Drug Abuse (2012). *Principles of drug abuse treatment for criminal justice populations: A research-based guide* (revised 2012). NIH Publication No. 11-5316. Available at: www.nida.nih.gov/PODAT_CJ

Portillo, S., Rudes, D. S., & Taxman, F. S. (2014). The transportability of contingency management in problem-solving courts. *Justice Quarterly*, DOI:10.1080/07418825.2014.902490

Robinson, C. R., Lowenkamp, C. T., Holsinger, A. M., VanBenschoten, S, Alexander, M., & Oleson, J. C. (2012). A random study of Staff Training Aimed at Reducing RE-arrest (STARR): Using core correctional practices in probation interactions. *Journal of Crime and Justice, 35*(2), 167–188.

Robinson, C. R., VanBenschoten, S., Alexander, M., & Lowenkamp, C. T. (2011). A random (almost) study of Staff Training Aimed at Reducing Re-Arrest (STARR): Reducing recidivism through intentional design. *Federal Probation, 75,* 57.

Sacks, S., Chapel, M., Sacks, J. Y, McKendrick, K., & Cleland, C. M. (2012). Randomized trial of a re-entry modified therapeutic community for offenders with co-occurring disorders: Crime outcomes. *Journal of Substance Abuse Treatment, 42,* 247–259.

Sacks, S., Banks, S., McKendrick, K., & Sacks, J. Y. (2008). Modified therapeutic community for co-occurring disorders: A summary of four studies. *Journal of Substance Abuse Treatment, 34*(1), 112–122.

Skeem, J. L., Encandela, J., & Louden, J. E. (2003). Perspectives on probation and mandated mental health treatment in specialized and traditional probation departments. *Behavioral Sciences & the Law, 21*(4), 429–458.

Skeem, J. L., Winter, E., Kennealy, P. J., Eno Louden, J., & Tatar, J. R., II (2013, December 30). Offenders with mental illness have criminogenic needs, too: Toward recidivism reduction. *Law and Human Behavior,* Advance online publication. doi:10.1037/lhb0000054

Taxman, F. S., & Belenko, S. (2012). *Implementing evidence-based practices in community corrections and addiction treatment.* New York: Springer.

Wilson, A. B., Farkas, K., Ishler, K. J., Gearhart, M., Morgan, R., & Ashe, M. (2014, April 7). Criminal thinking styles among people with serious mental illness in jail. *Law and Human Behavior.* Advance online publication. http://dx.doi.org/10.1037/lhb0000084

Wolff, N., Frueh, B. C., Shi, J., & Schumann, B. E. (2012). Effectiveness of cognitive-behavioral trauma treatment for incarcerated women with mental illnesses and substance abuse disorders. *Journal of Anxiety Disorders, 26,* 703–710.

CHAPTER 46

Pharmacotherapy for substance use disorders within correctional facilities

Sarah E. Wakeman and Josiah D. Rich

Introduction

The percentage of incarcerated individuals convicted of drug-related offenses varies by country, with rates as high as 53% among US sentenced federal prisoners and 58% of Thai prisoners (Bewley-Taylor, Hallam, & Allen, 2009). Roughly half of prisoners have an active substance use disorder (SUD; Mumola & Karberg, 2006), with even higher rates among women (78%). Alcohol use disorders (AUDs) are also overrepresented; 73% of UK prisoners are hazardous drinkers and 36% are dependent (MacAskill, Parkes, Brooks, et al., 2011). Given the prevalence of these disorders and the treatment needs of this population, this chapter presents the background, best practices, and evidence basis for the use of pharmacotherapy for SUD treatment within correctional settings.

Background

Despite the prevalence of SUDs, few prisoners who need treatment actually receive it while incarcerated. Among US prisoners, only 15% to 17% received SUD treatment from a trained professional (Mumola & Karberg, 2006). For those correctional facilities that do offer SUD treatment, it rarely includes medically indicated pharmacotherapy. Most often, correctional substance use treatment consists of psychoeducation or group counseling, with fewer facilities offering therapeutic communities (TCs). Traditional TCs are residential drug-free programs that focus on behavioral and psychosocial skill building. These programs often actively discourage pharmacological treatment and have been inaccurately embraced as the only model for treatment in many correctional settings (Bruce, Smith-Rohrburg, & Altice, 2007). The success of TCs is dependent on linkage to community aftercare programs, with no difference in outcomes between those who participate in an in-prison TC without aftercare linkage and controls (Vanderplasschen, Colpaert, Autrique, et al., 2013).

The lack of efficacy in the absence of effective postrelease linkage is not surprising. Addiction is a chronic relapsing disease, and the incarcerated setting is an artificial environment (Chandler, Fletcher, & Volkow, 2009). Although there is wide variability in the nature of correctional settings, some general observations can be made. Drug use behind bars occurs but is generally much

less frequent than for the same population in the community (see Chapters 24 and 31). There is decreased drug access, increase in prices, and, for most people behind bars, less opportunity to generate income to pay for drugs. Upon release there are many stressors, frustrations, triggers/cues, and an environment with much greater access to drugs that results in many relapsing to substance use. This challenging combination makes treatment during the reentry period crucial, and programs that lack that continuity are unlikely to be successful (see Chapter 47).

In addition to treatment during the transition out of incarceration, detoxification upon incarceration is also important (see Chapter 17). The World Health Organization (WHO), in their integrated alcohol care pathway, recommends that all affected prisoners be treated for alcohol withdrawal, yet detoxification is not uniform across US correctional facilities. Only 5% of prisons and 34% of jails offer any detoxification services, and only 1% of jails offer methadone for opioid withdrawal (Oser, Knudsen, Staton-Tindall, et al., 2009). An estimated 756,000 arrestees are at risk for untreated alcohol withdrawal and 277,000 for untreated opioid withdrawal annually in the United States (Fiscella, Pless, Meldrum, & Fiscella, 2004).

While only a small percentage of correctional facilities provide detoxification services, even fewer facilities offer pharmacotherapy for AUDs or SUDs despite the tremendous evidence base supporting the use of medications to treat addiction. Although there are limited studies on the outcomes of drug treatment during incarceration, there are nearly 50 years of evidence documenting the efficacy of methadone given in the community in reducing opioid use, drug-related health complications, overdose, death, criminal activity, and recidivism (Mattick, Breen, Kimber, & Davoli, 2003).

Buprenorphine is similarly an effective, safe, and cost-effective long-term treatment for opioid dependence that reduces other opioid use and improves health and quality-of-life outcomes. Internationally, there is growing experience with buprenorphine. In France there was a marked reduction in overdose following the widespread introduction of buprenorphine, as well as a reduction in HIV prevalence among injection drug users (Carrieri, Amass, Lucas, et al., 2006). The evidence supporting methadone and buprenorphine in the treatment of opioid dependence is so robust that WHO has added both to its list of essential medications. In keeping with the evidence base, WHO recommends that all prisoners with opioid use disorders should have access to methadone or other agonist treatment (UNODC-UNAIDS-WHO, 2006). WHO also recommends that following detoxification for alcohol withdrawal, further pharmacotherapy be offered to those with severe AUD. Yet, only 29 countries offer pharmacotherapy for opioid use disorders, and those that do are often limited to small pilot programs (Pecoraro & Woody, 2011). Pharmacotherapy for AUD is even less accessible, with few if any published reports of these medications being offered currently in any correctional facilities.

SUDs are highly prevalent worldwide among incarcerated populations; untreated addiction accounts for a significant portion of recidivism, morbidity, mortality, crime, and cost. Pharmacotherapy for opioid addiction and AUD is one of the most evidence-based treatments available for the devastating disease of addiction. While much of the research for pharmacological maintenance treatment comes from community studies, there is a clear evidence base suggesting benefit to prerelease pharmacotherapy with linkage to community treatments (McKenzie, Zaller, Dickman, et al., 2012). Given the artificial environment of incarceration and the decreased prevalence of drug use and availability, whether maintenance therapy throughout the duration of a lengthy sentence is indicated remains unclear. However, based on the existing evidence, all prisoners with active opioid addiction should be offered either detoxification or maintenance services when first entering corrections, a combination of education and counseling while incarcerated, and initiation of pharmacotherapy prior to release with direct linkage into community-based treatment. For those already on maintenance therapies who are incarcerated for short sentences, unless there are compelling reasons not to, treatment should be continued with linkage back into community-based treatment after release.

Detoxification

Medical detoxification refers to the use of pharmacological treatments to minimize the symptoms of drug withdrawal in the period immediately following cessation of use (Mattick & Hall, 1996). Detoxification alone is not treatment and by itself does not lead to any reduction in rates of relapse. While detoxification should not be viewed as a form of treatment, its worthy aim is to achieve a safe and humane withdrawal from a drug of dependence (American Society of Addiction Medicine, 2002; Mattick & Hall, 1996). Relevant basics of detoxification are reviewed here; more detailed information may be found in Chapter 17.

Opioid detoxification

Opioid withdrawal, while not usually life-threatening, can be a debilitating and painful syndrome of physiological and psychological symptoms. This constellation includes gastrointestinal distress, body aches, diaphoresis, piloerection, lacrimation, rhinorrhea, agitation, and anxiety. These may be objectively documented with clinical tools such as the Clinical Opiate Withdrawal Scale. The duration of withdrawal symptoms depends on the amount and type of opioid an individual is withdrawing from, with higher doses leading to more severe symptoms. Short-acting opioids such as heroin typically result in symptoms that last days;

longer-acting opioids such as methadone result in protracted withdrawal syndromes of several weeks or longer.

Medications used to treat opioid withdrawal include opioid agonists (methadone or buprenorphine) or alpha 2-adrenergic receptor agonists (e.g., clonidine or lofexidine). A metaanalysis of 22 studies compared treatment with methadone, buprenorphine, clonidine, or lofexidine and determined that methadone and buprenorphine were the most effective treatments for managing withdrawal symptoms. While methadone and buprenorphine were equally effective, buprenorphine resulted in a shorter duration of withdrawal (Gowing, Ali, & White, 2009).

In the absence of appropriate medical detoxification for opioids, ethnographic studies demonstrate that prisoners will attempt to get relief through other means. Their methods include complaining of fictitious alcohol withdrawal or psychiatric symptoms, intentionally injuring themselves, or getting medications from other inmates. Such behavior may be unsafe to the patient and both costly and burdensome to medical and security staff (Mitchell, Kelly, Brown, et al., 2009).

Alcohol detoxification

Alcohol withdrawal generally begins developing within hours of the last drink, peaks within 24 to 48 hours, and generally resolves in five to seven days (Mattick & Hall, 1996). The clinical syndrome of alcohol withdrawal includes symptoms related to autonomic nervous system hyperactivity, neuronal excitation, and alcohol withdrawal delirium (AWD), also known as delirium tremens. The initial signs and symptoms of alcohol withdrawal include restlessness, diaphoresis, hyperpyrexia, tachycardia, hypertension, tremors, nausea, vomiting, and anxiety. Seizures are rare and generally occur within 24 hours of cessation. AWD, while most severe, occurs only among 5% of alcohol-dependent patients within two to three days of cessation and is defined by impaired consciousness, cognitive changes, and perceptual disturbances. While initial studies found mortality rates to be as high as 15%, more recent studies indicate that between 1% and 5% of patients with AWD have a fatal outcome (Hasin, Stinson, Ogburn, & Grant, 2007; Mayo-Smith, Beecher, Fischer, et al., 2004).

Benzodiazepines have well-proven efficacy in reducing withdrawal severity, delirium, and seizure. While all benzodiazepines appear to be equally efficacious, longer-acting choices appear more effective in reducing seizures and preventing rebound symptoms, while shorter-acting agents may result in less oversedation. Structured assessment tools such as the Clinical Institute Withdrawal Assessment for Alcohol (CIWA) and symptom-triggered dosing (as opposed to fixed-schedule dosing) result in a more rapid detoxification and less total medication (Mayo-Smith, 1997). Agents such as beta blockers, clonidine, anticonvulsants, and neuroleptics may be used as adjunctive therapy but are not recommended as monotherapy for alcohol withdrawal.

Detoxification from other substances

Cessation of other drugs such as stimulants can cause a withdrawal syndrome. However, these symptoms are rarely life-threatening and there is no clear treatment beyond any required supportive care. Benzodiazepine withdrawal, however, can be severe and potentially fatal; prompt recognition and treatment are important. Benzodiazepine withdrawal is treated with a tapering schedule of benzodiazepines. Similar to alcohol detoxification, a clinical assessment tool such as CIWA can be used, and symptom-triggered taper methods that incorporate flexible dosing and duration are as effective as fixed-dose taper methods (McGregor, Machin, & White, 2003).

Pharmacological treatments for opioid use disorders

There are an estimated 13 million injection drug users in the world, the majority of whom inject heroin. In addition, opioids are the largest contributor to the global burden of disease from addiction, resulting in an estimated 9.2 million disability-adjusted life years and 55% of drug-related deaths in 2010 (Degenhardt, Whiteford, Ferrari, et al., 2013). Decades of evidence has demonstrated that detoxification strategies, regardless of duration or type of medication used, result in the same dismal outcome of 70% to 90% of people relapsing to drug use within one to two years. Additionally, only 5% to 30% of people with longstanding heroin addiction succeed with abstinence-based treatment. In contrast, both methadone and buprenorphine have been shown to be more clinically effective and cost-effective than no pharmacotherapy (Connock, Juarez-Garcia, Jowett, et al., 2007). Adequately dosed opioid agonist therapy results in treatment retention rates of 60% to 80%, with only 20% of those treated using any heroin at one year. An alternative pharmacological treatment is with the opioid antagonist naltrexone.

Agonist therapy

Methadone

Methadone, a full opioid agonist, was first demonstrated in 1965 to be effective with marked reductions in heroin use (Dole & Nyswander, 1965). Since then, evidence has confirmed methadone's effectiveness at reducing heroin use and other adverse consequences, including reductions in incarceration, HIV, and death (Dolan, Shearer, White, et al., 2005; Kimber, Copeland, Hickman, et al., 2010; Mattick et al., 2003). In 1997, the National Institutes of Health declared methadone maintenance to be the gold standard of treatment for opioid dependence (National Institutes of Health, 1998).

Methadone's high oral bioavailability, long half-life, and slow onset of action make once-daily oral dosing feasible with less euphoria than other opioids. Higher dosages (60–100 mg or more) are associated with increased treatment retention, reduced heroin use, decreased withdrawal symptoms, and increased abstinence from cocaine (Faggiano, Vigna-Taglianti, Versino, & Lemma, 2003). A minority of opioid-dependent people are on methadone maintenance treatment (MMT; National Institutes of Health, 1998). Stigma for MMT persists with some members of the public, medical community, and government. In addition, federal and state regulations have limited access to methadone largely due to fear of diversion. Although the US Office of National Drug Control Policy and the US Department of Justice adopted a policy position in support of MMT, similar fears of diversion and stigma around methadone maintenance exist within corrections (National Association of State Alcohol & Drug Abuse Directors, 2006). Only half of US correctional facilities use any methadone at all, primarily for detoxification or treatment of pregnant women admitted on methadone, and only one facility, Riker's Island, uses

methadone for maintenance (Nunn, Zaller, Dickman, et al., 2009; Rich, Boutwell, Shield, et al., 2005; Tomasino, Swanson, Nolan, & Shuman, 2001).

Worldwide there have been numerous successes instituting MMT within correctional facilities. In Australia, where a prison methadone program has existed since 1986, 9% of inmates were on methadone by 1997 (Dolan, Shearer, MacDonald, et al., 2003). Those treated with methadone maintenance had lower rates of heroin use upon release, mortality following release, and reincarceration (Dolan et al., 2003, 2005). In Canada, reduced drug use and recidivism among prisoners on continued methadone during incarceration prompted MMT for all opioid-dependent prisoners (Sibbald, 2002). In France, 77% of opioid-dependent prisoners are on methadone or buprenorphine (Marzo, Rotily, Meroueh, et al., 2009). New York City has been the exception in the United States, offering jail MMT with reduced recidivism and high postrelease treatment retention (Tomasino et al., 2001). Opioid agonist therapy in correctional facilities is associated with decreased heroin use, injection, and syringe-sharing while in prison (Hedrich, Alves, Farrell, et al., 2012).

Prerelease opioid agonist treatment is associated with increased treatment entry and retention after incarceration (Hedrich et al., 2012). Initiation of methadone during incarceration and prior to release is significantly more effective for increasing treatment retention, reducing drug use, and reducing criminal activity than either counseling alone or referral to MMT upon release (Gordon, Kinlock, Schwartz, & O'Grady, 2008; McKenzie et al., 2012). Additionally, the efficacy of prerelease methadone treatment appears to be dose-dependent, with daily doses greater than 80 mg resulting in markedly improved treatment retention (Wickersham, Zahari, Azar et al., 2013). However, prerelease methadone remains rare, and only 8% of US prisons refer opioid-dependent inmates to methadone programs at the time of release (Nunn et al., 2009; Rich et al., 2005).

Buprenorphine

Buprenorphine is a partial mu-opioid agonist first developed in the 1960s for analgesia and subsequently determined to be an effective pharmacotherapy for the treatment of opioid dependence (Bart, 2012). Buprenorphine reduces cravings and other opioid use. Its partial agonist effect results in less euphoria and a ceiling effect for respiratory depression that, combined with its long half-life, make it an ideal agent for management of opioid dependence (Bruce et al., 2007).

Broad international experience has demonstrated the benefit of buprenorphine treatment, with substantial reductions in overdose death and HIV infection with concomitant improvement in social functioning (Carrieri et al., 2006). The efficacy of buprenorphine is dose-dependent. Most patients stabilize on 12 to 16 mg daily, although higher dosages of 16 to 32 mg may improve treatment retention (Bart, 2012; Fareed, Vayalapalli, Casarella, & Drexler, 2012). While a systematic review demonstrated methadone to be superior overall, buprenorphine dosages in the studies reviewed were less than 16 mg. With flexible dosing, buprenorphine is as effective as methadone in reducing other opioid use and retaining people in treatment (Mattick, Breen, Kimber, & Davoli, 2014). Importantly, buprenorphine is viewed more favorably than methadone by people with opioid dependence (Schwartz, Kelly, O'Grady, et al., 2008). Buprenorphine is associated with substantial social benefits, including an increased number of sober relationships and reduced criminal activity. Buprenorphine has also reduced drug-related hospitalizations, potentially due to the mainstreaming of treatment into primary care, with a resultant decrease in stigma and increase in patient autonomy (Carrieri et al., 2006).

Within correctional facilities, there is growing experience with buprenorphine. In French prisons, 74% of opioid-dependent prisoners on agonist therapy are on buprenorphine (Marzo et al., 2009). In Puerto Rico, buprenorphine started during incarceration decreased illicit drug use and crime following release (Garcia, Correa, Viver, et al., 2007). In New York City, buprenorphine was more acceptable than, and as effective as, methadone in reducing self-reported relapse to opioid use, reincarceration, and criminal activity (Magura, Lee, Hershberger, et al., 2009). In Alabama, prerelease buprenorphine decreased opioid use and increased treatment retention among women (Cropsey, Lane, Hale, et al., 2011). Prerelease buprenorphine in Rhode Island demonstrated reasonable retention rates six months after release (Zaller, McKenzie, Friedmann, et al., 2013). Buprenorphine has an advantage over methadone for prerelease populations who are not opioid-tolerant; buprenorphine can be safely titrated to a blocking dose within a week (Zaller et al., 2013), whereas methadone can take months (Gordon et al., 2008).

Antagonist therapy

Naltrexone

Naltrexone, a semisynthetic mu- and kappa-opioid receptor antagonist, was first synthesized in the 1960s and can be administered in oral or intramuscular formulation. As an antagonist, it blocks the effects of opioids for 24 to 48 hours following oral administration and 28 days following an intramuscular long-acting dose of 380 mg. As a treatment for opioid dependence, naltrexone's ability to block the reinforcing effects of opioids seemed promising as a means of extinguishing the reward associated with ongoing opioid use (Bart, 2012). In practice, the results have been less impressive. For oral naltrexone, few patients are retained in treatment. However, in Russia, where methadone and buprenorphine are not available, intramuscular naltrexone has demonstrated efficacy as a treatment for opioid dependence, with increased abstinence rates and improved treatment retention compared to placebo (Krupitsky, Nunes, Ling, et al., 2011).

There has been no direct comparison of extended-release naltrexone to opioid agonist therapy; retention in treatment with long-acting naltrexone appears comparable to methadone maintenance (Bart, 2012). Among correctional populations, extended-release naltrexone has also shown some promise. A study of 61 individuals with a history of opioid dependence who were under community correctional supervision (probation, parole, or a diversion program) found that those who completed treatment with intramuscular naltrexone had reduced rates of other opioid use, reduced recidivism, and improved likelihood of employment (Coviello, Cornish, Lynch, et al., 2012). The evidence for oral naltrexone is conflicting. One study of 52 federal probationers in 1997 demonstrated improved treatment retention (52% versus 33%), decreased opioid use (8% versus 30%), and decreased return to prison (26% versus 56%) among those treated with naltrexone compared to counseling alone (Cornish, Metzger, Woody, et al., 1997). However, a subsequent study of oral naltrexone

compared to no pharmacotherapy for opioid-dependent individuals under community correctional supervision found low treatment retention rates and no differences in drug use (Coviello, Cornish, Lynch, et al., 2010). The use of injectable or implantable naltrexone for various populations is an area of active research, and more information should be available in the coming years. Many in the criminal justice field believe that providing agonist therapy is "giving them what they want" and is tantamount to rewarding bad behavior, whereas antagonist therapy, a blocking agent that does not provide euphoria, is inherently more in line with a correctional mindset.

Pharmacological treatments for alcohol use disorders

As with opioid use disorders, detoxification from alcohol alone rarely results in long-term sobriety. Unlike opioid use disorders, pharmacotherapy for AUDs is less efficacious but still offers meaningful benefit and is widely underused. Three medications approved by the US Food and Drug Administration for the treatment of AUD are naltrexone, acamprosate, and disulfiram. Evidence suggests that naltrexone reduces both the risk of relapse to heavy drinking and the frequency of drinking compared with placebo but does not significantly improve rates of abstinence. Acamprosate similarly reduces drinking frequency and also significantly increases the total duration of abstinence (Garbutt, West, Carey, et al., 1999). There are no placebo-controlled studies to suggest disulfiram improves continuous abstinence, but some evidence suggests a reduction in drinking frequency, particularly when dosing is supervised (Garbutt et al., 1999).

Summary

SUDs are highly prevalent among prisoners, and the relapsing nature of these disorders within the context of the criminalization of drug use results in high rates of recidivism, cost, spread of disease, and mortality. Pharmacotherapy for SUDs, in particular for opioids, has a robust evidence base. Untreated opioid dependence both within corrections and in the community is associated with HIV, hepatitis C, crime, and death by overdose. Substantial evidence argues that these risks are reduced through long-term treatment with agonist medications such as methadone and buprenorphine. A minority of prisoners receive addiction treatment while incarcerated. Those who do receive treatment are usually offered behavioral interventions, which have extremely poor outcomes when used alone.

Despite convincing evidence from years of research that shows the efficacy of buprenorphine and methadone for the treatment of opioid dependence, the vast majority of correctional facilities do not offer these life-saving medications. Lack of understanding about the disease model of addiction, persistent stigma that pharmacotherapy is simply a "substitute," the challenging logistics of administering medications, fear of diversion, and the punitive philosophy of corrections have limited the dissemination of pharmacotherapy. Given the differences in environment and drug use patterns between the prison setting and the community, we cannot simply extrapolate from community-based studies about the efficacy of maintenance therapy. Maintenance therapy for the duration of a prolonged prison sentence should be offered depending on the prevalence of illicit opioid use within a given facility. Prerelease pharmacotherapy with direct linkage to community treatment programs is an evidence-based intervention that should be offered to all opioid-dependent prisoners.

Pharmacotherapy for AUDs is also highly underused. While the evidence base is modest, it is clear that medications are an important tool in the treatment package for alcohol dependence. Additional well-designed studies are needed to better assess the impact of naltrexone and acamprosate within this population.

While detoxification alone is not treatment, it is an important and humane first step. The current lack of standardization of medical detoxification services within correctional facilities is distressing. Unassisted withdrawal not only inflicts undue suffering but can be life-threatening. In addition, fear of withdrawal may prevent individuals from seeking appropriate treatments such as methadone in the community and may encourage deceptive behavior while incarcerated in an effort to get relief.

The time has come to reexamine addiction treatment practices within corrections. Incarceration offers an opportunity to engage a highly marginalized population with a disproportionate burden of disease, particularly addiction. Using this opportunity to screen, diagnose, treat, and connect them with community treatment programs would improve not only the health of incarcerated populations but also the public health of the communities to which they will return.

Disclosure: One of the authors (J.D.R.) is a stockholder in Alkermes, which makes Vivitrol, a long-acting intramuscular naltrexone formulation.

References

American Society of Addiction Medicine (2002). *Access to appropriate detoxification services for persons incarcerated.* Available at: http://asam.org/docs/publicy-policy-statements/1detox--incarceration-7-02.pdf

Bart, G. (2012). Maintenance medication for opiate addiction: the foundation of recovery. *Journal of Addictive Diseases, 31*(3), 207–225.

Bewley-Taylor, D., Hallam, C., & Allen, R. (2009). *The incarceration of drug offenders: an overview.* Report Sixteen. The Beckley Foundation Drug Policy Programme. Available online at: http://www.beckleyfoundation.org/pdf/BF_Report_16.pdf

Bruce, R. D., Smith-Rohrburg, D., & Altice, F. L. (2007). Pharmacological treatment of substance abuse in correctional facilities; prospects and barriers to expanding access to evidence-based therapy. In R. Greifenger (Ed.), *Public health behind bars; from prisons to communities* (pp. 385–411). New York, NY: Springer.

Carrieri, M. P., Amass, L., Lucas, G. M., Vlahov, D., Wodak, A., & Woody, G. E. (2006). Buprenorphine use: the international experience. *Clinical Infectious Diseases, 43*(Suppl 4), S197–215.

Chandler, R. K., Fletcher, B. W., & Volkow, N. D. (2009). Treating drug abuse and addiction in the criminal justice system: improving public health and safety. *Journal of the American Medical Association, 301*(2), 183–190.

Connock, M., Juarez-Garcia, A., Jowett, S., Frew, E., et al. (2007). Methadone and buprenorphine for the management of opioid dependence: a systematic review and economic evaluation. *Health Technology Assessment, 11,* 9.

Cornish, J. W., Metzger, D., Woody, G. E., Wilson, D., et al. (1997). Naltrexone pharmacotherapy for opioid dependent federal probationers. *Journal of Substance Abuse Treatment, 14*(6), 529–534.

Coviello, D. M., Cornish, J. W., Lynch, K. G., Boney, T. Y., et al. (2010). A randomized trial of oral naltrexone for treating opioid-dependent offenders. *American Journal on Addictions, 19*(5), 422–432.

Coviello, D. M., Cornish, J. W., Lynch, K. G., Boney, T. Y., et al. (2012). A multi-site pilot study of extended-release injectable naltrexone treatment for previously opioid-dependent parolees and probationers. *Journal of Substance Abuse. 33*(1), 48–59.

Cropsey, K. L., Lane, P. S., Hale, G. J., Jackson, D. O., et al. (2011). Results of a pilot randomized controlled trial of buprenorphine for opioid dependent women in the criminal justice system. *Drug and Alcohol Dependence, 119*(3), 172–178.

Degenhardt, L., Whiteford, H. A., Ferrari, A. J., Baxter, A. J., et al. (2013). Global burden of disease attributable to illicit drug use and dependence: findings from the Global Burden of Disease Study 2010. *Lancet, 382*(9904), 1564–1574.

Dolan, K. A., Shearer, J., MacDonald, M., Mattick, R. P., et al. (2003). A randomized controlled trial of methadone maintenance treatment versus wait list control in an Australian prison system. *Drug and Alcohol Dependence, 72*(1), 59–65.

Dolan, K. A., Shearer, J., White, B., Zhou, J., et al. (2005). Four-year follow-up of imprisoned male heroin users and methadone treatment: mortality, re-incarceration and hepatitis C infection. *Addiction, 100*(6), 820–828.

Dole, V. P., & Nyswander, M. (1965). A medical treatment for diacetylmorphine (heroin) addiction: a clinical trial with methadone hydrochloride. *Journal of the American Medical Association, 193*(8), 646–650.

Faggiano, F., Vigna-Taglianti, F., Versino, E., & Lemma, P. (2003). Methadone maintenance at different dosages for opioid dependence. *Cochrane Database of Systematic Reviews, 3.* Art. No.: CD002208.

Fareed, A., Vayalapalli, S., Casarella, J., & Drexler, K. (2012). Effect of buprenorphine dose on treatment outcome. *Journal of Addictive Diseases, 31*(1), 8–18.

Fiscella, K., Pless, N., Meldrum, S., & Fiscella, P. (2004). Alcohol and opiate withdrawal in US jails. *American Journal of Public Health, 94,* 1522–1524.

Garbutt, J. C., West, S. L., Carey, T. S., Lohr, K. N., & Crews, F. T. (1999). Pharmacological treatment of alcohol dependence: A review of the evidence. *Journal of the American Medical Association, 281*(14), 1318–1325.

Garcia, C. A., Correa, G. C., Viver, A. D., Kinlock, T. W., et al. (2007). Buprenorphine-naloxone treatment for pre-release opioid-dependent inmates in Puerto Rico. *Journal of Addiction Medicine, 1*(3), 126–132.

Gordon, M. S., Kinlock, T. W., Schwartz, R. P., & O'Grady, K. E. (2008). A randomized clinical trial of methadone maintenance for prisoners: findings at 6 months post-release. *Addiction, 103*(8), 1333–1342.

Gowing, L., Ali, R., & White, J. M. (2009). Buprenorphine for the management of opioid withdrawal. *Cochrane Database of Systemic Reviews, 3,* CD002025.

Hasin, D. S., Stinson, F. S., Ogburn, E., & Grant, B. F. (2007). Prevalence, correlates, disability, and comorbidity of DSM-IV alcohol abuse and dependence in the United States: results from the National Epidemiologic Survey on Alcohol and Related Conditions. *Archives of General Psychiatry, 64,* 830–842.

Hedrich, D., Alves, P., Farrell, M., Stover, H., et al. (2012). The effectiveness of opioid maintenance treatment in prison settings: a systematic review. *Addiction, 107*(3), 501–517.

Kimber, J., Copeland, L., Hickman, M., Macleod, J., et al. (2010). Survival and cessation in injecting drug users: prospective observational study of outcomes and effect of opiate substitution treatment. *British Medical Journal, 341,* c3172.

Krupitsky, E., Nunes, E. V., Ling, W., Illeperuma, A., et al. (2011). Injectable extended-release naltrexone for opioid dependence: a double-blind, placebo-controlled, multicentre randomised trial. *Lancet, 377*(9776), 1506–1513.

MacAskill, S., Parkes, T., Brooks, O., Graham, L., et al. (2011). Assessment of alcohol problems using AUDIT in a prison setting: more than an 'aye or no' question. *BMC Public Health, 11,* 865.

Magura, S., Lee, J. D., Hershberger, J., Joseph, H., et al. (2009). Buprenorphine and methadone maintenance in jail and post-release: A randomized controlled clinical trial. *Drug and Alcohol Dependence, 99*(1-3), 222–230.

Marzo, J. N., Rotily, M., Meroueh, F., Varastet, M., et al. (2009). Maintenance therapy and 3-year outcome of opioid-dependent prisoners: a prospective study in France (2003–06). *Addiction, 104*(7), 1233–1240.

Mattick, R. P., Breen, C., Kimber, J., & Davoli, M. (2003). Methadone maintenance therapy versus no opioid replacement therapy for opioid dependence. *Cochrane Database of Systemic Reviews, 2,* CD002209.

Mattick, R. P., Breen, C., Kimber, J., & Davoli, M. (2014). Buprenorphine maintenance versus placebo or methadone maintenance for opioid dependence. *Cochrane Database of Systematic Reviews, 2,* CD002207.

Mattick, R. P., & Hall, W. (1996). Are detoxification programmes effective? *Lancet, 347*(8994), 97–100.

Mayo-Smith, M. F. (1997). Pharmacological management of alcohol withdrawal: a meta-analysis and evidence-based practice guideline. *Journal of the American Medical Association, 278*(2), 144-151.

Mayo-Smith, M. F., Beecher, L. H., Fischer, T. L., Gorelick, D. A., et al. (2004). Management of alcohol withdrawal delirium; An evidence-based practice guideline. *Archives of Internal Medicine, 164*(13), 1405–1412.

McGregor, C., Machin, A., & White, J. M. (2003). In-patient benzodiazepine withdrawal: comparison of fixed and symptom-triggered taper methods. *Drug and Alcohol Review, 22*(2), 175–180.

McKenzie, M., Zaller, N., Dickman, S. L., Green, T. C., et al. (2012). A randomized trial of methadone initiation prior to release from incarceration. *Substance Abuse, 33*(1),19–29.

Mitchell, S. G., Kelly, S. M., Brown, B. S., Reisinger, H. S., et al. (2009). Incarceration and opioid withdrawal: The experiences of methadone patients and out of treatment heroin users. *Journal of Psychoactive Drugs, 41*(2), 145–152.

Mumola, C. J., & Karberg, J. C. (2006). *Drug use and dependence, State and federal prisoners, 2004.* Bureau of Justice Statistics, NCJ 213530.

National Association of State Alcohol and Drug Abuse Directors (April 2006). *Methadone maintenance treatment and the criminal justice system.* Available online at: http://www.nasadad.org/resource.php?base_id=650 (accessed December 11, 2013).

National Institute of Health (1998). National Consensus Development Panel on Effective Medical Treatment of Opiate Addiction. *Journal of the American Medical Association, 280,* 1936–1943.

Nunn, A., Zaller, N., Dickman, S., Trimbur, C., et al. (2009). Methadone and buprenorphine prescribing and referral practices in US prison systems: results from a nationwide survey. *Drug and Alcohol Dependence, 105*(1-2), 83–88.

Oser, C. B., Knudsen, H. K., Staton-Tindall, M., Tasman, F., & Leukefeld, C. (2009). Organizational-level correlates of the provision of detoxification services and medication-based treatments for substance abuse in correctional institutions. *Drug and Alcohol Dependence, 103*(Suppl 1), S73–81.

Pecoraro, A., & Woody, G. E. (2011). Medication-assisted treatment for opioid dependence: Making a difference in prisons. *F1000 Medicine Reports, 3,* 1.

Rich, J. D., Boutwell, A. E., Shield, D. C., Key, R. G., et al. (2005). Attitudes and practices regarding the use of methadone in US state and federal prisons. *Journal of Urban Health, 82,* 411–419.

SAMHSA (2000). *Substance abuse treatment in adult and juvenile correctional facilities: findings from the Uniform Facilities Data Set 1997 Survey of Correctional Facilities.* Rockville, MD: Substance Abuse and Mental Health Services Administration, Office of Applied Studies.

Schwartz, R. P., Kelly, S. M., O'Grady, K. E., Mitchell, S. G., et al. (2008). Attitudes toward buprenorphine and methadone among opioid-dependent individuals. *American Journal of Addiction, 17*(5), 396.

Sibbald, B. (2002). Methadone maintenance expands inside federal prisons. *Canadian Medical Association Journal, 167*(10), 1154.

Tomasino, V., Swanson, A. J., Nolan, J., & Shuman, H. I. (2001). The Key Extended Entry Program (KEEP): a methadone treatment program for opiate-dependent inmates. *Mount Sinai Journal of Medicine, 68*(1), 14–20.

UNODC-UNAIDS-WHO (2006). *Framework for HIV AIDS prevention, treatment, and care in prison.* Available online at: https://www.unodc.org/pdf/HIV-AIDS_prisons_July06.pdf (accessed January 21, 2014).

Vanderplasschen, W., Colpaert, K., Autrique, M., Rapp, R. C., et al. (2013). Therapeutic communities for addictions: A review of their effectiveness from a recovery-oriented perspective. *Scientific World Journal, 2013,* 427817.

Wickersham, J. A., Zahari, M. M., Azar, M. M., Kamarulzaman, A., & Altice, F. L. (2013). Methadone dose at the time of release from prison significantly influences retention in treatment: implications from a pilot study of HIV-infected prisoners transitioning to the community in Malaysia. *Drug and Alcohol Dependedence, 132*(1-2), 378–382.

Zaller, N., McKenzie, M., Friedmann, P. D., Green, T. C., et al. (2013). Initiation of buprenorphine during incarceration and retention in treatment upon release. *Journal of Substance Abuse Treatment, 45*(2), 222–226.

CHAPTER 47

Transition to the community

Jaimie P. Meyer and Frederick L. Altice

Introduction

Reincarceration of former prisoners is commonly associated with relapse to drug and alcohol use because of ineffective treatment of substance use disorders (SUDs) after release. Although substantial efforts have focused on providing support for those with SUDs as they make the transition back to the community, evidence-based interventions are not commonly deployed. This chapter discusses best practice and evidence-based models in use for jails and prisons to support successful community reentry.

Epidemiology of substance use disorders

High entry rates of people who use drugs into prisons or jails results in the criminal justice system bearing a disproportionate burden of the epidemic of people with SUDs. In contrast to 8% of US adults in the general population (SAMHSA, 2012), up to 65% of prisoners meet *Diagnostic and Statistical Manual of Mental Disorders*–IV criteria for having an SUD (Mumola & Karberg, Revised 2007), and, depending on the geographic location, 70% of HIV-infected prisoners meet criteria for opioid dependence (Springer, Qiu, Saber-Tehrani, & Altice, 2012). In jails, two thirds of inmates report regular alcohol or drug use prior to incarceration (James, 2004), and women report higher rates of SUDs than their male counterparts (Binswanger, Merrill, Krueger, et al., 2010). Nearly half of jail inmates report preincarceration symptoms consistent with alcohol abuse or dependence (James & Karberg, 2005). These factors suggest a pressing need to identify and treat SUDs during incarceration and prior to community release.

Despite this demonstrated need, evidence-based SUD treatment programs during incarceration are relatively nonexistent (Meyer, Althoff, & Altice, 2013). Only 11% of US state or federal correctional facilities offer methadone or buprenorphine as medication-assisted therapies during detention, mostly for pregnant women or short-term detoxification (Nunn, Zaller, Dickman, et al., 2009; Rich, Boutwell, & Shield, 2005). Many facilities rely instead on behavioral programs that promote education, detoxification, and abstinence; these do not achieve the same level of benefit in SUD outcomes compared to medication-assisted therapy for either HIV-infected (Springer, Chen, & Altice, 2010) or uninfected prisoners (Kinlock, Gordon, Schwartz, et al., 2009).

After a period of detoxification and (enforced) abstinence from drugs or alcohol during incarceration, prisoners are often released to the same communities and risk environments from which they came, with little plan to support continuity of health care or persistent sobriety. Chronic and often untreated SUDs play a major role in prison recidivism and likely contribute to poor health outcomes after release (Meyer, Chen, & Springer, 2011). In the immediate postrelease period, prisoners are at high risk for relapse to drugs or alcohol (van Olphen, Freudenberg, Fortin, & Galea, 2006), with associated drug-related recidivism to prison (Freudenberg, Daniels, Crum, et al., 2008) and excess mortality due to drug overdose (Binswanger, Stern, Deyo, et al., 2007). In contrast, medication-assisted therapy that is provided either during incarceration or immediately after release reduces substance use relapse and prison recidivism, increases retention in drug treatment, and improves HIV treatment outcomes after release.

Addressing substance use disorders before release

Given the high prevalence of SUDs among prisoners and the relative undermanagement of SUDs during incarceration, evidence-based strategies are needed to effectively address SUDs among individuals who cycle through the criminal justice system and to curb postrelease drug-related recidivism, morbidity, and mortality. To ensure that persons who use drugs make a successful transition back to the community, prerelease discharge planning that incorporates several key components is required (Fig. 47.1): transitional case management that includes access to medical and social entitlement programs; screening for SUDs, briefly intervening, and referring to or directly providing evidence-based treatment (SBIRT) as needed; and adherence support. Comprehensive transitional programs for prisoners with SUDs should also incorporate diagnosis and treatment of psychiatric disorders during incarceration, with transition to integrated community mental health treatment programs (Lincoln, Kennedy, Tuthill, et al., 2006). Examples of jail and prison release programs for PWUDs are shown in Table 47.1.

Transitional case management

Transitional case management involves coordinating medical and psychosocial care for individuals with complex medical needs such as persons who use drugs (Springer, Spaulding, Meyer, & Altice, 2011). Case management services are currently the mainstay of prisoner release programs for HIV-infected inmates, with the goal of providing a seamless system of care to reduce recidivism, maintain overall health, and avert drug use. Community linkages differ by state and facility and sometimes only involve passive referrals. Transitional case management can play a key role in assisting soon-to-be-released prisoners with accessing medical and social entitlement programs. In the absence of evidence-based SUD treatment, however, transitional case management alone is

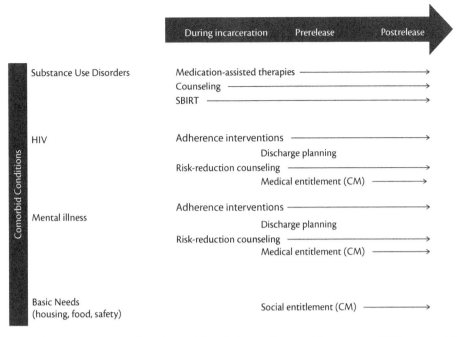

Fig. 47.1 Public health implications for adequate transitional care for HIV-infected prisoners: five essential components. SBIRT, screening, brief intervention, referral to treatment; CM, case management. Adapted from Springer, Spaulding, et al. (2011).

insufficient for fostering optimal treatment outcomes (Wohl, Scheyett, & Golin, 2011).

Despite advocacy for costly intensive case management interventions (Zaller, Holmes, & Dyl, 2008), a randomized controlled trial found that standard prerelease discharge planning was as effective at linking subjects to HIV care as intensive case management provided before and after prison release, although coordination of care involved only passive referrals to medical and social services (Wohl et al., 2011). A recent multisite prospective cohort study of jail detainees with HIV transitioning to the community assessed new methods for linking people living with HIV/AIDS to medical and ancillary services after release from jail, of which transitional intensive case management was a central component (Draine, Ahuja, Altice, et al., 2011a). Despite receiving a comprehensive package of transitional services, the cohort experienced high rates of relapse to cocaine and opioids in the six months following jail release. Relapse was directly associated with homelessness and baseline SUD severity; postrelease receipt of health insurance, however, mitigated against relapse to drug use (Krishnan, Wickersham, & Chitsaz, 2012).

Prerelease treatment for substance use disorders

Although best evidence for SUD treatment is with medication-assisted therapy (see Chapter 46), health care providers in the criminal justice system can, at a minimum, screen regularly for problematic drug or alcohol use and briefly intervene via SBIRT (Meyer et al., 2013). SBIRT is an evidence-based algorithm used to reduce negative consequences of alcohol or drug use that may be delivered in diverse clinical settings by treating clinicians or case managers or as computer modules (Madras, Compton, Avula, et al., 2009). SBIRT facilitates both routine screening for

problematic substance use and linkages between primary care and addiction specialty care. It was recently adapted for people transitioning from the criminal justice system (Prendergast & Cartier, 2013).

When given alone or with counseling, prerelease medication-assisted therapy is most physiologically and psychologically beneficial for relapse prevention and can secondarily improve postrelease care engagement (Bruce, Kresina, & McCance-Katz, 2010). Two recent interventions (Rich, McKenzie, Shield, et al., 2005; Springer et al., 2010) demonstrated that opioid agonist therapies initiated upon release are effective at preventing relapse to opioid use and, for persons living with HIV/AIDS, secondarily maintain antiretroviral therapy-related benefits achieved during incarceration (Meyer et al., 2011). Since persistent HIV viral suppression is associated with a decreased risk of HIV transmission, treatment of SUDs can be an effective secondary prevention measure for HIV as part of the "treatment as prevention" paradigm (Wilson, Law, Grulich, et al., 2008). Methadone and buprenorphine are the most effective medication-assisted therapies for treating opioid dependence (Amato, Davoli, Perucci, et al., 2005), although naltrexone has achieved some success in highly motivated patients (Lobmaier, Kornor, Kunoe, & Bjorndal, 2008).

Methadone, when initiated before community reentry, is more effective than referrals to postrelease methadone at preventing drug relapse and retention in drug treatment among prisoners making the transition to the community (Kinlock et al., 2009; Springer, Spaulding, et al., 2011). Retention on methadone maintenance after release was lower than retention rates in community settings, perhaps because the methadone dose was substantially lower than that needed to facilitate retention (Wickersham, Zahari, Azar, et al., 2013). While methadone is time-tested and cost-effective, implementation in correctional settings is limited by the fact that it is highly federally regulated and structured,

Table 47.1 Characteristics of Jail and Prison Release Programs

State or City	California (Cloutier, 2002)	Connecticut (Altice & Khoshnood, 1997)	North Carolina (Wohl et al., 2011)	New Jersey (Laufer, Arriola, & Dawson-Rose, 2002)	New York (Richie, Freudenberg, & Page, 2001)	Massachusetts (Conklin, Lincoln, & Flanigan, 1998; Lincoln et al., 2006)	Rhode Island (Zaller et al., 2008; Rich, Holmes, & Salas, 2001; Holmes, Dranioni, & Rich, 2002)	Virginia (Kaplowitz, Kaatz, & Weir-Wiggins, 2002)	Multisite[1] (Draine et al., 2011b)
Prison or Jail	Jail	Prison	Prison	Jail	Prison	Jail	Prison	Prison	Jail
Worked with prisoner before release	ü	ü	ü	ü	ü	ü	ü	ü	ü
Worked with prisoner after release	ü	ü	ü			ü	ü	ü	ü
Services Provided									
Case management and advocacy	ü	ü	ü	ü	ü	ü	ü		ü
Assistance with social and medical entitlements	ü	ü	ü	ü	ü	ü	ü	ü	ü
Medical and/or HIV care	ü						ü		ü
Nursing assistance	ü			ü	NR		ü		
Drug treatment services	ü				ü		ü		ü
Medication adherence interventions	ü			ü	NR		NR		ü
Housing	ü				NR	NR	NR	NR	ü
Mental health	ü				NR	NR	NR	NR	ü
Type of evaluation	Observational study	Observational study	RCT	Demonstration project	Observational study	Demonstration project	Observational study	Demonstration project	Demonstration project
Sample size	172	269	104	NR	700	NR	97	NR	1270

RCT, randomized controlled trial; NR, not reported.

[1]Involved 10 program sites in the following states: Connecticut, Georgia, Illinois, Massachusetts, New York, Ohio, Pennsylvania, South Carolina, and Rhode Island.

Source: Springer, Spaulding, et al., 2011.

requiring directly observed therapy and other measures to prevent diversion.

Buprenorphine, with its excellent safety profile, few drug interactions, and relative lack of federally legislated constraints, provides new possibilities for treating released prisoners who have opioid dependence (Smith-Rohrberg, Bruce, & Altice, 2004). Buprenorphine has recently been adopted in several jail settings and is safe and effective for sustaining HIV treatment outcomes in transitioning persons living with HIV/AIDS (Springer et al., 2010). Although US correctional settings have yet to see the benefits of buprenorphine treatment, among French prisoners it has been proven effective since 1996 (Levasseur, Marzo, Ross, & Blatier, 2002). The few programs in the correctional system that do initiate buprenorphine before release have shown feasibility, with sustained retention in buprenorphine treatment following release (Cropsey, Lane, & Hale, 2011; Garcia, Correa, Viver, et al., 2007; Magura, Lee, & Hershberger, 2009). The initiation and up-titration dosing of buprenorphine in correctional settings can be challenging among patients who are not in acute opioid withdrawal; these issues have been well described elsewhere (Kinlock, Gordon, Schwartz, & Fitzgerald, 2010; Smith-Rohrberg et al., 2004).

Extended-release naltrexone (XR-NTX), a complete opioid antagonist and once-monthly injectable medication, provides new evidence-based treatment options for prisoners with opioid dependence who are making the transition to the community. XR-NTX has important potential applications for correctional populations because of a lack of pharmacokinetic interactions with antiretroviral therapy (Altice, Kamarulzaman, Soriano, et al., 2010), ability to treat both opioid and alcohol dependence, adherence advantages over daily tablet formulations, and antagonistic properties that make overdose or diversion unlikely (Gastfriend, 2011). Although XR-NTX has been effective for treating alcohol use disorders, it has not been critically evaluated among HIV-infected individuals, either in community or correctional settings, although randomized controlled trials are ongoing (Springer, Altice, Herme, & Di Paola, 2013; Springer, Azar, & Altice, 2011). Methadone, buprenorphine, and XR-NTX, along with relevant pharmacokinetic drug interactions, have been reviewed for the treatment of SUDs in persons living with HIV/AIDS (Altice et al., 2010) and in those with psychiatric disorders (Saber-Tehrani et al., 2011).

Because many individuals who interface with the criminal justice system often use several mind-altering substances, multiple intervention modalities may be needed, including medication-assisted therapy and behavioral and cue-based therapies (Springer, Spaulding, et al., 2011). Behavioral interventions are most effective when delivered within therapeutic communities that are provided over a sustained period and continued after release (see Chapter 44); they are therefore labor-intensive and costly (Inciardi, Martin, & Butzin, 2004). Therapeutic communities and medication-assisted therapies that use methadone and buprenorphine (Smith-Rohrberg et al., 2004) and treatment of alcohol use disorders within correctional settings have been reviewed elsewhere (Springer, Azar, & Altice, 2011).

Adherence support

Transitional programs can incorporate effective ways to overcome problematic medication adherence that is common among persons who use drugs (Anand, Springer, Copenhaver, & Altice, 2010; Springer, Spaulding, et al., 2011). Cues and reminders may be useful for patients for whom a major reason for missed doses is "forgetting" because of chaotic lifestyles, comorbid mental illness, or HIV- or SUD-associated cognitive impairment. The simplicity and cost-effectiveness of reminders enables integration with other adherence interventions as part of transitional programs, but their impact on adherence is modest (Thompson, Mugavero, Amico, et al., 2012).

Adherence counseling strategies have been shown to change patients' knowledge, attitudes, and beliefs about medical treatment and to improve their adherence to complicated medication regimens (Leeman, Chang, Lee, et al., 2010; Springer, Spaulding, et al., 2011). Peer-driven counseling interventions can be affordable and acceptable; however, professionally trained counselors might, despite their added cost, be more effective and replicable, especially if they deliver validated and manualized interventions.

Contingency management has its roots in the mental health treatment community, where it has been used to manage SUDs (Stitzer & Petry, 2006). Participants are rewarded for positive health behaviors (e.g., excellent adherence) and sanctions are imposed for negative health behaviors (e.g., substance use or treatment nonadherence). Contingency management interventions may include direct financial compensation, token economy systems such as vouchers (Sorensen, Haug, & Delucchi, 2007), positive and negative reinforcing medications (Sorensen et al., 2007), and material incentives. Preliminary data support the use of contingency management for HIV treatment adherence (Rosen, Dieckhaus, & McMahon, 2007), but randomized controlled trials have not been conducted. Although contingency management has proven to be cost-effective in some settings, the absolute costs involved may be prohibitive to bring to scale. Moreover, the benefits of such interventions disappear immediately after cessation of the rewards/punishments, making treatment for lifelong chronic diseases unsustainable.

Directly administered antiretroviral therapy (DAART), which derived from the successes of directly observed therapy in tuberculosis treatment, has long been used in correctional settings to promote medication adherence and has documented efficacy (Babudieri, Aceti, D'Offizi, et al., 2000). A metaanalysis of DAART suggests it is not beneficial overall (Ford, Nachega, Engel, & Mills, 2009); however, individuals who were at particular risk for nonadherence (e.g., persons who use drugs or prisoners) were not differentially examined. A subsequent metaanalysis did, however, support the use of DAART among individuals at high risk for nonadherence, especially persons who use drugs (Hart, Jeon, & Ivers, 2010). In one randomized controlled trial of released HIV-infected prisoners, those receiving DAART were significantly more likely to maintain viral suppression than their counterparts (Altice, Tehrani, Qiu, et al., 2011), and DAART is now an evidence-based adherence strategy for postrelease care (Thompson et al., 2012). In a recent study of 882 HIV-infected prisoners and jail detainees (Meyer, Cepeda, Wu, et al., 2014), receipt of DAART was not significantly associated with achieving HIV viral suppression by the time of release, which may be explained by medication adherence (Wohl, Stephenson, & Golin, 2003) or facility resource availability. Patient and provider preferences likely also play a role in directly observed therapy selection: patients may opt out of directly observed therapy because of concerns about inadvertent disclosure of HIV status (Altice, Mostashari, & Friedland, 2001), and providers may triage patients whom they perceive as being nonadherent for directly observed therapy (Saberi, Caswell, Jamison, et al., 2012). Alternatively, directly observed therapy may have limited additional benefit when medication regimens are well tolerated and provided within a highly structured correctional setting, where patients have considerable access to psychiatric medications and less access to mind-altering substances such as alcohol or drugs that are associated with decreased adherence. In community settings, however, directly observed therapy has a clearly documented beneficial effect on treatment outcomes for certain populations, especially those with SUDs, for whom treatment nonpersistence is associated with high addiction severity and ongoing injection drug use (Altice, Maru, Bruce, et al., 2007; Berg, Litwin, Li, et al., 2010; Ing, Bae, Maru, & Altice, 2013). The major challenge to adherence interventions, including DAART, among transitioning prisoners and other persons who use drugs is the sustainability of benefit following the intervention (Binford, Kahana, & Altice, 2012).

Summary

Despite scientific evidence that supports transitional programs for prisoners with SUDs, there are significant logistical constraints to introducing evidence-based interventions into correctional systems and delivering them to prisoners prior to release. Innovative solutions that involve partnerships between all existing stakeholders, including individual patients with SUDs, the criminal justice system, and communities, are urgently needed to overcome existing impediments.

Acknowledgments

We acknowledge career development funding from the National Institute on Drug Abuse (K23 DA033858 for J.P.M. and K24 DA017072 for F.L.A.). The funding sources played no role in study design; data collection, analysis, or interpretation; writing of the chapter; or the decision to submit the chapter for publication. Portions of this chapter were excerpted from manuscripts previously published by J.P.M. and F.L.A., referenced herein, and used with permission from the authors.

References

Altice, F., Kamarulzaman, A., Soriano, V., Schechter, M., & Friedland, G. (2010). Treatment of medical, psychiatric, and substance-use comorbidities in people infected with HIV who use drugs. *Lancet*, *376*(9738), 367–387.

Altice, F. L., & Khoshnood, K. (1997). *Transitional case management as a strategy for linking HIV-infected prisoners to community health and social services (Project TLC)*. Hartford, CT: Connecticut Department of Public Health.

Altice, F. L., Maru, D. S., Bruce, R. D., Springer, S. A., & Friedland, G. H. (2007). Superiority of directly administered antiretroviral therapy over self-administered therapy among HIV-infected drug users: a prospective, randomized, controlled trial. *Clinical Infectious Diseases*, *45*(6), 770–778.

Altice, F. L., Mostashari, F., & Friedland, G. H. (2001). Trust and the acceptance of and adherence to antiretroviral therapy. *Journal of Acquired Immune Deficiency Syndrome*, *28*(1), 47–58.

Altice, F. L., Tehrani, A. S., Qiu, J., Herme, M., & Springer, S. A. (2011). *Directly administered antiretroviral therapy (DAART) is superior to self-administered therapy (SAT) among released HIV+ prisoners: results from a randomized controlled trial*. Presented at 18th Conference on Retroviruses and Opportunistic Infections, Boston, MA, February 27–March 2, 2011, Abstract K-131.

Amato, L., Davoli, M., Perucci, C. A., Ferri, M., Faggiano, F., & Mattick, R. P. (2005). An overview of systematic reviews of the effectiveness of opiate maintenance therapies: available evidence to inform clinical practice and research. *Journal of Substance Abuse and Treatment*, *28*(4), 321–329.

Anand, P., Springer, S. A., Copenhaver, M. M., & Altice, F. L. (2010). Neurocognitive impairment and HIV risk factors: a reciprocal relationship. *AIDS and Behavior*, *14*(6), 1213–1226.

Babudieri, S., Aceti, A., D'Offizi, G. P., Carbonara, S., & Starnini, G. (2000). Directly observed therapy to treat HIV infection in prisoners. *Journal of the American Medical Association*, *284*(2), 179–180.

Berg, K. M., Litwin, A., Li, X., Heo, M., & Arnsten, J. H. (2010). Directly observed antiretroviral therapy improves adherence and viral load in drug users attending methadone maintenance clinics: A randomized controlled trial. *Drug and Alcohol Dependence* (Epub September 14, 2010).

Binford, M. C., Kahana, S. Y., & Altice, F. L. (2012). A systematic review of antiretroviral adherence interventions for HIV-infected people who use drugs. *Current HIV/AIDS Report*, *9*(4), 287–312.

Binswanger, I. A., Merrill, J. O., Krueger, P. M., White, M. C., Booth, R. E., & Elmore, J. G. (2010). Gender differences in chronic medical, psychiatric, and substance-dependence disorders among jail inmates. *American Journal of Public Health*, *100*(3), 476–482.

Binswanger, I. A., Stern, M. F., Deyo, R. A., et al. (2007). Release from prison—a high risk of death for former inmates. *New England Journal of Medicine*, *356*(2), 157–165.

Bruce, R. D., Kresina, T. F., & McCance-Katz, E. F. (2010). Medication-assisted treatment and HIV/AIDS: Aspects in treating HIV-infected drug users. *AIDS*, *24*(3), 331–340.

Cloutier, G. (2002). *Strategies to support treatment adherence in newly released HIV-positive prisoners*. Presented at 14th International AIDS Conference, Barcelona, Spain, International AIDS Society.

Conklin, T. J., Lincoln, T., & Flanigan, T. P. (1998). A public health model to connect correctional health care with communities. *American Journal of Public Health*, *88*(8), 1249–1250.

Cropsey, K. L., Lane, P. S., Hale, G. J. (2011). Results of a pilot randomized controlled trial of buprenorphine for opioid-dependent women in the criminal justice system. *Drug & Alcohol Dependence*, *119*(3), 172–178.

Draine, J., Ahuja, D., Altice, F. L., et al. (2011). Strategies to enhance linkages between care for HIV/AIDS in jail and community settings. *AIDS Care*, *23*(3), 366–377

Ford, N., Nachega, J. B., Engel, M. E., & Mills, E. J. (2009). Directly observed antiretroviral therapy: A systematic review and meta-analysis of randomised clinical trials. *Lancet*, *374*(9707), 2064–2071.

Freudenberg, N., Daniels, J., Crum, M., Perkins, T., & Richie, B. E. (2008). Coming home from jail: The social and health consequences of community reentry for women, male adolescents, and their families and communities. *American Journal of Public Health*, *98*(9 Suppl), S191–S202.

Garcia, C. A., Correa, G., Viver, A. D., et al. (2007). Buprenorphine-naloxone treatment for pre-release opioid-dependent inmates in Puerto Rico. *Journal of Addiction Medicine*, *1*(3), 126–132.

Gastfriend, D. R. (2011). Intramuscular extended-release naltrexone: Current evidence. *Annals of the New York Academy of Sciences*, *1216*, 144–166.

Hart, J. E., Jeon, C. Y., & Ivers, L. C. (2010). Effect of directly observed therapy for highly active antiretroviral therapy on virologic, immunologic, and adherence outcomes: a meta-analysis and systematic review. *Journal of Acquired Immune Deficiency Syndrome*, *54*(2), 167–179.

Holmes, L., Drainoni, M., & Rich, J. (2002). *Harm reduction focused case-management for multiply diagnosed HIV-positive ex-offenders*. Presented at 14th International AIDS Conferences, Barcelona, Spain, International AIDS Society.

Inciardi, J. A., Martin, S. S., & Butzin, C. A. (2004). Five-year outcomes of therapeutic community treatment of drug-involved offenders after release from prison. *Crime & Delinquency, 50*(88), 88–107.

Ing, E. C., Bae, J. W., Maru, D. S., & Altice, F. L. (2013). Medication persistence of HIV-infected drug users on directly administered antiretroviral therapy. *AIDS Behavior, 17*(1), 113–121.

James, D., & Karberg, J. (2005). *Substance dependence, abuse, and treatment of jail inmates.* Available online at http://bjs.ojp.usdoj.gov/index.cfm?ty=pbdetail&iid=1128.

James, D. J. (2004). *Bureau of Justice Statistics Special Report: profile of jail inmates, 2002.* Available online at: http://bjs.ojp.usdoj.gov/.

Kaplowitz, L., Kaatz, J., & Weir-Wiggins, C. (2002). *Seamless transition of HIV+ inmates into community care in Virginia.* Presented at 14th International AIDS Conference, Barcelona, Spain, International AIDS Society.

Kinlock, T. W., Gordon, M. S., Schwartz, R. P., & Fitzgerald, T. T. (2010). Developing and implementing a new prison-based buprenorphine treatment program. *Journal of Offender Rehabilitation, 49*(2), 91–109.

Kinlock, T. W., Gordon, M. S., Schwartz, R. P., Fitzgerald, T. T., & O'Grady, K. E. (2009). A randomized clinical trial of methadone maintenance for prisoners: results at 12 months postrelease. *Journal of Substance Abuse Treatment, 37*(3), 277–285.

Krishnan, A., Wickersham, J. A., & Chitsaz, E. (2012). Post-release substance abuse outcomes among HIV-infected jail detainees: Results from a multisite study. *AIDS Behavior, 17* (Suppl 2), S171–180. doi:10.1007/s10461-012-0362-3

Laufer, F., Arriola, K., & Dawson-Rose, C. (2002). From jail to community: Innovative strategies to enhance continuity of HIV/AIDS care. *Prison Journal, 82,* 84–100.

Leeman, J., Chang, Y. K., Lee, E. J., Voils, C. I., Crandell, J., & Sandelowski, M. (2010). Implementation of antiretroviral therapy adherence interventions: A realist synthesis of evidence. *Journal of Advanced Nursing, 66*(9), 1915–1930.

Levasseur, L., Marzo, J. N., Ross, N., & Blatier, C. (2002). Frequency of re-incarcerations in the same detention center: role of substitution therapy. A preliminary retrospective analysis. *Annales de Médecine Interne (Paris), 153*(3 Suppl), 1S14–19.

Lincoln, T., Kennedy, S., Tuthill, R., Roberts, C., Conklin, T. J., & Hammett, T. M. (2006). Facilitators and barriers to continuing healthcare after jail: A community-integrated program. *Journal of Ambulatory Care Management, 29*(1), 2–16.

Lobmaier, P., Kornor, H., Kunoe, N., & Bjorndal, A. (2008). Sustained-release naltrexone for opioid dependence. *Cochrane Database Systematic Review, 2,* CD006140.

Madras, B. K., Compton, W. M., Avula, D., Stegbauer, T., Stein, J. B., & Clark, H. W. (2009). Screening, brief interventions, referral to treatment (SBIRT) for illicit drug and alcohol use at multiple healthcare sites: comparison at intake and 6 months later. *Drug and Alcohol Dependence, 99*(1-3), 280–295.

Magura, S., Lee, J. D., & Hershberger, J. (2009). Buprenorphine and methadone maintenance in jail and post-release: A randomized clinical trial. *Drug and Alcohol Dependence, 99*(1-3), 222–230.

Meyer, J., Cepeda, J., Wu, J., Trestman, R., Altice, F., & Springer, S. (2014). Viral suppression at the prison gate: optimizing HIV treatment during incarceration. *JAMA Internal Medicine, 174*(5), 721–729. PMID: 24687044 PMCID: PMC4074594.

Meyer, J. P., Althoff, A. L., & Altice, F. L. (2013). Optimizing care for HIV-infected people who use drugs: Evidence-based approaches to overcoming healthcare disparities. *Clinical Infectious Diseases, 57*(9), 1309–1317.

Meyer, J. P., Chen, N. E., & Springer, S. A. (2011). HIV treatment in the criminal justice system: Critical knowledge and intervention gaps. *AIDS Research and Treatment, 2011,* Article ID 680617.

Mumola, C., & Karberg, J. (Revised 2007). *Drug use and dependence, state and federal Prisoners, 2004.* NCJ 213530

Nunn, A., Zaller, N., Dickman, S., Trimbur, C., Nijhawan, A., & Rich, J. D. (2009). Methadone and buprenorphine prescribing and referral practices in US prison systems: results from a nationwide survey. *Drug and Alcohol Dependence, 105*(1-2), 83–88.

Prendergast, M. L., & Cartier, J. J. (2013). Screening, brief intervention, and referral to treatment (SBIRT) for offenders: protocol for a pragmatic randomized trial. *Addiction Science and Clinical Practice, 8*(1), 16.

Rich, J. D., Boutwell, A. E., & Shield, D. C. (2005). Attitudes and practices regarding the use of methadone in US state and federal prisons. *Journal of Urban Health, 82*(3), 411–419.

Rich, J. D., Holmes, L., & Salas, C., (2001). Successful linkage of medical care and community services for HIV-positive offenders being released from prison. *Journal of Urban Health, 78*(2), 279–289.

Rich, J. D., McKenzie, M., Shield, D. C., et al. (2005). Linkage with methadone treatment upon release from incarceration: a promising opportunity. *Journal of Addictive Diseases, 24*(3), 49–59.

Richie, B. E., Freudenberg, N., & Page, J. (2001). Reintegrating women leaving jail into urban communities: a description of a model program. *Journal of Urban Health, 78*(2), 290–303.

Rosen, M. I., Dieckhaus, K., & McMahon, T. J. (2007). Improved adherence with contingency management. *AIDS Patient Care STDS, 21*(1), 30–40.

Saber-Tehrani, A. S., Bruce, R. D., & Altice, F. L. (2011). Pharmacokinetic drug interactions and adverse consequences between psychotropic medications and pharmacotherapy for the treatment of opioid dependence. *American Journal of Drug & Alcohol Abuse, 37*(1), 1–11.

Saberi, P., Caswell, N. H., Jamison, R., Estes, M., & Tulsky, J. P. (2012). Directly observed versus self-administered antiretroviral therapies: preference of HIV-positive jailed inmates in San Francisco. *Journal of Urban Health, 89*(5), 794–801.

Smith-Rohrberg, D., Bruce, R. D., & Altice, F. L. (2004). Review of corrections-based therapy for opiate-dependent patients: Implications for buprenorphine treatment among correctional populations. *Journal of Drug Issues, 34*(2), 451–480.

Sorensen, J. L., Haug, N. A., & Delucchi, K. L. (2007). Voucher reinforcement improves medication adherence in HIV-positive methadone patients: A randomized trial. *Drug Alcohol Depend, 88*(1), 54–63.

Springer, S., Chen, S., & Altice, F. (2010). Improved HIV and substance abuse treatment outcomes for released HIV-infected prisoners: the impact of buprenorphine treatment. *Journal of Urban Health, 87*(4), 592–602.

Springer, S., Qiu, J., Saber-Tehrani, A., & Altice, F. (2012). Retention on buprenorphine is associated with high levels of maximal viral suppression among HIV-infected opioid dependent released prisoners. *PLoS ONE, 7*(5), e38335.

Springer, S. A., Altice, F. L., Herme, M., & Di Paola, A. (2013). Design and methods of a double blind randomized placebo-controlled trial of extended-release naltrexone for alcohol dependent and hazardous drinking prisoners with HIV who are transitioning to the community. *Contemporary Clinical Trials, 37*(2), 209–218.

Springer, S. A., Azar, M. M., & Altice, F. L. (2011). HIV, alcohol dependence, and the criminal justice system: A review and call for evidence-based treatment for released prisoners. *American Journal of Drug and Alcohol Abuse, 37*(1), 12–21.

Springer, S. A., Spaulding, A. C., Meyer, J. P., & Altice, F. L. (2011). Public health implications for adequate transitional care for HIV-infected prisoners: five essential components. *Clinical Infectious Diseases, 53*(5), 469–479.

Stitzer, M., & Petry, N. (2006). Contingency management for treatment of substance abuse. *Annual Review of Clinical Psychology, 2,* 411–434.

SAMHSA (Substance Abuse and Mental Health Services Administration) (2012). *Results from the 2011 National Survey on Drug Use and Health: summary of national findings.* Series H-44, HHS Publication No. (SMA) 12-4713. Available online at: http://www.samhsa.gov/data/NSDUH/2k11Results/NSDUHresults2011.htm#Ch7.

Thompson, M. A., Mugavero, M. J., Amico, K. R., et al. (2012) Guidelines for improving entry into and retention in care and antiretroviral adherence for persons with HIV: evidence-based recommendations from an International Association of Physicians in AIDS Care panel. *Annals of Internal Medicine, 156*(11), 817–833.

van Olphen, J., Freudenberg, N., Fortin, P., & Galea, S. (2006). Community reentry: perceptions of people with substance use problems returning home from New York City jails. *Journal of Urban Health, 83*(3), 372–381.

Wickersham, J. A., Zahari, M. M., Azar, M. M., Kamarulzaman, A., & Altice, F. L. (2013). Methadone dose at the time of release from prison significantly influences retention in treatment: Implications from a pilot study of HIV-infected prisoners transitioning to the community in Malaysia. *Drug and Alcohol Dependence, 132*(1-2), 378–382.

Wilson, D., Law, M., Grulich, A., Cooper, D., & Kaldor, J. (2008). Relation between HIV viral load and infectiousness: A model-based analysis. *Lancet, 372*(9635), 314–320.

Wohl, D. A., Scheyett, A., & Golin, C. E. (2011). Intensive case management before and after prison release is no more effective than comprehensive pre-release discharge planning in linking HIV-infected prisoners to care: A randomized trial. *AIDS Behavior, 15*(2), 356–364.

Wohl, D. A., Stephenson, B. L., & Golin, C. E. (2003). Adherence to directly observed antiretroviral therapy among human immunodeficiency virus-infected prison inmates. *Clinical Infectious Diseases, 36*(12), 1572–1576.

Zaller, N. D., Holmes, L., & Dyl, A. C., (2008). Linkage to treatment and supportive services among HIV-positive ex-offenders in Project Bridge. *Journal of Health Care for the Poor and Underserved, 19*(2), 522–531.

Aggression, self-injury, and misconduct

CHAPTER 48

Aggression

Robert L. Trestman

Introduction

Managing aggression is a challenge for psychiatry in all settings. Recognizing opportunities for appropriate assessment and intervention in correctional settings is an important component of correctional psychiatry. Studies reflect significant risks of violence for both correctional officers and inmates. Although prison homicides occur at rates (4 per 100,000 inmates; Mumola, 2005) lower than estimated community homicide rates (6.1 per 100,000 persons; Xu, Kockanek, Murphy, & Tejada-Vera, 2010), the rate of nonlethal violence is substantial. The data for assault are less clear, as definitions of what constitutes assault vary. The Bureau of Justice Statistics estimates the rate of assault on correctional staff at 155 per 1,000 persons (Duhart, 2001). For context, the same methodology estimates the rate of assault on police officers (the highest-risk occupation) at 261 per 1,000 officers and community-based mental health clinicians at 68 per 1,000 clinicians. Inmate-on-inmate assault has been estimated to range from 2 per 1,000 inmates (Bryne & Hummer, 2007) to as high as 200 per 1,000 inmates (Wolff, Blitz, Shi, et al., 2007). However assault is defined, correctional officers who have been the target of offender violence have an elevated risk of emotional exhaustion and burnout (Boudoukha, Hautekeete, Abdellaoui, et al., 2011). This chapter reviews the factors that contribute to the broad range of assaultive behaviors observed in correctional settings and some of the pragmatic issues and opportunities for assessment, diagnosis, and treatment of aggressive behaviors, both impulsive and predatory.

Definitions

Aggression is an integral part of the human experience. Understanding the motivations and types of aggressive behavior underpins the ability to prevent, manage, or mitigate it. In broad terms, aggression is typically defined in terms of either predatory/instrumental or impulsive acts of violence. Predatory aggression most often consists of premeditated behavior with a specific goal. Such goals might include robbery, intimidation, or revenge. In contrast, impulsive aggression is usually reactive in nature, responsive to an immediate stress or provocation. This simple dichotomy between predatory and impulsive aggression reasonably categorizes about 79% of aggressive behavior in violent offenders (Tapscott, Hancock, & Hoaken, 2012).

Making such a categorization has important value. It helps in determining how to manage the sequelae of the violence. In practice, though, the overlap of behaviors and motivations often seems to blur these descriptive boundaries. Some characteristics to consider in making this determination include the proximity of the triggering event (was there a planned delay between the triggering event and the assault, or was it immediately before the assault?), the activities immediately prior to the assault (was it a calm, controlled attack, or was there agitation and yelling?), an assessment of the motivation behind the assault (was there a motive such as revenge or dominance, or was it a reaction with no secondary gain?), and the level of insight into the consequences of the assaultive behavior (was there an absence or superficial expression of remorse, or was there meaningful remorse/recognition of overreaction?; Scott, Quanbeck, & Resnick, 2008).

Within this dichotomy, subtypes exist. For example, aggression that stems from intoxication or during detoxification is usually considered impulsive. Aggression due to psychotic paranoia or in response to command auditory hallucinations would be considered planned or instrumental, but logically would be managed very differently from predatory aggression intended to exact revenge.

Assessment

Many approaches have been devised to measure the nature of aggressive behaviors and their types, severity, frequency, and future risks. These include self-report questionnaires and structured interviews that fall into descriptive and predictive groupings. Relevant descriptive instruments include measures of impulsivity, aggression, and personality. One broadly used and well-validated assessment instrument for impulsivity is the Barratt Impulsiveness Scale (BIS 11; Barratt, 2000), which includes subscales for attention, lack of planning, and motor impulsivity. Measures of aggression per se typically target either lifetime history of aggression or current levels of aggression. Lifetime measures are useful for baseline assessment but less sensitive to change (e.g., the Life History of Aggression; Coccaro, Berman, & Kavoussi, 1997). Such instruments may be useful for making initial therapeutic recommendations. Other instruments that are sensitive to change over time include the well-researched Buss–Perry Aggression Questionnaire (BPAQ; Buss & Perry, 1992), with subscales measuring physical aggression, verbal aggression, hostility, and anger. The BPAQ is well suited to measuring the effectiveness of clinical treatment over time, with repeated measurements before, during, and after the intervention.

Instruments widely used to predict relative risks of future aggression include actuarial assessments such as the Level of Service Inventory-R (LSI-R) and the Psychopathy Check List-R (PCL-R; Andrews & Bonta, 1995; Hare, 2003) and structured clinical interviews such as the Historical Clinical Risk Management-20V3

(HCR-20) (Douglas, Hart, Webster, et al., 2013; Webster, Douglas, Eaves, & Hart, 1997). Metaanalysis suggests that the positive predictive validity of almost all instruments (including the LSI-R, PCL-R, and HCR-20) is strongest for low-risk individuals and at best moderate for high-risk offenders (Fazel, Singh, Doll, & Grann, 2012; Singh, Grann, & Fazel, 2011). The rapid expansion of this area of study includes initiatives to define standards for risk assessment tools, allowing for a more meaningful evaluation of the validity and reliability of legacy and proposed instruments and interviews (Singh, Yang, Bjorkly, et al., 2013).

Demographic risk factors for violence in correctional settings

Several demographic variables have been associated with a risk of violent behavior in correctional settings. By far the strongest predictor of violence is age; younger offenders are more likely to demonstrate aggression. Compared to inmates 31 to 35 years old, the likelihood of violent behavior is 3.5 times greater for those younger than 21 and 63% greater for those 21 to 25 years old (Cunningham & Sorensen, 2007). Level of education also predicts aggression during incarceration, with less education associated with greater risk (Berg & DeLisi, 2006). Gang membership also increases the risk of violence (Gaes, Wallace, Gilman, et al., 2002). Based on demographic factors alone, the individuals at highest risk of violent behavior are younger than 21, without high school diplomas or equivalents, and gang members. While minority status has been associated with an increased risk of violent behavior in jail or prison, the relationship is complex (Schenk & Fremouw, 2012).

Differential diagnosis

Not every act of aggression is due to a diagnosable mental illness. The likelihood of a contributing diagnosis increases with the frequency of aggressive behavior and with the consistency of the nature of the aggression.

The largest group of potential diagnoses includes disorders that have poor impulse control as one of their defining features. These disorders include borderline personality disorder, antisocial personality disorder, and intermittent explosive disorder (IED). While they share impulsivity as a characteristic, the manner of presentation varies dramatically among them. In general, the aggressive behaviors found in borderline personality disorder tend to be emotionally reactive to perceived threats (see Chapter 36). Such threats may derive from misperceived behavior or motivation of those near them. Individuals with antisocial personality disorder, by definition, have a pattern of behavior that violates social norms and usually includes premeditated, impulsive, or mixed violence. The aggressive behaviors tend to serve an instrumental purpose of furthering the person's goals (monetary, status, or otherwise). Individuals with IED, again by definition, overreact to a situation with explosive violence. While they typically have remorse subsequent to the event, that remorse does not prevent recurrence of overreactive aggression.

Schizophrenia has been associated with aggressive behavior, but the specifics have only recently been more clearly defined. The conditions under which individuals with schizophrenia are more likely to become aggressive include periods of no treatment, persecutory delusions, or active comorbid substance abuse (Fazel, Långström, Hjern, et al., 2009; Hodgins, 2008; Keers, Ullrich, DeStavola, & Coid, 2013).

Traumatic brain injury, a broad category associated with a host of potential injuries (Vaishnavi, Rao, & Fann, 2009; Warden, Gordon, McAllister, et al., 2006), can cause impulsive aggression if the damage includes areas of the prefrontal cortex. Related impairments in executive function can result in disinhibition and serious violence (Fazel, Lichtenstein, Grann, & Långström, 2011).

Traumatic life experiences may also play a role in aggression. One study of adult male offenders found a strong relationship between self-reported childhood trauma and scores on a lifetime aggression questionnaire (Sarchiapone, Carli, Cuomo, et al., 2009). A separate study of offenders found a similar relationship between childhood trauma and aggression (Swogger, You, Cashman-Brown, & Conner, 2011). That study also found a history of suicide attempts accompanying elevated lifetime aggression in offenders with a history of significant childhood trauma. The authors suggested a potential benefit of suicide risk reduction in this population by targeting aggression for treatment (Swogger et al., 2011).

Neurobiology

There has been a real interest in looking for neuropathological causes for serious aggression for decades. Recent work, much of it specifically with violent offenders, has focused on functional and structural neuropathology in neuroimaging studies, neurotransmitter and neuroendocrine research, and the potential contribution of epigenetics (Blair, 2008; Keune, van der Heiden, Varkuti, et al., 2012; Schiltz, Witzel, Bausch-Holterhoff, & Bogerts, 2013; Siever, 2008; Tremblay, 2008). The collective findings suggest abnormalities but do not identify direct causative neuropathological lesions leading to violent behavior.

Differential therapeutics

Depending on the environment, resources, and diagnosis, differential therapeutics and management of the patient follow the assessment. In correctional settings milieu management, psychotherapy, behavior management plans (covered in Chapter 50), and psychopharmacology each has a role to play.

Milieu management

Milieu management is not that different than what would occur on an inpatient psychiatric unit, with overall and individualized considerations made for the environment, potential stressors, and provocations related to aggression. Evidence suggests that effective milieu design and management are the most important factors in preventing aggression in correctional settings (Cooke, Wozniak, & Johnstone, 2008). This is particularly an issue in units or environments with higher-than-expected overall levels of aggression. Such considerations include proper environment management (e.g., regular and random custody searches to eliminate weapons), appropriate grievance resolution protocols, humane conditions of confinement, and respectful treatment (Welsh, Bader, & Evans, 2013). Perceptions of disrespectful treatment have a direct correlation with increased risk of violent thoughts (Butler & Maruna, 2009). After addressing unnecessary provocations and distressing situations, levels of aggressive behavior drop significantly (Cooke et al., 2008). Relevant concerns include staffing ratio, management of interpersonal grievances, fairness of the assignment of opportunities, and access to privileges, among other factors (Wortley, 2002). Treating the inmate population with dignity and respect and providing a safe environment substantially reduces the amount of violence on any correctional unit (Wortley, 2002). Of note, milieu management is an excellent approach for reducing both premeditated and impulsive aggression, while simultaneously improving staff morale (Cooke et al., 2008). A structured approach to reviewing the correctional milieu for violence risk factors has been developed and tested with positive results (Cooke et al., 2008; Johnstone & Cooke, 2010). Another substantial concern in correctional settings, particularly prisons, is gang aggression. Chapter 58 reviews this specialized and challenging topic.

Psychotherapy

Psychotherapies have been developed or adapted for use in offender rehabilitation. While targeted psychotherapies in correctional settings have a limited evidence base, a range of cognitive-behavioral therapies (CBT) have application to the reduction of violence and aggressive behavior. In a recent review of the literature, several randomized clinical trials and quasi-experimental studies supported the efficacy of CBT interventions in reducing violent behavior and reincarceration for violent offences (Ross et al., 2013). Although only a modest number of studies met review criteria, none looked at comparative effectiveness, and most took place in Europe or New Zealand, they found small (10% to 20%) but clinically and statistically significant reductions in violent behavior and reincarceration. When the outcome measure is reduction in recidivism rather than violence per se, an extensive review of available interventions demonstrates clear support for CBT programs and argues against the effectiveness of sanctions and deterrence-based programs (Duggan, 2008). One of the best-studied CBT programs, used both in institutional and community correctional settings, is Reasoning and Rehabilitation (R&R; Ross, Quayle, Newman, & Tansey, 1988). In a review of 16 experimental and quasi-experimental studies in Canada, the United States, and Great Britain, the results supported the use of R&R to reduce recidivism in both high- and low-risk offender populations (Tong & Farrington, 2006).

The commonalities among the interventions with positive findings include manual-based design with fidelity monitoring; skills-based training that includes emotion management, interpersonal relatedness, and impulse control; adequate duration to allow for skill acquisition through practice; and a reasonably supportive, reinforcing environment. Other CBT skills-based programs designed to meet these needs in correctional settings have been developed and are being evaluated (e.g., START NOW; Shelton & Wakai, 2011). As a clear caveat for all such structured interventions, manual-guided treatment provides critical consistency in treatment programming; however, success requires therapeutic alliance and motivational engagement (Day, Kozar, & Davey, 2013). In parallel to CBT-based research findings, studies with mindfulness-based treatment paradigms have demonstrated positive but similarly modest benefits (Fix & Fix, 2013).

Psychopharmacology

In the 1980s, there was an attempt to develop a class of medications called serenics, medications targeted specifically at the reduction of aggressive behavior. While no new medication resulted from that attempt (Umukoru, Aladeokin, & Eduviere, 2013), a range of potential medications warrant consideration. Based on the assessment and differential diagnosis, these medications include selective serotonin reuptake inhibitors (SSRIs), lithium, anticonvulsants, antipsychotics, and beta blockers.

Several studies have shown SSRIs to reduce impulsive aggression in patients with personality disorders (Goodman & New, 2000) and in those with traumatic brain injury (Warden et al., 2006). Fluoxetine has been the most studied agent in those with personality disorders, including double-blind randomized controlled studies, with effective doses ranging from 40 to 60 mg daily (Goodman & New, 2000). Open-label studies using other SSRIs have generally found similar results.

Lithium has a very interesting history in the treatment of aggression, with clinical trials dating back as far as the 1970s. In two populations of aggressive prisoners, lithium was shown to reduce violent aggression (as measured by disciplinary infractions) over 3 months (Sheard, Marini, Bridges, & Wagner, 1976) and 18 months (Tupin, Smith, Clanon, et al., 1973). A recent review of the literature found substantial consistency supporting lithium's effectiveness in the treatment of aggression in multiple settings (Müller-Oerlinghausen & Lewitzka, 2010). Arguably, one reason that lithium has not been used more extensively is the need for therapeutic monitoring to avoid toxicity, particularly for renal function. However, with patients who allow appropriate monitoring, a therapeutic trial of lithium is an excellent consideration.

Anticonvulsants have also been used in the treatment of aggression for several decades. For offenders with impulsive aggression secondary to traumatic brain injury, valproate preparations have shown effectiveness in multiple case studies (Geracioti, 1994; Warden et al., 2006). One large, multisite, randomized clinical trial of divalproex studied patients with a history of impulsive aggression (46% with prior incarcerations) and *Diagnostic and Statistical Manual of Mental Disorders*–IV Cluster B personality disorders, IED, or posttraumatic stress disorder (PTSD; Hollander, Tracey, Swann, et al., 2003). The patients with Cluster B personality disorder, not those with PTSD or IED, experienced substantial clinical and statistical improvement in impulsive aggression, irritability, and overall illness severity in a 12-week study. More limited data also exist supporting the use of carbamazepine (Warden et al., 2006), lamotrigine (Leiberich, Nickel, Tritt, & Gil, 2008), and oxcarbazepine (Bellino, Paradiso, & Bogetto, 2005). These studies used doses generally consistent with established therapeutic use in seizure or bipolar disorders.

Antipsychotics are commonly used in the management of acute aggression and agitation. Randomized clinical trials show inconsistent evidence that antipsychotic medications reduce violence in an unselected population (Volavka & Citrome, 2008). Even within the schizophrenic spectrum of disorders, heterogeneity of etiology may differentiate appropriateness of treatment with an antipsychotic, with some evidence supporting both positive psychotic symptom-driven aggression (e.g., persecutory delusions) and aggression secondary to cognition-impaired disinhibition

(Volavka & Citrome, 2008). Among the antipsychotics, clozapine may be more effective at treating aggression in schizophrenia (and perhaps other psychiatric disorders) than other antipsychotics (Frogley, Taylor, Dickens, & Picchioni, 2012; Krakowski, Czobor, & Nolan, 2008). With the exception of clozapine, most other antipsychotics (whether first or second generation) appear similar and more modestly effective in the treatment of aggression. This is likely due to a general effect of treatment through better control of the psychotic disorder or associated persecutory delusions (Keers et al., 2013), although that view is not universally held (Frogley et al., 2012).

Beta blockers, most commonly propranolol, have demonstrated significant benefit in treating impulsive aggression in both case studies and randomized clinical trials (Scott et al., 2008). In doses ranging from 40 to 520 mg/day, positive results have been obtained in patients experiencing impulsive aggression secondary to traumatic brain injuries (Warden et al., 2006), psychotic disorders, and personality disorders (Scott et al., 2008; Silver, Yudosky, Slater, et al., 1999). In one randomized study, two case examples are illustrative. Despite multiple previous clinical trials on other medications, these two individuals were chronically aggressive in a forensic psychiatry unit, with 7 and 21 aggressive episodes during the baseline assessment week, respectively. Following a month on propranolol, the frequency of aggressive outbursts dropped to an average of 1.5 and 1.75 per week, respectively (Silver et al., 1999).

Management of aggression

After assessment, differential diagnosis, and selection of therapeutic interventions, the real work may begin. Communicating the proposed interventions to all stakeholders, building support where needed (e.g., where milieu changes involve correctional staff), and gaining engagement of the patient are all required elements in this next phase. Sometimes it may be as simple as recommending participation in a therapy group or taking a new medication; often, it may require more extensive consensus building with a seriously challenging patient. Developing a methodology to measure improvement in targeted behaviors has equal importance to proposing interventions and engaging stakeholders. The time frame for measurement may range from weeks to months before significant improvement is seen in chronic disruptive or violent behavior. That time frame should be shared with the treatment team and the patient in order to avert expectations of unrealistically rapid responses and avoid disappointment.

Summary

Aggressive behavior is a common and challenging problem in correctional settings. To effectively address aggression, a thoughtful and comprehensive approach that may incorporate elements of environmental management, evaluation of potential motivating factors, differential diagnosis, and a coordinated intervention is needed. This always involves effective communication among stakeholders, including the patient. Recommended milieu changes and psychotherapeutic and/or pharmacological interventions need to be explicit. Consistent oversight and follow-up to measure the effects of each component of the intervention(s) are critical, as aggressive behavior may be both habitual and episodic.

References

Andrews, D. A., & Bonta, J. (1995). *LSI-R: The Level of Service Inventory-Revised*. Toronto, Canada: Multi-Health Systems

Barratt, E. S. (2000). Barratt Impulsiveness Scale, Version 11 (BIS 11). In American Psychiatric Association, *Handbook of psychiatric measures* (pp. 691–693). Washington, DC: American Psychiatric Association.

Berg, M. T., & DeLisi, M. (2006). The correctional melting pot: Race, ethnicity, citizenship, and prison violence. *Journal of Criminal Justice, 34*, 631–642.

Bellino, S., Paradiso, E., & Bogetto, F. (2005). Oxcarbazepine in the treatment of BPD: a pilot study. *Journal of Clinical Psychiatry, 66*, 1111–1115.

Blair, R. J. R. (2008). The amygdala and ventromedial prefrontal cortex: Functional contributions and dysfunction in psychopathy. *Philosophical Transactions of the Royal Society B, 363*, 2557–2565. doi:10.1098/rstb.2008.0027

Boudoukha, A. H., Hautekeete, M., Abdellaoui, S., Groux, W., & Garay, D. (2011). Burnout and victimisation: impact of inmates' aggression towards prison guards. *Encephale, 37*(4), 284–292. doi:10.1016/j.encep.2010.08.006

Bryne, J. M., & Hummer, D. (2007). Myths and realities of prison violence: A review of the evidence. *Victims and Offenders, 2*(1), 77–90.

Buss, A. H., & Perry, M. (1992). The Aggression Questionnaire. *Journal of Personality and Social Psychology, 63*, 452–459.

Butler, M., & Maruna, S. (2009). The impact of disrespect on prisoners' aggression: Outcomes of experimentally inducing violence-supportive cognitions. *Psychology, Crime & Law, 15*(2&3), 235–250.

Coccaro, E., Berman, M. E., & Kavoussi, R. J. (1997). Assessment of life history of aggression: development and psychometric characteristics. *Psychiatry Research, 73*(3), 147–157. doi:10.1016/S0165-1781(97)00119-4

Cooke, D., Wozniak, E., & Johnstone, L. (2008). Casting light on prison violence in Scotland: Evaluating the impact of situational risk factors. *Criminal Justice and Behavior, 35*, 1065–1078. doi:10.1177/0093854808318867

Cunningham, M. D., & Sorensen, J. R. (2007). Predictive factors for violent misconduct in close custody. *The Prison Journal, 87*(2), 241–253.

Day, A., Kozar, C., & Davey, L. (2013). Treatment approaches and offender behavior programs: Some critical issues. *Aggression and Violent Behavior, 18*, 630–635.

Douglas, K. S., Hart, S. D., Webster, C. D., Belfrage, H., & Eaves, D. (2013). *HCR: V3 Historical. Clinical, Risk, Management (Version 3): Assessing risk for violence*. Burnaby: Mental Health, Law, and Policy Institute, Simon Fraser University.

Duggan, C. (2008). Why are programmes for offenders with personality disorder not informed by the relevant scientific findings? *Philosophical Transactions of the Royal Society B, 363*, 2599–2612. doi:10.1098/rstb.2008.0025

Duhart, D. T. (2001). *Violence in the workplace, 1993–99*. Bureau of Justice Statistics, NCJ190076. Available at: http://bjs.ojp.usdoj.gov/content/pub/pdf/vw99.pdf

Fazel, S., Långström, N., Hjern, A., Grann, M., & Lichtenstein, P. (2009). Schizophrenia, substance abuse, and violent crime. *Journal of the American Medical Association, 301*(19), 2016–2023. doi:10.1001/jama.2009.675

Fazel, S., Lichtenstein, P., Grann, M., & Langstrom, N. (2011). Risk of violent crime in individuals with epilepsy and traumatic brain injury: A 35-Year Swedish population study. *PLoS Med 8*: e1001150. doi:10.1371/journal.pmed.1001150.

Fazel, S., Singh, J. P., Doll, H., & Grann, M. (2012). Use of risk assessment instruments to predict violence and antisocial behaviour in 73 samples involving 24,827 people: systematic review and meta-analysis. *British Medical Journal, 345*, e4692 doi:10.1136/bmj.e4692

Fix, R. L., & Fix, S. T. (2013). The effects of mindfulness-based treatments for aggression: A critical review. *Aggression and Violent Behavior, 18*(2), 219–227.

Frogley, C., Taylor, D., Dickens, G., & Picchioni, M. (2012). A systematic review of the evidence of clozapine's anti-aggressive effects. *International Journal of Neuropsychopharmacology, 15*(9), 1351–1371. doi:10.1017/S146114571100201X

Gaes, G. G., Wallace, S., Gilman, E., Klein-Saffran, J., & Suppa, S. (2002). The influence of prison gang affiliation on violence and other prison misconduct. *The Prison Journal, 82*(3), 359–385.

Geracioti, T. D. (1994).Valproic acid treatment of episodic explosiveness related to brain injury. *Journal of Clinical Psychiatry, 55*(9), 416–417.

Goodman, M., & New, A. (2000). Impulsive aggression in borderline personality disorder. *Current Psychiatry Reports, 2*, 56–61.

Hare, R. D. (2003). *Manual for the Revised Psychopathy Checklist* (2nd ed.). Toronto, Canada: Multi-Health Systems.

Hodgins, S. (2008). Violent behavior among people with schizophrenia: a framework for investigations of causes, and effective treatment, and prevention. *Philosophical Transactions of the Royal Society B, 363*, 2505–2518. doi:10.1098/rstb.2008.0034

Hollander, E., Tracey, K. A., Swann, A. C., et al. (2003). Divalproex in the treatment of impulsive aggression: efficacy in Cluster B personality disorders. *Neuropsychopharmacology, 28*, 1186–1197.

Johnstone, L., & Cooke, D. (2010). PRISM: A promising paradigm for assessing and managing institutional violence: Findings from a multiple case study analysis of five Scottish prisons. *International Journal of Forensic Mental Health, 9*, 185–191. doi:10.1080/14999013.2010.526477

Keers, R., Ullrich, S., DeStavola, B., & Coid, J. W. (2013). Association of violence with emergence of persecutory delusions in untreated schizophrenia. *American Journal of Psychiatry in Advance*, AiA, 1–8. doi:10.1176/appi.ajp.2013.13010134

Keune, P. M., van der Heiden, L., Varkuti, B., Konicar, L., Veit, R., & Birbaumer, N. (2012). Prefrontal brain asymmetry and aggression in imprisoned violent offenders. *Neuroscience Letters, 515*, 191–195. doi:10.1016/j.neulet.2012.03.058

Krakowski, M. I., Czobor, P., & Nolan, K. (2008). Atypical antipsychotics, neurocognitive deficits, and aggression in schizophrenic patients. *Journal of Clinical Psychopharmacology, 28*, 485–493.

Leiberich, P., Nickel, M. K., Tritt, K., & Gil, F. P. (2008). Lamotrigine treatment of aggression in female borderline patients, Part II: an 18-month follow-up. *Journal of Psychopharmacology, 22*, 805–808. doi:10.1177/0269881107084004

Müller-Oerlinghausen, B., & Lewitzka, U. (2010). Lithium reduces pathological aggression and suicidality: A mini-review. *Neuropsychobiology, 62*, 43–49. doi:10.1159/000314309

Mumola, C. J. (2005). *Suicide and homicide in state prisons and local jails.* Bureau of Justice Statistics, NCJ 210036.

Ross, R. R., Fabiano, E. A., & Ewles, C. D. (1988). Reasoning and rehabilitation. *International Journal of Offender Therapy and Comparative Criminology, 32*, 29–35.

Ross, J., Quayle, E., Newman, E., & Tansey, L. (2013). The impact of psychological therapies on violent behaviour in clinical and forensic settings: A systematic review. *Aggression and Violent Behavior, 18*(6), 761–773.

Sarchiapone, M., Carli, V., Cuomo, C., Marchetti, M., & Roy, A. (2009). Association between childhood trauma and aggression in male prisoners. *Psychiatry Research, 165*, 187–192. doi:10.1016/j.psychres.2008.04.026

Schenk, A. M., & Fremouw, W. J. (2012). Individual characteristics related to prison violence: A critical review of the literature. *Aggression and Violent Behavior, 17*, 430–442. doi:10.1016/j.avb.2012.05.005

Schiltz, K., Witzel, J. G., Bausch-Holterhoff, J., & Bogerts, B. (2013). High prevalence of brain pathology in violent prisoners: a qualitative CT and MRI scan study. *European Archives of Psychiatry and Clinical Neuroscience, 263*, 607–616. doi:10.1007/s00406-013-0403-6

Scott, C. L., Quanbeck, C. D., & Resnick, P. J. (2008). Assessment of dangerousness. In R. E. Hales, S. C. Yudofsky, & G. Gabbard (Eds.), *The American Psychiatric Publishing textbook of psychiatry* (pp. 1655–1672). Arlington VA: American Psychiatric Publishing.

Sheard, M. H., Marini, J. L., Bridges, C. I., & Wagner, E. (1976). The effect of lithium on impulsive aggressive behavior in man. *American Journal of Psychiatry, 133*(12), 1409–1413.

Shelton, D., & Wakai, S. (2011). A process evaluation of START NOW skills training for inmates with impulsive and aggressive behaviors. *Journal of the American Psychiatric Nurses Association, 17*(2), 148–157. doi:10.1177/1078390311401023

Siever, L. J. (2008). Neurobiology of aggression and violence. *American Journal of Psychiatry, 165*, 429–442. doi:10.1176/appi.ajp.2008.07111774

Silver, J. M., Yudovsky, S. C., Slater, J. A., et al. (1999). Propranolol treatment of chronically hospitalized aggressive patients. *Journal of Neuropsychiatry and Clinical Neurosciences, 11*, 328–335.

Singh, J. P., Grann, M., & Fazel, S. (2011). A comparative study of violence risk assessment tools: A systematic review and metaregression analysis of 68 studies involving 25,980 participants. *Clinical Psychology Review, 31*(3), 499–513.

Singh, J. P., Yang, S., Bjorkly, S., et al. (2013). *Reporting standards for risk assessment predictive validity studies: The Risk Assessment Guidelines for the Evaluation of Efficacy (RAGEE) Statement.* Tampa, FL: University of South Florida.

Swogger, M. T., You, S., Cashman-Brown, S., & Conner, K. R. (2011). Childhood physical abuse, aggression, and suicide attempts among criminal offenders. *Psychiatry Research, 185*, 363–367. doi:10.1016/j.psychres.2010.07.036

Tapscott, J., Hancock, M., & Hoaken, P. (2012). Severity and frequency of reactive and instrumental violent offending: Divergent validity of subtypes of violence in an adult forensic sample. *Criminal Justice and Behavior, 39*, 202–219.

Tong, L. S. J., & Farrington, D. P. (2006). How effective is the "Reasoning and Rehabilitation" programme in reducing reoffending? A meta-analysis of evaluations in four countries. *Psychology, Crime & Law, 12*(1), 3–24, doi:0.1080/10683160512331316253

Tremblay, R. E. (2008). Understanding development and prevention of chronic physical aggression: towards experimental epigenetic studies. *Philosophical Transactions of the Royal Society B, 363*, 2613–2622. doi:10.1098/rstb.2008.0030

Tupin, J. P., Smith, D. B., Clanon, T. L., et al. (1973). The long-term use of lithium in aggressive prisoners. *Comprehensive Psychiatry, 14*(4), 311–317.

Umukoro, S., Aladeokin, A., & Eduviere, A. T. (2013). Aggressive behavior: A comprehensive review of its neurochemical mechanisms and management. *Aggression and Violent Behavior, 18*(2), 195–203.

Vaishnavi, S., Rao, V., & Fann, J. R. (2009). Neuropsychiatric problems after traumatic brain injury: Unraveling the silent epidemic. *Psychosomatics, 50*(3), 198–205.

Volavka, J., & Citrome, L. (2008). Heterogeneity of violence in schizophrenia and implications for long-term treatment. *International Journal of Clinical Practice, 62*(8), 1237–1245. doi:10.1111/j.1742-1241.2008.01797

Warden, D. L., Gordon, B., McAllister, T. W., et al. (2006). Guidelines for the pharmacologic treatment of neurobehavioral sequelae of traumatic brain injury. *Journal of Neurotrauma, 23*(10), 1468–1501.

Webster, C. D., Douglas, K. S., Eaves, D., & Hart, S. D. (1997). *HCR-20: Assessing Risk for Violence (version 2).* Simon Fraser University, Mental Health, Law and Policy Institute.

Welsh, E., Bader, S., & Evans, S. E. (2013). Situational variables related to aggression in institutional settings. *Aggression and Violent Behavior, 18,* 792–796.

Wolff, N., Blitz, C. L., Shi, J., Siegel, J., & Bachman, R., (2007). Physical violence inside prisons: Rates of victimization. *Criminal Justice and Behavior, 34*(5), 588–599.

Wortley, R. (2002). *Situational prison control: Crime prevention in correctional institutions.* Cambridge, United Kingdom: Cambridge University Press.

Xu, J., Kockanek, K. D., Murphy, S. L., & Tejada-Vera, B. (2010). *Deaths: final data for 2007.* Hyattsville, MD: US Department of Health and Human Services, CDC, National Center for Health Statistics. National Vital Statistics Report, 58, (19). Available at: http://www.cdc.gov/NCHS/data/nvsr/nvsr58/nvsr58_19.pdf

CHAPTER 49

Self-injurious behaviors

Kenneth L. Appelbaum

Introduction

Self-injurious behaviors (SIB) in correctional facilities have similarities and differences with the phenomena in community settings. Along with some common precipitants, associated diagnoses, and helpful interventions, the behavior in jails and prisons has unique aspects compared to other environments. This chapter provides an overview of SIB, with special focus on correctional considerations and challenges.

Definition

Diverse terminology and definitions have been used to describe SIB. In addition to "self-injury," commonly used terms have included "nonsuicidal self-injury," "self-harm," "self-mutilation," and "parasuicide." The terms "self-injury" and "SIB" in this chapter refer to acts intended to cause bodily harm but not death. These acts typically involve cutting, burning, self-hitting, self-biting, hair pulling, head banging, and ingesting or inserting foreign objects. The definition does not include damaging or risky behaviors that do not have the primary intent of causing harm, such as tattooing, body piercing, substance abuse, autoerotic acts, or implantation of foreign bodies under the skin of the penis (Yap, Butler, Richters, et al., 2013) in an attempt to enhance sexual performance.

Although the distinction between SIB and suicidal behaviors has important conceptual and management implications, the boundary between them does not always have a bright line. Determinations of intent rely primarily on self-reports, which have limited reliability. Some individuals have ambivalence about the possibility of dying, along with occasional deliberately misleading self-reports. Even a true absence of suicidal intent does not eliminate potential lethality.

Reasons for self-injurious behaviors

In the broadest terms, SIB may be viewed as a response either to an internal state or external circumstances. The behavior provides relief from unpleasant emotions or cognitions in the former and from adverse environments or interpersonal interactions in the later. Regulation of negative affect such as anxiety and anger typically serves as the most prevalent function of SIB (Klonsky, 2007). Although interpersonal factors usually play less of a role, they likely have greater significance in correctional settings for reasons described later. Identifying behavioral precipitants helps clarify assessment and aids in management.

Epidemiology

In community samples, about 4% of adults report a history of SIB, with no significant gender differences in rate (Briere & Gil, 1998; Klonsky, Oltmanns, & Turkheimer, 2003). Despite its serious consequences in jails and prisons, reliable data on self-injury in those settings remain sparse. A survey of the 51 state and federal directors of correctional mental health services in the United States found that less than 2% of inmates per year self-injure (Appelbaum, Savageau, Trestman, et al., 2011). Although relatively few inmates engage in this behavior, they do so often enough that almost all systems that responded to the survey reported at least weekly incidents, and more than 70% of systems had episodes occurring several times per week to more than once per day. The survey also found, however, that almost half of the prison systems maintain no data related to SIB and the remainder track only limited information. A quarter of the responding systems do not attempt to distinguish between SIB and suicide attempts when self-injury occurs. Based on diagnostic impressions provided by the mental health system directors, more than half of self-injuring inmates have Cluster B personality disorders, followed by approximately 15% with mood disorders, 12% with mixed personality disorders, 8% with psychotic disorders, and 3% with cognitive and developmental disorders. A separate national survey in the United States found an average prevalence of 2.4% for inmate self-injury and 0.7% prevalence for serious SIB events (Smith & Kaminski, 2011). Many of the facilities that responded to this survey used their standard suicide treatment protocols for all self-injuries, without an attempt to provide interventions more specific to SIB. Another study of SIB in a single state prison system also found that although very few inmates engage in the behavior, some of them do so frequently. They are more likely to be young, white, and recently incarcerated, and they disproportionately consume resources and risk fatal injuries (Smith & Kaminski, 2010). Similar findings have been reported among inmates in England and Wales, including an association between self-harm and subsequent suicide (Hawton, Linsell, Adeniji, et al., 2013).

Assessment

SIB can occur in the context of several diagnoses or in the absence of an underlying psychiatric disorder. The *Diagnostic and Statistical Manual of Mental Disorders*, 5th edition (American Psychiatric Association, 2013) does not recognize SIB as its own diagnostic category but does include "nonsuicidal self-injury" as a condition for further study and research. The same diagnostic considerations apply to inmates as to people in community settings; however, aspects of jail and prison environments often play a disproportionate role as triggers for these behaviors.

The most common psychiatric conditions associated with SIB include psychotic, personality, cognitive, and mood disorders. Other chapters in this book address the general presentation, assessment, and management of these disorders in correctional settings. Self-injury that occurs in the context of these disorders, however, often has distinguishing characteristics.

Extreme acts of self-injury that result in significant tissue damage or permanent loss of functioning of a body organ occur most commonly in association with psychosis (Large, Babidge, Andrews, et al., 2009). These acts include damage to or enucleation of the eye, amputation of a digit or limb, and genital mutilation unrelated to gender dysphoria. The psychiatrist should respond to such behaviors as psychiatric emergencies due to a psychotic disorder until proven otherwise.

Borderline personality disorder is the diagnosis most commonly associated with self-injury. The behavior often serves to relieve dysphoria or anger; for some individuals, pain or the sight of blood counteracts dissociative states.

Self-injury among individuals with "intellectual disability (intellectual developmental disorder)," the terminology that has replaced mental retardation, typically presents as scratching, head banging and hitting, and hand biting (Furniss & Biswas, 2012). Other developmental conditions that may present with repeated, stereotypic self-injurious behaviors include Cornelia de Lange, fragile X, and Prader–Willi syndromes.

Examples of self-injury associated with other diagnoses include hair pulling in trichotillomania, skin picking in excoriation disorder, and acts that foster a sick role or hospital admission in factitious disorder. Obsessive–compulsive disorder can also involve behaviors that result in harm, such as excessive hand washing. Among affective disorders, depression has a greater association with deliberate self-harm, primarily poisoning, than does bipolar disorder (Haw, Houston, Townsend, et al., 2002).

Inmates, however, often have motives for self-harm that have little to do with symptoms of a primary psychiatric disorder. Thus, the psychiatric assessment must focus on more than just diagnosis. Without an understanding of other factors driving behavior, the medical, mental health, and custody staff cannot formulate effective interventions or management plans. Adequate assessment requires sensitive but frank and direct history-taking. Available evidence does not suggest that suicide attempts or self-injury increase in response to questioning about those behaviors (Gould, Marrocco, Kleinman, et al., 2005; Reynolds, Lindenboim, Comtois, et al., 2006).

Several self-report scales and structured interviews exist for assessment of self-injury but mostly as research tools, and none has been developed for use with incarcerated adults (Muehlenkamp, 2012). Whether through questionnaires or structured or unstructured interviews, the correctional psychiatrist needs to understand the history of the behavior and the purpose that it serves. Basic elements of history include age of onset, frequency, methods used, location of events, social context, severity, and outcomes.

Precipitants for self-harm in correctional settings

Environmental factors, which include behavioral triggers and responses, often play a key role in SIB, especially in jails and prisons. Self-injury can return a degree of control and autonomy to inmates who otherwise have limited means to affect their environment, cope with stress, or get what they want. Triggers, or antecedents, include interpersonal conflict, social isolation, relationship problems, and unmet needs. Environmental responses that reinforce the behaviors can include attention, change in housing, diversion (e.g., trip to infirmary or hospital), access to medications (e.g., analgesics), and staff annoyance.

The highest rate of SIB occurs in segregation and other lockdown units—settings that impose substantial deprivations (Appelbaum et al., 2011; Jones, 1986). As a group, inmates placed in segregation may have a predisposition toward these behaviors, including an increased prevalence of serious psychiatric disorders compared to inmates in general population units (Lovell, 2008; O'Keefe & Schnell, 2007). Nevertheless, the environment typically plays an aggravating role. The extreme conditions of confinement, including limited time out-of-cell, restricted privileges, and sensory overload, can result in significant psychological distress (Grassian, 1983; Pizarro & Stenius, 2004; Rhodes, 2005; Smith, 2006). For some individuals, physical pain provides a distraction and relief from mounting and intolerable psychological pain. The response by officers and medical and mental health staff provides human contact, lessens the boredom and monotony of life in lockdown, and temporarily moves the inmate to a less harsh setting when transfer to an infirmary, emergency room, or hospital results. Such social reinforcement also contributes to stereotypic self-harm that can arise under conditions of reduced social contact for inmates with neurodevelopmental disorders (Furniss & Biswas, 2012). Additional reinforcement occurs if inmates obtain access to sought-after medications such as narcotic analgesics.

The most vexing situations for correctional staff arise when inmates use self-injury in response to interpersonal conflicts and anger, with a goal of retaliation for perceived insults or unjust sanctions. Self-injury events impede normal operations and divert staff from other activities. Inmates have complete control over timing and severity, which can ensure maximum disruption for the facility. For example, nighttime incidents increase the likelihood of expensive and risky trips to an emergency room in facilities with limited after-hours medical coverage. Such trips will disturb the sleep and home life of administrators when policy requires their immediate notification of critical events. These disruptions effectively communicate anger and restore a sense of empowerment to the inmate.

Management of self-harm in correctional settings

Staff partnership

Effective management of self-injurious behaviors in correctional settings almost always requires partnership and cooperation between health care and custody staff. Disputes over who bears responsibility to address the problem serve little purpose, create discord, and impede progress. Custody staff may respond with understandable incredulity if told that extreme forms of self-injury do not indicate the presence of a mental health problem. Behaviors that I have encountered include insertion of double-A and larger batteries through the urethra and into the bladder, dismantling and consumption of components of a portable television, regurgitation of multiple doses of liquid medication into a plastic bag for later consumption in potentially toxic amounts, and disembowelment. Almost all experienced correctional psychiatrists can attest to similar cases. Whatever else these behaviors may represent, they are not signs of mental health, and correctional psychiatrists need to participate actively in assessment and management of inmates who act this way. At the same time, however, custody staff evade their own responsibility if they expect mental health professionals to address the situation on their own. The demonstrably disturbed nature of the behavior, no matter how extreme or bizarre, does not make the matter a problem for mental health staff alone to solve. Effective interventions sometimes require creative use of privileges, property, or housing placement, none of which psychiatrists can write prescriptions for.

Treatment interventions

When psychiatric disorders contribute to self-injurious behavior, inmates should receive appropriate treatment. Those who appear to have underlying depression may benefit from trials of antidepressant medications. Behavioral interventions may succeed for many individuals with neurodevelopmental disabilities. However, correctional psychiatrists need also to identify and treat depression and other psychiatric disorders that contribute to self-injury in this population (Tsiouris, Cohen, Patti, et al., 2003). Dialectical behavior therapy (DBT), the most widely studied psychotherapeutic intervention for patients with borderline personality disorder, has shown efficacy in reducing self-harm and improving functioning (Stoffers, Vollm, Rucker, et al., 2012), including in correctional settings (Shelton, Sampl, Kesten, et al., 2009). In some instances, such as antipsychotic medications for a delusional inmate, standard treatments by themselves may effectively extinguish the behaviors. Management, however, is rarely that simple. As noted, inmates tend to have other motives for self-harm, and the correctional environment often precipitates or reinforces those behaviors.

When a primary psychiatric disorder does not contribute to self-injury, pharmacotherapy has only a limited role (Harper, 2012; Sandman, 2009). Some evidence supports the use of several classes of medications for SIB per se, primarily opioid blockers, antipsychotics, antidepressants, and anticonvulsants. Benzodiazepines can also help with self-injury associated with anxiety; however, the potential to cause disinhibition that worsens behavior and the risk of medication diversion warrant caution in their use. Choice of agent relies on careful assessment of an individual's reasons for self-injury, which are not always clear. In addition, medication rarely resolves the problem and, at best, serves as an adjunct to environmental, interpersonal, and behavioral interventions described elsewhere in this chapter. The more challenging task for the correctional psychiatrist may entail tempering expectations of others for a simple pharmacological answer and resisting pressures to medicate inappropriately. Polypharmacy without compelling justification poses a particular problem. Discontinuation of medications after unsuccessful trials usually makes the most sense.

The absence of a serious psychiatric disorder as the primary cause of self-injury does not mean that mental health professionals have no role to play, even when the root cause involves conflict between the inmate and custody staff. Dismissing the behavior as manipulative accomplishes nothing. It should come as no surprise that some inmates will resort to self-harm to achieve their goals when they have few other persuasive tools at their disposal. Identifying those goals as the purpose of the behavior actually provides the basis for structuring an intervention. In that regard, the presence of manipulation is both understandable on the part of the inmate and helpful information for custody staff to formulate a response with the assistance and guidance of mental health professionals. All staff should view detection of a motive for the behavior as an important insight and first step in management.

A key element of effective response for many self-injurious inmates involves behavioral interventions. This may include behavior therapy as part of individualized treatment plans or during placement on specialized residential treatment units (see Chapter 22, Levels of Care). Extinction of these behaviors, however, is not a realistic goal for some individuals. Staff need to view a lessening of the frequency or severity of events as a successful outcome. Achieving this requires patience. Behaviors can actually worsen, sometimes dramatically in an occurrence known as an extinction burst, during initial phases of intervention. Progress often takes months, even years, not days or weeks. The greatest likelihood of successful behavioral therapy occurs with the use of DBT principles, including patient agreement with specific goals and structured treatment strategies; close monitoring; skill enhancement; and a nonconfrontational, present-oriented approach (Lynch & Cozza, 2009). Treatment providers who work with this population need ready access to support, consultation, and supervision.

Concerns sometimes arise about using behavioral rewards that gratify inmate desires. Both custody and health care staff may fear outbreaks of contagion in which other inmates mimic self-injurious behaviors to achieve their own goals. Clinicians and administrators might also want to avoid appearing weak in the eyes of colleagues or inmates by giving in to a self-injurer's demands. My experience and that of others, however, does not warrant excessive fear of contagion (Fagan, Cox, Helfand, et al., 2010). Very few individuals have the resolve to imitate serious self-harm to achieve their ends, and most inmates will acknowledge this if asked. As for concerns about the appearance of weakness, correctional and mental health professionals need to carefully consider their priorities. Rejection of an effective intervention merely because others will perceive it as a weakness, or even as capitulation, is its own form of weakness. A more effective and professional strategy focuses on real victories, not perceived defeats. If a safer, more orderly facility results, what has been lost? Managing self-injury is not a zero–sum game; both sides can win. Getting there, however, may require the right motivation, and rewards almost always work better than punishments in shaping behaviors.

Staff reactions

Clinical and custody staff may face other personal and professional challenges when dealing with self-injurious inmates. Bizarre behaviors commonly encountered in correctional settings, such as foreign body insertion or ingestion, occur relatively infrequently in other settings and may unsettle some clinicians. The extent of self-inflicted tissue damage, disfigurement, and other injuries can shock even the most jaded observer. If not acknowledged and addressed, feelings of distress or powerlessness can contribute to a loss of professional perspective, including use of pejorative language about self-injuring inmates. Along with the word "manipulative," dismissive terms such as "attention-seeking" or "conning" may arise. As a dangerous subtext, such terms minimize potential lethality. Published studies and accounts by colleagues support my own experience that many, if not most, self-inflicted fatalities occur in the apparent absence of suicidal intent among inmates deemed manipulative (Dear, Thomson, & Hills, 2000; Haycock, 1989; Smith & Kaminski, 2010). With an awareness of personal distress and language use, the correctional psychiatrist can model appropriate responses and terminology for other staff.

Safety contracts

Safety contracts can have a limited role when a well-established therapeutic alliance exists with the inmate and when the contract identifies alternative coping strategies and achievable goals. However, a safety contract should never substitute for a comprehensive assessment and management plan. Contracts also pose significant risks when used inappropriately. As with no-suicide agreements, they can divert attention away from the root causes of the behavior, forestall more effective interventions, and provide false reassurance. Safety contracts may also be accompanied by a mistaken belief that they decrease potential liability for the clinician. They can paradoxically increase liability in some instances because their use clearly demonstrates that the clinician recognized the risk of harm and the contract by itself does not represent an effective intervention for safety or treatment.

Physical restraints

During an acute, ongoing episode of self-injury, an inmate may need physical restraint if other reasonable interventions do not provide sufficient safety. Custody staff can apply restraints for security reasons; in some systems, medical staff can order them as a mental health intervention. Mental health restraints require clinical justifications and procedures. Although rules exist for their use in hospitals and other clinical settings in the United States, these rules generally have not been enacted in correctional facilities. In response, the American Psychiatric Association issued a resource document to help guide the use of mental health restraints in jails and prisons (Metzner, Tardiff, Lion, et al., 2007). The proposed standards would allow jails and prisons to use restraints for mental health purposes in hospitals, infirmaries, and special mental health housing units. The standards mostly parallel those routinely used in clinical settings with a few exceptions, primarily loosening of the time parameters for initial face-to-face assessment of restrained inmates because correctional facilities typically lack the clinical staffing and coverage to make adherence to tighter timelines practical. Recognition of the nontherapeutic aspects of the correctional environment has led me to recommend the use of mental health restraints only while arranging for transfer to a psychiatric hospital (Appelbaum, 2007). For similar reasons, standards in the United Kingdom limit the application of restraints to nonclinical prison correctional staff with security and custody responsibilities (O'Grady, 2007).

Hospitalization

When an inmate engages in serious and ongoing SIB, transfer to a hospital may become necessary. This runs the risk of reinforcing the behaviors, especially for inmates who seek respite from segregation or other restrictive housing units. One recommended strategy involves providing inmates with hospital or infirmary placements as rewards for set amounts of time without SIB and trying to avoid such placements in response to SIB (Fagan et al., 2010). This approach reinforces healthier behaviors and can provide a sense of control to the inmate. As previously noted, however, some individuals have significant psychological distress during prolonged segregation. The correctional psychiatrist should not hesitate to arrange transfer under these circumstances or in other situations that require hospital admission to help ensure safety. Symptoms often rapidly dissipate after hospitalization. Nevertheless, this temporary intervention does not address the root cause of the problem when draconian conditions of isolation contribute to psychological decompensation. A longer-term solution involves the availability of housing units with less extreme isolation for inmates who need high security. As with other management strategies for SIB, shared responsibility and creative collaboration among custody, medical, and mental health staff offers the greatest likelihood of successful intervention.

Summary

SIB poses significant challenges for correctional facilities. Although relatively few inmates engage in these acts, they cause considerable disruption to operations, resources, and safety. The etiology and management of self-injury in jails and prisons have both similarities and differences with community settings. Effective management requires joint responsibility and a coordinated response by clinical and custody staff. In most instances, this calls for a flexible approach to the environmental factors that contribute to the behavior. Maintaining a professional perspective and an openness to creative use of behavioral interventions increases the likelihood of success in lessening the frequency and severity of SIB.

References

American Psychiatric Association (2013). *Diagnostic and statistical manual of mental disorders* (5th ed.). Arlington, VA: American Psychiatric Publishing.

Appelbaum, K. L. (2007). Commentary: the use of restraint and seclusion in correctional mental health. *Journal of the American Academy of Psychiatry & the Law, 35,* 431–435.

Appelbaum, K. L., Savageau, J. A., Trestman, R. L., et al. (2011). A national survey of self-injurious behavior in American prisons. *Psychiatric Services, 62,* 285–290.

Briere, J., & Gil, E. (1998). Self-mutilation in clinical and general population samples: prevalence, correlates, and functions. *American Journal of Orthopsychiatry, 68,* 609–620.

Dear, G. E., Thomson, D. M., & Hills, A. M. (2000). Self-harm in prison: manipulators can also be suicide attempters. *Criminal Justice and Behavior, 27,* 160–175.

Fagan, T. J., Cox, J., Helfand, S. J., et al. (2010). Self-injurious behavior in correctional settings. *Journal of Correctional Health Care, 16,* 48–66.

Furniss, F., & Biswas, A. B. (2012). Recent research on aetiology, development and phenomenology of self-injurious behaviour in people with intellectual disabilities: a systematic review and implications for treatment. *Journal of Intellectual Disability Research, 56,* 453–475.

Gould, M. S., Marrocco, F. A., Kleinman, M., et al. (2005). Evaluating iatrogenic risk of youth suicide screening programs: a randomized controlled trial. *Journal of the American Medical Assocation, 293,* 1635–1643.

Grassian, S. (1983). Psychopathological effects of solitary confinement. *American Journal of Psychiatry, 140,* 1450–1454.

Harper, G. P. (2012). Psychopharmacological treatment. In B. W. Walsh (Ed.), *Treating self-injury: A practical guide.* New York: Guilford Press.

Haw, C., Houston, K., Townsend, E., et al. (2002) Deliberate self harm patients with depressive disorders: treatment and outcome. *Journal of Affective Disorders, 70,* 57–65.

Hawton, K., Linsell, L., Adeniji, T., et al. (2013). Self-harm in prisons in England and Wales: an epidemiological study of prevalence, risk factors, clustering, and subsequent suicide. *Lancet,* DOI:10.1016/S0140-6736(13)62118-2

Haycock, J. (1989). Manipulation and suicide attempts in jails and prisons. *Psychiatric Quarterly, 60,* 85–98.

Jones, A. (1986). Self-mutilation in prison: a comparison of mutilators and nonmutilators. *Criminal Justice and Behavior, 13,* 286–296.

Klonsky, E. D. (2007). The functions of deliberate self-injury: A review of the evidence. *Clinical Psychology Review, 27,* 226–239.

Klonsky, E. D., Oltmanns, T. F., & Turkheimer, E. (2003). Deliberate self-harm in a nonclinical population: prevalence and psychological correlates. *American Journal of Psychiatry, 160,* 1501–1508.

Large, M., Babidge, N., Andrews, D., et al. (2009). Major self-mutilation in the first episode of psychosis. *Schizophrenia Bulletin, 35,* 1012–1021.

Lovell, D. (2008). Patterns of disturbed behavior in a supermax population. *Criminal Justice and Behavior, 35,* 985–1004.

Lynch, T. R., & Cozza, C. (2009). Behavior therapy for nonsuicidal self-injury. In M. K. Nock (Ed.), *Understanding nonsuicidal self-injury: Origins, assessment, and treatment.* Washington, DC: American Psychological Association.

Metzner, J. L., Tardiff, K., Lion, J., et al. (2007). Resource document on the use of restraint and seclusion in correctional mental health care. *Journal of the American Academy of Psychiatry & the Law, 35,* 417–425.

Muehlenkamp, J. J. (2012). Formal assessment of self-injury. In B. W. Walsh (Ed.), *Treating self-injury: a practical guide* (2nd ed., pp. 88–98). New York: The Guilford Press.

O'Grady, J. C. (2007). Commentary: A British perspective on the use of restraint and seclusion in correctional mental health care. *Journal of the American Academy of Psychiatry & the Law, 35,* 439–443.

O'Keefe, M., & Schnell, M. (2007). Offenders with mental illness in the correctional system. *Journal of Offender Rehabilitation, 45,* 81–104.

Pizarro, J., & Stenius, V. M. K. (2004). Supermax prisons: their rise, current practices, and effect on inmates. *The Prison Journal, 84,* 248–264.

Reynolds, S. K., Lindenboim, N., Comtois, K. A., et al. (2006). Risky assessments: Participant suicidality and distress associated with research assessments in a treatment study of suicidal behavior. *Suicide and Life-Threatening Behavior, 36,* 19–34.

Rhodes, L. A. (2005). Pathological effects of the supermaximum prison. *American Journal of Public Health, 95,* 1692–1695.

Sandman, C. A. (2009). Psychopharmacologic treatment of nonsuicidal self-injury. In M. K. Nock (Ed.), *Understanding nonsuicidal self-injury: Origins, assessment, and treatment.* Washington, DC: American Psychological Association.

Shelton, D., Sampl, S., Kesten, K. L., et al. (2009). Treatment of impulsive aggression in correctional settings. *Behavioral Sciences & the Law, 27,* 787–800.

Smith, H. P., & Kaminski, R. J. (2010). Inmate self-injurious behaviors: distinguishing characteristics within a retrospective study. *Criminal Justice and Behavior, 37,* 81–96.

Smith, H. P., & Kaminski, R. J. (2011). Self-injurious behaviors in state prisons: findings from a national survey. *Criminal Justice and Behavior, 38,* 26–41.

Smith, P. S. (2006). The effects of solitary confinement on prison inmates. a brief history and review of the literature. *Crime and Justice, 34,* 441–528.

Stoffers, J. M., Vollm, B. A., Rucker, G., et al. (2012). Psychological therapies for people with borderline personality disorder. *Cochrane Database of Systemic Reviews, 15,* 8. Art.No.: CD005652. DOI:10.1002/14651858.CD005652.pub2

Tsiouris, J. A., Cohen, I. L., Patti, P. J., et al. (2003). Treatment of previously undiagnosed psychiatric disorders in persons with developmental disabilities decreased or eliminated self-injurious behavior. *Journal of Clinical Psychiatry, 64,* 1081–1090.

Yap, L., Butler, T., Richters, J., et al. (2013). Penile implants among prisoners: a cause for concern? *PLoS One, 8,* e53065.

CHAPTER 50

Behavior management plans

Henry Schmidt III and André M. Ivanoff

Introduction

Research and theoretical literatures use the term "behavior management" interchangeably with "treatment." The processes in behavior management include many strategies and methods found in sound cognitive-behavioral clinical practice. Most modern facilities have been built to enhance behavior management of offenders by staff. Isolation rooms, suicide-resistant clothing and bedding, recessed doorknobs and showerheads, and closed-circuit video monitors all assist in controlling and responding to resident behavior. Common correctional practices such as room and resident sweeps to remove contraband (weapons, drugs), use of physical force, delivery of appropriate psychiatric medication, and separation of sexes and youth from adults all serve to manage resident behavior. Planning of the physical facility occurs prior to construction, and practices are generally codified in policy developed and overseen by facility administrators. While research may inform many aspects of corrections work (e.g., see Chapter 43; Konrad, Daigle, & Daniel, 2007), there is almost no research per se on overall systems of care in correctional residential settings. Therapeutic communities for substance-abusing inmates and "boot camp" programs are notable exceptions.

Broadly speaking, we define behavior management as the point of interaction between staff and inmate patients within the facility (or any other location in which they work together). It is always occurring, although not always planned or well executed. A behavior management plan (BMP) takes into consideration staff abilities, specific characteristics of the unit, and the capacity of the patient for whom the plan is developed. A well-constructed BMP specifies who will do what, for whom, and in what contexts. As such, it is an individual element of a broader intervention, designed to focus on specific patient behavior. BMPs are most often developed and implemented for behaviors that pose a high risk to inmate or staff health within the facility or a high risk to disrupt the safety and programming within the facility. Most low-level behaviors are simply dealt with via codes of sanction administered on an ad hoc basis by staff members who observe them.

"Behavior management," defined here as a series of interventions designed to reduce behaviors that destabilize unit or facility functioning, is distinguished from "treatment." Treatment is viewed as a series of interventions designed to reduce the future frequency, intensity, and/or severity of a given behavior in the unit and upon return to the community. Thus, while there may be treatment characteristics included in BMPs, the scope of the intervention is typically more limited. A BMP may focus on a particular disruptive behavior in the unit, for instance, without any consideration of whether the behavior may occur in the community following release.

This chapter includes a review of concepts related to behavior management and the creation of BMPs. As an example of a structured BMP, attention is drawn to what is consider to be a core element of behavior management and an example of a BMP in action, referred to here as the Egregious Behavior Protocol. It is important to note that this protocol is also a core aspect of sound treatment, designed not only to manage high-risk behavior but also to reduce the likelihood of its occurrence in the future.

Literature review with background

Most documentation of behavior management systems and planning occurs in specific unit program descriptions, broader organizational policy, or even government white papers. BMPs occur within specific and specialized settings and are products of the personnel and policies therein. In cases where data are collected and reviewed internally, this may be regarded as quality assurance or program evaluation rather than as research conducted for publication. Such internal reviews may use pre–post designs, focusing on a target behavior (e.g., fighting, use of isolation rooms, inmate injury), and assess whether instances of such behaviors decrease following a change in policy or practice. In rare instances, an outside entity may step in and require that the system change its policy and practice to address instances of harmful outcome (suicide, murder, rape; cf. *U.S. v. The NYS OCFS*, 2009).

Most published research examines aspects of care, such as a specific intervention offered within a corrections setting, rather than comparing systems to one another. Fortunately, enough carefully constructed studies now exist that metaanalyses of program elements have led to a series of "what works" articles and policy briefs specific to programs (Lipsey, Howell, Kelly, et al., 2010) and type of offender (e.g., juveniles, adults, sex offenders). Future research is required to extend guidance on effective work with more specialized populations (e.g., females, seriously mentally ill offenders) and to clarify optimal program delivery methods.

Empirically validated models of program delivery generally follow Risk-Needs-Responsivity principles (Bonta & Andrews, 2007; Lipsey et al., 2010). In brief, these programs direct services to the highest-risk offenders, focusing on criminogenic needs (i.e., risk factors for recidivism) in a manner that takes into account offender abilities and learning styles. Such studies focus on recidivism as the outcome. The literature examining outcomes within correctional settings is in its infancy, with most articles focusing on suicide (Barboza & Wilson, 2011).

Offender access to treatment and prosocial supports even while in the community are limited (Polaschek, 2011), and the concentration of serious mental illness continues to grow in prison populations. Further, gang affiliation and recruitment (see Chapter 58) create a climate of fear and resistance that inhibit staff from working collaboratively with inmates and proactively establishing rehabilitative, functioning residential climates.

Effective programs can be created by evaluating the "what works" treatment literature. Programs that reduce recidivism typically include strategies and methods found in comprehensive cognitive-behavioral intervention models. Psychodynamic, human-centered, and "scared-straight" programs do not fare as well, with some programs actually increasing recidivism after release (Lipsey et al., 2010; Vaske, Galyean, & Cullen, 2011). While some BMPs may rely almost exclusively on staff action and use of segregation to address high-risk behavior, such plans are largely reactive to resident behavior and do little to reduce the risk of future incidents of the targeted behavior. For example, breaking up a fight and then assigning the instigator to a period in restricted housing does little to reduce the likelihood of that same individual causing a fight once returned to general population. Indeed, for some offenders, being removed from the general population may strengthen the behavior by providing protection, relief from overcrowded conditions, more ready access to health care, or individual time with staff, all of which contradict effective practice. With limited resources, plans must be proactive in addressing current and future instances of targeted behavior; these elements of BMPs are discussed in the remainder of the chapter.

Several core elements that predict the ultimate success of a BMP have been identified. BMPs require staff members who are trained to implement the core components in a facility that provides sufficient structure and programming to support it. Patient engagement enhances the rate of change. For the process to work, staff need more than training in basic behavioral techniques. Staff should be hired, trained, and retained based on their ability to reliably demonstrate the "soft skills" of interpersonal work—that is, warmth, caring, fairness, and nonjudgmental attitudes. The ability to assist patients in examining and altering their antisocial cognitions is also key, as is the ability to structure the milieu to generally favor prosocial problem solving. A milieu that provides social reinforcement of aggression or self-injury makes it almost impossible to obtain significant reductions in these behaviors.

Ideally, BMPs will be tightly linked with skills curricula and practices that are actively incorporated into the offender rehabilitation program. It is safe to assume that offenders do not enter correctional facilities with the entire complement of skills needed to be successful in less-structured or free-world settings. Those who do have those skills may report thoughts that reduce their willingness to use the skills in the situations needed. A comprehensive rehabilitation approach will match interventions to the broad needs of the population being served. These interventions, primarily skills-based, should be well understood by the staff, modeled routinely by staff and more advanced patients, and reinforced by both staff and patients via social interactions as well as by more structured token economies (where feasible) and level systems. This creates a powerful mechanism of behavior change, enhancing the specific elements of a BMP intervention to address a given behavior. Thus, a BMP should include specific skills, terms, and language taught in groups offered to the residents.

Application of behavior modification procedures requires that staff focus on the behaviors that are the target of the intervention. This requires focused training and supervision, as staff typically speak of personality attributes rather than the behavior directly.

Staff are often distracted in discussions of antisocial characteristics, entitlement, power struggles, and other psychological constructs and are not able to focus on the behaviors of interest. Behavior management requires the ability to clearly identify a specific behavior, particularly its intensity and duration. Staff also need to recognize behavioral sequences and to be aware of what precedes and what follows the target behavior (cf. Ivanoff & Schmidt, 2010). For example, aggression (a class of behaviors) includes a variety of specific behaviors, including clenched fists; a hard stare; standing stiffly with squared shoulders directed toward another; verbal statements of intent to harm; and punching, tackling, or kicking. Importantly, staff should also be able to identify when patients are attempting to use skills (no matter how poorly). Recognizing reductions in the intensity or duration of target behaviors is important since these are successes that deserve reinforcement, even though the target behavior may not be eliminated entirely. Thus, an all-or-nothing approach (i.e., "any level of a targeted behavior must be punished") should be discouraged in favor of solid behavior modification practices.

Programming in correctional settings typically focuses on cognitive modification, identifying criminal thinking as the primary or sole determinant of criminal behavior. For medium- and high-risk offenders, criminal behavior is multiply determined; thoughts are just one variable influencing criminal activity. We recommend a contextual behavioral approach in which several variables are seen as directly or indirectly influencing behavior, including cognitions, emotions, action urges, physiological responding, and overlearned behavior (habits). BMP interventions include a focus on patient thinking as well as a heavy emphasis on classic behavioral interventions such as role play, contingency management, modeling of functional (noncriminal, non-high-risk) behavior, and manipulation of cues when possible (e.g., exposure procedures).

Behavior management plan specifics

The behavior modification strategies of reinforcement and punishment should be central to the creation of BMPs. Structured practice—that is, behavior rehearsal—should also be included. For lower-functioning inmates, a script may be developed and practiced and used with either staff or peers on the unit. Overlearning of the new behavior is the goal, which increases the likelihood that the individual can apply the skill when needed. Such situations are often emotionally charged or subject to powerful cue control (i.e., an unhealthy reaction is triggered without conscious thought). Specific skills (behaviors taught in the facility's clinical or classroom settings) should be identified for use in the presence of cues that typically elicit a dysfunctional response. BMPs may also include patients' reviews of their own behavior. These reviews may be written or discussed verbally with staff following an episode of dysfunctional behavior.

The majority of high-risk offenders have had multiple arrests and live broadly antisocial lifestyles. Their causal factors for behavior, alongside criminogenic thinking, include habitual ways of responding, emotion-driven decision making, and a lifetime of reinforcement for aggression and other dysfunctional behaviors. Discussions with patients about their behavior may occur in treatment sessions or groups focused on topics related to recidivism; BMPs should be heavy on "practice, practice, practice." There may be two paths for a plan, one for situations where the patient is motivated to work with staff and the other where the patient is not (e.g., emotionally or physiologically dysregulated or willfully refusing to consider term of art action).

BMPs should clearly identify the behavior(s) to be changed. First to be targeted are extreme behaviors that threaten the health and safety of the patient, other inmates, or staff, such as suicide or other self-injurious behaviors, aggression, or trading medications. BMPs also target behaviors that threaten other programming within the institution, for example refusing to follow staff directives and problematic interactions with staff (excessive requests, hostile responses, refusal to participate in programming) or peers. Initially, clinically trained professionals may create and oversee implementation of the plan. Early and informed involvement of correctional officers is key. Once they understand the principles and practices typically used in BMPs, trained and experienced staff will be able to create them independently for many common behaviors, consulting with clinicians for intractable or very complex cases.

Effective plans consider treatment-related characteristics of the individual patient. The design of the BMP should take into account the level of cognitive functioning and symptoms and characteristics related to mental illness (i.e., mood, anxiety, psychotic, or personality disorder). Environmental factors that may influence behavior (e.g., overcrowding, stressors of first days of incarceration or imminent release, gang tensions) should be integrated into the BMP. In some institutions, inmates are housed based on admission/incident characteristics such as sex offense, serious mental illness, or cognitive impairment. Staff who routinely work in these specialized treatment units learn the common aspects of BMP interventions with their population, thus improving patient outcomes.

An application of behavior management plans: the egregious behavior protocol

One formalized approach to the BMP is a structured sequence for responding to inmate high-risk behavior that has been taught for years in correctional settings—the Egregious Behavior Protocol. This protocol, as defined here, was initially discussed in an article on the application of dialectical behavior therapy in an inpatient setting (Swenson, Sanderson, Dulit, & Linehan, 2001) and has been elaborated by McCann, Ivanoff, Schmidt, and Beach (2007). This protocol is designed to address high-risk behavior in residential settings (although its principles and practices could also be used in outpatient settings). Reinforcement-rich programs and those that prioritize reinforcement of patient behaviors as the predominant approach to change are likely to benefit most from this protocol for reasons highlighted later in the chapter. Although easiest to carry out in settings where all inmates live under the same contingencies, many BMPs are implemented with individuals living in general housing units.

The protocol is a response to an identified target behavior. Inmates should be oriented to the protocol before it is used, if possible. Most facilities either distribute a manual or list of unit rules to inmates at admission. Ideally, it is part of the orientation to the institution/unit admission (i.e., if inmates engage in these behaviors, the protocol lists the consequences that will be implemented). Intake information or/and a patient interview may reveal inmates' individual behaviors that staff should monitor closely. As such, it is important to clearly label all observable actions that would count as occurrences of the behavior. Thus, an aggressive patient is told that verbal threats, threatening stares, closed fists, a fighting stance, and punching or other physical contact with another inmate or staff are considered aggressive acts. Possessing or manufacturing a weapon or encouraging others to fight are also behaviors that would lead to application of the protocol. Those with histories of self-injury or suicidal behavior are informed that statements, threats, notes or journal entries, or possession of contraband to use for self-harm are causes for placement on the protocol.

Once the patient is oriented to the protocol, normal programming begins. Privileges and rewards are earned based on the unit's merit (level) system or token economy, and the resident may be assigned to classes or work details. Ideally, staff provide regular feedback to inmates regarding their behavior while modeling skillful and prosocial interactions and speech. Staff resources are directed to coaching patients on the unit when they demonstrate distress or low-level rule violations. Such coaching identifies the observed behavior to which the staff is responding (e.g., "You look upset right now"), states the staff's concerns ("Are you able to calm yourself down? Do you need some help?"), and provides concrete skills coaching ("Would it help if you sat over here and took some deep breaths, or distract yourself with this puzzle?"). In many situations, once staff have established credibility as supportive and caring, these interventions head off a more serious crisis. In instances where it is not effective, the patient may exhibit a target behavior, in which case the Egregious Behavior Protocol is implemented.

Egregious behavior protocol

Jackson is a 24-year-old in detention charged with armed robbery and third-degree assault. He has a history of mental health concerns and infractions while incarcerated. He is housed on a general population unit of two tiers, with two men per room. He returns from court one day agitated and muttering to himself. His movements are jerky and choppy. He goes into his room to find that the picture of his infant daughter is not taped to the wall where he left it. He begins yelling loudly, "You G-------- m------------ SOB! If you touched my picture I'm gonna kill you right now!" Several other inmates in the area hear Jackson yelling and making threats toward his roommate. Jackson leaves his room and starts to scan the unit for his roommate. An officer intervenes: "Hey, Jackson, chill! What's going on?"

Following the behavior, the first intervention is to restore safety and security. Fighting patients are restrained, as necessary, and then separated; a self-injuring patient's actions are stopped, means to self-harm are removed, and the patient is placed in a setting with minimal means to self-harm. Medical attention is sought, if needed. The patient is then informed that he or she is "off program" while the protocol is completed. Importantly, regular programming continues for all inmates not involved in the incident. It is important, therefore, that a recognized and active program for residents is in place, including education, recreation, entertainment, social activities, and other appropriate privileges.

The officer takes Jackson aside. "Hey, Jackson, you gotta stop. You can't be yelling and threatening to kill folks here—that kind of talk can get you box days. Can you tell me what happened? We gotta sort this out. You okay to talk to me now or do you need some time to cool down?

Are you okay for this minute? You're really upset. Something bad must've happened. Come sit in the counselor's office."

The officer spends two to three minutes determining what happened. In this case, it was a bad day in court where other charges were added to his current charges. He was feeling hopeless. Finally, not finding his daughter's picture when he entered his cell set him off. The officer validates the difficulty and moves quickly to "We've gotta make things right here."

A series of tasks is set in order to put the individual on the pathway back to restoration of full privileges and programming. The first is a commitment to not engage in the egregious behavior(s). Conversations between staff and patient initially focus on this until commitment is obtained. Interactions between the patient and peers on the unit are restricted until this occurs.

"Jackson, going to the box right now isn't going to help anything. I gotta get your word that you won't threaten your roommate again first."

The next task is completion of a chain or behavioral analysis of the incident (Ivanoff & Schmidt, 2010). This analysis details the environmental cue that preceded the incident, thoughts/emotions/action urges that led to the behavior, and actual or expected outcomes that may have reinforced the behavior. Vulnerabilities (contextual variables that increase the likelihood of responding to the cue with the egregious behavior) are also identified. This information should be documented in the patient's chart and is used in the development of a treatment plan.

Staff then work with the patient to gain commitment to learning and practicing skills that are identified as directly applicable to preventing the recurrence of the egregious behavior. These may address vulnerabilities, tolerance of cues, or dysfunctional links (e.g., thoughts, emotions, urges) in the chain. A list of skills that inmates can practice when feeling distressed, angry, or anxious can be taught to officers and passed on to inmates.

Environmental reinforcers may be addressed as well. Skills should be selected from curricula offered within the offender treatment program. Thus, a comprehensive skills curriculum should address emotion regulation and cognitive restructuring, at a minimum. Patients show their commitment to the BMP by demonstrating to staff and clinicians how they will use the skills, describing the steps, and then participating in structured role plays (or they may use the skills in the normal course of their activities while on the protocol). Demonstration of proficiency (not perfection) in the skills, along with ongoing commitment to use them when needed, is required to move toward reinstatement of privileges.

If a fight was the behavior in question, then problem solving with all parties involved is necessary, with the parties coming to agreement that the issue is resolved and a shared commitment exists not to cause harm to the other. In all instances, a "correction–overcorrection" is developed by the patient to address any harm that may have been caused by the egregious behavior. This may begin with apologies to those affected but also would generally include some service project designed to improve the individual or unit experiences of others. This is not necessarily a grand project; rather, it is something significant and meaningful to those receiving it.

As the patient works through the Egregious Behavior Protocol, rewards or small privileges may be extended to reinforce his or her willingness and the steps he or she has taken. Full privileges are restored once patients have completed the protocol and as they demonstrate their ability to successfully implement skills to avoid egregious behavior in the presence of cues. For those who continue to engage in similar egregious behaviors, a return to full programming may require more time and demonstrated practice than for first-time offenders, given that earlier interventions were not successful. Clinicians and constructive staff together orchestrate the restrictions, practice opportunities, and ultimately determine when the patient is returned to full programming.

It is important with every patient to balance the change demanded from the patient with staff interventions designed to maintain the patient's motivation to complete the task at hand. Burying patients in sanctions or seemingly insurmountable lists of tasks may needlessly delay (or even prevent) patients from applying themselves to the process. Further, the removal from basic daily programming is likely to be most salient when daily programming is actually meaningful and rewarding for patients. To "climb the ladder" of the protocol, there needs to be something worth reaching at the top. Thus, a fully developed residential program will include elements that all inmates want to access, ensuring that removal from the program (response cost) will be meaningful and rejoining the program will be a goal worth striving for.

Summary

BMPs are most effective when incorporated as standard practice in a rehabilitation program that offers comprehensive cognitive-behavioral skills curricula in treatment and in which staff are trained to provide behavioral interventions in their interactions with patients. While the research literature on management plans per se is scant, their foundation in solid behavioral principles is supported by the vast empirical catalogue of behavioral changes seen in patients of all backgrounds (Bottoms, Hay, & Sparks, 1995; Helfand, 2011; Shelton, Sampl, Kesten, et al., 2009). To be effective, BMPs must be applied by well-trained staff who ensure a swift intervention, fairness, and predictability. A standard approach to seriously disruptive behavior, the Egregious Behavior Protocol, was described as an example of a BMP in action.

References

Bonta, J., & Andrews, D.A (2007). *Risk-Need-Responsivity model for offender assessment and rehabilitation* (No. 2007-06). Ottawa, Canada: Department of Public Safety and Emergency Preparedness, Canada.

Barboza, S., & Wilson, J. S. (2011). Behavior management plans decrease inmate self-injury. *Corrections Today*. American Correctional Association, available at: https://www.aca.org/fileupload/177/ahaidar/Barboza%20and%20Wilson.pdf (accessed February 10, 2014).

Bottoms, A. E., Hay, W., & Sparks, J. R. (1995). Situational and social approaches to the prevention of disorder in long-term prisons. In T. J. Flanagan (Ed.), *Long-term imprisonment: Policy, science, and correctional practice* (pp. 186–189). Thousand Oaks, CA: Sage.

Helfand, S. J. (2011). Managing disruptive offenders. In T. J. Fagan & R. K. Ax (Eds.), *Correctional mental health: From theory to best practice* (pp. 309–326). Thousand Oaks, CA: SAGE Publications, Inc.

Ivanoff, A., & Schmidt, H. (2010). Functional assessment in forensic settings: A valuable tool for preventing and treating egregious behavior. *Journal of Cognitive Psychotherapy: An International Quarterly, 24*(2), 81–91.

Konrad, N., Daigle, M. S., & Daniel, A. E. (2007). Preventing suicide in prisons, Part I: Recommendations from the International Association for Suicide Prevention Task Force on suicide in prisons. *Crisis. The Journal of Crisis Intervention and Suicide Prevention, 28*(3), 113–121.

Lipsey, M. W., Howell, J. C., Kelly, M. R., Chapman, G., & Carver, D. (2010). *Improving the effectiveness of juvenile justice programs: a new perspective on evidence-based programs.* Center for Juvenile Justice Reform, Georgetown University.

McCann, R., Ivanoff, A., Schmidt, H., & Beach, B. (2007). DBT in residential forensic settings. In L. Dimeff, K. Koerner, & C. Sanderson (Eds.), *Dialectical behavior therapy in clinical practice* (pp. 112–144). New York: Guilford Press.

Polaschek, D. L. L. (2011). Many sizes fits all: A preliminary framework for conceptualizing the development and provision of cognitive-behavioral rehabilitation programs for offenders. *Aggression and Violent Behavior, 16*, 20–35.

Shelton, D., Sampl, S., Kesten, K. L., Zhang, W., & Trestman, R. L. (2009). Treatment of impulsive aggression in correctional settings. *Behavioral Sciences and the Law, 27*, 787–800.

Swenson, C. R., Sanderson, C., Dulit, R. A., & Linehan, M. M. (2001). The application of dialectical behavior therapy for patients with borderline personality disorder on inpatient units. *Psychiatric Quarterly, 72*(4), 307–324.

Vaske, J., Galyean, K., & Cullen, F. T. (2011). Toward a biosocial theory of offender rehabilitation: Why does cognitive-behavioral therapy work? *Journal of Criminal Justice, 39*, 90–102.

SECTION XII

Distinct populations

CHAPTER 51

Gender-specific treatment

Catherine F. Lewis

Introduction

Despite a roughly equal number of men and women in the general population, women consistently have lower rates of incarceration than their male peers (Carson & Golinelli, 2013). The difference is not trivial; there are 10 times as many men as women incarcerated in the United States (Carson & Golinelli, 2013).

The US correctional system was confronted with issues specific to female inmates in part as a product of the War on Drugs from the mid-1980s to the mid-1990s. During that period, the number of women incarcerated rose 888 percent (Mauer et al., 1999). The bulk of the rise was attributable to arrests for nonviolent drug-related charges. As the correctional system began to experience an influx of women, it became clear that they were different from their male peers. The differences included epidemiology of psychiatric disorders, intensity of health service use, social stressors, and patterns of offending. The logical question arose as to whether women needed a different treatment approach in the correctional system than men. The term "gender-responsive programming" emerged and represented the idea that women have specific needs distinct from their male peers that could best be met with treatment designed for women (Covington & Bloom, 2006; Wright et al., 2012). This chapter describes, given the current knowledge base, the patterns of offending and arrests for women versus men, the sociodemographics of incarcerated women, the psychopathology exhibited by incarcerated women, and how best to treat incarcerated women and implement this treatment within jails and prisons.

Background

In 2012 there were 1,571,013 people incarcerated in the United States; 1,462,147 (93.1 percent) were men and 108,886 (6.9 percent) were women (Carson & Golinelli, 2013). The number of women incarcerated at the end of 2012 was the lowest since 2005 and represented a 2.3 percent decrease from 2011 (Glaze & Herberman, 2013).

It is not surprising that most inmates are male; men are arrested more often than women for most offenses except embezzlement, truancy, and prostitution. Men are significantly more likely to be arrested for violent crime. Men account for more than 99 percent of all arrests for rape, 89 percent for murder and manslaughter, 85 percent for robbery, and 75 percent for assault (Federal Bureau of Investigation, 2013). In short, violent offending is a predominately male affair. At the end of 2012, a higher percentage of men (54.3 percent) were incarcerated for violent offenses than women (36.8 percent; Carson & Golinelli, 2013). Women who commit violent offenses are more likely than men to have male accomplices, to victimize someone they know, and to offend at the victim's home or school. Women are less likely to use weapons and to seriously injure their victims (Greenfeld & Snell, 1999). Most women (63.2 percent) are incarcerated for nonviolent offenses, including property crime (28 percent) and drug-related charges (25 percent; Carson & Golinelli, 2013).

Minorities are overrepresented in correctional populations. Of women incarcerated at the close of 2012, 23.1 percent were black, 16.7 percent Hispanic, 48.7 percent white, and 11.4 percent other (Carson & Golinelli, 2013). These numbers stand in contrast to those of the national population of the United States (13.1 percent black, 16.9 percent Hispanic, 63.0 percent white, 5.1 percent Asian, 1.9 percent other; US Census, 2012). The disparity in race among female inmates, while still notable, actually decreased by 30.7 percent for black women from 2000 to 2009 (Mauer, 2013).

Female inmates are likely to be in their early 30s and to never have been married despite having lived with at least one common-law partner for at least one year. They are mothers to an average of at least two children. This statistic is striking and important; current data suggest that close to a quarter of a million children have incarcerated mothers (Greenfeld & Snell, 2003; Van Voorhis et al., 2010). Most of these mothers (60 percent) were caretakers for their children at the time of arrest. Female inmates are more likely to have a high school education than their male counterparts but more likely to live below the poverty line and to be unemployed. Most were not seeking work at the time of arrest. They are generally less likely to be recidivists than their male peers; 51 percent of incarcerated women have one or no prior offenses versus 39 percent of incarcerated men (Greenfeld & Snell, 1999; Wright et al., 2012).

Incarcerated women report victimization more often than men (Bloom et al., 2003; Browne et al., 1999). One survey of approximately 40,000 women in prison found that close to half had been assaulted, a third physically abused, and a third sexually abused before incarceration (Snell & Morton, 1991). A similar study of 2,000 female inmates found that more than half reported physical abuse and more than a third reported sexual abuse (American Correctional Association, 1990). Those who were sexually abused were most often victimized for the first time during childhood (at age 5 to 14). These rates for abuse and victimization are higher than those reported by women in noncorrectional populations and are triple that of incarcerated males (American Correctional Association, 1990). All of these factors have a critical impact on the psychopathology observed in this population, how it manifests, and how treatment should be approached.

Psychiatric epidemiology of incarcerated women

Incarcerated women are more likely to have psychiatric disorders than incarcerated men and are more likely to have comorbid diagnoses (DiCataldo et al., 1995; Maden et al., 1994; Trestman et al., 2007). Multiple studies now exist that used different validated and reliable research interviews to determine the prevalence of psychiatric disorders among female inmates. Some of these studies focused on women in jail, others on women in prison, and others on mixed populations; one summarized multiple studies (Fazel & Danesh, 2002, Jordan et al., 1996; Lewis, 2006; Lynch et al., 2014; Steadman et al., 2009; Teplin, 1994; Trestman et al., 2007). Table 51.1 summarizes the results of several studies regarding the prevalence of psychiatric disorders in incarcerated women.

Substance use disorders

Substance use disorders (SUDs) are the most common disorders among female correctional populations. This point is critical to remember because treatment for other disorders will likely fail if substance use is not addressed. Women are more likely than men to be intravenous drug users, to have been introduced to substance use by men, to have partners who abuse substances, and to prostitute themselves for drugs (Greenfeld & Snell, 1999; Hammett, 2001). The use of intravenous drugs places women at high risk for contracting infectious diseases. Women are also more likely to use "hard drugs" (heroin, cocaine) and to use a greater number of drugs than men (Greenfeld & Snell, 1999). With respect to alcohol, women experience a phenomenon called "telescoping" in which their symptom severity proceeds at a much more rapid rate than male peers. This puts them at higher risk for physical effects earlier in the course of addiction than men (Schuckit et al., 1995).

Figure 51.1 shows the prevalence of SUDs for clinical populations and incarcerated populations of men and women. What is clear is that as the severity of illness worsens, the gender gap erodes—that is, incarcerated women use substances at a level at least as high as incarcerated men (Jordan et al., 1996; Lewis, 2006; Teplin et al., 1996). This is a striking contrast from the data from the general population (Kessler et al., 1994). Incarcerated women

use multiple substances as a rule, and the load of symptoms for substance dependence is high (Lewis, 2006, 2010). Two thirds of women who enter the correctional system had used drugs in the months preceding incarceration, 50 percent were using daily, and 40 percent were using at the time of the alleged offense (Greenfeld & Snell, 1999).

In summary, SUDs are the most common diagnoses in incarcerated women. When present, the disorder is severe, as evidenced by high symptom counts, early age of onset, and multiple substances used (Lewis, 2006, 2010). SUDs are associated with higher health service use, worsened prognosis for comorbid disorders, physical problems, comorbidity, and death by completed suicide (Kessler et al., 1999; Roy, 2003; Teplin et al., 1997; Wu et al., 1999).

Posttraumatic stress disorder

Posttraumatic stress disorder (PTSD) is increasingly recognized as a highly prevalent diagnosis among incarcerated women. In many instances, their abuse occurred early in life (i.e., during childhood) and was severe and enduring. Exposure to severe trauma in childhood may result in repeated revictimization in adulthood subsequent to high-risk behaviors (e.g., prostitution, intravenous drug use, interaction with dangerous people and situations; Zlotnick, 1997). PTSD also is a potent risk factor for suicide and has a synergistic effect in the presence of major depression (Brodsky et al., 2001). Perhaps more importantly, women with comorbid PTSD and SUDs have more inpatient admissions, higher symptom counts, higher service use, and more psychosocial problems (e.g., homelessness, domestic violence, loss of child custody) than women with either problem alone (Najavits, 1998; Zlotnick, 1997).

The importance of sustained, repetitive trauma from which someone cannot escape is particularly important in determining the course of PTSD (Herman, 1992). Many women who are incarcerated have experienced such situations as children in their homes, as adults in abusive relationships, and as prostitutes engaging in high-risk behavior. They can have symptoms of PTSD that are more tenacious than usual and less responsive to treatment (e.g., somatization, dissociation, chronic suicidality). They can also have pathological changes in the ability to form relationships

Table 51.1 Psychiatric diagnosis: women in community versus female offenders—lifetime prevalence

Disorder (%)	Community		Corrections		
	Kessler et al.[*]	Lewis[†]	Teplin[‡]	Jordan et al.[§]	Lynch et al.[‖]
Substance use disorder	17.9	65.4	70.2	NR	82
Alcohol use disorder	8.2	43.8	32.3	38.0	NR
Drug use disorder	5.9	56.6	63.6	44.2	NR
Antisocial personality disorder	1.2	32.3	13.8	11.9	NR
Posttraumatic stress disorder	10.4	40.8	33.5	30.0	53
Major depressive disorder	21.3	36.2	16.9	13.0	28.0

[*] National Comorbidity Survey; a sample of women in the community.

[†] Mid-sentence female felons (N = 136).

[‡] Pretrial female detainees (N = 1,272).

[§] Convicted female felons entering prison (N = 805).

[‖] Female jail detainees, multisite (N = 491).

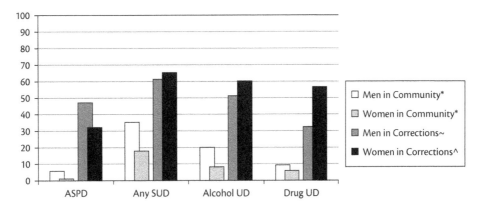

Fig. 51.1 Community and Correctional Mental Illness Prevalences are Different: Lifetime Prevalence, by Gender. *, National Comorbidity Survey (Kessler et al., 1994); ~, 728 jail detainees (Teplin et al., 1996); ^, 136 mid-sentence female felons (Lewis, 2006). ASPD, antisocial personality disorder; SUD, substance use disorder; UD, use disorder.

(e.g., intense, unstable relationships; boundary violations; formation of dependent relationships that place them at high risk for exploitation). Women who have been victimized as children are at risk for rape in adulthood, sexual harassment, battering, self-harm (e.g., cutting), and suicidality. While this construct of complex PTSD is an evolving one, it is important to consider for female inmates. Specifically, failure to correctly diagnose PTSD can lead to misapplication of a diagnosis of personality disorder, stigmatization, and incorrect treatment.

Antisocial personality disorder

Antisocial personality disorder (ASPD) is prevalent among female inmates, particularly convicted felons (Lewis, 2006; Warren et al., 2002; Zlotnick, 1999). ASPD is rare in clinical populations of women. As seen in Table 51.1 and Figure 51.1, the prevalence of ASPD in female correctional populations is much higher than that of women or men in the community. Among felons, the rate approaches that of males (Lewis, 2010; Lynch et al., 2014; Warren et al., 2002; Zlotnick, 1999). Once again, the severity of pathology erodes an expected gender gap. Women with ASPD (with onset of conduct disorder before age 10) have more severe addiction, higher risk of suicide, increased risk of violence, and poorer outcomes with treatment than do men in the community and approach the profile of incarcerated men with ASPD (Lewis, 2006).

Psychopathy has been found among female felons at prevalences approaching that of males (Warren, 2002). Psychopathy, which is refractory to treatment and an ominous prognosticator of outcomes, is rarely measured among incarcerated women. Despite this, when assessed for the presence of psychopathy, female felons have shown similar statistics as their male counterparts. These data are important because of implications for treatment.

Gender-responsive treatment

Examination of women within the correctional system as a discrete group is a relatively new phenomenon. In 1978, only 10,918 women were under the jurisdiction of correctional authorities; in 2011, there were 97,507 (Carson & Golinelli, 2013). Given the inflow of women into the correctional system and their complex needs, it is not surprising that it has taken some time to reflect on the correct way to address mental health issues for incarcerated

women. Given the complexity of the psychopathology exhibited by this population, it is highly unlikely that a one-size-fits-all approach will work. Indeed, some of the most severely ill women appear to have psychopathology resembling that of males, and it remains unclear what this means. While gender must be considered in all treatment for men and women, it is not yet time to call for "gender-responsive programming" for all women in corrections until there is evidence-based literature suggesting better outcomes (e.g., recidivism, morbidity, mortality) from the treatment. With these substantial caveats in mind, several basic tenets that could form a core to inform the treatment of incarcerated women are outlined here.

Steps toward a model treatment program for incarcerated women

Safety first: no treatment can occur in dangerous environments

A prerequisite for successful psychiatric treatment anywhere, but particularly salient in jails and prisons, is physical and emotional safety. Psychiatric staff working in correctional environments must recognize that there are times and situations that place safety and security above treatment (e.g., a patient may need to be strip-searched by Custody personnel). Women with PTSD are at heightened risk for revictimization by peers and staff. Management should include specific training for staff who work with female inmates, a mechanism for anonymous reporting of violations by staff, structured investigation procedures, provision of supervision to staff to assuage frustration and countertransference, and frequent external oversight of staff interactions with inmates.

Recognize psychopathy: women can victimize each other

Recent studies have shown that a high percentage of female felons meet the criteria for psychopathy (Lewis, 2006; Warren et al., 2002; Zlotnick, 1999). This subgroup is resistant to treatment and can disrupt groups and treatment units through contagion. While controversial, it is likely that these women would best be housed in a unit that addresses their specific issues. The emphasis in treatment should be on SUDs (often a harm-reduction rather than an abstinence model is most realistic), behavior management, addressing comorbid diagnoses such as major depression and PTSD, and offering support through case management. Women without substantial other pathology in these units would benefit from vocational programs with close oversight.

Concede limitations: equality is not equivalence

Research on women within the correctional system has grown significantly over the past 20 years. As appreciation of their complex comorbidity has grown, interest has logically risen in applying models successful in the community. The conundrum is that women who are incarcerated differ in many critical ways from their community peers, and most well-studied and validated treatment modules come from community samples. Currently, a variety of approaches are being attempted with incarcerated women, and evidence-based literature has modestly begun to emerge. As programs are evaluated, it is critical to recognize that incarcerated women have specialized profiles that set them apart from women in the community. Similarly, applications that appear to work in the community (e.g., motivational enhancement, contingency management) would be intriguing to integrate into correctional settings.

Don't discriminate: male staff can treat incarcerated women

Women who have experienced trauma do not necessarily require treatment and contact restricted to only women. Gender-responsive programming should not mean that women can demand only female treatment providers. That would be disruptive, unworkable, and not useful to ultimate recovery. In essence, it would also limit their access to providers, which is a bad idea. There is no robust literature that supports a claim that incarcerated women have better outcomes with female treatment providers. It is therefore important not to exclude male providers who are as likely to be effective, qualified, and helpful as female ones.

Coordinate your effort: have a case manager be "quarterback"

Incarcerated women have often struggled to receive services while in the community. They are not generally skilled self-advocates, and some do not know when to seek mental health or medical care. They have a host of worries outside of corrections, the most important of which is their children. Each woman in the system should ideally have a case manager, or "quarterback" (Lewis, 2006), whose job might include obtaining services while incarcerated and entitlements upon release (e.g., medical needs, mental health needs, vocational needs, concrete needs such as clothing/phone calls, contact with department of children and families).

Remember the next generation: motherhood is important

Because most incarcerated women are mothers, it is helpful to integrate parenting classes and vocational classes into treatment. Ideally, there would be child-friendly facilities for visits. For mothers incarcerated at a distance from their children, video visitation enabled by computer and appropriately supervised by correctional staff may be an option for maintaining and building these critical relationships.

Identify what you are treating: obtain detailed criterion-based diagnoses

Other than nonadherence, a major reason for treatment failure is inaccurate diagnosis or unrecognized comorbidity. This comorbidity includes other psychiatric diagnoses, medical conditions, and side effects from medications. Incarcerated women have complex pathology, which at times is overwhelming to the clinician. During a short, nonstructured interview, it is difficult to correctly diagnose women who have multiple issues. A structured interview offers the opportunity to assess the patient objectively, consider diagnoses that might not arise during an open-ended interview, quantify symptom counts, identify how many substances are used and severity of use, and have a reasoned assessment of often provocative, complex patients.

Use medication for a reason: adhere to practice guidelines whenever possible and practical

While there are best practice guidelines for many disorders, one of the difficulties confronting the clinician who treats a female inmate is that she may have so many disorders. One woman may have PTSD, major depression, panic disorder, multiple SUDs, ASPD, and side effects from medications for the treatment of HIV or hepatitis C. In these instances, it is not appropriate to withhold therapy because of a substance abuse history. The myth that "when they stop using, they will not be depressed" is not correct. Large prospective studies have shown definitively that women and men who use drugs and/or alcohol tend to have episodes of "clean" and "dirty" (i.e., when they are using) depression. Those with episodes of "dirty depression" are more likely to commit suicide and have higher morbidity (Schuckit, 1995). Thus, the history of addiction should not preclude aggressive treatment for depression. Other important issues in treating women are to be aware of body image issues (e.g., avoid medications that cause weight gain; avoid prescribing medications that women may abuse to lose weight) and to always know pregnancy status before prescribing.

Attack comorbidity head on: use integrated treatment

Treatments for SUDs are best integrated completely into treatment of other mental health disorders. The idea of integrated treatment for PTSD and SUD (the most common diagnoses for incarcerated women) has resulted in several programs, including Seeking Safety (Najavits, 2002), Helping Women Recover (Messina et al., 2010), and the Trauma Recovery and Empowerment Model (Fallot & Harris, 2002). Emerging literature suggests positive outcomes in correctional settings (McHugo et al., 2005; Zlotnick et al., 2003) and within the community (Messina et al., 2010).

Give women with the most severe disorders a "home base": use the therapeutic community

Many incarcerated women would benefit from highly structured housing with an integrated treatment program that addresses addiction, trauma, personality disorders including ASPD, and depression. The major advantage to a therapeutic community, coupled with personal case management, is a move toward stable, predictable, ongoing care rather than crisis-driven interventions in response to problem behaviors (e.g., cutting, attempting suicide, using drugs). Ideally, medical visits are coordinated for the therapeutic community so that physical problems are addressed. Few studies have formally examined health service use within prisons, but it is likely that a therapeutic community, as outlined here, would increase treatment adherence, decrease crisis-driven work, decrease exigent visits, and afford better outcomes (De Leon, 1995; Farabee et al., 1999; Roth & Presse, 2003).

Don't drop the ball: coordinate discharge care with an eagle eye

Discharge is a critical time for women who have been incarcerated. Many have limited resources (e.g., no home, no car, little money, no job) and some will have had entitlements cut off while incarcerated. The case manager is critical in ensuring that appointments are made that women are able to attend, that paperwork is filled out if necessary to reinstate entitlements, that medications for the waiting period before seeing a new provider are disbursed, and that appointments with new providers are made. If a woman has children, consideration should be given to a center that offers primary care as well as mental health to make attendance at appointments more likely.

Summary

Incarcerated women are a group with a high degree of psychiatric comorbidity. The most common diagnoses are SUD, PTSD, major depression, and ASPD. The profile of women in corrections is unique; it differs both from women in the community and from men in corrections. This renders the treatment mission difficult. There is little evidence-based literature on how to treat incarcerated women, in large part because there are so many more incarcerated men. Once the pathology of SUD and ASPD becomes severe, women have behaviors and outcomes similar to their male peers (e.g., suicide, violence, more severe substance use, recidivism). Applications of interventions developed for women in the community or for men are likely to be imperfect. Consequently, a therapeutic community for women with the most severe disorders (e.g., SUD, PTSD, self-injurious behavior) that is focused on treatment for trauma and SUD and with a strong focus on case management, cognitive-based psychotherapy, appropriate diagnoses, and evidence-based psychopharmacological treatment when necessary is potentially the best and most effective structure for service delivery to this challenging population (De Leon, 1995; Farabee et al., 1999; Roth & Presse, 2003).

References

American Correctional Association (1990). *The female offender.* Washington, DC: St. Mary's Press.

Brodsky, B. S., Oquendo, M., Ellis, S. P., et al. (2001). The relationship of childhood abuse of impulsivity and suicidal behavior in adults with major depression. *American Journal of Psychiatry, 158*, 1871–1877.

Browne, A., Miller, B., & Maguin E. (1999). Prevalence and severity of lifetime physical and sexual victimization among incarcerated women. *International Journal of the Law and Psychiatry, 22*, 2301–322.

Carson, S., & Golinelli, D. (2013). *Prisoners in 2012—advance counts.* Bureau of Justice Statistics. Washington, DC: Bureau of Justice.

Covington, S., & Bloom, B. (2006). Gender-responsive treatment and services in correctional settings. *Women and Therapy, 29*, 9–33.

De Leon, G. (1995). Therapeutic communities for addictions: a theoretical framework. *International Journal of Addiction, 30*, 1603–1645.

DiCataldo, F., Greer, A., & Profit, W. E. (1995). Screening prison inmates for mental disorder: and examination of the relationship between mental disorders and prison adjustment. *Bulletin of the American Academy of Psychiatry and the Law, 23*, 573–585.

Fallot, R. D., & Harris, M. (2002). The Trauma Recovery and Empowerment Model (TREM): Conceptual and practical issues in a group intervention for women. *Community Mental Health Journal, 38*, 475–485.

Farabee, D., Prendergast, M., Cartier, J., et al. (1999). Barriers to implementing effective correctional drug treatment programs. *Prison Journal, 79*, 150–162.

Fazel, S., & Danesh, J. (2002). Serious mental disorder in 23,000 prisoners: a systemic review of 62 surveys. *The Lancet, 359*, 545–550.

Federal Bureau of Investigation (2013). *Uniform Crime Reports.* Washington, DC: FBI.

Glaze, L. E., & Herberman, E. J. (2013). *Correctional populations in the United States, 2012.* Bureau of Justice Statistics. Washington, DC: Bureau of Justice.

Greenfeld, L. A., & Snell, T. L. (1999). *Bureau of Justice Statistics Special Report: Women Offenders.* Washington, DC: Bureau of Justice Statistics.

Hammett, T. M. (2001). Making the case for health interventions in correctional facilities. *Journal of Urban Health, 78*, 236–240.

Herman, J. L. (1992). Complex PTSD: a syndrome in survivors of prolonged and repeated trauma. *Journal of Traumatic Stress, 5*(3), 377–391.

Jordan, B. K., Schlenger, W. E., Fairbanks, J. A., et al. (1996). Prevalence of psychiatric disorders among incarcerated women, II: convicted felons entering prison. *Archives of General Psychiatry, 55*, 513–519.

Kessler, R. C., McGonagle, K. A., Zhao, S., et al. (1994). Lifetime and twelve-month prevalence of DSM-III-R psychiatric disorders in the United States: Results from the National Comorbidity Survey. *Archives of General Psychiatry, 51*, 8–19.

Kessler, R. C., Borges, G., & Walters, E. E. (1999). Prevalence of and risk factors for lifetime suicide attempts in the National Comorbidity Survey. *Archives of General Psychiatry, 56*, 617–626.

Lewis, C. F. (2006). Treating incarcerated women: gender matters. *Psychiatric Clinics of North America, 29*, 773–789.

Lewis, C. F. (2010). Childhood antecedents of adult violent offending in a group of female felons. *Behavioral Sciences and the Law, 28*, 224–234.

Lynch, S. M., DeHart, D. D., Beknap, J. E., et al. (2014). A multisite study of the prevalence of serious mental illness, PTSD, and substance use disorders of women in jail. *Psychiatric Services in Advance*, February 3, 1–5. (Accessed February 12, 2014, at http://ps.psychiatryonline.org/Article.aspx?ArticleID=1827875, doi:10.1176/appi.ps.201300172)

Maden, T., Swinton, M., & Gunn, J. (1994). Psychiatric disorder in women serving a prison sentence. *British Journal of Psychiatry, 164*, 44–54.

Mauer, M., Potler, C., & Wolf, R. (1999). *Gender and trust: women, drugs and the sentencing policy.* Washington, DC: The Sentencing Project.

Mauer, M. (2013). *The changing racial dynamics of women's incarceration.* Available at: www.sentencingproject.org

McHugo, G. J., Caspi, Y., Kammerer, N., et al. (2005). The assessment of trauma history in women with co-occurring substance abuse and mental disorders and a history of interpersonal violence. *Journal of Behavioral Health Services Research, 32*, 113–127.

Messina, N., Grella, C., Cartier, J., et al. (2010). A randomized experimental study of gender-responsive substance abuse treatment for women in prison. *Journal of Substance Abuse Treatment, 38*, 97–107.

Najavits, L. M., Weiss, R. D., Shaw, S. R., et al. (1998). Seeking Safety: outcome of a new cognitive-behavioral psychotherapy for women with PTSD and substance use disorder. *Journal of Trauma and Stress, 11*, 437–456.

Najavits, L. M. (2002). Seeking Safety: Therapy for trauma and substance abuse. *Corrections Today, 64*, 136–141.

Roth, B., & Presse, L. (2003). Nursing interventions for parasuicidal behaviors in female offenders. *Journal of Psychosocial Nursing Mental Health Services, 41*, 20–29.

Roy, A. (2003). Characteristics of drug addicts who attempt suicide. *Psychiatry Research, 103*, 121–199.

Schuckit, M. A., Andthenelli, R. M., Bucholz, K. K., et al. (1995). The time course and development of alcohol-related problems in men and women. *Journal of Studies on Alcohol, 56*, 218–225.

Snell, T. L., & Morton, D. C. (1991). *Survey of our state prison inmates 1991: women in prison.* Bureau of Justice Statistics, Office of Justice Programs. Washington, DC: Bureau of Justice.

Steadman, H. J., Osher, F. C., Robbins, P. C., et al. (2009). Prevalence of serious mental illness among jail inmates. *Psychiatric Services*, *60*(6), 761–765.

Teplin, L. A. (1994). Psychiatric and substance abuse disorders among urban jail detainees. *American Journal of Public Health*, *84*(2), 290–293.

Teplin, L. A., Abram, K. M., & McClelland, G. M. (1996). Prevalence of psychiatric disorders among incarcerated women, 1: pre-trial jail detainees. *Archives of General Psychiatry, 53.* 505–512.

Teplin, L. A., Abram, K. M., & McClelland, G. M. (1997). Mentally disordered women in jail, who receives services? *American Journal of Public Health, 87,* 604–609.

Trestman, R. L., Ford, J., Zhang, W. Z., et al. (2007). Current and lifetime psychiatric illness among inmates not identified as mentally ill at intake in Connecticut's jails. *Journal of the American Academy of Psychiatry and the Law, 35,* 490–500.

US Census Bureau: http://quickfacts.census.gov/qfd/states/00000.html

Van Voorhis, P., Salisbury, E. J., Wright, E. M., & Bauman, A. (2010). Women's risk factors and their contributions to existing risk/needs assessment: the current status of gender-responsive supplement. *Criminal Justice and Behavior, 37,* 261–288.

Warren, J. I., Hurt, S., Lopez, A. B., et al. (2002). Psychiatric symptoms, history of victimization, and violent behavior among incarcerated female felons: an American perspective. *International Journal of Law and Psychiatry, 25,* 129–149.

Wright, E., Van Voorhis, P., Salisbury, E. J., & Bauman, A. (2012). Gender-responsive lessons learned and policy implications for women in prison: a review. *Criminal Justice and Behavior, 39,* 1612–1632.

Wu, L. T., Kouzis, A. C., & Leaf, P.J. (1999). Influence of co-morbid alcohol and psychiatric disorders on utilization of mental health services in the National Comorbidity Survey. *American Journal of Psychiatry, 56*(8), 1230–1236.

Zlotnick, C. (1997). PTSD comorbidity and childhood abuse among incarcerated women. *Journal of Nervous and Mental Disorders, 185,* 761–763.

Zlotnick, C. (1999). Antisocial personality disorder, affective dysregulation and childhood abuse among incarcerated women. *Journal of Personality Disorders, 13,* 90–95.

Zlotnick, C., Najavits, L. M., Rohsenow, D.J., et al. (2003). A cognitive-behavioral treatment for incarcerated women with substance abuse disorder and posttraumatic stress disorder: Findings from a pilot study. *Journal of Substance Abuse Treatment, 25,* 99–105.

CHAPTER 52

Developmental disabilities

Barbara E. McDermott

Introduction

The US correctional system is vast and includes individuals incarcerated in jails and prisons, as well as those under the supervision of probation and parole. At year-end 2011, almost 7 million offenders were under the supervision of the adult correctional system, with 1 in every 107 adults incarcerated in jails or prisons (Glaze & Parks, 2012). While the purpose of the correctional system is multifaceted, including punishment and removal of the offender from society, one component is rehabilitation. With no offender does this seem more relevant than those with developmental disabilities. Although the research findings are inconsistent, most studies suggest that offenders with developmental delays commit fewer serious offenses yet serve more time in prison than offenders without such delays (MacEachron, 1979; Petersilia, 2000a). Talent and Keldgord (1975) opined, "Less effort has been expended in the United States to rehabilitate the mentally retarded offender than any other group of offenders." In 2000, Petersilia (2000a) noted that 25 years later this situation has remained essentially unchanged. This chapter outlines the progress that has been made in the identification and habilitation of individuals with developmental disabilities in the criminal justice system. Definitions and prevalence rates are discussed, as well as the vulnerabilities individuals with developmental delays present to the criminal justice system. Finally, screening, management, and programs designed to assist individuals with intellectual disabilities acquire skills (habilitation versus rehabilitation) necessary to moderate their vulnerabilities are discussed.

Definition of developmental disability/intellectual disability

Federal law has defined "developmental disability" via the Developmental Disabilities Assistance and Bill of Rights Act of 2000 (42 U.S.C. §§ 15001–15115). The legal standard required for an individual to be designated as having a developmental disorder includes the following:

◆ The disability is attributed to a mental or physical impairment or combination of the two;

◆ The disability manifested before the age of 22;

◆ The disability is likely to continue indefinitely;

◆ The disability results in functional limitations in three or more of the following areas:
   • Self-care,
   • Receptive or expressive language,
   • Mobility,
   • Self-direction,
   • Capacity for independent living,
   • Economic self-sufficiency; and

◆ Individualized support is of a lifelong or extended duration and is individually planned.

Many disorders meet these criteria, including physical disorders such as cerebral palsy and mental health disorders such as autism spectrum disorder. However, according to the Centers for Disease Control and Prevention (1996), intellectual disability is the most common developmental disability and individuals with intellectual disabilities are the most likely (of those with any developmental disability) to present to the criminal justice system. For this reason, persons with intellectual disabilities are the primary focus of this chapter.

The *Diagnostic and Statistical Manual of Mental Disorders*, fifth edition (DSM-5; American Psychiatric Association, 2013) has eliminated the diagnosis of mental retardation, consistent with Rosa's Law (Public Law 111-256), in favor of the diagnosis of intellectual disability. Although the criteria are essentially unchanged, the focus shifted from intelligence to adaptive skills and level of support necessary resulting from skills deficits. According to DSM-5, to receive a diagnosis of intellectual disability, the following criteria must be met:

◆ Deficits in intellectual functions confirmed by clinical assessment and standardized testing (removed the requirement for an IQ below 70);

◆ Deficits in adaptive functioning requiring ongoing support in one or more activities of daily living (removed requirement of deficits in two areas);

◆ Onset during the developmental period (removed onset before age 18, although the text notes that "developmental period" means childhood and adolescence).

The severity is coded based on functioning in three domains: conceptual (problem solving, reasoning ability), social (social and communicative behavior), and practical (self-care). DSM-5 defines four categories of severity—mild, moderate, severe, and profound—based on the extent of deficits in the above domains, noting that adaptive skills deficits dictate the level of support needed and that measured IQs in the lower levels are less accurate.

Prevalence of intellectual disability

Although reported prevalence rates of intellectual disability in the general population vary dependent on the method of assessment and age of the sample, the DSM-5 (American Psychiatric Association, 2013) indicates that the prevalence rate is estimated at about 1% of the population. Larson (2001), using the National Health Interview Survey—Disability Supplement, estimated that approximately 1.5% of noninstitutionalized Americans met criteria for either mental retardation or developmental disability.

The literature reporting the prevalence rates of incarcerated individuals with intellectual disability contains many methodological problems. As with the general population, differences in assessment, definition, and methodology, as well as regional differences, affect prevalence reports. Research has indicated that individuals with intellectual disabilities are overrepresented within the criminal justice system (e.g., Cockram, 1998; Petersilia, 1997; Santamour & West, 1982a), although some authors have found no differences from the general population (Conley et al., 1992; MacEachron, 1979; New York State Commission on Quality of Care for the Mentally Disabled, 1991). Santamour and West (1982a) reported that the rate of adults with intellectual disability in prison ranged from 8% to almost 30%. An estimated 4% to 10% of individuals in prison or jail in California are developmentally disabled (Petersilia, 2000a). However, some reports suggest that the prevalence of individuals with intellectual disability in corrections is comparable to the prevalence in the general population. For example, the New York State Commission on Quality of Care for the Mentally Disabled (1991) reported that 2% of approximately 53,400 inmates were developmentally disabled. Noble and Conley (1992) reported that approximately 14,000 to 20,000 inmates had developmental disabilities, constituting roughly 2% of all inmates in state and federal prisons. They also noted that rates of intellectual disability ranged from 0.5% to almost 20% within state and federal prisons, asserting that the differences are secondary to methods of assessment.

Approximately 89% of all individuals with intellectual disabilities fall within the mild range using the IQ criterion (Ellis & Luckasson, 1985). Consistent with the general population, the majority of inmates with intellectual disabilities are in the mild range (Noble & Conley, 1992). Given the shift in criteria in the DSM-5 from intelligence level to functional deficits, it is unknown whether these figures will change, although it is unlikely. Therefore, the particular vulnerabilities and habilitation issues present in an individual with mild intellectual disabilities are most relevant to those working with individuals with developmental disabilities within the correctional system; offenders with moderate to profound intellectual disabilities are unlikely to remain in the criminal justice system (Conley et al., 1992; Holland et al., 2002; Petrella, 1992).

Vulnerabilities leading to higher prevalence in corrections

Although the literature reflects controversy regarding the prevalence of offenders with intellectual disability in correctional facilities, if such individuals are overrepresented, several factors may explain this disparity. The definitions of intellectual disability and developmental disability require evidence of impairments in adaptive functioning. These impairments can span numerous areas, often resulting in cognitive limitations that affect their decision-making skills, communication skills, social understanding, moral reasoning, and ability to learn from past mistakes (McGee & Menolascino, 1992; Seay, 2006). Deficits in these areas may lead to increased criminal behavior. One such scenario is

when more functional friends or family members manipulate individuals with developmental disabilities into committing criminal acts (Ebert & Long, 2008; Jones, 2007; Linhorst et al., 2002).

Once arrested, offenders with intellectual disability may not understand their rights. For example, studies have shown that people with intellectual disability often do not understand the Miranda warning against self-incrimination (Cloud et al., 2002; Ellis & Luckasson, 1985; Everington & Fulero, 1999; Fulero & Everington, 1995; Petersilia, 2000a). Given this lack of knowledge, an individual with intellectual disability is more likely to waive his or her rights and provide incriminating information, increasing the likelihood of conviction and incarceration. Individuals with intellectual disability are more vulnerable during interrogations because they are more susceptible to suggestion, acquiesce more often, and have a desire to please authority figures (Cloud et al., 2002; Everington & Fulero, 1999; Jones, 2007; Matikka & Vesala, 1997; Pelka, 1997; Petersilia, 1997). These characteristics increase the likelihood of both false and legitimate confessions, increasing the likelihood of conviction.

Santamour and West (1982) proposed that probation is more likely given to individuals with higher intelligence, greater educational attainment, and an adequate work history. If this assertion is accurate, many people with intellectual disability would not be granted probation, as they often are less educated and may not have a stable work history. In a test of this concern, Mason and Murphy (2002) studied a group of 90 probationers in southeast England and found no significant differences in the number of probation violations between these two groups. This study suggests that if Santamour's supposition is accurate, the unwillingness to use probation is based on faulty beliefs about individuals with disabilities.

Impairments in decision making, communication, and moral reasoning, combined with susceptibility to suggestion and willingness to acquiesce, all coupled with a system that may be less inclined to release offenders with intellectual disability, cumulatively affect the number of incarcerated individuals with developmental disabilities. These factors may explain the disparity between the numbers of individuals with intellectual disability in the general population versus the numbers in jails and prisons. These same vulnerabilities lead to predictable problems in the correctional system.

Vulnerability of individuals with intellectual disability after incarceration

Clinical Vignette

Jerry was a 39-year-old who was arrested on a federal fraud charge. He was forced by his more functional brother to file a false claim with the Federal Emergency Management Agency following a flood. Although Jerry recognized that doing so was wrong, he wanted to please his brother and "fit in" with his brother's friends. His attorney expressed concerns about Jerry's judgment and intelligence and requested a competency evaluation. Jerry was described as a "slow learner" and had dropped out of school in the fifth grade. His mother described situations in which Jerry was teased, taken advantage of, and assaulted throughout his childhood. During the evaluation, Jerry became tearful, stating that he was tired of people "messing" with him. He described an incident while incarcerated where other inmates solicited him for oral sex.

Although he was able to resist, he described continued harassment by these individuals. He reported the behavior to the correctional officers but received no assistance. Ultimately, Jerry was "written up" for disruptive behavior when he became angry after continued solicitations.

People with developmental disabilities are 4 to 10 times more likely to be victims of crime than those who do not have disabilities. This trend holds true for persons with developmental disabilities in prison as well (Petersilia, 2000b). Prisoners with intellectual disability are more likely to be exploited, victimized, abused, and injured secondary to cognitive deficits (Ellis & Luckasson, 1985; Giamp & West, 2003; Müller-Isberner & Hodgins, 2000; Petersilia, 1997; Santamour & West, 1982a; Smith et al., 1990; Stavis, 1991; Table 52.1). Petersilia (1997) reported that offenders with intellectual disability housed with the general population are victimized in such ways as having their property stolen, being raped, or being manipulated by other inmates to violate the rules. They have difficulty understanding the rules, which also increases the likelihood of disciplinary action. In *Ruiz v. Estelle* (1980), the court opined, "Mentally retarded persons meet with unremitting hardships in prison. They are slow to adjust to prison life and its requirements, principally because they have almost insurmountable difficulties in comprehending what is expected of them. Not understanding or remembering disciplinary rules, they tend to commit a large number of disciplinary infractions."

Aside from the obvious consequences of such maltreatment (e.g., physical injury, emotional turmoil), there are more subtle consequences. Inmates who are developmentally disabled are likely to resolve conflicts with others by using physical aggression due, in part, to limitations in communication skills (Petersilia, 1997; Smith et al., 1990). Individuals with intellectual disability are more likely to have low frustration tolerance (Day, 1990) and

Table 52.1 Vulnerabilities of offenders with developmental disabilities pretrial and post-conviction

Cognitive limitations
- Mask their disability in order to understand more
- Difficulty understanding the adversarial nature of the criminal justice system
- Difficulty understanding Miranda warning and pleas
- Difficulty understanding and following rules

Adaptive skills deficits
- Difficulty following rules and routines
- More hygiene infractions
- Less likelihood of parole

Impaired social understanding
- Eager to please, may be more vulnerable to interrogations
- May interpret the actions of police officers as protective
- Vulnerable to manipulation and victimization
- May resolve conflicts with aggression

poor self-control (Benson, 1994; Cullen, 1993), increasing the likelihood of more disciplinary problems. Smith and colleagues (1990) found that youthful inmates who were mentally retarded received approximately three times as many disciplinary reports for noncompliant behavior and hygiene offenses and assaulted other inmates or correctional staff more than twice as often as other inmates. As a result of such disciplinary problems, inmates with intellectual disability may serve longer prison sentences, be denied parole, or be transferred to a more secure prison (Butwell et al., 2000; Ellis & Luckasson, 1985; Giamp & West, 2003; Petersilia, 1997; Santamour & West, 1982; Stavis, 1991). In *Ruiz v. Estelle* (1980), the court noted that

> It is common for mentally retarded inmates in TDC [Texas Department of Corrections] to serve longer sentences than inmates not fitting this category. Several reasons are evident. As previously noted, retarded inmates are more likely to have poor disciplinary records than their peers, which disqualify the former for early parole. They are frequently unable to succeed in institutional programs whose completion would increase their chances for parole, and they are also unlikely to be able to present well-defined employment and residential plans to the Parole Board.

Assessment procedures

The International Association for Correctional and Forensic Psychology has published standards for psychological services provided in jails, prisons, and other correctional facilities (2010). These standards include assessment of mental illness and cognitive function for each inmate at reception screening. The standards further state that all inmates receiving sentences of longer than one year be administered a "standard psychological evaluation within one month of admission," although they indicate such an evaluation may include group-administered intelligence assessments. Inmates requiring further assessment should be evaluated within two weeks of the initial assessment. While these standards are applicable to both jails and prisons, Scheyett (2009) found that in North Carolina, only 6% of surveyed jails used screening instruments for intellectual/developmental disabilities, suggesting that reception screening is less comprehensive in these shorter-term facilities. In contrast, most prison systems use reception and assessment procedures to identify any circumstance that would require specialized housing for the incoming inmate. During this classification process, some prisons attempt to identify offenders with intellectual disabilities. The National Commission on Correctional Health Care prison standards (2008) suggests that all inmates receive a brief intellectual assessment on admission. Megargee (2013) suggests either the Beta-III (Kellogg & Morton, 1999) or the General Ability Measure for Adults (Naglieri & Bardos, 1997) as screening tools for intelligence assessment, with follow-up using the Wechsler Adult Intelligence Scale (4th edition, 2008) when necessary. While Megargee's recommendations are ideal, many prisons administer screening assessments in groups, without a follow-up comprehensive assessment, reducing the validity of the results. MacEachron (1979) found that the prevalence of offenders with intellectual disability dropped significantly when individual (rather than group) assessments of intelligence were administered. McGee and Menolascino (1992) argue that even screening assessments should be administered individually and only by professionals trained in such administration.

These assessments are used primarily as a method for identifying inmates with deficits. Critical in formulating an individualized habilitation plan is a more comprehensive assessment that includes both strengths and deficit areas that may be most amenable to habilitation. Many jurisdictions use their own assessments to identify functional deficits (e.g., California, North Carolina); however, rarely are these assessments normed or standardized. The American Association on Intellectual and Developmental Disabilities has published a comprehensive assessment called the Supports Intensity Scale (SIS; Tassé et al., 2005). The SIS is designed to identify deficits in 57 life activities, 15 medical conditions, and 13 problem behaviors. Research has indicated that the SIS possesses good interrater reliability, especially if the raters are trained (Thompson et al., 2008).

Habilitation issues

The management of inmates with developmental disabilities has presented correctional systems with significant problems. One controversy has been whether inmates with developmental disabilities should be housed in the general prison population. Those in favor of housing with the general prison population adhere to the principal of normalization, suggesting that individuals with intellectual disability should be treated like others as much as possible (Santamour & West, 1982a). Critics argue that normalization does not take into account the disadvantages inmates with intellectual disabilities face. According to Petersilia (1997), "The emerging consensus within the profession seems to be that there are highly unique aspects to the correctional environment and that the normalization goals for the mentally retarded should not fully apply in this setting." Her statement suggests that specialized units may be more appropriate for such individuals.

Although court cases such as *Ruiz v. Estelle* (1980) established that individuals with intellectual or developmental disabilities have the right to treatment, Hall (1992) estimated that fewer than 10% of inmates with such deficits receive specialized services. Unlike programs for offenders with mental illness, the goals of specialized programs for offenders with developmental disabilities are not remediation of their disability. The goal of most programs is education, training, and skills enhancement tailored to the specific needs of the inmate. As with any other disorder, the diagnosis of intellectual disability provides no information about the needs of the specific individual. For these reasons, assessment is a critical component in any specialized program. Programs for offenders with intellectual disability generally focus on improving the functioning and adaptation of the inmate while incarcerated and upon release (Santamour, 1987). The vulnerabilities outlined in the previous sections lead to logical interventions and include skills training, educational/vocational habilitation, and counseling/treatment specific to the needs of each offender.

Skills training

Skills training for the offender with intellectual disability can encompass a wide variety of areas. The assessment process will help determine the areas that are most important for each individual, but they may include social skills training or training in areas of adaptive functioning. Corrigan (1991) conducted a meta-analysis of social skills training programs and found that individuals with developmental disabilities evidenced the greatest improvement. However, generalization of skills learned was lowest for this group. Social skills training was least effective for the offender group. Interestingly, although the offenders acquired the requisite skills, these skills did not translate into behavior change. This study suggests that social skills training may improve institutional behavior, at least with those individuals with developmental disabilities, but may not generalize to other settings.

Vocational training

Vocational training is an important aspect of a comprehensive program to treat inmates with developmental disabilities for several reasons. It teaches inmates the skills and information necessary to perform a job upon release and allows the inmate to work in a sheltered environment before reentry into the community (Santamour & West, 1982b). It also provides inmates with developmental disabilities the opportunity to engage in meaningful, productive work that decreases behavioral issues and increases feelings of self-worth (Shivley, 2004).

Treatment/anger management

Anger management is an important component in a treatment program for prisoners with intellectual disability (Hall, 1992). As previously noted, self-control and aggression can be a problem for some inmates (Shivley, 2004). Lack of self-control in a prison environment can lead to negative consequences such as increased disciplinary reports (Smith et al., 1990). The lack of communication and interpersonal skills can lead to frustration and an increased likelihood of conflict (Smith et al., 1990). Benson (1994) modified an anger management program for use with adults with intellectual disabilities. Although this program was not developed specifically for offenders, it may be useful in an overall habilitation program that includes individualized treatment. As Benson points out, self-control training may generalize more easily from one situation to another and can reduce incidents of aggression while incarcerated and enable the inmate to control his or her anger in the community.

Summary

The habilitation of individuals with developmental disabilities in the correctional system can no longer be ignored. While Hall (1992) noted that correctional facilities should not be viewed as treatment facilities, such institutions can no longer be "deliberately indifferent" to the needs of these offenders. Inmates with developmental delays may be more easily led, suggestible, and dependent. Lower levels of comprehension and poor adaptive skills can lead to more rule infractions and disciplinary action, leading to a decreased likelihood for parole. Research has indicated that these offenders serve more time for the same crime than do offenders without developmental disabilities (Petersilia, 2000a).

Opinions are mixed on whether appropriate services for such individuals should be provided on specialized units. Proponents of this approach cite the vulnerabilities of these offenders. However, all agree that specialized services must include appropriate assessment that takes into account culture and individualized approaches to habilitation. It cannot be presumed that services designed for inmates with mental illness will be appropriate for inmates with developmental disabilities.

Little research has been conducted on the efficacy of specialized services for offenders with developmental disabilities. As such, correctional facilities must take guidance from research based on nonoffender samples. An active collaboration between departments of corrections and agencies that provide services for individuals with developmental disabilities can enhance service delivery and improve the integration of the offender into the community. As courts continue to protect the rights of offenders with developmental disabilities, correctional facilities must explore creative ways to deliver appropriate services to these disadvantaged individuals.

References

American Psychiatric Association (2013). *Diagnostic and statistical manual of mental disorders* (5th ed.) Washington, DC: American Psychiatric Publishing.

Americans with Disabilities Act of 1990, 42 U.S.C. §§ 12101–12213.

Benson, B. A. (1994). Anger management training: a self-control programme for persons with mild mental retardation. In N. Bouras (Ed.), *Mental health in mental retardation: recent advances and practices* (pp. 224–232). New York: Cambridge University Press.

Butwell, M., Jamieson, E., Leese, M., & Taylor, P. (2000). Trends in special (high security) hospitals 2: Residency and discharge episodes, 1986-1995. *British Journal of Psychiatry, 176*, 260–265.

Centers for Disease Control and Prevention (1996). State-specific rates of mental retardation—United States, 1993. *Morbidity and Mortality Weekly Report, 45*, 61–65, 1996. Available at: http://www.cdc.gov/mmwr/preview/mmwrhtml/00040023.htm. (Accessed December 16, 2013.)

Clark v State of California, United States District Court of Northern California, No. C96-1486 FMS, 1998.

Cloud, M., Shepherd, G. B., Barkoff, A., & Shur, J. V. (2002). Words without meaning: the constitution, confessions, and mentally retarded suspects. *University of Chicago Law Review, 69*, 495–624.

Cockram, J., Jackson, R., & Underwood, R. (1998). People with an intellectual disability and the criminal justice system: the family perspective. *Journal of Intellectual & Developmental Disability, 23*, 41–56.

Conley, R. W., Luckasson, R., & Bouthilet, G. N. (1992). *The criminal justice system and mental retardation*. Baltimore, MD: Paul H. Brookes Publishing.

Corrigan, P. W. (1991). Social skills training in adult psychiatric populations: a meta-analysis. *Journal of Behavior Therapy and Experimental Psychiatry, 22*, 203–210.

Cullen, C. (1993). The treatment of people with learning disabilities who offend. In K. Howells & C. R. Hollin (Eds.), *Clinical approaches to the mentally disordered offender* (pp. 145–162). Chichester, West Sussex, UK: John Wiley & Sons Ltd.

Day, K. (1990). Mental retardation: clinical aspects and management. In R. Bluglass & P. Bowden (Eds.), *Principles and practice of forensic psychiatry* (pp. 399–418). Edinburgh, UK: Churchill Livingstone.

Developmental Disabilities Assistance and Bill of Rights Act of 2000, 42 U.S.C. §§ 15001–15115.

Ebert, R. S., & Long, J. S. (2008). Mental retardation and the criminal justice system: Forensic issues. In H. V. Hall (Ed.), *Forensic psychology and neuropsychology for criminal and civil cases* (pp. 375–392). Boca Raton, FL: CRC Press.

Ellis, J. W., & Luckasson, R. A. (1985). Mentally retarded criminal defendants. *The George Washington Law Review, 53*, 414–493.

Everington, C., & Fulero, S. M. (1999). Competence to confess: measuring understanding and suggestibility of defendants with mental retardation. *Mental Retardation, 37*, 212–220.

Fulero, S. M., & Everington, C. (1995). Assessing competency to waive Miranda rights in defendants with mental retardation. *Law and Human Behavior, 19*, 533–543.

Giamp, J. S., & West, M. E. (2003). Delivering psychological services to incarcerated men with developmental disabilities. In B. K. Schwartz (Ed.), *Correctional psychology: practice, programming, and administration* (pp. 8.1–8.29). Kingston, NJ: Civic Research Institute.

Glaze, L. E., & Parks, E. (2012). Correctional populations in the United States, 2011. NCJ 239972, 1–9.

Hall, J. N. (1992). Correctional services for inmates with mental retardation. In R.W. Conley, R. Luckasson, & G. N. Bouthilet (Eds.), *The criminal justice system and mental retardation: defendants and victims* (pp. 167–190). Baltimore, MD: Paul H. Brookes Publishing.

Holland, A. J., Clare, I. C. H., & Mukhopadhyay, T. (2002). Prevalence of "criminal offending" by men and women with intellectual disability and the characteristics of the "offenders": Implications for research and service development. *Journal of Intellectual Disability Research, 46*, 6–20.

International Association for Correctional and Forensic Psychology (2010). Standards for psychology services in jails, prisons, correctional facilities, and agencies. *Criminal Justice and Behavior, 37*, 749–808.

Jones, J. (2007). Persons with intellectual disabilities in the criminal justice system: Review of issues. *International Journal of Offender Therapy and Comparative Criminology, 51*, 723–733.

Kellogg, C. E., & Morton, N. W. (1999). *Beta III manual*. San Antonio, TX: The Psychological Corporation.

Larson, S. A., Lakin, K. C., Anderson, L., Kwak, L., Lee, J. H., & Anderson, D. (2001). Prevalence of mental retardation and developmental disabilities: Evidence from the National Health Interview Survey disability supplement. *American Journal on Mental Retardation, 106*, 231–252.

Linhorst, D. M., Bennett L., & McCutchen, T. (2002). Development and implementation of a program for offenders with developmental disabilities. *Mental Retardation, 40*, 41–50.

MacEachron, A. E. (1979). Mentally retarded offenders: prevalence and characteristics. *American Journal of Mental Deficiency, 84*, 165–176.

Mason, J., & Murphy, G. (2002). Intellectual disability amongst people on probation: prevalence and outcome. *Journal of Intellectual Disability Research, 46*, 230–238.

Matikka, L. M., & Vesala, H. T. (1997). Acquiescence in quality-of-life interviews with adults who have mental retardation. *Mental Retardation, 35*, 75–82.

McGee, J. J., & Menolascino, F. J. (1992). The evaluation of defendants with mental retardation in the criminal justice system. In R.W. Conley, R. Luckasson, & G. N. Bouthilet (Eds.), *The criminal justice system and mental retardation: defendants and victims* (pp. 55–77). Baltimore, MD: Paul H. Brookes Publishing.

Megargee, E. I. (2013). Psychological assessment in correctional settings. In J. R. Graham & J. A. Naglieri (Eds.), *Handbook of psychology, Volume 10: Assessment psychology* (pp. 394–424). Hoboken, NJ: John Wiley and Sons.

Müller-Isberner, R., & Hodgins, S. (2000). Evidence-based treatment for mentally disordered offenders. In S. Hodgins and R. Müller-Isberner (Eds.), *Violence, crime and mentally disordered offenders* (pp. 7–38). Chichester, West Sussex, UK: John Wiley & Sons Ltd.

Naglieri, J. A., & Bardos, A. (1997). *GAMA (General Ability Measure for Adults) manual*. Minneapolis, MN: Pearson.

National Commission on Correctional Health Care (2008). Standards for health services in prisons.

New York State Commission on Quality of Care for the Mentally Disabled (1992). Inmates with developmental disabilities in NYS correctional facilities, March 1991. Available at: http://www.justicecenter.ny.gov/sites/default/files/archivereports/Publications/00067.pdf. (Accessed December 16, 2013.)

Noble, J. H., & Conley, R. W. (1992). Toward an epidemiology of relevant attributes. In R. W. Conley, R. Luckasson, & G. N. Bouthilet (Eds.), *The criminal justice system and mental retardation: defendants and victims* (pp. 17–53). Baltimore, MD: Paul H. Brookes Publishing.

Pelka, F. (1997). Unequal justice: preserving the rights of the mentally retarded in the criminal justice system. *Humanist, 57,* 28–32.

Pennsylvania Department of Corrections v Yeskey, 524 U.S. 206 (1998).

Petersilia, J. (1997). Justice for all? Offenders with mental retardation and the California corrections system. *The Prison Journal, 77,* 358–381.

Petersilia, J. (2000a). *Doing justice? Criminal offenders with developmental disabilities.* California Policy Research Center Brief, Vol. 12, No. 4, University of California.

Petersilia, J. (2000b). Invisible victims: violence against persons with developmental disabilities. *Human Rights, 27,* 9–13.

Petrella, R. C. (1992). Defendants with mental retardation in the forensic services system. In R. W. Conley, R. Luckasson, & G. N. Bouthilet (Eds.), *The criminal justice system and mental retardation: defendants and victims* (pp. 79–96). Baltimore, MD: Paul H. Brookes Publishing.

Revised Beta Examination—Second Edition (Revised Beta-II) (1974). San Antonio, TX: Psychological Corporation.

Rosa's Law. Public Law 111-256, October 5, 2010.

Ruiz v Estelle, 503 F. Supp. 1265, (S.D. Tex), cert denied, 103 Ct 1438, 1980.

Santamour, M. B. (1987). The offender with mental retardation. *The Prison Journal, 66,* 3–18.

Santamour, M. B., & West, B. (1982a). The mentally retarded offender: presentation of the facts and a discussion of issues. In M. B. Santamour & P. S. Watson (Eds.), *The retarded offender* (pp. 7–36). New York: Praeger Publishers.

Santamour, M. B., & West, B. (1982b). Retarded offenders: Habilitative program development. In M. B. Santamour & P. S. Watson

(Eds.), *The retarded offender* (pp. 272–296). New York: Praeger Publishers.

Scheyett, A., Vaughn, J., Taylor, M., & Parish, S. (2009). Are we there yet? Screening processes for intellectual and developmental disabilities in jail settings. *Intellectual and Developmental Disabilities, 47,* 13–23.

Seay, O. J. (2006). Evaluating mental retardation for forensic purposes. *Applied Psychology in Criminal Justice, 2,* 52–81.

Shively, R. (2004). Treating offenders with mental retardation and developmental disabilities. *Corrections Today, 66,* 84–87.

Smith, C., Algozzine, B., Schmid, R. E., & Hennly, T. (1990). Prison adjustment of youthful inmates with mental retardation. *Mental Retardation, 28,* 177–181.

Stavis, P. F. (1991). Doing justice? The criminal justice system and persons with mental retardation. *New York State Commission on Quality of Care for the Mentally Disabled, Quality of Care Newsletter,* Issue 47, January-February.

Talent, A., & Keldgord, R. (1975). The mentally retarded probationer. *Federal Probation, 39,* 39–46.

Tassé, M. J., Schalock, R., Thompson, J. R., & Wehmeyer, M. (2005). *Guidelines for interviewing people with disabilities: Support Intensity Scale.* Washington, DC, AAMR.

Thompson, J. R., Tassé, M. J., & McLaughlin, C. A. (2008). Interrater reliability of the Supports Intensity Scale (SIS). *American Journal of Mental Retardation, 113,* 231–237.

Wechsler, D. (2008). *WAIS-4 Administration and Scoring Manual.* San Antonio, TX: Psychological Corporation.

CHAPTER 53

Traumatic brain injury

Pamela M. Diamond

Introduction

During the past decade, traumatic brain injury (TBI) has become a frequent topic in the media. The wars in Iraq and Afghanistan have brought home the realities of these injuries. Soldiers returning from war with nonfatal blast injuries have found adjustment to their previous lives to be very challenging and sometimes impossible. These men and women began to give a face to a problem previously unrecognized by the average person. Many of those who suffered from TBI in the war zones came home with no obvious injuries; their TBI was diagnosed as "mild" based on their reactions to the initial insult. Yet many with these "mild" injuries found they could no longer remember things they used to. They had trouble paying attention. They became easily irritated and sometimes struck out at those they loved. Their experiences helped to bring attention to what has been called the "invisible epidemic" of mild TBI.

Attention soon shifted to additional risks for this new sort of TBI that seemed to have the potential to disrupt a person's life disproportionately to the perceived injury. Athletes who experienced frequent injuries while engaging in football, hockey, or boxing began to share experiences similar to those identified by the returning soldiers. Parents and coaches became more concerned about the risks to children playing sports. New rules and regulations were developed to minimize the risk to those budding athletes while allowing them to continue to develop athletic skills. The National Football League was successfully sued by a group of retired players for not providing adequate protections.

It has been a decade of expanding awareness, increased research, and growing concern about TBI of all severity levels. From the shooting and long-term recovery efforts of Senator Gabrielle Giffords to the middle school football player who found himself dazed and dizzy after an unexpected hit during a game, TBI is no longer hidden from the general public. Consistent with this increased attention, researchers and policy makers have made strides toward greater understanding of the risks of TBI, the scope and complexity of the symptom profiles seen after TBI, and the types of treatments that optimize recovery. It has also been a time of increasing awareness of subgroups at high risk of TBI and TBI-related problems. Residents of prisons and jails are among those high-risk groups. This chapter reviews the prevalence of TBI in correctional settings; its impact on co-occurring mental illness and substance use; and opportunities to recognize, intervene, and treat patients with TBI.

Prevalence of traumatic brain injury in prisons—current research

TBI mortality and morbidity rates in the community are greater for males than females at all ages except for children age 4 and younger; incidence rates peak between ages 15 and 24 and at 65 years and above (Thurman et al., 1999). In general, TBI incidence is higher among low-income groups, and blacks are more likely to experience firearm-related head injury than are other populations in the United States (Hanks et al., 2003; Turkstra et al., 2003). Violence is one of the leading causes of TBI among young males (Thurman et al., 1999). Substance abuse also plays an important part in incidence and rehabilitation (Corrigan, 1995; Parry-Jones et al., 2006).

Because the demonstrated behavioral and contextual risk factors for TBI overlap with risk factors for incarceration, elevated prevalence of TBI is expected in prisoner populations. Prisoners are likely to have used both legal and illegal substances and to have engaged in activities that put them at risk of both unintentional and intentional injury. They are also very likely to be male and black (Carson & Golinelli, 2013). Inmate records contain many stories of bar fights, car wrecks, gang violence, and domestic abuse, more often than not accompanied by substance use. Most prisoners also come from financially impoverished situations, where mild to moderate injuries may have been undertreated.

Early in this century, the Centers for Disease Control and Prevention (CDC) began an initiative to determine the prevalence of TBI among institutionalized populations including those in prisons and jails. Previous research indicated that rates of TBI among those incarcerated ranged from 25 percent to 87 percent compared to about 8.5 percent in the general population (Wald et al., 2014). These early studies were criticized, however, for multiple reasons, including small samples, specialized groups (e.g., death row inmates, substance abusers), single gender, noncomparable facilities, and disparate countries. Perhaps more problematic, studies were done without standardization of TBI definition or measurement (Diamond et al., 2007). These limitations likely led to the wide range of estimates and made it difficult to generalize beyond the individual study.

A recent metaanalysis focused on 20 studies that reported lifetime TBI among incarcerated adults. Each study had clear definitions of TBI and described their assessment methods. The rate of TBI was approximately 60 percent with a range of ±12 percent. The rate of TBI with loss of consciousness (LOC) was somewhat lower at approximately 50 percent ±10 percent (Shiroma et al., 2010). These estimates are consistent with the findings of a CDC-funded epidemiological study conducted in the South Carolina prison system using a validated instrument to assess TBI among a stratified sample of inmates representative of the prison population. Rates in that study ranged from 50 percent to 70 percent depending on gender and release status (eligible for release versus not eligible). When restricted to TBI with LOC, the rates for inmates eligible for release were between

42 percent and 50 percent. Most inmates reported a history of multiple TBIs over their lifetime, with average age at first TBI of approximately 16 years. Ongoing symptoms related to TBI were commonly reported and covaried with the severity of the injury experience (Ferguson et al., 2012).

Cognitive dysfunction is an important factor linking TBI with many of the conditions already known to be associated with an increased risk of incarceration, poor prison adjustment, and recidivism. The following sections review and highlight what is known about some of the complex linkages between and among substance abuse, mental illness, TBI, and cognitive dysfunction. The goal is to clarify why TBI is an important factor for correctional management and to identify some common ground with other conditions currently addressed in most prison systems that may facilitate the development of TBI-specific enhancements to existing programming efforts.

Overview of symptoms and sequelae

TBI may result in cognitive, motor, or emotional problems that can impact an individual's ability to deal with the world around them. These sequelae vary from minor memory lapses to complete inability to speak or navigate without help. The extent and nature of the sequelae of TBI are generally associated with both the severity of the blow to the head and the location of the injury (Silver et al., 2005). Those who experience the most severe injuries often do not survive. Others are confined to rehabilitation facilities and require lifelong care (Thurman et al., 1999). There is another large group of people who have had a TBI associated with a more diffuse symptom profile; prisoners are more likely to be in this group. Symptoms may be temporary, delayed, or recurrent. They may affect many areas of cognition and behavior. Family, friends, and even the individual with the injury may not be aware of the linkage between what may have been perceived as a minor blow to the head and the difficulties they are having with attention, motor skills, impulse control, and so forth (Centers for Disease Control and Prevention, 2009; Langlois et al., 2005). These are the sorts of injuries that can place a person at increased risk of incarceration, homelessness, and other adverse outcomes. For those already incarcerated, many of these deficits can have a profound effect on their ability to adjust to the day-to-day demands of living in a prison environment.

The high rate of TBI in prison populations is a significant problem for correctional management because of the cognitive and behavioral sequelae of TBI, such as aggression and violence, and because of the common co-occurrence of TBI with alcohol or substance abuse. These sequelae and comorbidities may negatively impact offenders' ability to function within the prison and to reintegrate successfully into the community after release. Moreover, the sheer number of prisoners potentially affected by TBI is of concern, since the number of adults incarcerated just in US state and federal prisons continues to range around 1.5 million (Carson & Golinelli, 2013). As large numbers of people continue to be incarcerated—and as more inmates are released into the community—understanding and addressing the health needs of this diverse population becomes increasingly important for health and health care in both correctional and community settings (National Commission on Correctional Health Care, 2002).

Traumatic brain injury and mental health

Individuals who survive moderate to severe head injuries often deal with subsequent changes in cognition, motor ability, mood, and behavior. Irritability and aggression may result from TBI, and evidence suggests that frequency and/or severity of aggression may increase rather than decrease over time after a head injury (Brooks et al., 1986; Hall et al., 1994). There is suggestive evidence that TBI may play a role in violent crime by reducing impulse control and increasing aggressive tendencies. Studies have consistently indicated that the likelihood of arrest increases post-TBI and that the prevalence of head injury is higher among individuals incarcerated for violent crimes (Brewer-Smyth et al., 2004; Cohen et al., 1999; Miller, 1999). These findings may be linked to the changes in psychological functioning often seen in victims of TBI, such as increased verbal and physical aggression, low tolerance for frustration, and poor impulse control (Miller, 1999).

Depression is the mental disorder most commonly found following TBI. Studies have used structured diagnostic instruments and self-report scales; they have taken their measures at differing times after the injury; and they have looked at both severe and mild TBI. Consistently, these studies have found rates of depression among those with TBI significantly higher than those of the general public (Deb et al., 1999; Mooney & Speed, 2001; Rapoport et al., 2003; Seel et al., 2003; Seel & Kreutzer, 2003). Furthermore, those with TBI who experience post-injury depression tend to have poorer outcomes and more difficulty with day-to-day functioning. The findings of these studies are also consistent with the conclusions of a systematic review of studies of depression and TBI (Rosenthal, Christensen, & Ross, 1998). While depression seems to be the most commonly noted mental disorder following TBI, studies also have identified elevated rates of comorbid anxiety disorders (Mooney & Speed, 2001) and personality disorders due to head trauma (Hibbard et al., 2000). Overall, findings seem to consistently show that those who experience even mild TBI are at high risk for mood and behavioral disorders post-injury, which impedes progress toward recovery and may increase the risk of a repeat TBI resulting from their aggressive behavior, incarceration, and other problems with impulse control.

Traumatic brain injury and substance abuse

The relationship between TBI and substance abuse is complex. Evidence suggests that persons with TBI are more likely to have alcohol or substance abuse problems (Moore et al., 1994; Silver et al., 2001). Studies also suggest that one third to one half of persons presenting to hospitals with TBI were alcohol intoxicated at the time of their injury, and roughly the same proportions indicated general misuse of alcohol prior to the injurious incident (Corrigan, 1995; Parry-Jones et al., 2006). In a large study of 550 voluntary participants in substance abuse treatment, 40 percent reported a history of TBI. Those with TBI also had elevated rates of concomitant anxiety and depressive disorders and more severe substance use disorders (Felde et al., 2006). Those in integrated treatment for substance abuse and mental disorder (dually diagnosed) appear to have an even higher rate of TBI. In a study published in 2008, Corrigan (Corrigan & Deutschle, Jr., 2008) found that 72 percent of the patients in a dual-diagnosis program had a history of TBI. Further, those individuals diagnosed with substance abuse, mental disorder, and TBI had poorer current functioning, were more likely to have a personality disorder, and initiated their substance use at an earlier age.

Additionally, in most studies, history of alcohol or illicit substance use was associated with poorer neurological, medical, neuropsychological, and functional outcomes (Corrigan, 1995; Parry-Jones et al., 2006). It has been suggested that TBI history may affect the ability of those who are incarcerated to recover from substance abuse, to successfully reintegrate into the community, and to avoid recidivism (Corrigan, 1995; US DHHS, 1998; Valliant et al., 2003). Identifying and understanding TBI-related problems in persons with substance abuse issues may help to guide treatment efforts (US DHHS, 1998).

Screening for traumatic brain injury

Several screening instruments for TBI have been developed and validated for use in corrections over the past decade. These instruments include the Traumatic Brain Injury Questionnaire (TBIQ; Diamond et al., 2007), the Traumatic Brain Injury Identification (Bogner & Corrigan, 2009) tool, and the Brain Injury Screening Questionnaire (BISQ; Cantor et al., 2004). All assess lifetime TBI, provide some indication of severity, allow for reporting multiple injuries, and differentiate among those injuries associated with LOC and/or posttraumatic amnesia. They differ somewhat in their scoring and reporting; however, all have been assessed psychometrically. Although there are generally benefits associated with short screening instruments, the literature has been consistent in finding that tools that ask only one or two questions about head injury embedded in a larger self-report or interview instrument badly underestimate the prevalence of TBI. Diamond and colleagues (2007) compared results from the TBIQ, an interview-based instrument, to inmate responses to an item asking about head injury on a standard screening tool used in the federal prison system. Only 19 percent of the inmates who reported a TBI on the TBIQ had responded positively to the embedded screening question. The Health Resources Services Administration (HRSA; 2006) provides links to a wide range of TBI screening instruments that have been adapted for use in settings that range from preschools to prisons. There are also several new instruments being developed for use with returning military personnel that are likely to add to the choices available for a screening program in a jail or prison system.

Screening for TBI among inmate populations is not routinely done in most correctional systems despite the availability of validated tools. HRSA has supported pilot screening programs in different states over the past several years. These included a project in Minnesota that screened approximately 1000 inmates for TBI using the TBIQ and a project in Wyoming that used the BISQ. These studies found prevalence rates consistent with the studies already mentioned (Brain Injury Association of Wyoming, 2008; Wald et al., 2014). One of the concerns expressed by prison administrators when asked about the feasibility of routine screening for TBI in their facility is the cost associated with both the screening and the subsequent treatment programs. Others have raised concerns about routine screening because of the lack of tested, specific, and effective treatments (Vanderploeg & Belanger, 2013). Given that the current epidemiological evidence points to high rates of TBI and related symptoms among prison populations (i.e.,

60 percent or greater), perhaps it would be best to focus on developing and/or modifying programs routinely provided in prisons to better meet the needs of those with concomitant cognitive deficits regardless of origin.

Programs and services for traumatic brain injury–related symptoms

Much of the research on TBI rehabilitation is focused on the more severe forms of TBI and may not be applicable to those with milder forms, especially those housed in secure prison facilities. The cognitive deficits associated with TBI, regardless of etiology, are similar to those of many mental and substance use disorders. They often affect an individual's ability to process information, attend to incoming messages, and interact with others. Perhaps it would be helpful to adapt current programs based on our knowledge of the likely deficits shared by those with TBI, mental illness, and substance abuse. Current approaches to substance abuse treatment are often based on cognitive behavior theory and use a standard protocol developed for use with individuals who do not have impaired cognitive processes. In fact, these methods rely heavily on the person's ability to "think" about his or her condition and develop solutions. For example, most inmates who might benefit from substance abuse treatment have impaired cognitive functioning. Clinicians may use information about the nature of these deficits in order to modify protocols and, in turn, more effectively meet the needs of these individuals. Simple changes (e.g., shorter sessions, more repetition, and simple directions) could make a big difference in enhancing treatment effectiveness. Such changes might also reduce premature treatment dropout through enhanced engagement. These modifications should be carefully designed and piloted prior to widespread use. Currently, however, nothing in the published literature describes prison-based programs specifically designed or modified for offenders with mild TBI and its related symptoms. Such programs may exist in individual settings; it still remains to validate and disseminate such initiatives.

In addition to the development of programs designed to directly help offenders deal more effectively with cognitive deficits in their day-to-day lives, educational interventions are likely to help reduce the impact of these symptoms on the prison environment. Because individuals who suffer from these cognitive deficits tend to follow directions poorly and wander off task, staff may interpret these behaviors as oppositional and react with anger and/or accuse the person of "breaking the rules." In fact, these individuals may not be able to appropriately process the multistep or affect-laden information presented to them. Training staff to be sensitive to these impairments may lead to more responsive service systems and fewer incidents of misunderstanding between staff and the persons they manage. Educational interventions designed to raise awareness for TBI and its symptoms have been developed for law enforcement and for corrections, but they are not yet widely disseminated. They also tend to focus on the more severe symptoms associated with moderate to severe TBI rather than the more diffuse symptom pattern found among those with mild TBI. This is an area where interventions could be designed and implemented in prisons without great cost, and the results could potentially be very positive for the system and its inmates.

Summary

Recent studies have confirmed a 50 percent to 60 percent prevalence of TBI among prisoners. Most prisoners have experienced multiple injuries and had their first TBI in their mid-teens. Routine screening for TBI is rarely done in these settings despite the availability of tested instruments. The cognitive deficits associated with mild to moderate TBI are often indistinguishable from those associated with many mental illnesses and substance abuse. Etiology is difficult to establish; nevertheless, the common symptom patterns often make adjustment to jail or prison difficult. Educational interventions designed to improve staff knowledge of the prevalence of TBI and frequent symptom patterns are important first steps. Training staff to modify their behavior and facilitate communication with symptomatic inmates may reduce episodes of misunderstanding and potential aggression. Similarly, current programming may be modified to accommodate the cognitive deficits of inmates with TBI and other disorders.

References

Bogner, J., & Corrigan, J. D. (2009). Reliability and predictive validity of the Ohio State University TBI identification method with prisoners. *Journal of Head Trauma Rehabilitation*, 24(4), 279–291.

Brain Injury Association of Wyoming (2008). *Study of undiagnosed brain injuries in Wyoming's prison population*. The Wyoming Department of Health Division of Developmental Disabilities, Wyoming. Accessed February 18, 2014, at: http://www.wybia.org/documents/document_display-DocID-Prison%20study%20final.pdf.cfm

Brewer-Smyth, K., Burgess, A. W., & Shults, J. (2004). Physical and sexual abuse, salivary cortisol, and neurologic correlates of violent criminal behavior in female prison inmates. *Biological Psychiatry*, 55, 21–31.

Brooks, N., Campsie, L., Symington, C., Beattie, A., & McKinlay, W. (1986). The five-year outcome of severe blunt head injury: A relative's view. *Journal of Neurology, Neurosurgery and Psychiatry*, 49, 764–770.

Cantor, J. B., Gordon, W. A., Schwartz, M. E., Charatz, H. J., Ashman, T. A., & Abramowitz, S. (2004). Child and parent responses to a brain injury screening questionnaire. *Archives of Physical Medicine and Rehabilitation*, 85(4 Suppl 2), S54–S60.

Carson, E., & Golinelli, D. (2013). *Prisoners in 2012: Trends in admissions and releases, 1991–2012*. Bureau of Justice Statistics, NCJ243920.

Centers for Disease Control and Prevention (2009). *Traumatic brain injury (TBI): Topic home*. Accessed February 18, 2014, at: http://www.cdc.gov/TraumaticBrainInjury/index.html

Cohen, R. A., Rosenbaum, A., Kane, R. L., Warnken, W. J., & Benjamin, S. (1999). Neuropsychological correlates of domestic violence. *Violence and Victims*, 14(4), 397–411.

Corrigan, J. D. (1995). Substance abuse as a mediating factor in outcome from traumatic brain injury. *Archives of Physical Medicine and Rehabilitation*, 76(4), 302–309.

Corrigan, J. D., & Deutschle, J. J., Jr. (2008). The presence and impact of traumatic brain injury among clients in treatment for co-occurring mental illness and substance abuse. *Brain Injury*, 22(3), 223–231.

Deb, S., Lyons, I., Ali, I., & McCarthy, G. (1999). Rate of psychiatric illness 1 year after traumatic brain injury. *American Journal of Psychiatry*, 156, 374–378.

Diamond, P. M., Harzke, A. J., Magaletta, P. R., Cummins, A. G., & Frankowski, R. (2007). Screening for traumatic brain injury in an offender sample: A first look at the reliability and validity of the Traumatic Brain Injury Questionnaire. *Journal of Head Trauma Rehabilitation*, 22(6), 330–338.

Felde, A. B., Westermeyer, J., & Thuras, P. (2006). Co-morbid traumatic brain injury and substance use disorder: Childhood predictors and adult correlates. *Brain Injury*, 20(1), 41–49.

Ferguson, P. L., Pickelsimer, E. E., Corrigan, J. D., Bogner, J. A., & Wald, M. (2012). Prevalence of traumatic brain injury among prisoners in South Carolina. *Journal of Head Trauma Rehabilitation*, 27(3), E11–E20.

Hall, K., Karzmark, P., Stevens, M., Englander, J., O'Hare, P., & Wright, J. (1994). Family stressors in traumatic brain injury: A two-year follow-up. *Archives of Physical Medicine and Rehabilitation*, 75, 876–884.

Hanks, R. A., Wood, D. L., Millis, S., et al. (2003). Violent traumatic brain injury: Occurrence, patient characteristics, and risk factors from the Traumatic Brain Injury Model Systems project. *Archives of Physical Medicine and Rehabilitation*, 84(2), 249–254.

Health Resources and Services Administration (2006). *Traumatic brain injury screening: An introduction*. US Department of Health and Human Services.

Hibbard, M. R., Bogdany, J., Uysal, S., et al. (2000). Axis II psychopathology in individuals with traumatic brain injury. *Brain Injury*, 14(1), 45–61.

Langlois, J. A., Marr, A., Mitchko, J., & Johnson, R. L. (2005). Tracking the silent epidemic and educating the public: CDC's traumatic brain injury-associated activities under the TBI Act of 1996 and the Children's Health Act of 2000. *Journal of Head Trauma Rehabilitation*, 20(3), 196–204.

Miller, E. (1999). Head injury and offending. *Journal of Forensic Psychiatry*, 10(1), 157–166.

Mooney, G., & Speed, J. (2001). The association between mild traumatic brain injury and psychiatric conditions. *Brain Injury*, 15(10), 865–877.

Moore, D., Greer, B. G., & Li, L. (1994). Alcohol and other substance use/abuse among people with disabilities. *Journal of Social Behavior and Personality*, 9(5), 369–382.

National Commission on Correctional Health Care (2002). *The health status of soon-to-be-released inmates: A report to Congress*, Vol. 1. Chicago, IL: NCCHC. Accessed on February 18, 2014, at: http://www.ncchc.org/health-status-of-soon-to-be-released-inmates

Parry-Jones, B. L., Vaughan, F. L., & Miles Cox, W. (2006). Traumatic brain injury and substance misuse: a systematic review of prevalence and outcomes research (1994–2004). *Neuropsychological Rehabilitation*, 16(5), 537–560.

Rapoport, M., McCullagh, S., Streiner, D., & Feinstein, A. (2003). The clinical significance of major depression following mild traumatic brain injury. *Psychosomatics*, 44, 31–37.

Rosenthal, M., Christensen, B. K., & Ross, T. P. (1998). Depression following traumatic brain injury. *Archives of Physical Medicine and Rehabilitation*, 79(1), 90–103.

Seel, R. T., & Kreutzer, J. S. (2003). Depression assessment after traumatic brain injury: an empirically based classification method. *Archives of Physical Medicine and Rehabilitation*, 84(11), 1621–1628.

Seel, R. T., Kreutzer, J. S., Rosenthal, M., Hammond, F. M., Corrigan, J. D., & Black, K. (2003). Depression after traumatic brain injury: a National Institute on Disability and Rehabilitation Research Model Systems multicenter investigation. *Archives of Physical Medicine and Rehabilitation*, 84(2), 177–184.

Shiroma, E. J., Ferguson, P. L., & Pickelsimer, E. E. (2010). Prevalence of traumatic brain injury in an offender population: a meta-analysis. *Journal of Correctional Health Care*, 16(2), 147–159.

Silver, J. M., Kramer, R., Greenwald, S., & Weissman, M. (2001). The association between head injuries and psychiatric disorders: Findings from the New Haven NIMH Epidemiologic Catchment Area Study. *Brain Injury*, 15(11), 935–945.

Silver, J. M., McAllister, T. W., & Yudofsky, S. C. (2005), *Textbook of traumatic brain injury*, 2nd ed. Washington, DC: American Psychiatric Publishing, Inc.

Thurman, D. J., Alverson, C., Dunn, K. A., Guerrero, J., & Sniezek, J. E. (1999). Traumatic brain injury in the United States: A public health perspective. *Journal of Head Trauma Rehabilitation*, 14(6), 602–615.

Turkstra, L., Jones, D., & Toler, H. L. (2003). Brain injury and violent crime. *Brain Injury*, 17(1), 39–47.

US DHHS (1998). *Substance use disorder and treatment for people with physical and cognitive disabilities: Treatment improvement protocol*. US DHHS, MD, Series 29 (SMA) 98–3249. Accessed February 18, 2014, at: http://www.ncbi.nlm.nih.gov/books/ NBK64881/?term=substance%20use%20disorder%20treatment%20 for%20people%20with%20physical%20and%20cognitive%20 disabilities

Valliant, P. M., Freeston, A., Pottier, D., & Kosmyna, R. (2003). Personality and executive functioning as risk factors in recidivists. *Psychological Reports*, 92, 299–306.

Vanderploeg, R. D., & Belanger, H. G. (2013). Screening for a remote history of mild traumatic brain injury: when a good idea is bad. *Journal of Head Trauma Rehabilitation*, 28(3), 211–218.

Wald, M. M., Helgeson, S. R., & Langlois, J. A. (2014). Traumatic brain injury among prisoners. *Brain Injury Professional*. Accessed on February 18, 2014, at: http://www.brainline.org/content/2008/11/ traumatic-brain-injury-among-prisoners_pageall.html

CHAPTER 54

A roadmap for providing psychiatric services to incarcerated veterans
A challenging subspecialty

James F. DeGroot

Introduction

The field of correctional psychiatry has grown and rates of incarceration have risen over the past 35 years. Significant subgroups within the incarcerated population include an increasing number of veterans with issues specific to their past military service. The correctional landscape was transformed from a somewhat homogeneous group of male convicts to a more heterogeneous group of many traumatized men, women (see Chapter 51), and adolescents (see Chapter 56). With civil rights litigation, correctional budgets ballooned not only to pay for correction's core mission of security but also to pay for the required medical and mental health care services (see Chapters 3 and 10).

Several subspecialties emerged and continue to emerge because of this expansion. One of these subspecialties is the provision of mental health services to veterans. The success of mental health care providers with this population depends on their understanding of where these traumatized veterans "come from and are going to," recognizing that military and correctional cultures have distinct languages, laws, and ethical standards. For example, providers should realize that both military and correctional cultures are dominated by males who value physical strength, independence, and courage while devaluing cowardice, dependence, and help-seeking behavior. Both worlds also value the ability to defend one's self and devalue violence against women and children. In contrast, correctional patients tend to be undisciplined and stigmatized, while military patients tend to be disciplined and admired. Historically, the correctional and military worlds rarely interacted except during times of war, when some military veterans are convicted of felonies and incarcerated. These veterans fall from grace and become disenfranchised inmates who struggle to explain their behavior. Society also struggles with the ambivalence of wanting to simultaneously punish and rescue them; mental health care providers struggle with their own emotional responses as they treat these distressed people.

To help mental health care providers meet their personal and professional challenges in working with this complex population, an informational roadmap is presented in this chapter in order to navigate difficult terrain. The goal in using this map is to help providers avoid potholes (of burnout, cynicism, and malevolence) and head-on collisions with prison leadership and/or offenders, resulting in a loss of credibility.

Demographics of incarcerated veterans

A review of data from the Bureau of Justice Statistics reveals that the percentage of inmates who were veterans increased during and after the Vietnam War until 1985 when it reached a high of 20 percent. By 1997 the percentage fell to 12 percent and by 2004 it fell to 10 percent (Bureau of Justice Statistics, 2004). As an aggregate, they are not overrepresented in the criminal justice system; however, the trend observed with Vietnam veterans suggests that there is a gap between the time veterans are discharged from the military and the time they are incarcerated. With more than 2 million personnel having served in Iraq and Afghanistan, the number of incarcerated veterans is likely to rise unless community resources are increased (Institute for Veteran Policy, 2011).

Data from Georgia Department of Corrections (GDC) indicated that during November 2013 the system count was 54,443 inmates, which included 50,835 (93 percent) males and 3,608 (7 percent) females. The total number of self-identified incarcerated veterans was 3,552 (6.5 percent) of the total inmate population. The number of incarcerated male and female veterans was 3,479 and 73, respectively. The total number of inmates receiving mental health services was 9,782, with 8,020 males and 1,762 females. Analyses revealed somewhat greater percentages of veterans receiving mental health care than nonveterans: 19.2 percent versus 15.5 percent males and 52.1 percent versus 48.8 percent females, respectively. An examination of inmate diagnoses revealed 102 male and 5 female veterans were diagnosed with posttraumatic stress disorder (PTSD) along with 688 male and 337 female nonveterans. Of the 102 male veterans diagnosed with PTSD, 64 agreed to participate in an ongoing treatment outcome study. Unless otherwise stated, the GDC data discussed in a later section are from the 64 male veterans diagnosed with PTSD.

The number of veterans in GDC, 3,552 or 6.5 percent of the total inmate population, may be an underestimation of the actual number of incarcerated veterans. It is difficult to identify veterans because many veterans do not believe they are veterans unless they served in combat. Others deny having been in the military because they do not want "to lose their service-connected disability checks." Some don't want their families to lose their benefits while they are in prison and some are embarrassed by their situation.

Veteran demographics

The demographics of incarcerated veterans differ from those of the general inmate population in several ways. For example, veterans tend to be white males who are older than nonveteran inmates, better educated, and either currently or formerly married. They also tend to be convicted of violent crimes more frequently than nonveterans (57 percent and 47 percent, respectively) and receive longer sentences (Bureau of Justice Statistics, 2004). Domestic violence is a common problem among veterans, especially those who have been deployed for an extended period of time and are having difficulty reintegrating into their family. Data reveal that 4 in 10 veterans feel as if they are "a guest in their own home," 1 in 4 believe their children are afraid of them, 3 in 5 disagree with their spouses about their family responsibilities, and 3 in 5 believe their marital relationship is in trouble. The number of veterans convicted of assaulting women was significantly greater than nonveterans, 60 percent and 41 percent, respectively (Bureau of Justice Statistics, 2004). Likewise, veterans were convicted at a greater rate than nonveterans for assaulting minors (40 percent and 24 percent, respectively) or for sex crimes (23 percent and 9 percent, respectively; Substance Abuse Mental Health Services Administration, 2013a).

Wartime, combat, and discharge status among incarcerated veterans are also significant factors. For example, 54 percent of the veterans incarcerated in state prisons and 64 percent of the veterans incarcerated in federal prisons served during wartime; only 20 percent had been in combat. Incarcerated veterans who received a less-than-honorable discharge totaled 38 percent (Bureau of Justice Statistics, 2004). In GDC's select PTSD sample, 70 percent were in combat, which means 30 percent (19 of the 64 incarcerated veterans) developed PTSD from traumas other than combat. In this sample, 67 percent received an honorable discharge and 33 percent received a less-than-honorable discharge. Further analyses did not find a relationship between the type of discharge and whether a veteran was in combat. Similarly, there was no relationship between the type of discharge and the number of times these veterans were incarcerated.

Prevalence and impact of trauma and stress

Prevalence of trauma

Trauma is not a rare phenomenon, with more than 50 percent of the veteran population experiencing at least one significant trauma in their lives (Department of Veteran Affairs, 2013). Traumas differ in that some are experienced directly, some indirectly, and some vicariously. Regardless of how it is experienced, trauma is a significant event. People's vulnerability to trauma and the expression of their distress is variable. Vulnerability to trauma-based disorders varies as a function of risk and protective factors, the intensity of

the trauma, and its duration. Risk factors include prior trauma, mental health problems, little support from family and friends, the recent loss of a loved one, recent stressful life changes, a history of alcohol and/or drug abuse, limited education, and age. Protective factors include the absence of early life-threatening events, an optimistic outlook on life, resourcefulness, and a strong social support network (Clark, 2013). Expressions of distress include internalizing symptoms such as anxiety, dysphoria, and isolating behavior or externalizing symptoms such as disinhibition, anger, and aggressive/impulsive behavior. Most people who experience trauma and become symptomatic do not develop PTSD. The National Co-Morbidity Survey Replication revealed that 7 percent to 8 percent of the population will develop PTSD at some point in their lives, with women being more likely to develop it than men. Approximately 10 percent of the female population in comparison to 5 percent of the male population develops PTSD, often accompanied by depression, substance abuse, emotional dysregulation, and behavioral problems (Kessler, Berglund, Demler, et. al., 2005).

The prevalence of trauma among offenders incarcerated in US jails, state prisons, and federal prisons is high. The Bureau of Justice Statistics (1999) reports that 19 percent of state prisoners, 10 percent of federal prisoners, and 16 percent of those in local jails report a history of physical and/or sexual abuse. Histories of childhood abuse are more common among incarcerated males and females than in the community. Bureau of Justice Statistics (2006) reports that in the community 5 percent to 8 percent of adult males and 12 percent to 17 percent of adult females report a history of childhood abuse; in prison 6 percent to 14 percent of adult males and 23 percent to 37 percent of adult females report a history of childhood abuse. A review of GDC's database during a class-action lawsuit (*Cason v. Seckinger*, 1984), which included allegations of sexual misconduct, revealed that mentally ill inmates had a much higher incidence of childhood abuse than inmates who were not receiving mental health services. The database also revealed that the incidence of abuse increased with the severity of mental illness for both males and females.

Active-duty military personnel and veterans are at increased risk of developing posttraumatic stress symptoms and PTSD because of wartime stressors and sexual misconduct (Litz & Schlenger, 2009; Wood, 2012a). The Veterans Administration estimated 11 percent to 20 percent of veterans of the Iraq and Afghanistan wars developed PTSD as compared to 30 percent of Vietnam veterans who developed PTSD. Among Iraq and Afghanistan veterans, PTSD is often linked to traumatic brain injury caused by blast waves from explosions (NIH Medline Plus, 2009). The US Department of Veterans Affairs (VA) also noted that among veterans using VA health care, 23 percent and 55 percent of the women reported being sexually assaulted or harassed, respectively, while on active duty. Additionally, 38 percent of the men experienced sexual harassment while on active duty (New York State Office of Mental Health, 2008).

Impact of trauma

The Adverse Childhood Experiences (ACE) research was conducted by the Centers for Disease Control and Prevention in collaboration with Kaiser Permanente. Over a 10-year period, 17,421 people were screened to identify the effects of adverse childhood experiences (trauma) over the lifespan. The adverse experiences that were studied consisted of five household categories (substance abuse, divorce, mental illness, domestic violence, and criminal behavior), three abuse categories (emotional, physical, and sexual), and two neglect categories (emotional and physical). The results revealed that as the number of adverse events increases, the probability of medical, emotional, behavioral, interpersonal, educational, and arousal problems also increases (Centers for Disease Control and Prevention, 2013).

The impact of these adverse childhood experiences is reflected in subsequent risk of attempting suicide. The ACE study discovered that 1 percent of people who have no adverse childhood experiences attempt suicide, 10 percent of people who have three adverse experiences attempt suicide, and 20 percent of people who have seven adverse experiences attempt suicide (Centers for Disease Control and Prevention, 2008). The impact of trauma on veterans may be similarly illustrated (Wood, 2012b; Wortzel et al., 2009). The number of veterans who died from suicide ranged from 18 to 22 every day between 1999 and 2011 (Department of Veterans Affairs, 2013b). During 2012, a military veteran committed suicide every 65 minutes and 349 active-duty personnel committed suicide (Basu, 2013). The number of attempted and completed suicides is higher in jails and prisons than in the community, which should come as no surprise given the high incidence of trauma among inmates (Bureau of Justice Statistics, 2005). For example, an analysis of GDC's selected veteran population revealed that 70 percent had at least four adverse experiences in comparison to the those in the community where only 12.59 percent had at least four adverse experiences (Centers for Disease Control and Prevention, 2013).

Challenges and strategies in the provision of services to incarcerated veterans

Challenges

The biggest challenge facing the criminal justice system at this time is to reduce the number of incarcerated offenders. Criminal justice reinvestment and justice reform initiatives are focused on diverting and releasing nonviolent offenders to more cost-effective treatment in the community. Examples of such initiatives include mental health courts and drug courts, which divert nonviolent offenders from prison to more appropriate community-based mental health programs and substance abuse programs. Other diversion programs include day reporting centers and integrated treatment facilities, which were created for probationers who are on the verge of having their probation revoked. Veteran courts have also been created within the past five years, primarily to divert nonviolent combat veterans from incarceration. Additionally, more than 30 states have initiated legislative efforts to provide alternative treatment for veterans with psychological trauma and/or substance abuse issues resulting from their military service (Institute for Veteran Policy, 2011).

Over the past 25 years, treatment programs have been developed for incarcerated mentally ill and chemically dependent offenders whose crimes are related to their illness. Programs for incarcerated, traumatized veterans are also being developed. For example, some state prisons and county jails have created veteran dorms/units where combat and noncombat veterans can again experience camaraderie and participate in rigid daily programs that help them adapt to prison and prepare to reenter the community. One of these veteran's units opened in

Muscogee County Jail in Georgia, just a few miles away from the home of the US Army Airborne and Ranger training brigades. In order to facilitate successful community reentry from both the county jail and the US Army, the Muscogee County Jail program began working closely with the community, connecting veteran offenders with appropriate services such as the VA, Community Service Board, Alcoholics Anonymous, and organizations that help with supportive housing and supportive employment (Salahi, 2012).

The GDC is actively involved in developing and maintaining diversion and reentry programs, especially for mentally ill, chemically dependent, and veteran offenders. Mental health professionals have been actively participating in these initiatives by identifying, assessing, and treating them. These efforts have recently included veterans. The data from this effort have revealed that a higher percentage of male and female veterans receive mental health services than male and female nonveterans (i.e., 19.2 percent and 15.5 percent for males and 52.1 percent and 48.7 percent for females, respectively). It also revealed that male veterans are more often diagnosed with PTSD than nonveterans; however, female veterans are less likely to be diagnosed with PTSD than nonveterans. Additionally, veterans are more likely to have comorbid diagnoses including a substance use disorder, major depressive disorder, and/or a personality disorder. Furthermore, the assessments revealed that the severity of untreated chronic PTSD fluctuates over time; both the severity and chronicity appear to be exacerbated by adverse childhood experiences and being retraumatized in prison.

Evaluating and diagnosing traumatized veterans is a challenge because the clinician must distinguish the symptoms from those of traumatic brain injury, a personality disorder, and other comorbid disorders. Two common diagnostic errors include over- and underdiagnosing PTSD. Many correctional clinicians often overdiagnose PTSD when evaluating combat veterans who have multiple "military" risk factors (i.e., a description of weak unit leadership, deployments of long duration, a history of multiple deployments, and the experience of intense combat) and externalizing symptoms (i.e., sleep disturbance, reckless behavior, irritability, and aggressive behavior). However, the combat veteran may have few if any intrusive symptoms (i.e., distress during repetitive reviews of traumatic memories and trauma related situations). Clinicians, rather than observing distress among these veterans in group therapy, often see them relishing the opportunity to tell their stories. In fact, one clinician observed a veteran describe his traumatic experiences as "exhilarating."

In contrast, PTSD is often underdiagnosed during the diagnosis of comorbid disorders in noncombat veterans who have few if any "military" risk factors and externalizing symptoms. However, the noncombat veteran may have intrusive symptoms that result in dysphoria, fear, distractibility, and/or depersonalization. Rather than being directly exposed to the threat of being killed in combat, these veterans have been indirectly exposed to violence by treating injured veterans in an army medical center or by gathering dead veterans' personal effects. Clinicians need to maintain objectivity in diagnosing veterans with PTSD. The challenge is to not place too much weight on the presence of "military" risk factors, direct exposure to combat, or externalizing symptoms while minimizing indirect exposure to combat and internalizing symptoms.

Strategies

GDC's veterans have traditionally been integrated into the general inmate population and mentally ill veterans have received mental health services with nonveterans. Unfortunately, due to large mental health caseloads, the type, frequency, and intensity of therapy tends to be generic. In order to develop an effective mental health treatment program for these incarcerated veterans, a team of clinicians conducted a survey and performed individual interviews. The results indicated that veterans were dissatisfied with their mental health treatment. Most veterans said that they wanted more frequent and intense therapy. They also wanted to participate in homogeneous groups where they could talk about their traumatic combat experiences with people who have similar experiences. After reviewing these results, the clinical team reviewed practice guidelines (Department of Veterans and Department of Defense, 2010; Foa et al., 2009; Substance Abuse and Mental Health Services Administration, 2013b), trauma-informed care models (Miller & Najavits, 2012), and several evidence-based interventions to include cognitive processing therapy, mindfulness practices in treating traumatic stress, prolonged exposure therapy, stress inoculation training, eye movement desensitization and reprocessing therapy, and yoga. GDC resources were assessed, leadership was briefed, and community partners (vocational rehabilitation and community service boards) were contacted.

Lessons learned during the implementation of this veterans' PTSD treatment program include the following:

◆ Read practice guidelines in order to develop selection criteria and determine needed resources;

◆ Develop program values that overlap with the practice guidelines, military values, and correctional procedures (i.e., safety, loyalty, mutual respect, team cohesion, respect for leadership, mission, structure, and training);

◆ Clearly identify the program's mission, treatment goals, and strategies;

◆ Identify a program leader in whom staff and veterans have confidence;

◆ Develop cohesive treatment teams;

◆ Train veterans and staff to include correctional officers in trauma-informed care. Appropriate models may include cognitive-based therapies such as prolonged exposure therapy and cognitive processing therapy (Brim, Ermold, & Riggs, 2013; Copeland & Schulz, 2012);

◆ Emphasize safety, which is important for anyone in therapy, especially for traumatized veterans who left an unsafe environment and entered another threatening environment.

Summary

The demographics and life experiences of incarcerated veterans, both combat and noncombat, differ substantially from those of nonveteran offenders. Additionally, their criminogenic risk factors and mental health needs also differ from other incarcerated mental health consumers. Nonveterans are being treated with evidence-based correctional mental health and substance abuse treatment programs; however, similar programs have not been developed with the unique characteristics of veterans in mind. There is a critical need to create and implement evidence-based programs to treat the emotional, behavioral, and neurological needs of mentally ill and traumatized veterans. Psychiatry needs to be at the table along with an interdisciplinary team to ensure the best possible treatment for the men and women who were injured while fighting for their country.

References

Basu, M. (2013, Nov. 14). *Why suicide rate among veterans may be more than 22 a day.* CNN. Available at: http://www.cnn.com/2013/09/21/us/22-veteran-suicides-a-day/. Accessed on October 29, 2013.

Brim, W., Ermold, J., & Riggs, D. (2013). *Prolonged exposure therapy for PTSD for veterans and military personnel.* Relias Learning. Available at: http://www.essentiallearning. net/student/content/sections/lectora/ProlongedExposureTherapyVets/index.html

Bureau of Justice Statistics (1999). *Prior abuse reported by inmates and probationers.* Available at: http://www.wcl.american.edu/faculty/smith/0303conf/article2.pdf

Bureau of Justice Statistics (2004). *Veterans in state and federal prison.* Available at: http://www.bjs.gov/content/pub/pdf/p04.pdf.

Bureau of Justice Statistics (2005). *Suicide and homicide in state prisons and local jails.* Available at: http://www.bjs.gov/content/pub/pdf/shsply:pdf.

Bureau of Justice Statistics (2006). *Mental health problems of prison and jail inmates.* Available at: http://www.bjs/content/pub/pdf/mhppji.pdf.

Cason, et al., Plaintiffs, v. Seckinger, et al., Defendants (1984). No. 84-313-1-MAC. Available at: http://www.ada.gov/briefs/casonbr.pdf. Accessed on November 26, 2013.

Centers for Disease Control and Prevention (2008). *The effects of childhood stress on health across the lifespan.* Available at: http://www.cdc.gov/ ncipc/pub-res/pdf/childhood_stress.pdf

Centers for Disease Control and Prevention (2013a). *Adverse Childhood Experiences (ACE) Study.* Available from: http://www.cdc.gov/ace/

Centers for Disease Control and Prevention (2013b). *Data and statistics: Prevalence of individual adverse childhood experiences.* Available at: http://www.cdc.gov/ace/prevalence/htm. Accessed on November 28, 2013.

Clark, J. (2013). *How post-traumatic stress disorder works.* How Stuff Works. Available at: http://science.howstuffworks.com/ptsd7.htm

Copeland, L., & Schulz, P. (2012). *Cognitive processing therapy for PTSD in veterans and military personnel.* Essential Learning. Available at: http:// www.essentiallearning.net/student/content/Lectura/CognitiveProcessing TherapyforPTSDin VeteransandMilitaryPersonnel/index.html

Department of Veterans Affairs—National Center for PTSD (2013a). *How common is PTSD?* Available at: http://www.ptsd.va.gov/public/pages/how-common-is-ptsd-asp

Department of Veterans Affairs—Office of Public and Intergovernmental Affairs (2013b). *VA issues new report on suicide data.* Available at: http://www.va.gov/opa/pressrel/pressrelease. ofm?id=24

Department of Veterans Affairs and Department of Defense (2010). *Clinical practice guideline for management of post-traumatic stress.* Available at: http://www.downloads.va.gov/

Foa, E., Keane, T., Friedman, M., & Cohen, J. (2009). *Effective treatment for PTSD: Practice guidelines from the International Society for Traumatic Stress.* New York: Guilford Press.

Georgia Department of Corrections (2013). *Inmate statistical profile.* Available at: http://www.dcor.state.ga.us/Reseaech/Monthly/Profile_all_inmates _2003_12.pdf

Institute of Veteran Policy (2011). *Veterans and criminal justice: A review of the literature.* Available at: http://www.swords-to-plowshares.org/wp-content/uploads/Veterans-and-Criminal-Justice-Literature-Review.pdf

Kessler, R. C., Berglund, P., Demler, O., et al. (2005). Lifetime prevalence and age-of-onset distributions of DSM-IV disorders in the National Comorbidity Survey Replication. *Archives of General Psychiatry, 62*, 593–602. Available at: http://www.ncbi.nlm.nih. gov/pubmed/15939837. Accessed on November 20, 2013.

Litz, B., & Schloenger, W. (2009). PTSD in service members and new veterans of the Iraq and Afghanistan wars: A bibliography and critique. *PTSD Research Quarterly, 20*(1), 1050–1835. Available at: http://www.ptsd.va.gov/ professional/newsletter/research-quarterly/V20N1.pdf. Accessed on October 22, 2013.

Miller, N., & Najavitis, L. (2012). Creating trauma-informed correctional care: a balance of goals and environment. *European Journal of Psychotraumatology, 3*, 17246-DOI:10:3402/eipt.v3i0.17246. Available at: http://www.ncbi.nlm.nih. gov/pmc/articles/pmc3402099/. Accessed on October 10, 2013.

New York State Office of Mental Health (2008). *Post-traumatic stress disorder.* Available at: http://www.omh.ny.gov/omhweb/booklets/ptsd.htm

NIH Medline Plus (2009). *PTSD: A growing epidemic.* Available at: http://www.n/m.nih.gov/medlineplus/magazine/issues/winter09/articles/winter09pg10-14.html

PEW Charitable Trusts (2008). *One in 100: Behind bars in America 2008.* Available at: http://www.pewstates.org/ uploadedFiles/PCS-Assets/2008/0ne%20in% percent20100.pdf. Accessed on October 29, 2013.

Salahi, L. (2012, April 26). *Growing number of prisons offer special dorms for military vets.* abc News. Available at: http://abcnews-go.com.Health/Wellness/ special-jail-housing-military-veterans/story?id=1622008. Accessed on September 27, 2013.

Sarteschi, C. (2013). *Mentally ill offenders involved with the U. S. criminal justice system.* Sage Open. Available at: http://sgo.sageepub.com/content/ 3/3/2158244013497029#sec-2. Accessed on November 21, 2013.

Substance Abuse and Mental Health Services Administration (2013a). *Co-occurring disorders in veterans and military service members.* Available at: http://www.samhsa.gov/co-occurring/topics/military/impact-of-deployment.aspx

Substance Abuse and Mental Health Services Administration (2013b). *Trauma-informed care and trauma services.* Available at: http://www.samhsa. gov/nctic/trauma.asp

Wood, D. (2012a, July 4). *Iraq, Afghanistan war veterans struggle with combat trauma.* Huffington Post. Available at: http://www.huffingtonpost. com/2012/07/04/iraq-afghanistan-war-veterans-combat-trauma_n_1645701.html. Accessed on October 19, 2013.

Wood, D. (2012b, October 2). *Veterans: Coming home.* Huffington Post. Available from: http://www.huffingtonpost.com/2012/10/02/veterans-coming-home_n_1932366.html. Accessed on October 19, 2013.

Wortzel, H., Binswanger, I. A., Anderson, C. A., et al. (2009). Suicide among incarcerated veterans. *Journal of the American Academy of Psychiatry and the Law, 37*, 82–91. Available at: http://www.ncbi.nlm.nih.gov/pubmed/19297638. Accessed on November 13, 2013.

CHAPTER 55

Lesbian, gay, bisexual, and transgendered inmates

Randi Kaufman, Kevin Kapila, and
Kenneth L. Appelbaum

Introduction

The lesbian, gay, bisexual, and transgender (LGBT) population has been, and remains, disenfranchised in many ways. Despite increasing acceptance of sexual orientation, evidenced by recent strides in legalizing gay marriage in several states, LGBT people continue to have a higher prevalence of mental illness due to minority stress than heterosexuals (Meyer, 2003). Factors such as stigma, prejudice, and discrimination lead to an increased incidence of mental suffering as a result of stressful, hostile, and often unsafe environments. Prejudice within the LGBT community around race, gender, disability, or mental illness also exists. Transgender individuals have a high risk of being targeted for violence and hate crimes, harassment and discrimination, unemployment and underemployment, poverty, homelessness, substance abuse, suicide, and self-harm (Grant et al., 2011). The stressors that LGBT individuals face likely contribute to their disproportionate risk of contact with the criminal justice system, beginning in adolescence and extending into adulthood (National Institute of Corrections, 2013b). Transgender individuals in particular have a risk for incarceration, for reasons ranging from imprisonment based on gender identity expression alone to the need to earn money through the underground economy due to difficulty finding employment (Grant et al., 2011).

In addition to homophobia and transphobia, LGBT individuals with mental illness experience further stigmatization. Clinicians need to understand the multiple stigmas that may affect an individual's willingness to seek mental health care. The unique needs of incarcerated LGBT individuals with mental illness are often invisible and generally misunderstood and underserved. This chapter seeks to add to the clinical knowledge of practitioners who work with this population, clarify legal precedent, and establish best practices.

General considerations of the lesbian, gay, bisexual, and transgendered experience in prison

Working with LGBT inmates poses special challenges to comprehensive care. Although all inmates experience loss of freedom and separation from loved ones, LGBT inmates face added burdens of discrimination, marginalization, and physical and sexual abuse. Important considerations that affect their incarceration experience include self-comfort with sexual orientation or gender identity, whether they are out or closeted, whether their appearance reveals sexual orientation or gender nonconformity, and their ability to portray the gender with which they identify. Correctional psychiatrists should inquire without assumption about these issues and let the patient lead the discussion. No uniform approach can address the mental health needs of all LGBT inmates. A safe, empathic alliance between clinician and patient combined with a balance between interest and respect about sexual and gender identity experiences has great importance in correctional settings where sex and gender stereotypes tend to pervade.

Inmates with sexual or gender minority status should have an evaluation of medical and mental health needs and assessment of victimization risk at initial reception and whenever transferred to another facility. Approximately 3.5% of heterosexual males report being sexually victimized by another inmate, but those rates soar to 34% for bisexual and 39% for homosexual or gay male inmates (Beck et al., 2012). Reported rates of victimization by staff were at least two to three times higher for gay, lesbian, and bisexual inmates compared to heterosexual counterparts. Fifteen percent of transgender inmates report sexual assault, with black transgender inmates reporting much higher assault rates by both other inmates and staff than their counterparts (Grant et al., 2011). Nevertheless, isolation for safety or placement in an LGBT segregated unit should occur only when individually necessary and not as a substitute for other protective interventions. According to the National Prison Rape Elimination Commission (NPREC), any form of isolation should remain a "last resort and interim measure only." The NPREC (2009) also "specifically prohibits housing prisoners based solely on their sexual orientation or gender identity because it can lead to demoralizing and dangerous labeling."

The National Institute of Corrections (2013a) has a website with guidelines and resources to help correctional institutions provide care and develop LGBT treatment policies. Initial steps may involve assessment of staff attitudes and knowledge, open and noncritical dialogue about knowledge gaps, and education for all members of the custody and clinical team. Education must include a clear message to treat LGBT inmates with respect and that harassment by staff will not be tolerated.

Coming out

Coming out refers to the process where the LGBT person accepts and discloses his or her sexual orientation or gender identity. How, when, and why to disclose is a highly personal decision. The process is not sequential and can be lifelong. Incarceration represents a new situation in which to come out or stay closeted. Despite previous choices, some people may choose differently in prison for reasons of safety, mental and emotional well-being, or fear of rejection. Remaining closeted can further isolate LGBT inmates by cutting them off from supports. Inmates who are transferred to a new facility may make different choices about coming out. For example, some who came out in a different prison where they felt safe and supported might decide not to do so after transfer. In this situation, they may still fear that inmates or correctional officers from their previous prison might reveal their status. Psychiatrists can help inmates cope with the emotional effects of remaining closeted and fearing discovery. When practical, clinicians can advocate for placement in settings where inmates can safely reveal their sexual orientation or gender identity. For inmates who lack sufficient emotional stability and coping skills, the clinician should initially limit the focus to stabilization.

Challenges around coming out for transgendered inmates include restricted access to clothing, make-up, accoutrements, hairstyle, and ability to "pass" (i.e., being seen as one's identified, not natal, gender) when housed in a prison that does not correspond to the person's gender identity. Inability to express gender identity may cause mental and emotional distress; however, being identified as transgender in prison may put the inmate at greater risk for physical or sexual assault. Discussing these issues in the safety of a therapeutic relationship can improve mental and emotional health and allow the person who decides to stay closeted to feel known authentically to someone safe in the prison setting.

Behavior versus identity

Complicating the picture, someone in prison might make different behavioral choices that may not be based on identity. Evidence suggests that the longer one spends in prison and the higher the security level, the greater the inclination to engage in same-sex sexual behavior, even for those who had not done so before incarceration (Garland et al., 2005). This can create confusion for inmates who have never considered themselves as gay, lesbian, or bisexual. They might question their sexual orientation for the first time and confront feelings of internalized homophobia. Behavior and identity, however, do not necessarily correspond. Same-sex behavior might represent a desire for love, pleasure, bonding, protection, or favors from another inmate rather than a change from heterosexual to homosexual (Garland et al., 2005). An informed, empathic mental health clinician can help inmates safely work through their feelings and provide education about safer sex practices, especially for heterosexual individuals who might not view themselves as at risk for sexually transmitted infections such as HIV while engaging in same-sex activities.

Family of choice

A healthy response to the high rate of family rejection that many LGBT people have experienced is to create a family of choice. Even if not explicitly rejected, some LGBT people decide to end relationships with unsupportive family members and look elsewhere for support. Creating a family of choice, even for those with good relationships with their biological families, is woven into the fabric of the LGBT community. A family of choice may include an extensive network of friends, partners, ex-partners, mentors, colleagues, clergy, and others. Families of choice often play an integral part in meaningful life events and developmental milestones such as school or career achievements, holidays, religious ceremonies, marriage, illness, and death and provide a network of support to turn to in times of crisis. The mental health clinician who works with incarcerated LGBT people should take chosen family into consideration when taking the social history, recognizing that family structure may not include the biological family or may be a combination of the biological family and family of choice.

Correctional systems that allow for conjugal visits or visits to sick or dying family members might not extend those rights to LGBT inmates. Clinical support to help cope with the distress of unfair policies and advocacy on their behalf may be indicated.

Understanding the differences in L, G, B, and T

Mental health issues of LGBT individuals have often been studied as if lesbians, gays, bisexuals, and transgender individuals are a homogeneous group. While LGB includes sexual orientation only, LGBT includes gender identity. Although homophobia and transphobia have similar effects, each group also faces unique issues and experiences. For example, the HIV epidemic has affected the health of gay and bisexual men more than lesbians, and sexism in our society more directly affects lesbian and bisexual women than gay men. Similarly, the lack of familiarity with transgender people and their issues puts them at much higher risk for societal discrimination and lack of access to appropriate and informed medical and mental health care.

Bisexuals

Bisexuality is the capacity for emotional, romantic, and physical attraction to more than one gender. Bisexuals frequently contend with incomplete acceptance by the heterosexual, lesbian, or gay communities. They are often incorrectly seen either as heterosexuals who want to appear edgy or trendy or as homosexuals unwilling to admit to being gay. They often do not volunteer their sexual orientation (Miller & Solot, 2000), allowing others to make assumptions. Although bisexuals have been part of the LGBT movement, their needs may go unaddressed, with negative health consequences (San Francisco Human Rights Commission, 2011). Although their visibility has increased, they continue to be seen through the lens of negative stereotypes, including myths about promiscuity or infidelity and false accusations of responsibility for transmitting HIV from the gay male community to the heterosexual community (Ekstrand et al., 1994). These stereotypes have mental health consequences that include higher rates of depression, anxiety, and suicidal ideation (Brennan et al., 2010; King et al., 2008; Koh, 2006; Miller, 2007) and higher rates of physical and sexual abuse than gay and lesbian communities (McCabe, 2010). Bisexual women have lower levels of education, more health problems, and higher levels of mental distress than lesbian women (Fredriksen-Goldsen et al., 2010). Resources appropriate for gays and lesbians may therefore not meet the needs of bisexuals.

Lesbians

Lesbians frequently contend with sexism as well as homophobia. Although they face typical women's health issues, the additional stressor of homophobia puts them at greater risk for mental health problems. They experience higher rates of depression and use more mental health services than the general population (Bradford, 1994; Cochran, 2009; Cochran, 2003; King et al., 2008; Koh, 2006) and have higher rates of obesity, which may derive from or contribute to mental distress (Valanis et al., 2000). Lesbians who are more open about their sexual orientation have lower rates of psychological distress (Bradford, 1994; Koh, 2006). Assisting an incarcerated lesbian may involve helping her with self-acceptance and with balancing the mental health benefits against the safety risks of coming out.

Gay men

Many gay men live with the specter of HIV. Older generations dealt with the devastating impact of the AIDS epidemic at a time when little was known, a diagnosis of AIDS was often a death sentence, and friends and partners died due to the absence of effective antiviral therapy. Younger gay men cope with the reality that sexual exploration could result in a serious medical illness. HIV is not the only sexually transmitted infection (STI) prevalent in the gay male community. STIs, syphilis in particular, have been increasing among gay and bisexual men. In 2008, men who have sex with men accounted for 63% of primary and secondary syphilis cases in the United States. Gonorrhea, chlamydia, and herpes also remain common (Centers for Disease Control and Prevention, 2013). Human papilloma virus, the most common STI in the United States, also affects gay men. Correctional psychiatrists need to be sensitive to issues of shame about STIs while reinforcing safer sex practices and screening.

Prevalent drug use in the gay community may result in incarceration. Ecstasy, crystal methamphetamine, gamma hydroxybutyrate, and ketamine are common at gay clubs and circuit parties. Crystal methamphetamine dependence in particular has grown in the past decade and is associated with more unprotected sexual encounters. Alcohol abuse also is prevalent among gay men. Not unlike their heterosexual counterparts, some younger gay men go through a period of exploration with these drugs but do not develop addiction. Gay men might also use drugs or alcohol for social acceptance, to reduce anxiety, or to cope with feelings of internalized homophobia or self-hatred.

Transgender individuals

"Transgender" is an umbrella term for people who experience or present their gender differently from their natal, or assigned, gender. Gender dysphoria, the *Diagnostic and Statistical Manual of Mental Disorders*–5 (American Psychiatric Association, 2013) diagnosis that replaced the previous diagnosis of gender identity disorder, describes emotional or cognitive discontent with the assigned gender. Gender and gender identity exist on a wide spectrum, and not everyone views his or her identity, anatomy, gender expression, and sexuality in ways that line up neatly in a traditional, conventional manner. Transgender is often used synonymously with "transsexual," which refers to a person who seeks, or has undergone, a transition from male to female or female to male, socially (coming out to others and/or changing clothing, hairstyle, grooming, name, or pronoun), medically (puberty blockers and/or cross-sex hormone therapy), or surgically. Because the meaning of terms such as "transgender," "transsexual," and "gender nonconforming" can differ, individuals should be asked to explain what they mean.

Transgender people commonly encounter discrimination, rejection, and isolation. They face personal intrusiveness when others stare, point, or laugh at them, call them names, or ask them inappropriate questions (e.g., "do you have a penis?"). Many transgender people desire sex-reassignment surgery, but others do not. Reasons for not having surgery include concern about a loss of sensation postoperatively, poor cosmetic result, desire to please a partner, fear of medical procedures, fear of losing custody of children, or enjoyment of one's original genitalia. Some individuals cannot afford surgery, have medical contraindications, have no one to assist them after surgery, or cannot take time off from work for recovery. Similarly, individuals differ regarding their preferred name and pronouns. Following their preferences helps create a safe and empathic alliance by indicating respect, a nonjudgmental attitude, and acceptance of the person's gender.

Assessment of lesbian, gay, and bisexual inmates

The correctional psychiatrist needs to be aware of personal bias, which might manifest through body language, nervousness in taking a sexual history, or poor eye contact. If necessary, the psychiatrist should seek supervision. It is best to use gender-neutral terminology when inquiring about sexual partners and to avoid assumptions about sexual orientation, even if an inmate discloses a same-sex relationship. The provider can express interest regarding how the patient's sexual orientation influences the chief complaint without assuming that this orientation accounts for the presenting problem. Social history should explore the effect sexual orientation has had on the inmate's relationship with family and friends or with experiences of discrimination.

Correctional psychiatrists need to screen for drug use and any perceived benefits that drugs have had for the individual. For example, does a particular drug seem to help the person deal with anxiety, feel like he or she fits in, improve self-esteem, or enhance or enable sexual ability? Such questions convey concern and knowledge of common issues in the gay male community.

LGB inmates who have symptoms of depression or anxiety will respond to pharmacotherapy and to the same modes of psychodynamic and cognitive-behavioral therapy as would any inmate. They will respond best to a therapist who understands how homophobia may affect their symptoms and who provides a safe space for them to engage in treatment.

The diagnosis of bipolar disorder can be made inappropriately in LGB inmates. A person who has repressed his or her sexual orientation and finally comes out and starts to accept it may do so with a mix of euphoria and shame and feel like he or she is on an emotional roller coaster. This is not a mixed manic state; rather, it is part of the normal coming-out process. A person who finally acts on sexual feelings he or she has long repressed may have multiple partners, which should not be interpreted as manic hypersexuality.

Transgender Inmates

Maria is a 32-year-old transwoman incarcerated for breaking and entering. Although she appears female, with long hair, breasts, feminine facial characteristics, and a feminine voice, she is housed in a male prison because she has male genitalia. Placement in the male prison immediately outed her as transgender. Prison staff refer to her by her legal male name and male pronouns. They have refused her requests for transfer to a female prison, for a private cell and shower, for a razor to shave, and to be called Maria. They view her as oppositional because she does not respond to the male name and pronouns, and some of them call her "faggot" or "she-male." Other inmates taunt and proposition her. Her assigned mental health provider has no experience with transgender individuals and falsely attributes her symptoms of posttraumatic stress disorder, anxiety, depression, and estrogen withdrawal to withdrawal from illegal substances. Her requests for hormones and cosmetics are denied.

Assessment of transgender inmates

When assessing a transgender person, the correctional psychiatrist needs either expertise in gender dysphoria or appropriate supervision. Inexperienced providers should seek education about gender identity issues and examine their own feelings, beliefs, and understanding of what gender and gender nonconformity means. If negative stereotypes or bias interfere with their ability to assess or treat the patient, they should refer the individual to another clinician. In Maria's case, the lack of knowledge, understanding, and respect for her experience and needs by her mental health provider ruptured their relationship, left her without clinical support, and contributed to her anxiety and distress.

Assessment of a gender-nonconforming individual includes a gender history. Table 55.1 includes suggested questions that can be used when taking a history. A helpful approach involves beginning with broad and general inquiries, with focused follow-up questions as indicated. The history includes questions about gender-related distress and how the person has dealt with it. Puberty represents a critical time for many transgendered individuals as they begin to have unwanted physical changes.

Maria, for example, played with her sister's toys and wore her clothing, which led to a beating from her father when he found out. This created a stressful dilemma in which she felt terrified of discovery if she dressed up but worsening dysphoria and anxiety if she did not. During puberty, she painfully tucked in her genitals and had fantasies of castration. She reported that her crime of breaking and entering occurred in an effort to get funds for sex-reassignment surgery.

Self-harm can result, especially focused on body parts that cause dysphoria. Transgender individuals often experience difficulty with dating and sexual relationships and commonly use fantasies of their desired body to enhance sexual arousal. They may avoid disrobing to keep unwanted body parts out of view. They may have confusion about sexual orientation, not knowing whether they are gay or transgender. The history should explore their understanding of their gender and any desire to transition. Individuals also may differ regarding which social, medical, and surgical options they seek.

Table 55.1 Taking a gender history

Developmental Period	Common Questions
General	When did you first realize there was something different about your gender?
	When did you first come out to someone about your gender?
Childhood	What is your earliest memory of your gender?
	What kinds of toys and activities did you like?
	Did you prefer male or female friends?
	What type of clothing did you prefer to wear? Were you allowed to wear this clothing?
	Did you sit or stand to urinate?
	When did you understand that people saw you as a boy/girl?
	How did your parents/siblings/peers relate to your gender?
	Did you ever wear clothing of the other sex?
	Did you ever get caught?
	How did you feel about your gender? How did you handle your feelings?
Puberty	When did you begin to experience physical changes?
	How did you feel about these changes? How did you handle your feelings?
Youth/Adulthood	Who are you attracted to? (males/females/transgender and/or gender-nonconforming people)
	(If you are sexual) How do you feel about your body during sex?
	Are there parts of your body that you don't feel comfortable having touched or things you are not comfortable doing?
	Are there parts of your body that you don't feel comfortable having visible during sex?
	How do your sexual fantasies relate to your gender?

Although rare, symptoms of gender dysphoria can derive from other mental health disorders. The differential diagnosis includes psychotic disorders, body dysmorphic disorder, trauma, transvestic fetishism, eating disorders, borderline personality disorder, obsessive–compulsive disorder, and nonconformity to stereotypical gender roles. In addition, other mental health disorders may co-occur with gender dysphoria, further complicating the diagnosis. The assessment should attempt to distinguish among mental health symptoms due to gender dysphoria itself, social stigmatization, distress over denial of appropriate medical care such as hormone therapy, or other unrelated reasons.

Transgender health in prison

Most state and federal prison systems in the United States have policies or other directives regarding health care for transgendered inmates. They vary, however, in whether they allow continuation or initiation of hormones, and none currently provides sex-reassignment surgery (Brown & McDuffie, 2009). Blanket restrictions on access to recognized medical care lack parallel with other medical conditions.

Professional organizations such as the American Medical Association (2008) and the American Psychiatric Association (2012) have approved policies that support insurance coverage for gender transition treatment as recommended by a physician. A position statement by the National Commission on Correctional Health Care (NCCHC; 2009) states that correctional health staff "should follow accepted standards developed by professionals with expertise in transgender health" and references the "Standards of Care for Gender Identity Disorders," available from the World Professional Association for Transgender Health (Coleman et al., 2012), as the source of those standards. NCCHC recommendations for health management and patient safety of transgender inmates include the following:

◆ Manage medical and surgical issues by accepted professional standards;

◆ Eliminate blanket policies that restrict medical treatment;

◆ A "freeze" frame approach is "inappropriate";

◆ Inmates on hormone therapy should continue to receive this therapy without interruption pending specialist evaluation, unless contraindicated by urgent medical reasons;

◆ Inmates not on hormone therapy should have an evaluation by a qualified health care provider to determine their medical necessity;

◆ Provide medically necessary treatment for genital self-harm or surgical complications;

◆ Provide patients with educational materials;

◆ Do not use psychotherapy to attempt to alter gender identity as this "inappropriately portrays [gender dysphoria] as a mental illness and not a medical condition";

◆ Consider inmate safety, due to being targets for violence; and

◆ Discharge planning should address continued care in the community.

Policies also need to ensure respect when conducting strip searches (e.g., using officers of the inmate's self-identified gender), privacy in bathrooms and showers, and appropriate access to gender-preferred canteen and toiletry items. Meeting a transgendered individual's medical and mental health needs in a manner that allows gender expression represents good clinical care, even in prison.

In recent years, lawsuits by transgendered inmates have resulted in expanded access to treatment. Courts in the United States have recognized gender dysphoria as a serious medical condition, and they generally defer to medical staff recommendations in determining Eighth Amendment violations for failure to treat (National Institute of Corrections, 2013b). Courts have increasingly rejected policies that have blanket prohibitions on continuation or initiation of hormones, restrict the professional judgment of clinical staff with expertise in gender dysphoria, and deny treatment based on unsubstantiated security concerns, expense, or public disfavor. In 2012, a court set precedent and ordered sex-reassignment surgery for an inmate; the state has appealed that decision (*Kosilek v. Spencer*).

Summary

Correctional psychiatrists need to understand the challenges faced by LGBT inmates, including those unique to each subgroup. Knowledgeable and sensitive clinical assessment can assist this population with their adjustment, safety, and mental health while incarcerated. Psychiatrists can also aid other correctional staff with their awareness of these issues and help ensure that these inmates have access to appropriate medical and mental health services consistent with prevailing standards.

References

American Medical Association (2008). *Removing financial barriers to care for transgender patients*, H-185.950. Available at: http://www.ama-assn.org//ama/pub/about-ama/our-people/member-groups-sections/glbt-advisory-committee/ama-policy-regarding-sexual-orientation.page.

American Psychiatric Association (2012). *Position statement on access to care for transgender and gender variant individuals*. Available at: www.psychiatry.org/file%20library/advocacy%20and%20newsroom/position%20statements/ps2012_transgendercare.pdf

American Psychiatric Association (2013). *Diagnostic and statistical manual of mental disorders* (5th ed.). Arlington, VA: American Psychiatric Publishing.

Beck, A. J., Johnson, C., & Statistics, U.S. Bureau of Justice (2012). *Sexual victimization reported by former state prisoners, 2008*. Available at: http://purl.fdlp.gov/GPO/gpo29057.

Bradford, J., Ryan, C., & Rothblum, E. (1994). National Lesbian Health Care Survey: implications for mental health. *Journal of Counseling and Clinical Psychology*, 62, 228–242.

Brennan, D. J., Ross, L. E., Dobinson, C., et al. (2010). Men's sexual orientation and health in Canada. *Canadian Journal of Public Health*, 101, 255–258.

Brown, G. R., & McDuffie, E. (2009). Health care policies addressing transgender inmates in prison systems in the United States. *Journal of Correctional Health Care*, 15, 280–291.

Centers for Disease Control and Prevention (2013). *Gay and bisexual men's health: sexually transmitted diseases*. Available at: http://www.cdc.gov/msmhealth/std.htm.

Cochran, S. D., & Mays, V. M. (2009). Burden of psychiatric morbidity among lesbian, gay, and bisexual individuals in the California Quality of Life Survey. *Journal of Abnormal Psychology*, 118, 647–658.

Cochran, S. D., Mays, V. M., & Sullivan, J. G. (2003). Prevalence of mental disorders, psychological distress, and mental health services use among lesbian, gay, and bisexual adults in the United States. *Journal of Consulting and Clinical Psychology*, 71, 53–61.

Coleman E., Bockting W., Botzer M., et al. (2012). Standards of care for the health of transsexual, transgender, and gender-nonconforming people, Version 7. *International Journal of Transgenderism*, 13, 165–232.

Ekstrand, M. L., Coates, T. J., Guydish, J. R., et al. (1994). Are bisexually identified men in San Francisco a common vector for spreading HIV infection to women? *American Journal of Public Health*, 84, 915–919.

Fredriksen-Goldsen, K. I., Kim, H. J., Barkan, S. E., et al. (2010). Disparities in health-related quality of life: a comparison of lesbians and bisexual women. *American Journal of Public Health*, 100, 2255–2261.

Garland, J. T., Morgan, R. D., & Beer, A. M. (2005). Impact of time in prison and security level on inmates' sexual attitude, behavior, and identity. *Psychological Services*, 2, 151–162.

Grant J., Mottet L., Tanis J., et al. (2011). *Injustice at every turn: A report of the National Transgender Discrimination Survey*. Available at: http://www.thetaskforce.org/reports_and_research/ntds.

King, M., Semlyen, J., Tai, S. S., et al. (2008). A systematic review of mental disorder, suicide, and deliberate self harm in lesbian, gay and bisexual people. *BMC Psychiatry*, 8, 70.

Koh, A. S., & Ross, L. K. (2006). Mental health issues: a comparison of lesbian, bisexual and heterosexual women. *Journal of Homosexuality, 51*, 33–57.

Kosilek v. Spencer. 889 F.Supp.2d 190 (D. Mass. Sept. 4, 2012).

McCabe, S., Bostwick, W. B., Hughes, T. L., et al. (2010). The relationship between discrimination and substance use disorders among lesbian, gay and bisexual adults in the Unites States. *American Journal of Public Health, 100*, 1946–1952.

Meyer, I. H. (2003). Prejudice, social stress, and mental health in lesbian, gay, and bisexual populations: conceptual issues and research evidence. *Psychological Bulletin, 129*, 674–697.

Miller, M., Andre, A., Ebin, J., & Bessonova, L. (2007). *Bisexual health: An introduction and model practices for HIV/STI prevention programming.* Available at: http://www.thetaskforce.org/downloads/reports/reports/bi_health_5_07_b.pdf.

Miller, M., & Solot, D. (2000). *Tips for health care providers when working with bisexually-identified and behaviorally-bisexual clients.* Available at: http://www.health.state.mn.us/divs/idepc/diseases/syphilis/eliminationproject/workingwithbisexual.pdf.

National Commission on Correctional Health Care Board of Directors (2009). *Transgender health care in correctional settings.* Available at: http://www.ncchc.org/transgender-health-care-in-correctional-settings.

National Institute of Corrections (2013a). *Lesbian, gay, bisexual, transgender and intersex offenders.* Available at: http://nicic.gov/LGBTI.

National Institute of Corrections (2013b). *Policy review and development guide: Lesbian, gay, bisexual, transgender, and intersex persons in custodial settings.* Available at: http://static.nicic.gov/Library/027507.pdf.

National Prison Rape Elimination Commission (2009). *National Prison Rape Elimination Commission Report.* Available at: https://www.ncjrs.gov/pdffiles1/226680.pdf.

San Francisco Human Rights Commission L.A.C. (2011). *Bisexual invisibility: Impacts and recommendations.* Available at: http://www.sf-hrc.org/modules/showdocument.aspx?documentid=989.

Valanis, B. G., Bowen, D. J., Bassford, T., et al. (2000). Sexual orientation and health: comparisons in the Women's Health Initiative sample. *Archives of Family Medicine, 9*, 843–853.

CHAPTER 56

Juveniles

Carl C. Bell

Introduction

The incarceration of juveniles occurs in both juvenile systems and adult correctional systems, depending on jurisdiction, age, and criminal charges. This chapter reviews the history of juvenile incarceration and best or evidence-based practices in the management and treatment of incarcerated juvenile offenders.

History of the juvenile court and juvenile detention centers

In 1871, the Chicago fire caused a great disruption in the city. Many Eastern and Southern European immigrants moved to Chicago to take advantage of the resulting opportunities, and Chicago became a city with a population that was 70% foreign-born or first-generation Americans. In such an upheaval, numerous families, due to poverty and unfamiliar community circumstances, could not provide stable environments and flourish. The reality that the new European immigrants were not doing well was also reflected in the extraordinarily high rates of domestic violence among this population in Chicago from 1875 to 1920 (Adler, 2003). Accordingly, in 1889 Jane Addams founded Hull House on Chicago's Near West Side as a social settlement house "to aid in the solution of the social and industrial problems which are engendered by the modern conditions of life in a great city" (Beuttler & Bell, 2010, p. 5). She was quoted as saying,

> Children over ten years of age were arrested, held in the police stations, tried in the police courts. If convicted they were usually fined and if the fine was not paid sent to the city prison. However, often they were let off because justices could neither tolerate sending children to Bridewell nor bear to be themselves guilty of the harsh folly of compelling poverty-stricken parents to pay fines. No exchange of court records existed and the same children could be in and out of various police stations an indefinite number of times, more hardened and more skillful with each experience. (Addams, 2004 p. 133)

In their efforts to change the harsh conditions besetting Chicago's European immigrant youth, in 1899 Addams and her colleagues worked to establish the first juvenile court in Illinois to distinguish between delinquency and criminality.

The procedures of the juvenile court were designed to be "primarily protective and educational rather than punitive, and the commission of a child to a correctional institution is deemed to be for his welfare and not for the sole purpose of inflicting penalty" (Beuttler & Bell, 2010, p. 5). Ten years later, in 1909, these foresighted women convinced Illinois to discover the cause of delinquency, and the Juvenile Psychopathic Institute (later called the Institute for Juvenile Research, IJR) was created. Neurologist

William Healy, MD, the first director, was charged with studying the delinquent's biological aspects of brain functioning and intelligence, social factors, attitudes, and motivations. Thus, the IJR was the birthplace of child psychiatry (Schowalter, 2000).

IJR's initial goal was to develop an understanding of the causes of behavioral disturbances in youth by doing research and providing services to delinquent youth while also developing strategies to prevent delinquency. Early studies found no relationship between genetics and criminality. IJR researchers Shaw and McKay (1942) noted that delinquency was less due to genetic, ethnic, or cultural factors and more due to social disruption, which eroded formal and informal social control in specific transitional neighborhoods ("delinquency areas") in a city. In an effort to prevent delinquency, the Chicago Area Project, designed to create social fabric in these "delinquency areas," was born. However, 50 years ago, the science was not as advanced as it is now. The research designs were empirical and qualitative instead of being quantitative, and much of the IJR's research was biographical. The statistical methodology was very primitive by today's standards, and multivariate influences could not be adequately studied. However, despite this lack of scientific methodology, the IJR's observations were consistent with the majority of recent findings. Their observations were that children's genetics did not cause delinquency, but rather the lack of social fabric was more directly linked to delinquency in the new immigrant communities. Of course, this finding predated by 50 years the seminal research of Sampson and colleagues (1997), who coined the term "collective efficacy," demonstrating more rigorously that formal and informal social controls reduce and may prevent delinquency.

Early juvenile court and detention center philosophy

Retrospectively, the early juvenile court and detention center philosophy centered on strengthening families. The early court sought to provide protective factors for families by increasing the social fabric around delinquent youth; increasing connectedness and social bonds between delinquent youth and adults; providing delinquent youth with opportunities (often in the form of vocational training) to give them a sense of self-esteem; providing opportunities to develop social and emotional skills; providing an adult protective shield to monitor situations that could result in risky behaviors; and helping youth transform the negative energy from traumatic life experiences into constructive energy. Looking back at the court's strategy and activities from today's perspective, the activities to strengthen families would fit nicely into a modern biopsychosocial model of behavior change, specifically the theory of triadic influence (TTI; Flay et al., 2009). TTI is an evidence-based theory of health behavior change (Flay et al., 2004) that has also been simplified to engage community participants (Bell et al., 2002) to enhance successful implementation.

Shift in juvenile court and detention philosophy

Social policy tends to swing back and forth like a pendulum. Consequently, this effective, century-old habilation approach to juvenile delinquency has slowly eroded. This movement from habilation to retribution was accelerated following the 1967 Gault case (Gault, 1967). Gerald Gault was a 15-year-old boy adjudicated a delinquent by an Arizona juvenile court for making "lewd" phone calls. As a result, he was committed to the Arizona State Industrial School until he turned 21. As was typical of juvenile court in those days, he was not afforded counsel or an opportunity to confront or cross-examine his accuser, nor was he offered privilege against self-incrimination. After the hearing, although he had no right to appeal to a higher court, the case reached the US Supreme Court. The maximum penalty Gault would have received if he were an adult was a $50 fine or two months in jail. Had he been 18, he would have had substantial constitutional and state statutory rights. The Supreme Court chided the juvenile court for its pretension of paternalism and blasted the juvenile court model as inadequate to dispense justice.

As a result of the Gault decision, juveniles began to be given their Miranda rights and access to counsel. Gradually, the juvenile court moved away from a system of habilation to one of due process, with resultant criminalization of delinquent juvenile behavior. The Gault decision, combined with public misperceptions of youthful "superpredators" and a perceived upsurge in violent juvenile offenders, created pressure to protect society that challenged the habilation model and favored punishment. Accordingly, "dangerous" juveniles are again increasingly being transferred to the adult criminal justice system, where the consequences are much harsher (National Academy of Sciences, 2012). Expansion of the juvenile correctional population has caused issues of juvenile competency, health care needs, and prevention strategies to surface as areas in need of immediate attention (National Academy of Sciences, 2012). As modern science has done a better job of understanding brain development (National Academy of Sciences, 2012, p. 96), it has become increasing clear that adolescents are at greater risk for being legally incompetent. Specifically, the MacArthur Foundation's 15-year research endeavor found that a significant proportion of adolescents age 15 or younger are probably incompetent to stand trial based on adult measures of legal competency. Further, a delinquent's age strongly influences his or her ability to consider the consequences of his or her behavior or to resist peer pressure (MacArthur Foundation, 2006).

Regarding the health and mental care of youth in the juvenile justice system, the American Academy of Pediatrics Committee on Adolescence Policy Statement (2011) makes it clear that youth in the system are a high-risk population that have unmet physical, developmental, and mental health needs and these issues occur at higher rates than in the general adolescent population. Lastly, "mental, emotional and behavioral disorders among young people burden . . . juvenile justice systems and, according to one estimate, more than a quarter of total service costs for children who have

these disorders are incurred in the school and juvenile justice systems" (National Research Council and Institute of Medicine, 2009, p. 5). Accordingly, mental health practitioners involved with juvenile confinement need to be acutely aware of these realities and take them under consideration to practice health care ethically (McBride & Bell, 2011).

The existing juvenile justice system

Recent estimates demonstrate that in 2009 the juvenile courts in the United States handled an estimated 1.5 million delinquency cases that involved criminal charges (Knoll & Sickmund, 2012). The trend, however, is not simply linear. From 1985 through 1997, the number of delinquency cases climbed steadily (63%), but from 1997 through 2009, the delinquency caseload then dropped 20%. In 2009, formal probation was the most severe disposition ordered in 60% of cases in which the juvenile was adjudicated delinquent, and 27% of cases were ordered to residential placement (e.g., a group home or juvenile correctional facility) as the most severe disposition. Thus, per the National Juvenile Court Data Archive, the number of youth entering corrections is now decreasing (Knoll & Sickmund, 2012).

The National Academy of Science's Reforming Juvenile Justice report maintains that confining youths away from their homes and communities interferes with three important social conditions that contribute to adolescents' healthy psychological development (National Academy of Science, 2012): the presence of a connected and concerned parent or a parent surrogate; the adolescent's association with prosocial peers who model positive social behavior and academic success; and activities that require autonomous decision making and critical-thinking skills. Unfortunately, despite some successful efforts aimed at juvenile justice reform, many juvenile justice detention and confinement centers do not provide these necessities for healthy development.

Making the care and management of incarcerated juveniles more complex is the fact that youth in the system have high rates of mental health problems (Cauffman & Grisso, 2005; Illinois Models for Change, 2010; Shufelt & Cocozza, 2006; Teplin et al., 2002). Nearly 70% have at least one diagnosable mental disorder (not counting conduct disorder) and more than 60% have comorbid diagnoses; the prevalence of mental disorders is 40% to 60% higher than that found in comparable community samples (approximately 17% to 22%; Cauffman & Grisso, 2005). Unfortunately, many states fail to provide adequate community mental health services for their youth. As a result, some parents actually seek mental health treatment for their children within the juvenile justice system (Grisso, 2006, 2008; Skowyra & Cocozza, 2006). One congressional report (Waxman & Collins, 2004) notes that more than half of states were detaining youth with mental health needs until services could be obtained in more appropriate community settings.

Based on clinical experience, Bell (2012, 2014) posits that many of the mental disorders observed in incarcerated youth are due to fetal alcohol exposure (FAE). FAE is the most common cause of intellectual deficiency (mostly mild), speech and language disorders, attention-deficit/hyperactivity disorders (ADHD), and specific learning disorders (Stratton et al., 1996). Youths with fetal alcohol spectrum disorder (FASD) are 19 times more likely to be incarcerated than are youths without FASD in a given year

(Popova et al., 2011). Woods and colleagues (2012) highlight the need to do a thorough neurobehavioral assessment of individuals in the correctional system, and Brown and colleagues (2012) outline treatment strategies for youth with FASD. It has been estimated that two thirds to three fourths of the youth in the Cook County (Illinois) Detention Center have problems with mild intellectual deficiency, speech and language disorders, ADHD, and specific learning disorders (e.g., inability to read; Earl Dunlap and Dave Roush, personal communication, 2010).

Finally, the American Bar Association (2012) has recognized FASD as a major issue in child welfare, juvenile justice, and adult justice systems. Most recently, the problem of FASD or, as it is referred to in *Diagnostic and Statistical Manual of Mental Disorders*–5 (DSM-5), neurobehavioral disorder associated with prenatal alcohol exposure (NDA-PAE), has been designated as a "condition for further study" (American Psychiatric Association, 2013). Considering that many youth with NDA-PAE or FASD have serious difficulties with affect regulation, the prevalence of NDA-PAE and FASD in these three public systems should not be a surprise. However, it is also clear that these systems are poorly prepared to appropriately manage these brain-injured youth. Recent research suggests that in addition to psychotherapeutic and social interventions, choline, vitamin A, and folate may reduce the morbidity from this neuropsychiatric disorder (Ballard et al., 2012; Monk et al., 2012; Otero et al., 2012). However, because the brain is always developing, it is unclear whether this intervention will have equivalent or diminishing efficacy in utero, in infancy, childhood, adolescence, and young adulthood, or, possibly, even in later years.

Another major psychiatric dynamic among youth in correctional settings is the extremely high rate of exposure to trauma and violence. Early work examining the exposure of incarcerated youth to traumatic violence in the United States revealed that in Pennsylvania more than one third had been stabbed, 60% had been shot at, one fourth reported seeing a family member stabbed, and 42% reported having seen a friend stabbed (DeFazio & Warford, 1993). In Illinois, two thirds had witnessed at least one killing and two fifths had seen a friend killed (Bell & Jenkins, 1995). More recently, Abram and colleagues (2004) found that more than half of their samples had been exposed to six or more traumatic events. Considering the high rates of trauma, neurodevelopmental disorders, and mental illness in corrections, current science and older wisdom suggest we begin to take a strength-based, prevention approach to the problem.

Fortunately, there are national juvenile detention and juvenile center health care standards promulgated by a collection of national health care organizations that seek to improve correctional health care (e.g., National Commission on Correctional Health Care, 2011). These standards address the day-to-day physical and mental health care practices for quality health care in juvenile confinement and detention facilities. Such standards require that all inmates be screened for physical and mental health problems on admission, receive a health assessment within a given period of time, and are informed about how to access health care (Cohen, 1998). Further, the standards require that regular sick-call services are in place, the correctional staff have first-aid and CPR training, and the facility has systems to respond to emergency health concerns (National Commission on Correctional Health Care, 2011).

A developmental approach to juvenile justice

Because we consider America to be an enlightened society and the subjects of the juvenile justice system are children, the overarching goal of this system should be to support the positive social, emotional, and intellectual development of its charges. In turn, this approach would enhance the safety of communities. Another major role of the system is to hold youth accountable for wrongdoing and prevent further offending while at the same time treating youth fairly and with justice. The former positive developmental approach does not conflict with the latter safety approach. Holding adolescents responsible for behavior that sometimes leads to juvenile crimes ensures that offenders will be held accountable and also provides justice to victims. However, children are still developing, and their brains develop from the "bottom up" and "inside out," causing their flight, fight, or freeze (limbic) systems to be fully engaged before their judgment and wisdom (frontal lobe) systems are in place to mediate their behavior. Children are not little adults (Bell & McBride, 2010). Put more simply, children are essentially "all gasoline and no brakes or steering wheel," and they need mature adults to provide "braking and steering" until they can develop their own internal control systems. Accordingly, the mechanisms of accountability for juveniles should not mimic adult punishments (National Academy of Sciences, 2012). Condemnation, control, and lengthy confinement are not ordinarily needed to ensure that juveniles are held accountable. The National Academy of Sciences report suggests that juvenile courts should provide an opportunity for youths to accept responsibility for their actions, make amends to victims and the community, and participate in programs that give them a sense of purpose, such as community service (National Academy of Sciences, 2012).

An aim of juvenile justice should be to prevent reoffending. The efficacy of prevention depends, in part, on how youth are treated while in juvenile justice and adult corrections facilities. However, a few youths are prone to be serious, chronic, violent offenders (Department of Health and Human Services, 2001). To identify those at risk for serious, chronic offenses, courts need to implement risk and need assessments. These tools provide some guidance in determining whether a youth is at a low, medium, or high risk of reoffending based on factors such as prior offending history and school performance. Research reveals that someone who presents with a high-risk profile can be effectively supported to reduce his or her risk with evidence-based interventions, community monitoring, or changes in life situation (Lipsey et al., 2010). Further, use of such interventions allows for better targeting of resources, focusing the more intense and costly interventions on those at greater risk of reoffending. Effectively implemented evidence-based interventions such as the Good Behavior Game (Kellam et al., 2008) or certain types of therapy such as aggression replacement therapy and cognitive-behavioral therapy have been shown to reduce reoffending (Mendel, 2000; Sherman et al., 1997). Well-organized community-based interventions show greater reductions in rearrests than programs offered in institutional settings (National Academy of Sciences, 2012). Furthermore, there is no convincing evidence that confinement of juvenile offenders beyond six months appreciably reduces the likelihood of subsequent offending (National Academy of Sciences, 2012, p. 6).

Treating youth fairly and with dignity can enhance moral development, legal behavior, and appropriate social control during adolescence. Although the judicial ideal is to have youth represented by properly trained counsel and to have an opportunity to participate in the proceedings, the reality is often different. Attorneys in juvenile courts are often poorly prepared and under-resourced (Wilson, 1999). Of course, if racial and ethnic disparities could be addressed, cultural, racial, and ethnic groups would feel more inclined to believe in the fairness of the US justice system (Alexander, 2010).

Assessment and treatment—best practices

Considering the complexity of the mental, emotional, and behavioral disorders of youth in corrections, there are several best-practice approaches to assessment and treatment. First, all juvenile correctional facilities should have receiving and screening health and mental health procedures; best-practice receiving and screening forms can be found in the National Commission on Correctional Health Care Juvenile Detention Standards (2011). Of note, due to the US prisoner research protection guidelines, it is difficult to develop or obtain practice guidelines that are evidence-based (see Chapter 70). Screening for suicidal ideation is especially important, as suicide rates in the corrections population have historically been higher than in the general population (Bell, 2005). Trained mental health workers can do screening and, when indicated, patients can be referred for psychiatric follow-up. It is also important to screen for developmental disabilities such as FASD; the appendix of DSM-5 has proposed criteria for neurobehavioral disorder associated with prenatal alcohol exposure that can be used for that purpose (American Psychiatric Association, 2013, p. 798). This is an important consideration, as the brain damage from FASD may be remediated using nutritional supplements (Ballard et al., 2012). In addition, it is important to ask questions about childhood trauma in this population; supportive guides are now available (Bell, 2013).

The future

The future of juvenile corrections holds some interesting challenges. The juvenile correctional population is shrinking, while the mental health needs of juveniles who still become incarcerated are getting more extensive. Administrators will be faced with decreasing budgets. The knowledge base of the mental health needs of juveniles in corrections will continue to increase, resulting in a demand for the provision of respectful and effective treatments for those in custody. We hope that a more strength-based approach will take hold once again, replacing the retribution/punishment approach that is currently the norm in many facilities. We also hope there will be greater recognition of the prevalence of fetal alcohol exposure in juvenile detainees, and research will have matured to the point of providing effective preventive interventions. Research science needs to step up and develop instruments that can identify this neuropsychiatric problem said to be a primary cause for the common mental health issues in juvenile corrections (i.e., speech and language disorders, mild intellectual deficiency, specific learning disorders, and ADHD). Further, more attention needs to be given to providing evidence-based, trauma-informed care for treating youth in juvenile corrections.

Summary

As our understanding of youth development becomes more sophisticated and our information technology develops more interconnectedness, we will be in a better position to coordinate the services (juvenile detention, special education, foster care, and mental health) that troubled youth need. When this occurs, the United States will be able to achieve the public health goal that the sixteenth US surgeon general outlined in his 2000 Youth Conference when he declared that to preserve our nation's public health, we would need to look to the youth involved with juvenile detention, special education, foster care, and mental health systems (US Public Health Service, 2000).

References

Abram, K. M., Teplin, L. A., Charles, D. R., et al. (2004). Post-traumatic stress disorder and trauma in youth in juvenile detention. *Archives of General Psychiatry, 61*, 403–410.

Addams, J. (2004). *My friend, Julia Lathrop.* Champlain, IL: University of Illinois Press.

Addler, J. S. (2003). "We've got a right to fight: We're married": Domestic homicide in Chicago, 1975–1920. *Journal of Interdisciplinary History, 34*(1), 27–48.

Alexander, M. (2010). *The new Jim Crow.* New York: The New Press.

American Academy of Pediatrics, Committee on Adolescence (2011). Policy statement—health care for youth in the juvenile justice system. *Pediatrics, 128,* 1219.

American Bar Association (2013). *FASD: Identification and advocacy.* Chicago, IL: American Bar Association. Available at: http://apps.americanbar.org/litigation/committees/childrights/content/articles/fall2012-0912-fasd-identification-advocacy.html

American Psychiatric Association (2013) *Diagnostic and statistical manual of mental disorders* (5th ed.). Washington, DC: American Psychiatric Press Inc.

Ballard, M. S., Sun, M., & Ko, J. (2012). Vitamin A, folate, and choline as possible preventive intervention to fetal alcohol syndrome. *Medical Hypotheses, 78*, 489–493.

Bell, C. C. (2005). Correctional psychiatry. In B. J. Sadock & V. A. Sadock (Eds.), *Comprehensive textbook of psychiatry* (8th ed., pp. 4002–4012). Baltimore, MD: Williams & Wilkins.

Bell, C. C. (2012) An ethical conundrum in correctional health care. *Correct Care, 26*(2), 3–4.

Bell, C. C. (2013). Trauma and living in violent neighborhoods. *Psychiatric Times, 30*(5), 16–19. Available at: http://www.psychiatrictimes.com/special-reports/content/article/10168/2141180

Bell, C. C. (2014). Taking issue—fetal alcohol exposure in the African-American community. *Psychiatric Services, 65*(5), 569–569.

Bell, C. C., Flay, B., & Paikoff, R. (2002). Strategies for health behavioral change. In J. Chunn (Ed.), *The health behavioral change imperative: Theory, education, and practice in diverse populations* (pp. 17–40). New York: Kluwer Academic/Plenum Publishers. Available at: http://people.oregonstate.edu/~flayb/MY%20PUBLICATIONS/Multiple%20behaviors/Bell,Flay,Paikoff.pdf

Bell, C. C., & Jenkins, E. J. (1995). Violence prevention and intervention in juvenile detention and correctional facilities. *Journal of Correctional Health Care, 2*(1), 17–38.

Bell, C. C., & McBride, D. F. (2010). Affect regulation and the prevention of risky behaviors. *Journal of the American Medical Association, 304*(5), 565–566.

Beuttler, F. W., & Bell, C. C. (2010). *For the welfare of every child—a brief history of the Institute for Juvenile Research, 1909—2010.* Chicago: University of Illinois.

Brown, N. N., Connor, P. D., & Adler, R. S. (2012). Conduct-disordered adolescents with fetal alcohol spectrum disorder: Intervention in secure settings. *Criminal Justice and Behavior, 39*, 770–793.

Cauffman, E., & Grisso, T. (2005). Mental health issues among minority offenders in the juvenile justice system. In D. F. Hawkins & K. Kempf-Leonard (Eds.), *Our children, their children: confronting racial and ethnic differences in American juvenile hustice* (pp. 390–412). Chicago, IL: University of Chicago Press.

Cohen, M. D. (1998). Special problems of health services for juvenile justice programs. In M. Puisis (Ed.), *Clinical practice in correctional medicine* (pp. 332–343). St. Louis, MO: Mosby.

Department of Health and Human Services (2001). *Youth violence: a report of the Surgeon General*. Rockville, MD: Department of Health and Human Services.

Flay, B. R., Graumlich, S., Segawa, E., et al. (2004). Effects of two prevention programs on high-risk behaviors among African American youth: a randomized trial. *Archives of Pediatrics and Adolescent Medicine, 158*(4), 377–384.

Flay, B. R., Snyder, F., & Petraitis, J. (2009). The theory of triadic influence. In R. J. DiClemente, M. C. Kegler, & R. A. Crosby (Eds.), *Emerging theories in health promotion practice and research* (2nd ed., pp. 451–510). New York: Jossey-Bass.

Grisso, T., & Grisso, T. (2006). *Double jeopardy: Adolescent offenders with mental disorders. Executive summary*. Available at: http://www.adjj. org/downloads/5314Double% 20Jeopardy.pdf; [accessed April 2012].

Grisso, T., & Grisso, T. (2008). Adolescent offenders with mental disorders. *Future of Children, 18*(2), 143–164.

Illinois Models for Change Behavioral Health Assessment Team (2010). *Report on the behavioral health program for youth committed to Illinois' Department of Juvenile Justice*. Available at: http://www. modelsforchange.net/publications/271 [accessed April 2012].

In re Gault, 387. U.S. 1 (1967).

Kellam, S. G., Brown, C. H., Poduska, J. M., et al. (2008). Effects of a universal classroom behavior management program in first and second grades on young adult behavioral, psychiatric, and social outcomes. *Drug and Alcohol Dependence, 95*, S5–S28.

Knoll, C., & Sickmumd, M. (2012). *Delinquency cases in juvenile court, 2009*. Washington, DC: U.S Department of Justice, Office of Justice Programs, Office of Juvenile Justice and Delinquency Prevention, NCJ 239081. Available at: http://www.ojjdp.gov/ pubs/239081.pdf

Lipsey, M. W., Howell, J. C., Kelly, M. R., et al. (2010). *Improving the effectiveness of juvenile justice programs: A new perspective on evidence-based practice* (pp. 21–28). Washington, DC: Center for Juvenile Justice Reform.

MacArthur Foundation Research Network on Adolescent Development and Juvenile Justice (2006). *Bringing research to policy and practice in juvenile justice*. Available at: http://www.adjj.org/ downloads/552network_overview.pdf

McBride, D. F., & Bell, C. C. (2011). Guest editorial: Is denial of evidence-based prevention a violation of human rights? *Journal of the National Medical Association, 103*(7), 618–619.

Mendel, R. A. (2000). *Less hype, more help: Reducing juvenile crime, what works—and what doesn't*. Washington, DC: American Youth Policy Forum.

Monk, B. R., Leslie, F. M., & Thomas, J. D. (2012). The effects of perinatal choline supplementation on hippocampal cholinergic development in rats exposed to alcohol during the brain growth spurt. *Hippocampus, 22*, 1750–1757.

National Academy of Science (2012). *Reforming juvenile justice: A developmental approach*, R. J. Bonnie, B. M. Chemers, & J. Schuck (Eds.), Committee on Law and Justice, Division of Behavioral and Social Sciences Education. Washington, DC: National Academy of Sciences Press. Available at: http://www.nap.edu/catalog. php?record_id=14685

National Drug Control Strategy (1989). Washington, DC: The White House. Available at: https://www.ncjrs.gov/pdffiles1/ondcp/119466. pdf 14.

National Commission on Correctional Health Care (NCCHC) (2011). *Standards for health services in juvenile detention and confinement facilities*. Chicago, IL: National Commission on Correctional Health Care.

National Research Council and Institute of Medicine (2009). *Preventing mental, emotional, and behavioral disorders among young people: Progress and possibilities*, M. E. O'Connell, T. Boat, & K. E. Warner (Eds.). Committee on Prevention of Mental Disorders and Substance Abuse Among Children, Youth, and Young Adults: Research Advances and Promising Interventions. Washington, DC: The National Academies Press.

Otero, N. K. H., Thomas, J. D., Saski, C. A., Xia, A., & Kelly, S. J. (2012). Choline supplementation and DNA methylation in the hippocampus and prefrontal cortex of rats exposed to alcohol during development. *Alcoholism: Clinical and Experimental Research, 36*(10), 1701–1709.

Popova, S., Lange, S., Bekmuradov, D., et al. (2011). Fetal alcohol spectrum disorder prevalence estimates in correctional systems: a systematic literature review. *Canadian Journal of Public Health, 102*, 336–340.

Sampson, R. J., Raudenbush, S. W., & Earls, F. (1997). Neighborhoods and violent crime: A multilevel study of collective efficacy. *Science, 277*, 918–924.

Schowalter, J. E. (2000). Child and adolescent psychiatry comes of age, 1944–1994. In R. W. Menninger & J. C. Nemiah (Eds.), *American psychiatry after World War II, 1944–1994* (pp. 461–480). Washington, DC: American Psychiatric Press.

Shaw, C. R., & McKay, H. (1942). *Juvenile delinquency and urban areas*. Chicago, IL: University of Chicago Press.

Sherman, L. W., Gottfredson, D., MacKenzie, D., Eck, J., Reuter, P., & Bushway, S. (1997). *Preventing crime: what works, what doesn't, what's promising*. Washington, DC: Office of Justice Programs, National Institute of Justice, U.S. Department of Justice.

Shufelt, J., & Cocozza, J. (2006). *Youth with mental health disorders in the juvenile justice system: results from a multi-state prevalence study*. Delmar, NY: National Center for Mental Health and Juvenile Justice.

Stratton, K., Howe, C., & Battaglia, F. C. (Eds). (1996). *Fetal alcohol syndrome: diagnosis, epidemiology, prevention and treatment*. Washington, DC: National Academy Press.

Teplin, L. A., Abram, K. M., McClelland, G. M., et al. (2002). Psychiatric disorders in youth in juvenile detention. *Archives of General Psychiatry, 59*(12), 1133–1143.

US Public Health Service (2000). *Report of the Surgeon General's Conference on Children's Mental Health: a national action agenda*. Washington, DC: Department of Health and Human Services.

Waxman, H. A., & Collins, S. (2004). *Incarceration of youth who are waiting for community mental health services in the United States*. Washington, DC: U.S. House of Representatives, Committee on Government Reform.

Wilson, R. J. (1999). *Improving criminal justice systems through strategies and innovative collaborations: report of the National Symposium on Indigent Defense*. Rockville, MD: US Department of Justice—Bureau of Justice Assistance. Available at: https://www.ncjrs. gov/app/publications/abstract.aspx?ID=181344

Woods, G. W., Freedman, D., & Greenspan, S. (2012). Neurobehavioral assessment in forensic practice. *International Journal of Law and Psychiatry, 35*(5-6), 432–439.

CHAPTER 57

Aging prisoners and the provision of correctional mental health

Kristin G. Cloyes and Kathryn A. Burns

Introduction

The US prison population is aging rapidly, and prison systems across the United States must now care for a growing number of inmates who are elderly, in poor physical and mental health, and significantly affected by age-related impairment (Binswanger, Kruger, & Steiner, 2009; Kuhlman & Ruddell, 2005; Loeb & AbuDagga, 2006; Rikard & Rosenberg, 2007; Williams, Stern, Mellow, et al., 2012). This situation creates critical challenges for state and federal corrections systems and correctional health professionals today. Human Rights Watch's 2012 report *Old Behind Bars* found that the number of US prisoners aged 65 or older grew at 94 times the rate of the overall prison population between 2007 and 2012 (Human Rights Watch, 2012). The Bureau of Justice Statistics reports that in 2011 7.9% of state and federal inmates were 55 or older; there were 26,700 over age 65 (Carson & Sabol, 2012).

This growth is complicated by the fact that chronological age does not necessarily match "health age" or health status in prison (Chiu, 2010). As a result, many prison systems have adjusted their definition of "elderly" down to age 55 (and some as low as 40) to reflect the relatively poor health status of aging men and women in their institutions (Binswanger et al., 2009; Chiu, 2010; Human Rights Watch, 2012). Typical correctional health services in prisons across the United States are already hard pressed to keep up with increasing demands for care of aging inmates. The responsibility to provide adequate health services for prisoners remains despite shrinking local, county, state, and federal budgets (Mitka, 2004; Snyder, van Wormer, Chadha, & Jaggers, 2009; Williams, Lindquist, Hill, et al., 2009).

Central issues for providers in psychiatric and psychosocial care of aging prisoners

Aging, life transitions, and grief

Elderly inmates do not fit normative psychological standards of healthy aging such as Erikson's psychosocial stages of life. Community-dwelling middle-aged adults (aged 40–65) are understood to be creating a positive legacy based on a subjective sense of usefulness and family or civic involvement, while adults over 65 are thought of as engaged in life review and assessment that leads to either fulfillment and wisdom or regret and despair. Inmates, especially those who are estranged from family and community, often do not experience normative lifespan progression; thus,

markers of success associated with healthy development and aging are often not part of the context of older incarcerated adults.

Normative models of age-associated grief, coping with loss, and bereavement also highlight risks specific to older incarcerated adults. Complicated grief is defined as getting "stuck" in the acute phases of grief and a failure to integrate the grief experience into ongoing life. Disenfranchised grief, a concept first developed by Doka (1989), is defined as an experience where one suffers from and mourns a loss, but loss, grief response, or both are not socially acknowledged or supported. While there are few scientific studies of complicated and disenfranchised grief among people who are incarcerated, rates of both are reasonably thought to be high because of the histories of inmates and the cultural context of prisons and jails (Olson & McEwen, 2004). If unrecognized and untreated, complicated and disenfranchised grief can lead to major depression, exacerbate underlying cognitive dysfunction (e.g., impaired memory and judgment), and result in significant disability. Untreated grief has also been identified as a risk factor for both suicide and recidivism, as it may underlie issues such as substance use that complicate transition to the community (Harner, Hentz, & Evangelista, 2011).

Normative lifespan and grief models may not easily accommodate the experiences of aging inmates; however, mental health professionals who work in corrections settings are developing programs that promote positive age-related life transitions and coping with loss. The True Grit program in Nevada, a cohort-based structured living program aimed at promoting healthier "aging in place" for prison inmates over the age of 60, provides participants daily opportunities for meaningful participation in physical, social, and spiritual activities. One evaluation of this program indicates that participants report high life satisfaction and low psychological distress (Kopera-Frye, Harrison, Iribarne, et al., 2013). Similarly, grief and coping interventions that focus on the specific challenges faced by older incarcerated men and women must emphasize and work toward the potential for healthy coping and transition within the context of incarceration. These challenges include loss of loved ones while incarcerated; loss of time, experience, and opportunity; lack of perceived safety and privacy in expression of grief; and the cumulative effects of multiple or serial losses.

Comorbidity, cognitive disorders, mental illness, and co-occurring disorders in elderly prisoners

Elderly prisoners, many of whom have poor physical and mental health, present a complex array of medical, psychological, and logistical needs that complicate the provision of psychiatric care for this group. Challenges to mental health treatment include complex interactions among chronic long-term physical illness, disabilities related to unhealthy aging, cognitive dysfunction, mental illness, substance abuse history, and significant psychological and social stressors related to aging while incarcerated. These stressors are exacerbated by the loss of social status, lack of protection, and the fear of dying in prison.

High prevalence of comorbidity and disability

Inmates experience higher rates of disease, comorbidity, long-term chronic illness, and age-related disability—at earlier ages—than their community-dwelling counterparts (Kuhlman & Ruddell, 2005; Loeb, Steffensmeier, & Lawrence, 2008; Mara, 2004; Williams, Lindquist, Sudore, et al., 2006). Older prisoners have a significantly higher prevalence of infectious disease, heart disease, lung disease, metabolic disorder, and cancers, including both higher rates of cancer overall and more aggressive forms of cancer, than the majority of elderly patients (Binswanger et al., 2009; Maruschak & Beavers, 2009; Mathew, Elting, Cooksley, et al., 2005).

Dementia and age-related cognitive disorders

To date, there are no national studies on the prevalence of dementia in US prisons, but extrapolations can be made from community data. The decade from 2000 to 2010 saw a 10% increase in the estimated incidence of Alzheimer's disease in the US population; estimates also predict a 30% increase in Alzheimer's among those over 65 in the next 20 years (Hebert, Scherr, Bienias, et al., 2003). Because incarcerated men and women have significantly poorer health than their free-world counterparts, including poorer outcomes on factors correlated with all forms of dementia, it stands to reason that rates of dementia and age-related cognitive dysfunction in incarcerated older adults would be even higher. Cognitive dysfunction of those at earlier stages of disease may easily be misdiagnosed or treated as "behavioral" in nature. Moreover, progression of dementia and increased confusion puts those affected at odds with other inmates and staff, creating serious challenges to accommodating their increasing frailty and providing for their safety (Fazel, McMillan, & O'Donnell, 2002).

Mental illness and co-occurring disorders

Older inmates are also at particular risk for anxiety related to aging in prison. Specific factors include fear of victimization, loss of social status, and loss of physical and social autonomy (Aday, 2003). Suicide is often overlooked among older adults; people over 65 now make up 12.5% of the US population but account for 15.7% of suicides. Many of the risk factors for later-life suicide, including male gender, depression, and cerebrovascular disease (Sneed & Culang-Reinlieb, 2011), are overrepresented among incarcerated older adults. Mental health risks are further complicated by current and historical substance use that are likely to represent years of cumulative effects of untreated disorders. One large sample study reported that 70% of older inmates report a history of substance use; while most used substances for more than four decades, more than one third never received treatment (Arndt, Turvey, & Flaum, 2002).

Mental health assessment for older prisoners

The interplay among these illnesses and risk factors creates the need for adapted, focused assessment and treatment. Providers should consider incorporating some modifications to the mental health and suicide risk screening and assessment process when evaluating older inmates. One such modification is the incorporation of measures to assess cognitive impairment or dementia. Instruments to consider include the Mini-Mental State Examination or the Montreal Cognitive Assessment (Folstein, Folstein, & McHugh, 1975; Nasreddine, Phillips, Bedirian, et al., 2005), which are both in the public domain and widely available. The instruments can also be used at periodic intervals to document and track cognitive ability and/or decline, if any.

Mental health care providers should also consider incorporating use of an activities-of-daily-living scale to assess functioning. The Older Americans Resources and Services Activities of Daily Living Scale may be helpful in this regard, but it has not been modified specifically for use with incarcerated persons (George & Fillenbaum, 1985). While some questions are not relevant, other items regarding ambulation, grooming and personal hygiene, and toileting issues are universally applicable. On a programmatic level, assessment of activities of daily living in a population of geriatric inmates permits a form of program needs assessment. For example, caregiver staffing levels may need to be adjusted if additional assistance with basic hygiene and grooming is necessary.

Consideration should be given to repeating the mental health cognitive and activities-of-daily-living assessment as part of the annual health appraisal many correctional facilities undertake for inmates older than 50. This would permit documentation of baseline functioning and serial reassessment to permit early intervention in individual cases. It also helps in monitoring the population to make the necessary adjustments to staffing, procedures, and environmental modifications, as discussed previously. Further, combining the annual physical and mental health assessment could serve as the springboard to ensure that mental health care and physical health care are coordinated. Formulating mental health diagnoses, physical examination, and laboratory testing to rule out (and treat) physical causes of the psychiatric dysfunction are important for patients of all ages but particularly so with the older correctional population, whose medical morbidity exceeds that of same-age peers in the community. Thyroid imbalance, infection, hypoglycemia, and hypoxia may present with confusion and impaired attention in an older population.

Comprehensive assessment may also require neurological consultation and brain imaging. Neuropsychological testing may provide useful baseline information and assist in distinguishing depression from dementia, as both share a number of symptoms, including impaired attention leading to memory deficits, anhedonia, diminished appetite, and sleep disturbance (Small, 2009). The distinction is important in order to begin the most appropriate and effective course of treatment.

Medication management for older inmates

It is important to recall the old adage "start low, go slow" when prescribing psychotropic medications to older inmates. Starting doses of psychotropic medications are generally much lower than those for adult patients, perhaps as little as one-quarter the usual starting dose, and a longer interval is required to permit accommodation to the medication before increasing the dose. Although it will take longer to achieve a therapeutic dose or level, the medication will be much better tolerated in the long run. Psychotropic medication management is another area that should be approached in consultation with physical health care providers and perhaps a pharmacist. This follows from the high prevalence of medical contraindications and the very real possibility of drug–drug interactions given the number of medications often prescribed to manage conditions requiring chronic care (e.g., hepatitis, chronic obstructive pulmonary disease, hypertension, and cardiac problems).

The difficulty in differentiating depression from dementia has been mentioned earlier. The distinction is important—unlike most forms of dementia, the symptoms of depression can resolve with appropriate treatment. With older inmate patients, prescribers should consider using one of the selective serotonin reuptake inhibitors due to their safety profile. Antidepressant medications that have anticholinergic side effects should be avoided as they may cause or increase confusion in the elderly (Blazer, 2013). Treatment response is improved by combining antidepressant medication with cognitive-oriented psychotherapy. Cognitive-behavioral therapy for late-life depression is one such evidence-based practice that is effective in the elderly. It may also be provided as the primary treatment for patients who cannot take medication due to intolerable side effects or secondary to a medical contraindication that precludes use of an antidepressant (Thompson, Coon, Gallagher-Thompson, et al., 2001).

For patients with a longstanding history of serious mental illness such as bipolar disorder or schizophrenia, medications that were previously effective in managing symptoms can be continued or restarted. It may be possible, even desirable, to taper or reduce the doses to the lowest effective doses to minimize the medication "burden" for patients taking medications for multiple conditions and to decrease the likelihood of drug interactions and side effects. Further, as people age, the severity and intensity of symptoms often remit so they can be maintained at lower medication doses.

Given the prevalence of dementia, particularly Alzheimer's disease, correctional facilities should consider adding a cholinesterase inhibitor to their psychotropic medication formulary if not already present. Four medications have been approved for treatment of Alzheimer's dementia: donepezil, rivastigmine, galantamine, and tacrine. Tacrine is not generally recommended due to its dose-related hepatotoxicity. The cholinesterase inhibitors have not been studied in a head-to-head comparison, but there is some evidence that they may stabilize current functioning and delay further cognitive loss. Actual improvement, if any, is modest (Gunther, 2013). However, stabilizing functioning and postponing decline are important goals in correctional facilities that aim to preserve independent functioning as long as possible in order to reduce the need for more intensive nursing and other supportive services. Civilian nursing home placements are difficult to secure with this population, and creating a nursing home level of care in correctional facilities is expensive.

The choice of agent(s) for formulary placement therefore can be based on weighing factors such as cost per dose and available preparations (e.g., tablet, sustained release, transdermal patch). Rivastigmine, for example, is available in tablet and transdermal patch preparations and is eliminated primarily via the kidneys rather than hepatic metabolism. Use of a patch can also minimize the side effects of cholinesterase inhibitors, which most commonly involve gastrointestinal symptoms (e.g., nausea and vomiting).

A fifth agent approved for treatment of dementia, memantine, is not a cholinesterase inhibitor but acts as an antagonist in the glutaminergic system. Use of memantine is generally reserved for cases of moderate to severe Alzheimer's disease. It is usually added to a regimen that includes continued prescription of a cholinesterase inhibitor, although it could be used as a first-line agent for patients who cannot tolerate a cholinesterase inhibitor. Memantine may prevent or at least slow the rate of further cognitive decline, although actual improvement, if any, is modest. It is well tolerated, but side effects may include headache, somnolence, dizziness, and confusion. Since memantine is a second-line agent, it is not a likely candidate for inclusion on the regular correctional formulary; clinical administrators may opt to make it available on a case-by-case basis through a nonformulary process.

There are no medications approved for treatment of agitation and psychotic symptoms in patients with dementia. The safety and efficacy of antipsychotic medications in the elderly have come under scrutiny in recent years (Kamble, Chen, Sherer, & Aparasu, 2009). New onset of agitation and psychosis may be manifestations of dementia and might improve with cholinesterase inhibitor treatment. If use of an antipsychotic medication is contemplated to treat agitation and psychotic symptoms, starting with a very low dose of a second-generation medication such as quetiapine is recommended. Any antipsychotic medication with significant anticholinergic effects should be avoided due to the potential impact on cognitive functioning. Benzodiazepines in the elderly are likely to cause adverse effects such as disinhibition and increase the risk for falls. If benzodiazepine use is contemplated, short-acting medications such as lorazepam or alprazolam should be considered over longer-acting medications (Madhusoodan & Bogunovic, 2004).

Environmental and system-level interventions for aging prisoners

Beyond the factors previously mentioned, the delivery of correctional health is also challenging because of the context of incarceration itself. In addition to lack of infrastructure, staff shortages, and staffing models that may not meet growing demands for geriatric care, gathering necessary data and recruiting qualified health professionals into corrections settings can be very difficult (Ahalt, Trestman, Rich, et al., 2013). Typical correctional practices related to housing, movement, meals, and daily schedule also introduce risks for elderly prisoners, including an increased risk for victimization (Aday, 2003; Stojkovic, 2007). Environment-related dysfunction may occur secondary to lack of adaptive equipment or the capacity to accommodate changing physical needs.

Need for specialized programs and staff education

Little if any corrections-specific training for geriatric and geropsychiatric issues and long-term chronic illness management exists. This has led correctional health programs to adapt training and education curricula and other resources designed and delivered for community-dwelling populations for use in prisons and jails. Other corrections administrations and health care programs have taken a more grassroots approach to increasing geriatric capacity and growing expertise "in place" among those staff already engaged in providing health care and security. However geriatric service capacity is increased, the provision of context-responsive correctional health care must consider the unique needs and, in some cases, conflicting goals of correctional settings. Design and implementation of new programs or units, adaptation of existing norms and policies, and delivery of specialized training all require careful attention to balancing both sides of the custody-versus-care dynamic within which all services are provided.

Long-term care units

Recent reports and position papers on the rising number of elderly inmates in US jails and prisons have called attention to the problematic nature of housing older, frail, medically or cognitively compromised inmates with younger, healthier inmates in general population (Kerbs & Jolley, 2009). Despite a growing number of arguments in favor of releasing elderly prisoners who are seriously ill, incapacitated, and no longer thought to pose risk (Chiu, 2010; Rikard & Rosenberg, 2007), the number of incarcerated men and women who require long-term care on an ongoing basis will continue to increase. Approaches to accommodating long-term care needs include separate housing for aging and ill inmates, increased staffing models, adaptions to unit policy that allow for more flexibility in daily structure (e.g., time allowed for movement, meals, or daily hygiene), and the use of orderlies or peer volunteer programs to provide direct care, support, and protection (Mara, 2002). Decisions about the focus and extent of such programs must be made. Do institutions provide specialized units and services for only the most disabled and ill inmates, or should a continuum of care be available? Moreover, heterogeneity among ill elderly inmates means that health care and security staff must have the training to address a wide variety of conditions—the needs of an ambulatory patient with severe dementia can be quite different than those of a patient with residual schizophrenia, chronic obstructive pulmonary disease, and acute pneumonia.

Palliative and end-of-life care

The need for palliative and end-of-life care for older adults in prison is also emerging for prison systems across the United States (Linder & Meyers, 2007). While one report documents that there are 69 formal prison hospice programs in the United States (Hoffman & Dickinson, 2011), the actual number is difficult to verify because of differences in how systems define what constitutes hospice and end-of-life care. Organizations such as the National Hospice and Palliative Care Organization, the National Prison Hospice Association, and the Guiding Responsive Action for Corrections in End-of-Life (GRACE) Project have promulgated broad standards for prison palliative and end-of-life care; however, the characteristics, policies, and practices of specific programs across institutions or states are neither consistently documented nor widely available.

Geriatric training for staff

Correctional systems often lack the resources to provide either health or custodial staff with appropriate geriatric training and education. This lack of knowledge and experience can lead to situations where symptoms and behaviors of older inmates with cognitive dysfunction or age-related debilitation may be misinterpreted. Both practice and policy experts now call for training programs for correctional staff that focus on common disorders of older inmates, changes in functional health status, and a working understanding of how underlying disease processes such as dementia may affect behavior or activity level (Aday & Krabill, 2013).

Adaptive equipment, practices, and policies to accommodate older inmates

Environmental factors may also require modification; examples include accommodating bed and commode height and installing handrails in hallways and showers. If a significant number of inmates cannot walk without assistance, some institutional procedures may require modification as well—for example, decentralizing medication administration, sick call, and chronic care clinic by holding these activities on the housing units. Such procedural modifications will have an impact on the demand for treatment space, equipment and supplies, unit policies, and staffing levels (health care and correctional staff).

Summary

The integration of geriatric and geropsychiatric treatment and care, derived from empirical data and practice-based evidence, is necessary for delivering adequate health care to incarcerated older adults (Aday & Krabill, 2013; Smyer, Gragert, & Martins, 2006). This chapter covers issues concerning the provision of such care, including those that stem from the aging and health status of this population and those that arise from the poor fit between the needs of aging inmates and correctional environments. The capacity for correctional health providers to meet the mental health needs of an exponentially growing group of older and sicker prisoners will depend on increased research and the dissemination of best-practice models that are specific to the correctional context.

References

Aday, R. H. (2003). *Aging prisoners: Crisis in American corrections.* Portsmouth, NH: Greenwood Publishing Group.

Aday, R. H., & Krabill, J. J. (2013). Older and geriatric offenders: Critical issues for the 21st century. In L. Gideon (Ed.), *Special needs offenders in correctional institutions* (pp. 203–231). Los Angeles: Sage.

Ahalt, C., Trestman, R. L., Rich, J. D., Greifinger, R. B., & Williams, B. A. (2013). Paying the price: The pressing need for quality, cost, and outcomes data to improve correctional health care for older prisoners. *Journal of the American Geriatrics Society, 61*(11), 2013–2019.

Arndt, S., Turvey, C. L. & Flaum, M. (2002). Older offenders, substance abuse, and treatment. *American Journal of Geriatric Psychiatry, 10*(6), 733–739.

Binswanger, I. A., Krueger, P. M., & Steiner, J. F. (2009). Prevalence of chronic medical conditions among jail and prison inmates in the USA compared with the general population. *Journal of Epidemiology and Community Health, 63*(11), 912–919.

Blazer, D. G. (2013). Psychiatric illness in the elderly. *The Carlat Report Psychiatry, 11*(10), 1–7.

Carson, E., & Sabol, W. (2012). *Prisoners in 2011.* U.S. Department of Justice, Office of Justice Programs, Bureau of Justice Statistics.

Chiu, T. (2010). *It's about time: Aging prisoners, increasing costs and geriatric release.* New York: Vera Institute of Justice.

Doka, K. (1989). *Disenfranchised grief: Recognizing hidden sorrow.* Lexington, MA: Lexington Books.

Fazel, S., McMillan, J., & O'Donnell, I. (2002). Dementia in prison: Ethical and legal implications. *Journal of Medical Ethics, 28,* 156–159.

Folstein Mini-Mental State Exam. Available at: http://www.utmb.edu/psychology/Folstein%20Mini.pdf (accessed December 9, 2013).

Folstein, M. F., Folstein, S. E., & McHugh, P. R. (1975). Mini-Mental State. A practical method for grading the cognitive state of patients for the clinician. *Journal of Psychiatric Research, 12*(3), 189–198.

George, L. K., & Fillenbaum, G.G. (1985). OARS methodology. A decade of experience in geriatric assessment. *Journal of the American Geriatrics Society, 33*(9), 607–615.

Gunther, C. S. (2013). Current pharmacologic treatment of dementia. *The Carlat Report Psychiatry, 11*(10), 1–8.

Harner, H. M., Hentz, P. M., & Evangelista, M. C. (2011). Grief interrupted: the experience of loss among incarcerated women. *Qualitative Health Research, 21*(4), 454–464.

Hebert, L. E., Scherr, P. A., Bienias, J. L., Bennett, D. A., & Evans, D. A. (2003). Alzheimer disease in the US population: prevalence estimates using the 2000 census. *Archives of Neurology, 60*(8), 1119–1122.

Hoffman, H. C., & Dickinson, G. E. (2011). Characteristics of prison hospice programs in the United States. *American Journal of Hospice & Palliative Care, 28*(4), 245–252.

Human Rights Watch (2012). *Old behind bars: The aging prison population in the United States.* Retrieved from http://www.hrw.org/sites/default/files/repotrs/usprisons01 12webcover_0.pdf

Kamble, P., Chen, H., Sherer, J. T., & Aparasu, R. R. (2009). Use of antipsychotics among elderly nursing home residents with dementia in the United States. *Drugs and Aging, 26*(6), 483–492.

Kerbs, J., & Jolley, J. (2009). A commentary on age segregation for older prisoners: Philosophical and pragmatic considerations for correctional systems. *Criminal Justice Review, 34*(1), 119–139.

Kopera-Frye, K., Harrison, M. T., Iribarne, J., et al. (2013). Veterans aging in place behind bars: a structured living program that works. *Psychological Services, 10*(1), 79–86.

Kuhlmann, R., & Ruddell, R. (2005). Elderly jail inmates: Problems, prevalence and public health. *Californian Journal of Health Promotion, 3*(2), 49–60.

Linder, J. F., & Meyers, F. J. (2007). Palliative care for prison inmates: 'don't let me die in prison'. *Journal of the American Medical Association, 298*(8), 894–901.

Loeb, S., & AbuDagga, A. (2006). Health-related research on older inmates: An integrative review. *Research in Nursing & Health, 29,* 556–565.

Loeb, S. J., Steffensmeier, D., & Lawrence, F. (2008). Comparing incarcerated and community-dwelling older men's health. *Western Journal of Nursing Research, 30*(2), 234–258.

Madhusoodanan, S., & Bogunovic, O.J. (2004). Safety of benzodiazepines in the geriatric population. *Expert Opinion on Drug Safety, 3*(5), 485–493.

Mara, C. M. (2002). Expansion of long-term care in the prison system: an aging inmate population poses policy and programmatic questions. *Journal of Aging & Social Policy, 14*(2), 43–61.

Mara, C. M. (2004). Chronic illness, disability and long-term care in the prison setting. In P. Katz, M. D. Mezey, & M. B. Kapp (Eds.), *Vulnerable populations in the long term care continuum* (vol. 5, pp. 39–56). New York: Springer.

Maruschak, L. M., & Beavers, R. (2009). HIV in prisons, 2007-08. *Bureau of Justice Statistics Bulletin*, Department of Justice, Office of Justice Programs, NCJ 228307.

Mathew, P., Elting, L., Cooksley, C., Owen, S., & Lin, J. (2005). Cancer in an incarcerated population. *Cancer, 104*(10), 2197–204.

Mitka, M. (2004). Aging prisoners stressing health care system. *Journal of the American Medical Association, 292*(4), 423–4.

Montreal Cognitive Assessment. Available at: http://www.mocatest.org (accessed December 9, 2013).

Nasreddine, Z. S., Phillips, N. A., Bedirian, V., et al. (2005). The Montreal Cognitive Assessment, MoCA: A brief screening tool for mild cognitive impairment. *Journal of the American Geriatrics Society, 53*(4), 695–699.

Olson, M. J., & McEwen, M. A. (2004). Grief counseling groups in a medium-security prison. *Journal for Specialists in Group Work, 29*(2), 225–236.

Rikard, R. V., & Rosenberg, E. (2007). Aging inmates: a convergence of trends in the American criminal justice system. *Journal of Correctional Health Care, 13,* 150–162.

Small, G. W. (2009). Differential diagnoses and assessment of depression in elderly patients. *Journal of Clinical Psychiatry, 70*(12), e47.

Smyer, T., Gragert, M., & Martins, D. C. (2006). Aging prisoners: Strategies for health care. In P. Burbank (Ed.), *Vulnerable older adults: Health care needs and intervention* (pp. 75–97). New York: Springer.

Sneed, J. R., & Culang-Reinlieb, M. E. (2011). The vascular depression hypothesis: an update. *American Journal of Geriatric Psychiatry, 19*(2), 99–103.

Snyder, C., van Wormer, K., Chadha, J., & Jaggers, J. W. (2009). Older adult inmates: the challenge for social work. *Social Work, 54*(2), 117–124.

Stojkovic, S. (2007). Elderly prisoners: A growing and forgotten group within correctional systems vulnerable to elder abuse. *Journal of Elder Abuse & Neglect, 19*(3-4), 97–117.

Thompson, L. W., Coon, D. W., Gallagher-Thompson, D., Sommer, B. R., & Koin, D. (2001). Comparison of desipramine and cognitive/behavioral therapy in the treatment of elderly outpatients with mid-to-moderate depression. *American Journal of Geriatric Psychiatry, 9*(3), 225–240.

Williams, B. A., Lindquist, K., Hill, T., et al. (2009). Caregiving behind bars: Correctional officer reports of disability in geriatric prisoners. *Journal of the American Geriatrics Society, 57*(7), 1286–1292.

Williams, B. A., Lindquist, K., Sudore, R. L., Strupp, H. M., Willmott, D. J., & Walter, L. C. (2006). Being old and doing time: functional impairment and adverse experiences of geriatric female prisoners. *Journal of the American Geriatrics Society, 54*(4), 702–707.

Williams, B. A., Stern, M. F., Mellow, J., Safer, M., & Greifinger, R. B. (2012). Aging in correctional custody: setting a policy agenda for older prisoner health care. *American Journal of Public Health, 102*(8), 1475–1481.

CHAPTER 58

Clinical and legal implications of gangs

Annette L. Hanson

Introduction

Gangs are a fact of life in jails and prisons. Psychiatrists need to be aware of the dynamics of gang leadership, membership, and involvement when working with any gang member, as that will affect his or her ability to participate in and interest in collaborative treatment. This chapter first presents a review of gang prevalence and the roles gangs play in the community and in correctional settings. Historical context, institutional management techniques, and approaches to therapeutic intervention are then discussed.

Background

According to the National Gang Intelligence Center, in 2010 there were approximately 1.4 million members of 33,000 street and prison gangs in the United States. This represents a 40% increase over gang membership reported by federal, state, and local law enforcement and correctional systems in 2009 (National Gang Intelligence Center, 2011). While the exact prevalence of gang affiliation in correctional facilities is not known, studies have shown that between 9% and 24% of prison inmates have affiliations to street or prison gangs (Gaes, Wallace, Gilman, et al., 2002; Griffin & Hepburn, 2006; Jackson & Sharpe, 1997; New Jersey Commission of Investigation, 2013). As many as 480 active prison gangs in the United States have been identified, including at least five that operate nationally (Boyd, 2010).

Prison gangs and the challenges they present are not unique to the United States (Coid, Ullrich, Keers, et al., 2013). In 2011 the Inter-American Commission on Human Rights called for reform after a clash between gangs in one Venezuelan prison left 19 prisoners dead and 25 seriously injured (Inter-American Commission on Human Rights, 2011). Similarly, a gang war in Brazil's fourth largest prison caused the deaths of 59 prisoners in a single year, some killed through beheading or torture (BBC, 2013). American prison and street gangs with Mexican, Caribbean, and South American connections such as MS-13, La Eme, Latin, Surenos, and Nortenos also have ties to international drug trafficking organizations.

Although there has been an increase in gang-affiliated female offenders, relatively less is known about this group than about male gang members. In one of the few studies of female prison inmates, Scott and Ruddell (2011) found that female gang members had more past convictions, were more likely to be assigned to a higher security level, and were more likely to have been incarcerated in the juvenile justice system than nongang members. There are several social theories to explain the motivation for joining a gang. One large random sampling of 7,212 adolescents drawn from a national longitudinal health study found little evidence that risk factors for gang involvement differed between teenage males and females. Neighborhood disadvantage, parent–child relationship factors, school safety, and exposure to violent peers were risk factors for both genders (Bell, 2009). Of more concern is the observation that female gang members are more likely to serve an intelligence-gathering function and may seek employment in law enforcement or government agencies for this purpose (Scott & Ruddell, 2011).

A gang has commonly been defined as a group of three or more individuals who engage in criminal activity and that identifies itself with a common name or sign (Martin, Gwynne, Parillo, et al., 2011). Within correctional facilities, the more generic term "security threat group" (STG) has been used to denote a group of two or more individuals who represent a threat to the security or orderly management of the facility and who act in concert to disrupt programs and activities. The STG designation recognizes that certain organized activities such as possession and distribution of tobacco would not be considered a crime in free society but would be considered a violation of correctional rules in some facilities. Regardless of designation, both prison gangs and STGs are often bound by common ideological, ethnic, or racial ties. They have an organizational structure that includes a leader, a council, a code of conduct, and oaths of loyalty and secrecy. Violence is a common price of admission to membership, as well as a consequence of disloyalty or withdrawal.

The first prison gangs arose in California in the 1950s and 1960s, and many of these early gangs are nationally known today, including the Crips, Bloods, Aryan Brotherhood, Black Guerrilla Family, MS-13, and Black Gangster Disciples. The boundaries of any given gang are fluid, and they may blend with regional chapters or groups that assume the name of a national organization but have no formal or official ties to it. New gangs have formed due to the resettlement of refugees, such as Somalian and Vietnamese street gangs in the Upper Midwest. Finally, gangs may form within a prison system for protection from a larger gang. In 2000, a group of white prisoners banded together in the Maryland prison system to form Dead Man Inc., which now has a national presence.

Community-based gangs are bound by a common antisocial interest or criminal activity, including drug distribution, weapons trafficking, prostitution, human smuggling, and violent crimes such as robbery. In jail and prison, by virtue of the more controlled environment, there is a shift toward acquisition of property or other privileges, such as cell phones, tobacco, sex, drugs, and extra food or clothing. Gangs have also been known to direct loan shark and gambling operations within a jail or prison. Gang-related violence is generally intended to protect territory and distribution channels rather than for direct financial gain. Gangs have been known to plan and carry out assaults on other inmates and to contract with another gang to carry out "hits" on officers, prisoners, or witnesses outside the facility. Witness intimidation is a necessary aspect of gang life, and a newly recruited member may be asked to take part in this as an initiation ritual. The financial side of gang business takes place mainly outside the facility between associates of the prison gang (typically the buyer) and the community-based gang (the seller or provider).

The extent and impact of gang activity on a facility will depend on the size and geographic location of the facility. Smaller jails and prisons and facilities in rural areas are more likely to be involved with local or regional groups, also known as street gangs, while large facilities in urban areas will be affected more by nationally known or connected gangs.

The impact of gangs within a facility is considerable. One survey of Florida prisoners found that inmates who were suspected or confirmed gang members were 35% more likely to commit violent acts than nonmembers (Cunningham & Sorensen, 2007). Similarly, a study of 82,504 Federal Bureau of Prison inmates found that gang membership was associated with increased violent behavior as well as less serious rule infractions. Further, the likelihood of violent misconduct was higher for members who were core to the organization rather than peripheral. However, even peripheral members were more likely to commit violence than nonmembers (Gaes et al., 2002). In a study of 2,158 male inmates in the Arizona Department of Corrections, gang-affiliated inmates were more than twice as likely as nonaffiliated inmates to commit an assault during the first three years of confinement, even when controlled for age, ethnicity, commitment offense, prior incarceration, sentence length, and security level (Griffin & Hepburn, 2006).

Since the terrorist attacks on September 11, 2001, prison gangs have also become a potential national security risk. Gangs espousing strong antigovernment, prorevolutionary views have drawn the attention of counterterrorism experts, particularly since some domestic terrorists are now housed in federal prison. The "radicalization" of prison gangs is an ongoing concern. To address this issue, the National Gang Intelligence Center (NGIC) was created in 2005 to establish information-sharing networks between the Federal Bureau of Investigation, the Drug Enforcement Administration, the Bureau of Alcohol, Tobacco, Firearms and Explosives, the Federal Bureau of Prisons, Immigrations and Customs Enforcement, and the Department of Defense. Law enforcement databases share information between these agencies and typically include identifying information, gang affiliation, known associates, as well as tattoos or other identifying characteristics of any confirmed gang member. The NGIC issues regular threat assessment reports to track gang trends and networks nationally.

Institutional management

The NGIC maintains a list of confirmed prison gangs and provides support for gang-related investigations within facilities. For more regionalized gangs, many institutions have a policy for establishing which group of individuals should be deemed an STG. An STG designation can be given based on involvement with or connection to a known, established organization or it may be an internal group identified by institutional intelligence-gathering methods.

Once a group is designated as an established gang or STG, newly received inmates are assessed for affiliation. The facility may have an STG specialist who interviews the inmate to determine if he or she actually is a gang member and to gather intelligence about gang structure, involved members, distribution, and activities. The STG officer may ask if the prisoner knows certain basic principles of a given gang, such as a gang credo, hand symbol, or other signs. He or she may be asked about participation in gang-related violence or institutional misconduct. Once this determination is made, the inmate is said to be a "validated" gang member. Validation allows the institution to manage the inmate with special security measures such as placing the inmate in a higher-security facility or in restricted housing or to restrict liberty within the facility. Fourteen states segregate prisoners who are validated gang members (Van Houten, 2009). Most prison systems use a variety of gang control and suppression strategies such as sharing intelligence with law enforcement, monitoring institutional mail and phone calls, and using modern data-mining approaches through the use of social media (Winterdyk & Ruddell, 2010). Jail and prison policies typically consider any attempt to recruit for a gang as a violation of institutional rules.

For inmates not identified at intake, gang validation may be made later during incarceration if the inmate participates in a gang-related crime or rule violation or is identified as an associate of a validated gang member. He or she could also be identified later through inclusion in a law enforcement gang database. Other identifiers could be authorship or possession of gang-related documents, pictures with validated members, or possession of gang-related books.

Over time, correctional strategies to control gangs have alternated between gang suppression and gang dispersal efforts. Dispersion, or transfer of gang leaders to out-of-state systems, eventually was shown to be ineffective in that it inadvertently provided an opportunity for a gang to establish itself in new territory. Suppression involved placing leaders in isolation through long-term segregation. Advocacy groups challenged this practice as being arbitrary and inhumane. More recently, prison systems have created policies that allow gang members to work their way out of long-term segregation or avoid it completely through a gang renunciation program.

The renunciation program used in the Texas prison system requires the inmate to be housed in a specialized unit for several weeks while completing several modules designed to help him manage life without a gang (Mandeville, 2004). Other renunciation programs provide anger management training, substance abuse treatment, and job skills training. During renunciation, the inmate is required to live on a tier with members of competing gangs for a period of time without sustaining any infractions. Once this process is complete, he is allowed to transfer to the general prison population in a regular facility without a gang-labeled status.

Legal aspects of gang management

Initially street and prison gangs were prosecuted under the federal Racketeer Influenced and Corrupt Organizations (RICO) Act, which designated certain crimes as racketeering offenses when committed for the purpose of furthering or supporting an existing criminal enterprise (RICO, 1970). Any money gained through this organized illegal activity was considered "unlawful debt" subject to seizure, and the participant could be sentenced to 20 years to a life sentence depending on the underlying offense. RICO was used to prosecute Mafia families in the 1970s, as well as certain outlaw motorcycle gangs involved in interstate trafficking of weapons.

The limitation of RICO for prison gang prosecution was that the law could only be used if there was proof of money-laundering activities or interstate crime. For a prison-based gang, financial transactions are often conducted through the use of disposable prepaid cell phones or through cash transfers made by telephone using the number on a prepaid debit card. Although the debit cards (sometimes called "green dot" cards) have monetary value, they are not subject to the same money-laundering laws as traditional financial instruments.

To address this problem, many states adapted variations of RICO in local antigang legislation. The goal of state legislation was to punish recruitment of youth into gangs as well as the gang's criminal activity. Antigang legislation allowed prosecution for a criminal act with additional criminal liability under state racketeering laws if the act was committed to further the goals of the organization. The laws allowed for enhanced sentencing and for expert testimony at trial regarding the nature, culture, and symbols or signs of known gangs. By 2005 only 13 states had no antigang legislation (Thompson, 2005).

Legal efforts to break up and control gangs have not gone unchallenged. Since institutional management often involves restriction of privileges, placement on long-term segregation, or transfer to a control unit prison, advocacy groups and individual inmates have filed suit against these policies based on First and Eighth Amendment, religious freedom, and antidiscrimination claims. Gang validation procedures have been challenged as arbitrary and inaccurate, leading to inappropriate segregation or restrictions on prisoners who have exhibited no institutional violence.

Unfortunately, religious services have been used to facilitate gang meetings, promote extremism, and plan criminal activity. The Civil Rights of Institutionalized Persons Act protects the religious freedom of prisoners under the section known as the Protection of Religious Exercise in Land Use and by Institutionalized Persons Act (RLUIPA, 2000). Any effort to investigate gang activity by monitoring religious services or to control gang communication by restricting religious services or practices would likely fall within the reach of a RLUIPA claim. Religious affiliation alone has also been barred as a basis for inmate gang validation.

Housing assignments used to prevent intragang violence or to suppress gang leadership have been challenged under both Eighth Amendment and antidiscrimination laws. In *Johnson v. California* (2005), an inmate sued the California Department of Corrections over a policy that segregated inmates by race temporarily pending a regular housing assignment. This policy was defended as nondiscriminatory since all prisoners were subject to it and because it was reasonably related to institutional security. The US Supreme Court reversed the lower court's judgment that upheld the policy and ruled that any prison policy based solely on race should be held to a strict scrutiny standard rather than following traditional deference to the judgment of prison officials. Similarly, Eighth Amendment claims against the use of long-term solitary confinement have been brought when the sole reason for the segregation was to separate a gang leader from the general population, absent proof of institutional rule-breaking or violence.

Aside from body cavity searches, courts have generally held that prisoners do not have a right to privacy. Gang control policies often include the examination of mail for coded communication and the monitoring of phone calls between identified gang members. Property such as gang-related reading material may be seized if the seizure is reasonably related to a legitimate penological purpose. Since some gangs are quasireligious in nature, reading material can only be banned if it encourages violence, undermines offender rehabilitation, or represents a threat to institutional security.

Implications for the clinician

Case Vignette

The patient is a 23-year-old man incarcerated for a misdemeanor theft. As a prison maintenance worker, he had access to tools and locations in the facility that would allow for an escape. Gang members on the tier attempted to coerce him into the plan, but he resisted and reported the plan to the security chief. While the investigation was pending, he was moved to segregation for protective custody. Gang-affiliated officers there made implied threats and warned him not to cooperate. On segregation rounds, he asked to be seen in the psychology department, where he expressed fear for his safety but exhibited no signs of clinical depression or other evidence of mental illness. He asked the institutional clinician to contact the security chief so that he could reveal the names of the gang-involved officers. He had no external family or relationships to rely on for support.

In this vignette, the patient revealed the presence of gangs to the correctional psychiatrist. While at present it is not a standard of clinical care to question correctional patients about gang involvement or gang activity on a tier, this knowledge can inform the clinician's assessment of a patient's mental state and safety risk. Unfortunately, there is little information available in the literature regarding how to do this, and gang assessment is not part of traditional psychiatric training or correctional orientation.

In most situations, this information can be obtained by directly questioning patients periodically about safety concerns on the tier and about their own observations. An inmate may observe that access to the telephone is controlled by a group of prisoners or that there are rivalries on the unit between factions of inmates. An inmate may report that he has been asked to hold contraband or keep quiet about smuggling or other illicit activity. He may express frustration that volunteer jobs on the unit are given preferentially to gang members, a sign that the gang may be colluding with correctional staff. He may report pressure from others to join a gang. An inmate who frequently seeks psychiatric admission or repeatedly requests protective custody should raise a concern about gang influence.

The correctional psychiatrist who learns of gang activity in the facility has a duty to help the patient negotiate the risks this situation poses to him or her but also has a duty to ensure institutional safety. Reporting gang members to custody could place the patient in danger since an investigation can only take place based on information from an identified reliable informant. The principles of nonmalfeasance and respect for patient confidentiality dictate that the clinician explore the potential ramifications of disclosure with the patient and act in accordance with the inmate's wishes. An inmate who wants to cooperate with an investigation should be offered the option of protective housing, if such an offer is within the clinician's authority. Involuntary protective custody should be avoided since this could bar the patient from jobs, programs, and activities he or she would normally have access to. If the gang activity presents a serious enough risk of imminent danger to the unit or institution, such as an impending riot or planned violence, the traditional duty to warn or protect third parties would apply. The advantage of cooperation would be to clear the patient of any potential connection or involvement with the gang and to avoid the risk of guilt by association.

There is evidence to suggest that gang members are more likely to suffer from mental disorders and to use psychiatric services than other prisoners. A 2013 study of 4,664 men in Great Britain compared prevalence of mental disorders, mental health service use, and suicide attempts among violent men according to gang membership. The gang members were more likely to have seen a psychiatrist or psychologist, to have been admitted to a psychiatric hospital, and to have attempted suicide (Coid et al., 2013).

When assessing a correctional patient who is also a gang member, several additional questions should be asked to inform treatment. Box 58.1 includes a list of suggested questions. The answers to these questions will reveal potential vulnerability to victimization or coercion, potential for violence, and the strength of gang affiliation. While a prisoner may join a gang for protection, gang membership actually increases the risk of being a victim of violence. While there are no published studies, in my experience, fear of retaliatory violence can also be a risk factor for self-injury, particularly when the intended target is an outside family member or loved one. Retaliatory violence can also take place when a member decides to leave a gang, and the risk can carry over into the community following release. The strength of gang affiliation and the degree of involvement are relevant in that more peripherally involved gang members are more likely to renounce and leave the group than key members.

Documenting the answers to these questions poses another dilemma for the correctional clinician. In a system that uses a combined medical and psychiatric record system, the correctional psychiatrist should be circumspect about documenting specific information regarding a patient who reports corruption, who cooperates with internal gang prevention efforts, or who frankly acknowledges involvement in illegal gang activities.

Correctional psychiatrists should also be aware that prisoners can use an institutional mental health system to facilitate gang business. In a facility that uses a "pill line" to pass medication, the pharmacy window can become an unofficial gang meeting place. Medication passes have been stolen or forged because they give

---

Box 58.1. Suggested assessment questions for gang members

1. Which gang are you part of?
2. How long have you been a member?
3. Did you join in the community or in the facility?
4. What led you to join?
5. What role do you play in the gang?
6. Have you ever thought about leaving the gang or have you tried to leave?
7. What happened when you tried to leave?
8. Is anyone harassing you or threatening you here?
9. Do you owe anybody money?
10. Have you been asked to hold contraband?
11. Are you being pressured to do something you don't want to do?
12. What have they said would happen if you don't go along with them?
13. Is your family safe? Do you have concerns about friends, family, or children on the outside?
14. If you move to another facility, will this problem follow you?
15. How long has this been going on?
16. Do you want to report this activity to the security chief?

---

relative freedom of movement through a facility at specified times of the day. For this reason, a medication pass is sometimes called a "skate" in prison slang. A prisoner may press a psychiatrist to prescribe medication in order to get a medication pass.

Gangs have also used the psychiatric infirmary. A gang member may seek admission in order to follow or get close to an intended target. A psychiatric unit may be used as a meeting place for gang members from separate tiers. When a prisoner seeks frequent admission, the clinician should ask the tier officer about any gang-related connections between admitted patients or about gang conflicts that might be a factor in the admission.

Psychiatric medications may be traded and sold as a commodity to support gang business. Any medication with sedative effects has economic value within a jail or prison and will support a gang's underground or black market trade. Also, vulnerable psychiatric patients may be coerced or intimidated into giving up their prescribed medication. Judicious use of medication with abuse potential will decrease the likelihood of this activity.

Gang-led, organized hunger strikes will require the involvement of an institutional psychiatrist. Hunger strike policies typically require that the striker's competency be assessed on a regular basis in order to determine the striker's understanding of the effects of starvation and to determine if the decision to strike is free of coercion. If the tier and the hunger strike were under the control of a gang, an unaffiliated prisoner would likely feel a high degree of coercion to cooperate with the strike.

All gang influence is not negative, however. I have seen inmates organize themselves into protective groups centered on religious studies—a self-labeled "God gang." And even a hardened gang once banded together to make sure a formerly manic prisoner took his medication when he was known to become violent when ill.

Summary

Gang management is a challenge for correctional institutions; treating gang members with psychiatric illness is a challenge for psychiatry. Understanding the background, motivation, and dynamics of gangs is an important aspect of psychiatric practice in jails and prisons. Psychiatric care is best when it is informed by sensitivity to the culture, environmental effects, and individual impact of gangs on the correctional patient.

References

BBC. Gang war in Brazil's Pedrinhas jail kills 59 in 2013. Available at http://www.bbc.co.uk/news/world-latin-america-25536187 (accessed January 5, 2014).

Bell, K. (2009). Gender and gangs: a quantitative comparison. *Crime and Delinquency, 55,* 363–387.

Boyd, S. (2010). Implementing the missing peace: reconsidering prison gang management. *Quinnipiac Law Review, 28,* 969–1018.

Coid, J., Ullrich, S., Keers, R., Bebbington, P., DeStavola, B., Kallis, C., et al. (2013). Gang membership, violence, and psychiatric morbidity. *American Journal of Psychiatry, 170,* 985–993.

Cunningham, M., & Sorensen, J. (2007). Predictive factors for violent misconduct in close custody. *The Prison Journal, 87,* 241–253.

Gaes, G., Wallace, S., Gilman, E., Klein-Saffran, J., & Suppa, S. (2002). The influence of prison gang affiliation on violence and other prison misconduct. *The Prison Journal, 82,* 359–385.

Griffin, M., & Hepburn, J. (2006). The effect of gang affiliation on violent misconduct among inmates during the early years of confinement. *Criminal Justice and Behavior, 33,* 419–448.

Inter-American Commission on Human Rights. IACHR Deplores Violent Deaths in Venezuelan Prison. Available at http://www.oas.org/en/iachr/media_center/PReleases/2011/057.asp (accessed January 5, 2014).

Jackson, M., & Sharpe, E. (1997). Prison gang research: preliminary findings in eastern North Carolina. *Journal of Gang Research, 5,* 1–7.

Johnson v. California (2005) 543 U.S. 499.

Mandeville, M. (2004). Leaving Gang Life Behind in Texas. Corrections.com. Available at http://www.corrections.com/news/article/3071 (accessed November 11, 2013).

Martin, R., Gwynne, J., Parillo, R., Younker, B., & Carter, R. (2011). Alabama prison gang survey. *Journal of Gang Research, 18,* 1–19.

National Gang Intelligence Center. National gang threat assessment: emerging trends 2011. Available at: http://www.fbi.gov/stats-services/publications/2011-national-gang-threat-assessment (accessed November 10, 2013).

New Jersey Commission of Investigation (NJCI). Gangland behind bars: how and why organized criminal street gangs thrive in New Jersey's prisons. Available at: http://nicic.gov/Library/025742 (accessed November 24, 2013).

Protection of Religious Exercise in Land Use and by Institutionalized Persons Act 2000. Title 42, USC Section 2000.

Racketeer Influenced and Corrupt Organizations Act (RICO) 1970. Title 18, USC Chapter 96.

Scott, T., & Ruddell, R. (2011). Canadian female gang inmates: risks, needs, and the potential for prison rehabilitation. *Journal of Offender Rehabilitation, 50,* 305–326.

Thompson, J. (2005). South Carolina or South Central? Proposing comprehensive criminal gang prevention legislation for the palmetto state. *South Carolina Law Review, 56,* 735–750.

Van Houten, B. (2009) Security classification and gang validation. In *A jailhouse lawyer's manual.* New York: Columbia Human Rights Law Review. Available at: http://www3.law.columbia.edu/hrlr/jlm/chapter-31.pdf (accessed November 14, 2013).

Winterdyk, J., & Ruddell, R. (2010). Managing prison gangs: results from a survey of U.S. prison systems. *Journal of Criminal Justice, 38,* 730–736.

CHAPTER 59

Treatment of incarcerated sex offenders

Fabian M. Saleh, Albert J. Grudzinskas, and H. Martin Malin

Introduction

The treatment of sex offenders in correctional contexts is arguably one of the most challenging undertakings for psychiatrists. Sex offenders are a highly stigmatized population that typically engenders intense negative feelings in both the professional and lay communities. This chapter reviews some of the clinical and legal issues relevant to the care of convicted sex offenders in correctional settings.

Incidence of sex offending

The growing number of sex offenses in recent years, "overdramatized by print and video media that overvalue sensationalism" (LaFond & Winick, 1998), has had a profound impact on public perception. While the number of sex offenses committed in the United States on an annual basis is significant, the figure is not astronomical. In 2012, the latest year for which comprehensive data have been compiled, there were 73,080 incidents of sex "crimes against persons" in the United States; these crimes involved 79,625 individual victims and 76,927 offenders according to the Federal Bureau of Investigation's National Incident-Based Reporting System (NIBRS; 2012). The 2012 figures include 67,861 incidents of "forcible" sex offenses (rape, sodomy, assault with an object, or forcible fondling) and 6,137 "nonforcible" sex offenses (incest and statutory rape). There were an additional 15,335 incidents of sex "crimes against society," comprising 9,309 prostitution offenses and 6,026 offenses involving pornography/obscene material. Thus, all sex crimes against persons or society accounted for about 1.7% of the more than 5 million incidents of crime reported in the 2012 NIBRS data, and sex crimes against persons accounted for about 6.3% of the more than 1 million reported crimes against persons.

The rate of recidivism over 25 years among sex offenders has been estimated to be as high as 52% (Prentky, Knight, & Lee, 1997, p. 11). However, recent analysis of the data has shown that while persons incarcerated for sex offenses are rearrested at high rates, it is (with a few notable exceptions) seldom for a new sexual offense. In a large study of 272,111 prisoners, 68% of whom were rearrested during a three-year follow-up, 43% of the 9,691 male sex offenders released (two thirds of all male sex offenders released in 1994) were rearrested for another crime within three years of release. More specifically, the released sex offenders were rearrested for a new sex crime at a rate of 5.3%, only 10% of the overall recidivism rate (Langan, Schmitt, & Durose, 2003).

The law, however, is "a reflection of the society that generates it. The current attitudes, fears, and beliefs of the community about the world around it, accurate or not, are reflected in the law that governs at any given time" (Hafemeister & Petrila, 1994). In 1997, child pornography offenders who possessed, received, or distributed child pornography but did not produce or attempt production received a mean sentence of 20.59 months of confinement. In 2007, defendants sentenced for the same conduct received a mean sentence of 91.30 months, an increase of 443% over the past 10 years (Stabenow, 2009). The behaviors did not change; society's perception of and response to them did.

Medical–legal considerations

Sex offenders are a heterogeneous clinical population. Mental health professionals must not conflate whatever psychiatric diagnoses might be assigned to a given patient with the legal designation of that same patient as a "sex offender." The legal designation is based on the fact that the patient has transgressed against society and/or one or more of its members by violating culturally defined rules governing permissible sexual behavior. The psychiatric diagnosis addresses the issue of what underlying vulnerabilities might be causative or contributory to such transgression.

Sex offending is a legal construct without clinical significance, and debate surrounding the management of the "sex offender" is seldom well informed by medical knowledge. The lay perception and, to some degree, the legal construct of the sex offender is one of an evil person or at least a person who has done evil things, causing undeserved pain to others by behaving badly. Society's understanding of sex offending is further clouded by the use of such pseudo-psychiatric terminology as "mentally disordered sex offender," "sexually violent person," and the more commonly used pejorative "sexual predator." Such terms are in widespread parlance and frequently encountered in judicial proceedings. These terms may be seen to justify the civil commitment of sex offenders who have served their penal sentences. "Sexually violent person" laws take it as a given that many sex offenders have a mental condition that predisposes them to commit sex offenses. Indefinite civil commitment might then be justifiable since they are perceived as being at high risk of reoffending due to a serious impairment in the ability to control their dangerous behavior (Elwood, 2009).

The legality of any given sexual behavior is culture-bound—what is legal at one time may not be legal at another. What constitutes a sex offense also differs from jurisdiction to jurisdiction. The term provides no context regarding the offender's motivation and does not, by itself, indicate any underlying psychopathology. Illegal sexual behavior, however, is different from most other illegal behavior in that it may occur in the context of a strong, biologically mediated drive (Saleh, Grudzinskas, Malin, & Dwyer, 2010).

There is no single motivation for engaging in sexual behavior or committing sex offenses. The psychiatrist, as part of assessment for treatment, wants to know what has motivated a patient who may otherwise be a law-abiding citizen to engage in illegal behavior. Conversely, the psychiatrist who encounters a patient who has made a life career of antisocial behavior will not be greatly surprised to learn that the patient has simply added illegal sexual behavior to his or her repertoire (Saleh et al., 2010).

Sex offenders and mental illness

People may commit sex offenses in the context of a psychiatric condition. These conditions include developmental disorders, depression, mania, intoxication with psychoactive substances, and altered mental states associated with delusions, hallucinations, and compulsions. While there are clearly sex offenders whose illegal behavior is rooted in refractory personality disorders, others just as clearly commit their offenses in the context of serious mood or psychotic disorders (Berlin, Saleh, & Malin, 2009). An altered state of consciousness with impaired reality testing appears to be an important contributor to illegal behavior in some sex offenders. For example, Berlin (1986) documented the case of a patient with bipolar disorder who raped several women during a prolonged manic episode; he believed they were seeking him out, having been sent as sacrificial lambs in a cosmic battle between good and evil. While he had previously run naked through a canteen during a similar manic state while stationed overseas in the military, he had no prior history of criminal behavior outside of such altered mental states. While the cognitive-behavioral and moral habilitation strategies that form the core of typical offender treatment programs may be adjunctively useful in such cases, pharmacotherapy clearly plays a central role for individuals who suffer from perceptual disorders.

The same can likely be said for sex offenses committed in the context of paraphilic disorders. The imagery pathognomonic of the paraphilic disorders is enmeshed with the biology of sexual desire and may impair the ability to conform sexual behavior to accepted norms. Paraphilias therefore form a class of disorders qualitatively different from other mental disorders (Fagan, Lehne, Strand, & Berlin, 2005). As is the case with perceptual disorders, treatment strategies that involve pharmacological blunting of the sex drive may enhance the effectiveness of more conventional cognitive-behavioral treatment strategies. In addition, paraphilic-like behavior that results from general medical disorders, including traumatic brain injury, is sometimes ameliorated by medical therapy (Lehne, 1986).

Of course, not all sex offenders have paraphilias and not all patients with paraphilias commit sex offenses. In addition, the consensual expression of some paraphilias (e.g., the cross-dressing associated with transvestic fetishism) is not currently illegal in the United States but may be in some other countries. Similarly, until the mid-1970s, child pornography was openly and legally displayed for sale on the shelves of adult booksellers in most major US cities. Such a practice today would certainly lead to prosecution.

Ethical concerns with sex offender treatment

As noted earlier, sex offenders are an exceptionally heterogeneous group. Some, but not all, will eventually come to be seen as legitimate psychiatric patients. Some of those will be seen while incarcerated. Incarcerated persons are owed a basic duty of care (see Chapter 3; *DeShaney v. Winnebago Dept. of Social Services*, 1989). The US Supreme Court has grounded this right in the Eighth Amendment proscription on cruel and unusual punishment (*Estelle v. Gamble*, 1976) and the Fourteenth Amendment due process clause (*Bell v. Wolfish*, 1979). The duty to "avoid deliberate indifference" (see *Farmer v. Brennan*, 1994) to the inmate's medical or psychological needs is seen as an obligation to "avoid the needless infliction or prolongation of pain and suffering" (Cohen, 2003). While the civil rights of those persons who are being treated while incarcerated are similar to the rights of other persons in treatment, and are protected by the US Constitution (and, in many instances, by additional state laws and judicial decisions), there are differences. "Correctional clinicians work with the offender, but for the department, facility, or agency, and must be able to differentiate and balance the ethical/legal obligations owed to the correctional organization or agency and the community and the offender client" (American Association for Correctional Psychology, 1999, p. 456; see also American Psychiatric Association, 2000; Pinta, 2009).

The nature of the prison environment and the need to secure the safety of staff, visitors, and inmates affect mental health care in important ways (see Chapter 7; Pinta, 2009). The American Psychiatric Association's task force on jails and prisons recognizes, for example, that there are numerous instances where confidentiality must "be weighed against institutional needs for safety and security" (American Psychiatric Association, 2000). The concepts of confidentiality and privilege are grounded in a person's expectation of privacy. Full disclosure of the limits of privacy and the nature of the clinician's agency, particularly in instances of diagnosis, evaluation, and classification in incarcerated settings, helps clinicians avoid conflicts as treatment proceeds (see Chapter 8).

Additional privacy issues arise in the treatment of sex offenders since treatment is often mandated (Clayton, 2002). This can lead to significant risks for the offender when coupled with the belief among many clinicians that sex offenders must "acknowledge their responsibility for the offense and their problematic sexual behavior before they can fully participate in treatment and work toward change" (Farkas & Miller, 2008). Such risks for the inmate may go beyond concerns of threats from other inmates if their sex offender status becomes known. The US Supreme Court in *McKune v. Lile* (2002) found that the admission of guilt required for participation in treatment programs, even when coupled with loss of privileges and transfer to a higher security level, was not "compelling enough" to be unconstitutional.

Assessment

The clinical response to sex offending properly begins with thorough and accurate differential diagnosis. In the differential diagnostic process, the clinician will collect the usual medical and psychosocial historical data and attempt to synthesize an explanation for the behavior as a function of the patient's life story (Fagan, Lehne, Strand, & Berlin, 2005). While terms having legal significance may well be left to the legislature (see *Kansas v. Hendricks*, 1997), without a medical diagnosis to inform the specific treatment needs of a specific patient, there can be no treatment. The days of relying on the "great professor principle" paradigm of psychiatric nosology described by Kendler (1990) have given way to the "consensus of the experts" paradigm of diagnosis for the *Diagnostic and Statistical Manual of Mental Disorders*–5. Today, a differential diagnosis should take into account global patterns of behavioral problems; pervasive impairments in interpersonal relationships; isolated, opportunistic, or impulsive sexual problem behaviors; time-limited, reactive patterns of oversexualized behaviors; and psychiatric, neuropsychiatric, and/or neurological disorders, including paraphilic disorders such as pedophilia. Only then can treatment goals be established. Such goals typically include risk reduction of future sexual misconduct/sexual-offending behavior, improvement in quality of life, decreased personal distress, increased patient autonomy and independency, and reintegration into the community if appropriate and possible.

Psychotherapeutic interventions

Psychotherapy with sex offenders typically involves some form of highly structured cognitive-behavioral therapy program. Some states (e.g., California, Texas) prohibit general psychotherapists without specialized training, certification, or subspecialty licensure in sex offender management from treating convicted sex offenders. It has become common to refer to mental health interventions with sex offenders as "treatment" or "management" rather than "psychotherapy." The underlying assumption of this philosophy is that the primary beneficiary of sex offender treatment should be society, not the individual offender, and that community safety takes precedence over the mental health needs of any individual offender. To that end, treatment is highly directive and focuses on taking full responsibility for the offending behavior and the cognitive restructuring of thinking errors and deficiencies in moral judgment that led to the behavior. Such treatment seeks to identify high-risk situations in which behavioral control might fail and attempts to teach cognitive and behavioral strategies that would help the offender avoid high-risk situations that could lead to reoffending.

Sex offender treatment in correctional settings is highly proscriptive. The state of Texas, for example, asserts that

> Sex offender treatment is different than traditional psychotherapy in that treatment is mandated, structured, victim centered, and the treatment provider imposes values and limits. Providers cannot remain neutral because of the risk of colluding with, adding to, and/or contributing to the offender's denial. In sex offender treatment, confidentiality is not maintained due to the enormous public safety issues. Because secrecy is the lifeblood of sexual offending, treatment providers cannot guarantee confidentiality. Treatment providers must not solely rely on self-report because sex offenders see

> trust as abuseable. . . . Sex offender treatment requires the offender to face the consequences of their behavior on their victims and society. (Anonymous, 2014)

Sex offender treatment is not typically aimed at reducing sexual arousal, although it may address deviant arousal patterns through such cognitive-behavioral strategies as covert sensitization and olfactory conditioning (Corabian, Dennett, & Harstall, 2011). It is more common to teach techniques for behavioral management of sexual arousal patterns.

Treatment with testosterone-lowering medications

Androgen-lowering medications should be considered the treatment of choice for symptomatic paraphilic sex offenders (Saleh, et al., 2010). Consistent with community treatment standards, incarcerated sex offenders should be afforded anti-androgens to decrease the likelihood of sexual recidivism while decreasing paraphilic symptomatology. The case of *Osheroff v. Chestnut Lodge* (1985) emphasizes that a failure to use all available and appropriate treatments could be grounds for malpractice. Dr. Osheroff, a nephrologist with a two-year history of anxiety and depressive symptoms, was treated for seven months with psychotherapy alone without improvement at Chestnut Lodge, a prestigious psychoanalytically oriented psychiatric hospital in Rockville, MD. He was then transferred to another facility, where he was treated with medications and rapidly improved. He then sued Chestnut Lodge and received a settlement (Klerman, 1990).

Prescribing androgen-lowering medications to incarcerated individuals raises complex legal and ethical concerns (Mellela, Travin, & Cullen et al., 1989; Miller, 1998; Ward, Gannon, & Birgden, 2007). In the United States, at this writing, nine states authorize some form of mandated surgical or pharmacological sex drive–reduction treatment (commonly but erroneously referred to as "castration") as an adjunct to parole or probation supervision for certain sex offenders for whom release to the community from incarceration is being contemplated. The term "chemical castration" is a misnomer since "castration" necessarily refers to the surgical removal of gonads. Thus, in sex offenders, castration involves mutilation, including the irreversible destruction of healthy reproductive tissue, and renders the patient sterile as well as hormonally altered. Pharmacotherapy, by contrast, is nonmutilating and preserves healthy gonadal tissue while altering hormonal balance to decrease sexual drive. Pharmacological drive reduction does not typically interfere with spermatogenesis or the ability to reproduce.

Jurisdictions vary in the permissibility of surgical or pharmacological drive reduction (Scott & Holmberg, 2003). Texas (Tex. Gov't Code Ann., 2003) provides for voluntary surgical castration as the only treatment option. California (Cal. Penal Code, 2003), Florida (Fla. Stat. Ann., 2002), Iowa (Iowa Code, 2003), and Louisiana (La. Rev. Stat. Ann., 2003) allow for some provision of either pharmacotherapy or voluntary surgical castration. Georgia (Ga. Code Ann, 2002), Montana (Mont. Code Ann., 2002), Oregon (Ore. Rev. Stat., 2001), and Wisconsin (Wis. Stat. Ann., 2002) permit the use of pharmacotherapy only. Numerous other states have either considered such laws or have judicial decisions that address the process without legislative authority (see *State v. Brown*, 1985; *People v. Gauntlett*, 1984). The practice has also been sanctioned in Canada and, at various times, in Denmark, Germany, Norway, Sweden, and Switzerland (Druhm, 1997).

Although full consideration of the legal and ethical issues involved in this topic is beyond the scope of this chapter, an overview of the issues is provided later. In the various state actions and in numerous commentaries (see Druhm, 1997; Miller, 1998; Rice & Harris, 2011; Winslade, Stone, Smith-Bell, & Webb, 1998), challenges are usually organized on Eighth Amendment (i.e., that the forced treatment is cruel and unusual punishment) or Fourteenth Amendment grounds (i.e., the process is not sufficiently spelled out to satisfy due process concerns). These are usually counter to the argument that this is a treatment with therapeutic value. Further complicating the issue is the fact that the medications have demonstrated efficacy only for offenders whose behavior is based on sex drive; they have not shown efficacy for offenders whose behavior derives from anger or a hostile disposition.

Finally, the courts will have to resolve the issue that the statutes mentioned do not all provide for discrimination among offenders to ensure that only those who would benefit from treatment are actually receiving the treatment if forced treatment is to proceed within the dictates of constitutional law as we know it. Clinicians also have to consider the consequences of withholding a medication that may help decrease a person's tormented, out-of-control feelings or impulses; lessen the intensity of paraphilic fantasies and urges, in turn facilitating fuller participation in a cognitive-behavioral program; and reduce the risk of reoffending.

Summary

The potential contributions of psychiatry to sex offender management span a considerable segment of the patient's life, from post-arrest evaluation and emergent care, through adjudication in the courts, incarceration, possible civil commitment, and supervised release. Nevertheless, as physicians and healers, psychiatrists bring much-needed medical expertise to the discussion. Foremost is the ability of psychiatry to demonstrate that sex offenders are not a homogeneous population. Further, a rational, effective, and humane approach to the social problem of sex offending depends on accurate assessment, diagnosis, and treatment approaches for the offender. Psychiatrists can also inform the ongoing debate about competency, dangerousness, the appropriateness of civil commitment, life-long sex offender registration, compulsory medication, and other medically relevant issues in sex offender management.

References

American Association for Correctional Psychology (1999). Standards for psychological services in jails, prisons, correctional facilities and agencies. *Criminal Justice and Behavior 27*(4), 433–494.

American Psychiatric Association (2000). *Psychiatric services in jails and prisons*. Task force to revise the APA guidelines on psychiatric services in jails and prisons. Washington, DC: American Psychiatric Association.

Anonymous (2014). Texas Department of State Health Services, Counsel on sex offender treatment—treatment of sex offenders—difference between sex offender treatment and psychotherapy. Available at https://www.dshs.state.tx.us/csot/csot_tdifference.shtm (accessed February 22, 2014).

Bell v. Wolfish, 441 U.S. 520 (1979).

Berlin, F. (1986). Interviews with five rapists. *American Journal of Forensic Psychiatry, 41*, 11–41.

Berlin, F. S., Saleh, F. M., & Malin, H. M. (2009). Mental illness and sex offending. In F. M. Saleh, A. J. Grudzinskas, Jr., J. M. Bradford, & D. J. Brodsky (Eds.), *Sex offenders: identification, risk assessment, treatment, and legal issues*. New York: Oxford University Press.

California Penal Code § 645 (West 2003).

Clayton, S. L. (2002) Sex Offenders, 27 Corrections Compendium 8.

Cohen, F. (2003). Correctional mental health law & policy: A primer. *District of Columbia Law Review, 7*(1), 117–142.

Corabian, P., Dennett, L., & Harstall, C. (2011). Treatment for convicted adult male sex offenders: An overview of systematic reviews. *Sexual Offender Treatment, 6*, 1.

DeShaney v. Winnebago Dept. of Social Services, 489 U.S. 189 (1989).

Druhm, K. W. (1997). Comment: A welcome return to Draconia: California Penal Law 645, the castration of sex offenders and the Constitution. *Albany Law Review, 61*, 285.

Elwood, R. W. (2009). Mental disorder, predisposition, prediction, and ability to control: evaluating sex offenders for civil commitment. *Sexual Abuse: A Journal of Research and Treatment. 21*(4), 395–411.

Estelle v. Gamble, 429 U.S. 97 (1976).

Fagan, P. J., Lehne, G., Strand, J., & Berlin, F. (2005). Paraphilias. In G. O. Gabbard, J. S. Beck, & J. Holmes (Eds.), *Oxford textbook of psychotherapy* (pp. 215–227). Oxford: Oxford University Press.

Farkas, M. A., & Miller, G. (2008). Sex offender treatment: Reconciling criminal justice priorities and therapeutic goals. *Federal Sentencing Reporter, 21*, 78.

Farmer v. Brennan, 511 U.S. (1994).

Federal Bureau of Investigation (2012). *Data tables: National Incident-Based Reporting System*. Washington, DC: FBI.

Florida Statutes Annotated §§ 794.011-0235 (West 2002).

Georgia Code Annotated § 16-6-4 and §42-9-44.2 (2002).

Hafemeister, T. L., & Petrila, J. (1994) Treating the mentally disordered offender: Society's uncertain, conflicted, and changing views. *Florida State University Law Review, 21*, 731.

Iowa Code § 903B. 1 (2003).

Kansas v. Hendricks, 521 U.S. 346, 359 (1997).

Kendler, K. S. (1990). Toward a scientific psychiatric nosology. *Archives of General Psychiatry, 47*, 969–973.

Klerman, G. L. (1990). The psychiatric patient's right to effective treatment: implications of Osheroff v. Chestnut Lodge. *American Journal of Psychiatry, 147*(4), 409–418.

LaFond, J. Q., & Winick, B.J. (1998). Special Theme: Sex offenders: scientific, legal, and policy perspective. Foreword: Sex offenders and the law. *Psychology, Public Policy, and Law, 3*, 3.

Langan, P. A., Schmitt, E. L., & Durose M. R. (2003). *Recidivism of sex offenders released from prison in 1994*. Washington, DC: U.S. Department of Justice.

Lehne, G. K. (1986). Brain damage and paraphilia: Treated with medroxyprogesterone acetate. *Sexuality and Disability, 7*, 145–158.

Louisiana Revised Statutes Annotated § 15:538 (West 2003).

McKune v. Lile, 536 U.S. 24 (2002).

Mellela, J. T., Travin, S., & Cullen, K. (1989). Legal and ethical issues in the use of antiandrogens in treating sex offenders. *Bulletin of American Academy of Psychiatry and Law 17*(3), 222–233.

Miller, R. D. (1998). Forced administration of sex-drive-reducing medication to sex offenders: Treatment or punishment? *Psychology, Public Policy, and Law, 4*(1/2), 175–199.

Montana Code Annotated § 45-5-512 (2002).

Oregon Revised Statutes §§ 144.625–631 (2001).

Osheroff v. Chestnut Lodge, Inc., Maryland Court of Special Appeals, 490 A. 2d 720 (1985).

People v. Gauntlett, 352 N.W.2d 310 (Mich. Ct. App. 1984).

Pinta, E. R. (2009). Decisions to breach confidentiality when prisoners report violations of institutional rules. *Journal of the American Academy of Psychiatry and the Law, 37*, 150–154.

Prentky, R., Knight, R., & Lee, A. (1997). *Child sexual molestation: Research issues*. Washington, DC: U.S. Department of Justice.

Rice, M. E., & Harris, G. T. (2011). Is Androgen deprivation therapy effective in the treatment of sex offenders? *Psychology, Public Policy, and Law, 17*, 315.

Saleh, F. M., Grudzinskas, A. J., Malin, H. M., & Dwyer, G. (2010). The management of sex offenders: Perspectives for psychiatry. *Harvard Review of Psychiatry, 18*(6), 359–368.

Scott, C. L., & Holmberg, T. (2003). Castration of sex offenders: Prisoners' right versus public safety. *Journal of the American Academy of Psychiatry and the Law, 31*, 502–509.

Stabenow, T. (2009). Deconstructing the myth of careful study: A primer on the flawed progression of the child pornography guidelines 2-3.

Available at http://www.fd.org/pdf_lib/child%20porn%20july%20revision.pdf (accessed January 16, 2014).

State v. Brown, 326 S.E.2d 410 (S.C. 1985).

Texas Government Code Annotated § 501.061 & § 508.226 (2003).

Ward, T., Gannon, T. A., & Birgden, A. (2007). Human rights and the treatment of sex offenders. *Sexual Abuse, 19*(3), 195–216.

Winslade, W., Stone, T. H., Smith-Bell, M., & Webb, D. M. (1998). Castrating pedophiles convicted of sex offenses against children: New treatment or old punishment? *SMU Law Review, 51*, 349.

Wisconsin Statutes § 304.06 & §§ 980.08-12 (2002).

CHAPTER 60

Cultural competence

Reena Kapoor and Ezra E. H. Griffith

Introduction

Cultural competence is an essential aspect of providing mental health care in any setting. An understanding of culture is even more important in correctional settings, as several unique factors may lead to conflict and misunderstanding if not adequately addressed. First, minority ethnic groups are vastly overrepresented in prisons and jails, so a familiarity with the predominant culture of those groups is necessary to engage inmates in treatment and diagnose them accurately. Second, mental health clinicians may be unfamiliar with law enforcement culture, which heavily influences the practices of corrections officers and differs significantly from health care culture. Third, many correctional psychiatrists grow up and train outside the United States, bringing their own cultural beliefs about crime and punishment into the American health care system. These factors—and others—add to the complexity of providing culturally competent care in correctional facilities. This chapter addresses these issues, the perspectives that contribute to diverse cultural distinctions, and details many of the processes and procedures that lead to culturally competant care delivery in jails and prisons.

Recognition of the importance of cultural competance

The field of correctional psychiatry has formally acknowledged the importance of cultural awareness since the publication of the American Psychiatric Association's standards for psychiatric services in jails and prisons in 2000 (American Psychiatric Association, 2000). These standards articulated the need to provide training in important areas of cultural awareness, including ethnicity, gender, religious/spiritual, sexual orientation, and family factors that influence expression of mental illness or psychological distress in correctional settings. The goals of this training were to improve tolerance of diverse populations, empathy for the minority experience, and understanding of ethnocentric bias and its potential effects.

Outside of corrections, psychiatry has experienced a massive growth of interest in cultural issues during the past few decades. The *Diagnostic and Statistical Manual of Mental Disorders* (DSM) first included guidance about the cultural formulation in its fourth edition, published in 1994 (American Psychiatric Association, 1994). Since then, the field of cultural psychiatry has only continued to expand, with agencies such as the National Center for Cultural Competence and the US Department of Health and Human Services developing resources for clinicians and health care agencies to improve their understanding of culture (National Center for Cultural Competence, 2004; US Department of Health and Human Services, 2013b). The DSM-5 has also carried this mission forward, revising the cultural formulation and providing clinicians with a semistructured interview format to assess important cultural areas, such as definitions of the presenting problem, perceptions of the cause and context, and factors that affect coping and help-seeking (American Psychiatric Association, 2013).

As the field of cultural psychiatry has developed, scholars have attempted to apply its principles to the correctional setting. This work is still in its infancy, but several recent articles and book chapters have addressed the task of providing culturally competent care in prisons and jails (Kapoor, Dike, Burns, et al., 2013; Ortega, 2011; Tseng, Matthews, & Elwyn, 2004). These resources provide guidance to correctional mental health clinicians on matters such as immigrant populations, language barriers, the validity of psychological testing in different ethnic groups, the stigma of mental illness in prison, religion's role in coping with the stress of incarceration, and many others. While more research remains to be done, correctional psychiatrists today have more resources at their disposal to educate themselves about culture than at any time in history.

Current standards for cultural competence

Cultural competence is defined as "a set of congruent behaviors, attitudes, and policies that come together in a system, agency, or among professionals that enables effective work in cross-cultural situations" (US Department of Health and Human Services, 2013b). Stated another way, cultural competence involves building understanding and tolerance of diverse cultures in the service of providing better patient care. Although many methods for achieving cultural competence in health care have been described in the literature (National Center for Cultural Competence, 2004; US Department of Health and Human Services Office of Minority Health, 2000), they generally have some features in common, including improving self-awareness and valuing diversity, communicating effectively, acquiring cultural knowledge, managing the dynamics of difference, and adapting to the changing cultural needs of the community being served. These standards do not address the correctional setting, but the values and methods they advocate are no less applicable in prisons and jails than in the community.

Self-awareness and commitment to diversity

The first step toward cultural competence includes assessing one's own cultural awareness. Cultural self-awareness involves "recognition of one's own cultural influences upon values, beliefs, and judgments, as well as the influences derived from the professional's work culture" (Winkelman, 2005). For example, at the individual level, culturally aware correctional psychiatrists may recognize the difference in ethnic background between themselves and most of their patients and the difference in socioeconomic class between themselves and other correctional staff. In addition, they may understand that medicine has its own culture, which is different from the law enforcement culture in which corrections professionals were educated.

At a correctional systems level, valuing diversity involves a commitment to maintaining a diverse workplace in which many viewpoints are valued. Correctional facilities, like all health care settings, are expected to maintain a workforce that is diverse in gender, ethnic background, age, religion, and sexual orientation. The commitment to diversity includes security, health care, and ancillary staff such as spiritual advisers and education professionals.

Language and communication

Language is often the first barrier that mental health professionals face when trying to provide culturally competent care. When a correctional system or individual health care practitioner cannot speak an inmate's language, clinical assessment or treatment may be extremely limited. Therefore, access to language assistance for inmates with limited English proficiency is essential (US Department of Health and Human Services, 2013a). Given the remote locations of many prisons and jails, these services can be provided through the use of telephone interpreters as long as access to health care services is not unduly delayed. As in other health care settings, maintaining confidentiality is of the utmost importance; the use of untrained interpreters such as family members and other patients should be avoided. In areas where languages other than English are commonly spoken, facilities should also provide written materials and signage in the common languages of the community. For example, in some parts of the United States, medication consent forms and facility policies should be translated into Spanish.

The problem of communication does not end with translation of foreign languages; cultural competence requires consideration of other aspects of the communications process. For example, some inmates have had limited education, and communication must be tailored to their reading level. In addition, correctional professionals should strive to ask open-ended, judgment-free questions to convey respect and tolerance for diverse viewpoints.

Cultural knowledge

Health care professionals, including those who work in correctional settings, should be familiar with the different norms of the cultures commonly found in the community they serve. In prisons and jails, essential knowledge includes an understanding of the minority ethnic populations that are overrepresented in the criminal justice system. It also includes an understanding of special populations of prisoners such as women, juveniles, geriatric inmates, transgender individuals, and immigrants.

Health care providers and security staff should also be familiar with the cultural differences between their professions. Many correctional systems provide education about mental illness, such as crisis intervention team training, to security officers so that they recognize signs and symptoms of illness and can respond appropriately (Hicks, 2011). In addition, mental health professionals must undergo training to understand the unique security aspects of the correctional setting—for example, use of force, searches, lockdowns, counts, and safety procedures.

Managing differences and adapting to change

Health care systems are responsible for creating culturally appropriate goals and policies and also for assessing how well these goals are being met over time. Correctional systems are no different; they must maintain data about initiatives such as workforce diversity and access to language assistance. When significant problems or disparities are identified, for example delays in access to treatment for non-English speakers, systems must take steps to rectify these problems. These steps can include reallocation of resources, policy revision, grievance procedures, and other quality improvement measures. Finally, correctional systems are responsible for communicating the efficacy of these improvement efforts to all stakeholders, including inmates, security staff, and health care providers.

Essential cultural knowledge for clinicians in correctional settings

An exhaustive discussion of all aspects of culture in prison settings is beyond the scope of this chapter. Essential knowledge for correctional mental health professionals includes an understanding of race/ethnicity, religion, age, sexual orientation, religion/spirituality, gender, and other factors that affect the experience of incarceration. Other chapters in this text address some of these subjects in detail, so this chapter touches on only two areas not mentioned elsewhere—cultural beliefs about the criminal justice system and the culture of prisons themselves.

Cultural beliefs about the criminal justice system

Blacks and Hispanics are significantly overrepresented in correctional settings compared to the general population. According to 2010 census data, blacks represented 12.2% of the US population, Hispanics 16.3%, and non-Hispanic whites 63.7% (US Census Bureau, 2011). By contrast, data about prisons in the same year indicate that blacks made up 37.9% of the population, Hispanics 22.3%, and non-Hispanic whites 32.2% (Bureau of Justice Statistics, 2010). The Bureau of Justice Statistics (2010) estimated that 7.3% of all black men ages 30–34 were incarcerated—a figure that dwarfed the incarceration rate of other ethnic groups. Furthermore, 41.8% of the inmates on death row are black (Fins, 2013), and blacks were more likely to receive a death sentence if their victims were white (US General Accounting Office, 1990).

In this context of extremely disproportionate involvement of ethnic minorities with the criminal justice system, it is no surprise that cultural beliefs about crime and punishment have developed in communities of color. Some scholars have gone so far as to call our system of mass incarceration "slavery" and "the new Jim Crow," drawing a link between historical means of control over minority populations and our modern criminal justice practices (Alexander, 2010; Wacquant, 2002). Recent policies such as stop-and-frisk in New York City have further inflamed the debate about whether police unfairly target ethnic minorities, as the overwhelming number of persons stopped—approximately 85%—are black or Latino (New York Civil Liberties Union, 2013; Peters,

2013). The end result is that in many communities of color, incarceration is viewed not as a personal failure or source of shame but as the most recent battle in the ongoing struggle for civil rights.

The high rates of incarceration in minority communities also have effects on family structure and role modeling for young men. When so many adult males are in prison, many children are raised without fathers and must seek alternative sources of guidance and support. For many boys in urban communities, gang leaders fill that role (Morris, 2012). Gang leaders are respected, and time spent in prison is often seen as an initiation into the group rather than as a punishment for an unlawful act. Bravado, even pride, in incarceration is not uncommon (Morris, 2012).

For the mental health professional working for the first time with black and Hispanic patients, particularly those from impoverished or urban areas, an understanding of cultural beliefs about the criminal justice system in these communities can be invaluable. Clinicians from a middle-class, white background may interpret an inmate's statements about the unfairness of the criminal justice system as evidence of callousness or lack of responsibility for actions. Clinicians may also view discussions about growing up fatherless or without positive role models as excuses for bad behavior. Without an understanding of the norms in the inmate's culture of origin, the inmate may be labeled inappropriately as having paranoid ideation or antisocial personality disorder. Of course, these diagnoses may be appropriate; however, the clinician must use caution and interpret the patient's statements through a culturally informed lens before reaching such a conclusion, as the patient may simply be expressing community beliefs.

Understanding a patient's beliefs about the criminal justice system is essential when working with black and Hispanic populations, but it is also important when working with immigrant and refugee populations, which make up more prisoners each year. In 2010, more than 400,000 immigrants were detained in jails, prisons, and private detention centers (Bernstein, 2011). While most immigrants in detention are from Mexico and Central America, detainees also include asylum seekers from nearly every country in the world (Shah, 2013). Therefore, correctional mental health professionals are likely to encounter patients from many foreign cultures.

A common thread among many detained immigrants is that they come from countries in which the rule of law is not enforced consistently. Corruption, bribery, political retaliation, and extremely harsh punishments can be common in other countries. For example, Mexico has experienced tremendous violence related to drug trafficking in recent years, and unscrupulous law enforcement officials have at times been complicit in allowing the lawlessness to continue (Hernandez, 2013). In totalitarian societies, the opposite situation occurs: Secrets must be kept from government officials who rule with an iron fist. In many countries around the world, nobody—not judges, lawyers, or even doctors—can be trusted to engage honestly in professional activities. Immigrants may therefore have a deeply held mistrust of government agencies, including the criminal justice system and corrections officials.

This skepticism can often be mistaken for frank paranoia and is difficult for some mental health professionals to understand. For example, a prisoner from China may be accustomed to an authoritarian government in which people with views opposing the state can be imprisoned or even "disappeared" simply because of their political beliefs (Kline, 2011). Similarly, a prisoner from India may believe that the government is inherently corrupt and that a favorable outcome in court is not possible for a person without the means to pay bribes. While it is impossible for a prison psychiatrist to become familiar with every culture in the world, let alone its political problems, it is important to keep in mind that individuals from other countries may have a very different understanding of the criminal justice system from that of the average American. What may appear to be paranoia (and therefore a sign of a psychotic illness) may actually be a culturally appropriate belief about the rule of law in the patient's home country.

The culture of prisons

Social scientists have studied prison culture for decades, long before the creation of popular books and television shows made the subject trendy. Initial studies of prisons from the 1940s described the process of "prisonization" in which inmates assimilated the norms and behavioral expectations of life within the institution (Clemmer, 1940). Prison culture was described as harsh and predatory, with frequent threats of violence, an emphasis on showing respect, and a rigidly enforced hierarchy of power and control. In traditional prison culture, any sign of weakness would be exploited, gang affiliations were obligatory, and inmates were at constant risk of violence.

In attempting to explain how this culture developed in prisons, sociologists initially postulated two competing theories—the deprivation model and the importation model. In the deprivation model, the culture of prisons arose from the many "pains of imprisonment," including the deprivation of liberty, material goods, autonomy, heterosexual relationships, and security (Sykes, 1958). The predatory aspects of prison life were seen to be adaptive responses to an environment of severe deprivation. By contrast, the importation model proposed that prisoners brought the violent features of their culture into the institution from the outside world. Inmates were thought to adhere to the same social norms, some of which were antisocial, to which they subscribed prior to being incarcerated (Irwin & Cressey, 1962).

Modern theorists have integrated these two models, stating that inmate culture is influenced by both the shared experience of deprivation and by individual characteristics such as stability of personality, the culture in which the inmate was raised, and length of incarceration (Hochstetler & DeLisi, 2005). There is no one-size-fits-all culture of prisons, although the stereotype of prisons as hypermasculine environments in which power struggles are common still applies in some settings. The proliferation of women's prisons has further complicated matters, as women often approach the experience of incarceration differently from men, creating romantic relationships and pseudo-families rather than gang affiliations (Forsyth & Evans, 2003). As prison populations have grown exponentially since the 1980s, so, too, have the number of subcultures within prisons.

For the correctional mental health professional, a working knowledge of the institution's culture can be very helpful. Clinicians can learn most about prison culture from the inmates, typically by inquiring about interpersonal relationships in the cell block, tattoos, meals, and recreational activities. In addition, inmate letters and artwork are often evocative, describing the experience of deprivation and "killing time." Security officers can be a helpful source of information about subcultures that inmates may not be willing to share with a clinician, such as gang affiliations or the prevalence of illicit drugs.

Once mental health clinicians have acquired a basic understanding of prison subcultures, they must assess the degree to which inmates have assimilated into one (or more) of these cultures. First, clinicians must inquire about a patient's culture outside of the correctional environment and then inquire about how cultural beliefs and practices have changed since incarceration. In addition, clinicians should try to evaluate the extent to which a patient's adaptation to prison culture has been healthful or unhealthful. Has the patient found prosocial peers, or has behavior regressed in response to others? For example, some inmates learn maladaptive coping mechanisms such as smearing body fluids or self-injury from others whom they perceive as receiving more attention or care after engaging in these behaviors. Other inmates may react to prison culture in just the opposite way, seeing mental illness as a stigma and experiencing shame or fear about asking for help from mental health professionals.

Culturally competent practice in correctional settings

Correctional mental health professionals practicing in isolation cannot achieve cultural competence; it requires a systemwide commitment to diversity and cultural awareness. Corrections officers, administrators, and other professionals must also support culturally competent care, which can be challenging in the chronically understaffed and overburdened environment of corrections. Simply put, attending to the cultural needs of inmates can seem like a luxury. Furthermore, some perceive cultural competence as a niche interest of scholars rather than a serious concern for practitioners, who would much rather avoid the additional paperwork generated by a systemwide effort to improve cultural awareness.

Nonetheless, cultural competence is an essential aspect of providing good mental health care to inmates, in part because an understanding of culture can lead to concrete improvements in patient outcomes. For example, an inmate may find the experience of speaking with a mental health professional stigmatizing, so allowing him to keep up a "public" face of bravado while privately encouraging him to speak freely may provide a mechanism through which he can ask for help (Ortega, 2011). In another example, the gregarious manner in which Hispanic inmates communicate with each other may be perceived as a security threat unless properly understood as part of their culture (Packard, 2005); mental health professionals can help communicate this cultural nuance to security officers and prevent potential sanctions

Table 60.1 Important areas of consideration for cultural formulation in correctional settings

Cultural Identity Before and After Incarceration

- With what cultural group(s) did the patient identify before entering the prison system?
- With what culture/subgroup does the patient associate within the prison?
- To what extent has the patient continued to associate with his culture of origin versus assimilated with prison culture?
- How is the patient adjusting to the experience of isolation, loss, and deprivation common in all prisons?
- Does the patient's current cultural association represent an adaptive or maladaptive response to imprisonment?

Cultural Beliefs About Mental Illness

- How is mental illness experienced/expressed/explained in the patient's culture of origin? To what degree is there stigma (or not)?
- How is mental illness perceived in the patient's prison subculture? By the custody staff?

Cultural Beliefs About Criminal Justice System

- How are incarceration and the criminal justice system explained in that culture? To what degree is there stigma (or not)?
- How is the patient's crime (such as sex offense, violence against child) perceived in the prison subculture? By the custody staff?

Cultural Factors Between Patient and Clinician

- What are the differences between the patient's cultural identity (both before and after prison) and the clinician's?
- Is the clinician able to appreciate the effect of the cultural influences on the interactions with the patient?
- What effect does the prison environment have on the clinician? Is the repeated exposure to manipulation and malingering causing burnout in the clinician or perhaps adversely affecting perceptions of the patient?
- Is the clinician overidentifying with custody staff or with the patient (especially if one or the other is of the same culture as the clinician)?
- Is the physical plant or presence of other people such as custody officers affecting the patient's expression of symptoms or trust of the clinician?

Cultural Factors Affecting Treatment Planning

- Is the prison environment masking or exacerbating particular symptoms of mental illness? For example, is prolonged solitary confinement exacerbating psychosis or depression?
- Can the clinician appreciate differences between the culture of the mental health staff and correctional officers?
- How can the clinician's understanding of cultural factors be translated into correctional language and made acceptable in a correctional culture? How can culturally aware treatment best be explained to officers focused on safety and security?
- To what extent can custody officers be involved in treatment planning, particularly when they share aspects of the patient's culture?

Adapted from Kapoor, R., Dike, C., Burns, C., Carvalho, V., & Griffith, E.E. (2013). Cultural competence in correctional mental health. *International Journal of Law and Psychiatry*, 36(3–4), 273–280.

for misconduct. In a third example, medication doses may need adjustment during Ramadan for Muslim inmates who fast during the daylight hours.

In addition to resulting in better patient outcomes, culturally competent care adheres to the important ethics principle of respect for patients. Individuals involved with the criminal justice system are often treated with disdain or hostility, both inside prisons and in the community. Furthermore, individuals who suffer from mental illness are also often marginalized and treated as second-class citizens in society. Therefore, incarcerated persons who seek treatment for mental illness are doubly stigmatized. Their potential to feel devalued and dehumanized is high. Working with a mental health professional who has demonstrated a commitment to learning about them as individuals, including their individual cultural background, can help build a therapeutic alliance and a relationship of mutual respect.

In considering how best to include an understanding of culture into mental health assessments and treatment, a list of important areas to consider can be very helpful. DSM-5 provides a semi-structured cultural formulation interview that guides clinicians through the process of obtaining culturally relevant information from the patient (Table 60.1; American Psychiatric Association, 2013). After obtaining this information, clinicians can assess to what extent cultural factors play a role in the patient's presentation. They can also formulate a treatment plan that is specific to both the patient and the correctional setting.

Of course, correctional settings can pose numerous challenges to providing culturally competent care. As mentioned previously, one barrier is that prisons and jails often lack sufficient staff to facilitate engagement in the detailed application of the cultural formulation. Another major problem is that in a correctional environment, the mental health professional may not control decisions made about what happens to an inmate. Security officers ultimately may decide whether a treatment plan is implemented, so including them in treatment planning is an additional task faced by correctional mental health professionals. In some cases, this can be quite a challenge, as corrections officers generally do not approach inmates with a therapeutic mentality. Therefore, mental health professionals in prisons and jails must use their understanding of correctional culture to translate patient formulations and treatment plans into language that security staff can understand. When this explanation is done effectively, security staff can serve as valuable partners and advocates in treatment planning or communicating with the patient, as they often share important aspects of the patient's culture and understand how best to convey information.

Summary

Creating the cultural formulation and executing treatment planning in the correctional setting should be a collaborative effort between mental health and security staff. Some cultural competence principles are common to all health care settings, including valuing diversity, communicating effectively, acquiring knowledge of different cultures, and adapting to changes in the cultural environment. However, the correctional setting requires additional knowledge and skills. First, correctional mental health professionals must become familiar with cultural factors that affect the individual's experience of incarceration, such as ethnicity, gender, age, sexual orientation, and socioeconomic status. In addition, mental health professionals must learn about the culture of prisons. Finally, mental health professionals in jails and prisons must be skilled in translating their ideas into correctional language so that security officers will understand and implement treatment plans. When effective collaboration is achieved, tangible benefits such as a safer prison and healthier inmates can follow.

References

Alexander, M. (2010). *The new Jim Crow: Mass incarceration in the age of colorblindness*. New York: The New Press.

American Psychiatric Association (1994). *Diagnostic and statistical manual of mental disorders* (4th ed.). Washington, DC: American Psychiatric Association.

American Psychiatric Association (2000). *Psychiatric services in jails and prisons* (2nd ed.) Washington, DC: American Psychiatric Association.

American Psychiatric Association (2013). *Diagnostic and statistical manual of mental disorders* (5th ed.). Arlington, VA: American Psychiatric Association.

Bernstein, N. (2011, September 29). Getting tough on ommigrants to turn a profit. *New York Times*, pp. A1.

Bureau of Justice Statistics (2010). Prisoners in 2010. Available at: http://www.bjs.gov/content/pub/pdf/p10.pdf (accessed November 30, 2013).

Clemmer, D. (1940). *The prison community*. Boston: Christopher.

Fins, D. (2013). Death row U.S.A., Spring 2013. Available at: http://www.naacpldf.org/death-row-usa (accessed November 30, 2013).

Forsyth, C. J., & Evans, R. D. (2003). Reconsidering the pseudo-family/gang distinction in prison research. *Journal of Police and Criminal Psychology, 18*(1), 15–23.

Hernandez, A. (2013). *Narcoland: The Mexican drug lords and their godfathers*. Brooklyn, NY: Verso.

Hicks, E. (2011, August 10). Crisis intervention in a correctional setting. Available at: http://www.correctionsone.com/jail-management/articles/4206236-Crisis-intervention-in-a-correctional-setting/ (accessed December 1, 2013).

Hochstetler, A., & DeLisi, M. (2005). Importation, deprivation, and varieties of serving time: An integrated-lifestyle-exposure model of prison offending. *Journal of Criminal Justice, 33*, 257–266.

Irwin, J., & Cressey, D. (1962). Thieves, convicts, and the inmate subculture. *Social Problems, 54*, 590–603.

Kapoor, R., Dike, C., Burns, C., Carvalho, V., & Griffith, E. E. (2013). Cultural competence in correctional mental health. *International Journal of Law and Psychiatry, 36*(3-4), 273–280.

Kline, P. (2011). Why are people disappearing in China? Available at: http://www.hrw.org/news/2011/09/22/why-are-people-disappearing-china-0 (accessed November 30, 2013).

Morris, E. J. (2012). Respect, Protection, Faith, and Love Major Care Constructs Identified Within the Subculture of Selected Urban African American Adolescent Gang Members. *Journal of Transcultural Nursing, 23*(3), 262–269.

National Center for Cultural Competence (2004). Cultural competence health practitioner assessment. Available at: http://nccc.georgetown.edu/features/CCHPA.html (accessed December 1, 2013).

New York Civil Liberties Union. Stop-and-frisk data. Available at: http://www.nyclu.org/content/stop-and-frisk-data (accessed November 30, 2013).

Ortega, C. N. (2011). Issues in multicultural assessment and treatment. In T. J. Fagan & R. F. Ax (Eds.), *Correctional mental health: from theory to best practice* (pp. 125–144). Thousand Oaks, CA: SAGE Publications.

Packard, E. (2005, November). Cultural education goes both ways in U.S. prisons. Available at: http://www.apa.org/monitor/nov05/prisons.aspx (accessed December 6, 2013).

Peters, J. (2013). Yes, Mr. Bloomberg, stop-and-frisk is really, really racist. Available at: http://www.slate.com/blogs/crime/2013/07/01/

mayor_bloomberg_stop_and_frisk_yes_the_controversial_policy_is_really_really.html (accessed November 30, 2013).

Shah, S. (2013, Nov. 22). Immigration detention quotas must be stopped. *Houston Chronicle*. Available at: http://www.chron.com/opinion/outlook/article/Shah-Immigration-detention-quotas-must-be-stopped-5002771.php (accessed November 30, 2013).

Sykes, G. M. (1958). *The society of captives*. Princeton, NJ: Princeton University Press.

Tseng, W., Matthews, D., & Elwyn, T. S. (2004). *Cultural competence in forensic mental health*. New York: Brunner-Routledge.

US Census Bureau (2011). Overview of Race and Hispanic Origin: 2010. 2010 Census Briefs. Available at: http://www.census.gov/prod/cen2010/briefs/c2010br-02.pdf (accessed October 9, 2014).

US Department of Health and Human Services (2013a). National standards for culturally and linguistically appropriate services (CLAS) in health and health care. Available at: http://minorityhealth.hhs.gov/templates/browse.aspx?lvl=2&lvlID=15 (accessed December 1, 2013).

US Department of Health and Human Services (2013b). What is cultural competency? Available at: http://minorityhealth.hhs.gov/templates/browse.aspx?lvl=2&lvlID=11 (accessed November 30, 2013).

US General Accounting Office (1990). Death penalty sentencing: Research indicates pattern of racial disparities. Available at: http://www.gao.gov/assets/220/212180.pdf (accessed November 30, 2013).

US Department of Health and Human Services, Office of Minority Health. (2000). Assuring Cultural Competence in Health Care: Recommendations for National Standards and an Outcomes-Focused Research Agenda. 65 Federal Register 80865.

Wacquant, L. (2002). From slavery to mass incarceration. *The New Left Review, 13*, 41–60.

Winkelman, M. (2005). *Cultural awareness, sensitivity & competence*. Peosta, IA: Eddie Bowers Publishing Co., Inc.

SECTION XIII

Special topics

CHAPTER 61

Forensic issues

Erik J. Roskes and Donna Vanderpool

Introduction

This chapter focuses on common forensic issues that a psychiatrist working in a correctional setting may have to manage. These issues include detainees found incompetent to stand trial (IST) and liability exposures that a correctional psychiatrist may face. State and local laws vary widely, and different problems may arise depending on the location in which the psychiatrist works. Examples used may not generalize to all settings. This chapter provides correctional psychiatrists with grounding in the nature of forensic challenges that they may face. Psychiatrists practicing in correctional settings should become familiar with relevant federal, state, and local laws that may impact correctional practice.

Competency restoration and the correctional psychiatrist

Approximately 60,000 competency evaluations are ordered in the United States every year, with about one fifth of these defendants being found IST (National Judicial College, 2012). Upon adjudication as IST, a criminal case is stayed while the defendant is treated, with the goal of rendering that defendant competent to stand trial (CST) so that the criminal case may proceed. In general, this does not involve correctional psychiatrists; in most states, the IST finding permits the court to place the defendant in a clinical setting for treatment to restore competency. Such orders, however, do not by themselves permit treatment over the objection of a defendant. In *Sell v. United States* (2003), the US Supreme Court found that

> . . . the Constitution permits the Government involuntarily to administer antipsychotic drugs to a mentally ill defendant facing serious criminal charges in order to render that defendant competent to stand trial, but only if the treatment is medically appropriate, is substantially unlikely to have side effects that may undermine the fairness of the trial, and, taking account of less intrusive alternatives, is necessary significantly to further *important governmental trial-related interests*. This standard will permit involuntary administration of drugs *solely for trial competency purposes* in certain instances. But those instances may be rare [emphasis added].

These instances will be rare because most criminal cases involve minor charges that do not rise to the level of "important governmental trial-related interests." Unfortunately, many of these detainees spend long periods of time incarcerated in local jails awaiting transfer to a state hospital facility due to significant shortages of forensic beds for competency restoration purposes. It is frequently not legally permissible to involuntarily medicate these persons on a nonemergency basis in a jail setting due to state law and/or regulations (see Chapter 26). In most jurisdictions, the procedure outlined by the US Supreme Court in *Washington v. Harper* (1990) is interpreted as applying to prison settings in contrast to jails, which limits the ability to use nonemergency involuntary psychotropic medications in many jails. The Court held that the due process clause permits a state to treat an inmate based solely on determinations by medical professionals that the inmate is dangerous and treatment is in the inmate's medical interest. Some states, however, use stricter criteria such as full judicial review, findings of incompetence, and the appointment of a guardian or substituted decision maker; psychiatrists need to know the procedural requirements in their own jurisdictions.

Where treatment is provided depends entirely on local resources. Ideally, such defendants would be transferred to a hospital for treatment, and this occurs in many states. For example, in Maryland, a defendant found IST and dangerous to self, others, or the property of others due to mental disorder is committed to a state psychiatric hospital until that defendant is no longer IST or dangerous due to mental disorder or until "there is not a substantial likelihood that the defendant will become competent to stand trial in the foreseeable future" (*Jackson v. Indiana*, 1972). Alternatively, a defendant found IST and dangerous due to "mental retardation" (many state statutes continue to use this term) is committed to a facility for people with intellectual disabilities until reaching similar endpoints (Annotated Code of Maryland, 2013, Crim. Proc., §3–106). Thus, Maryland provides all treatment pursuant to a finding of IST and dangerousness due to mental disorder or mental retardation in clinical settings. Some judges in Maryland have interpreted the law as requiring the immediate transfer of the defendant from court to the hospital upon the finding of IST and dangerousness due to mental disorder.

In many states, a finding of IST alone is sufficient to commit the defendant (personal communication, W. Lawrence Fitch, JD, November 24, 2013). In Maryland, the dangerousness requirement leaves a potential gap in that, by law, defendants found IST but not found dangerous due to mental illness or mental retardation may not be committed to a hospital or a facility for people with intellectual disability for treatment or habilitation to restore competency. Such defendants, if remanded or unable to make bail, would remain incarcerated, and the jail would remain legally obligated to provide constitutionally adequate mental health services to the detainee in the context of his/her serious mental illness (see Chapter 3). If treatment is refused and the detainee does not meet criteria for involuntary treatment, the treatment plan should be revised to encourage treatment adherence. However, at present, jails in Maryland have no ability to provide treatment for competency restoration purposes.

For example, consider a defendant arrested for drug possession. The defendant is a young man with an IQ in the mid-70s and with no apparent mental illness. He cooperates with the police, presenting no resistance upon arrest. The court finds that he does not understand the charges and cannot work with his attorney. Yet, he remains cooperative and compliant with all proceedings. This defendant's crime is not dangerous in the common sense of the term, and even if the crime is legally presumed to be dangerous (*Jones v. US*, 1983), that dangerousness has no obvious connection to mental illness or intellectual disability. In some states, such as New York, defendants found IST for misdemeanor crimes cannot be criminally committed but instead must have their charges dismissed; if such defendants do not meet civil commitment criteria, they must be released (New York CPL §730.70, undated).

In some states, the available hospital resources do not meet the demand, and defendants found IST must be managed in detention (GAINS, 2007). Jennings and Bell (2012) describe the jail-based competency restoration program used in one Virginia county. Kapoor (2011) reported that defendants in Texas found IST and committed for treatment waited between 72 and 180 days to be admitted to the hospital. Texas recently examined alternative strategies toward resolving cases halted due to the defendant's incompetence to proceed. In an issue brief, the Hogg Foundation (2013) compared the costs, length of stay, and restoration rates of the following four competency restoration models: state psychiatric hospital, community/private hospital, outpatient, and jail based. The review found that jail-based and community-based restoration programs are generally far less costly for defendants who do not require hospitalization based on either clinical need or the severity of the offense.

The National Judicial College (2012) conducted a review of competency restoration practices and provided a set of best practice recommendations. Their overarching recommendation was that restoration be carried out "in the least-restrictive treatment setting or facility consistent with the public safety and treatment needs of the defendant." The review concluded that hospital-based competency restoration should be reserved only for incompetent defendants who

◆ Present with imminent risk toward themselves or others,

◆ Are at risk of significant self-neglect,

◆ Require a comprehensive diagnostic assessment including an assessment for potential malingering,

◆ Lack the capacity to provide consent for treatment, or

◆ May require involuntary or emergency treatment.

Based on available data, best practice, and the authors' experience, restoration may occur in jail for defendants who do not fall into these categories but who require ongoing detention on public safety grounds. Defendants who are not remanded or who can make bail should have access to community-based competency restoration programs.

While each venue for competency restoration has its strengths and weaknesses, the utility of jail- or community-based restoration programs is predicated on the availability of adequate and specialized staffing and on the separation of evaluators and treatment staff to avoid conflict of interest (Chapter 8 has further discussion of role conflicts). Thus, in jails already stretched thin due to overcrowding and inadequate staffing, competency restoration is not recommended as a solution to the lack of availability of hospital beds or community-based resources unless new staff and adequate programming space are specifically allocated. However, if there is adequate staffing, both in numbers and in training and experience, a jail-based competency restoration program could be considered where there are inadequate hospital-based resources and where relevant statutes and regulations permit this approach. Psychiatrists working in correctional institutions that treat defendants found IST are strongly encouraged to become familiar with competency restoration, education, and habilitation procedures beyond psychopharmacology. In addition, psychiatrists in these situations should advocate for a clear separation between the two potentially conflicted roles of treatment (which may include restoration techniques) and forensic evaluation and reporting that keeps the court apprised of the defendant's competency status. Finally, corrections managers are encouraged to advocate for adequate resources for defendants found IST and in clinical need of hospitalization; the adoption of jail-based restoration programs does not negate the need for other mental health resources including hospital- and community-based competency restoration programs.

Liability risk in correctional care

Psychiatrists working in correctional settings face increased litigation risks regarding professional negligence and other forms of liability. They need to review the categories of claims covered by their insurance policies. Especially important is understanding whether the insurer covers forensic and correctional work.

Correctional psychiatrists also need to consider the standard of care that they deliver to their patients. A resource document of the American Psychiatric Association (2000) states that

> [t]he fundamental policy goal for correctional mental health care is to provide the same level of mental health services to each patient in the criminal justice process *that should be available in the community*. This policy goal is deliberately higher than the "community standard" that is called for in various legal contexts [emphasis added].

At times, there may be restrictions on care, such as medication formularies or volume-based expectations regarding the number of cases seen per unit time. These are common management strategies in many settings and, as a matter of principle, should be included in the conceptual standard of care, but they may not be acceptable reasons for failing to engage in proper clinical management. For example, when viewed through the lens of malpractice or other litigation, questions may be raised regarding the psychiatrist's failure to seek a formulary exception or to spend adequate time assessing or providing treatment to a patient in crisis. It is imperative to document effectively and completely, to manage known risks of medications, and to engage in and document routine informed consent discussions with patients. As in all settings, communication with other providers helps ensure appropriate care; working with the correctional staff who know the patients well is also advisable (see the rest of this chapter and Chapter 9). Finally, becoming familiar with relevant guidelines and accreditation standards promulgated by organizations such as the American Psychiatric Association (2000), the American Correctional Association (2009), and the National Commission on Correctional Health Care (2008) can be useful.

Correctional psychiatry is accompanied by increased professional liability exposure when compared with general psychiatric practice in the community due to unique risks for the following reasons:

◆ *Inmates in the United States have a constitutional right to receive medical care (see Chapter 3), allowing them to claim civil rights violations in addition to claims for medical malpractice.* Courts have held that deliberate indifference to serious medical and mental health needs violates the Eighth Amendment. Federal law (42 US Code §1983) imposes liability on government employees—or those linked to the government (such as private contractors)—for violation of a citizen's constitutional rights including those covered by the Eighth Amendment. As discussed in *Estelle v. Gamble* (1976), deliberate indifference to serious medical needs of prisoners constitutes the unnecessary and wanton infliction of pain proscribed by the Eighth Amendment, which is actionable against correctional psychiatrists under §1983.

◆ *The rate of suicide is high in correctional settings, although it has fallen dramatically in the past three decades* (see Chapter 43). As of 2011, there were 43 suicides per 100,000 population in local jails and 16 per 100,000 in state prisons (Noonan & Ginder, 2013); for comparison, the overall US suicide rate in 2010 was 12 per 100,000 (Centers for Disease Control and Prevention, 2013). Suicides in correctional settings often result in a claim against the psychiatrist for medical malpractice (i.e., professional negligence) and may also result in a claim of deliberate indifference under §1983.

◆ *There is the potential for class action exposure.* Advocacy groups may file class action litigation against the correctional facility for alleged problems such as overcrowding, violence, and substandard health care. Correctional psychiatrists may be named in these cases against correctional facilities.

◆ *The correctional psychiatrist lacks full control of the treatment environment.* Inmates are in the custody of the corrections staff, who may impede access to necessary treatment. Additionally, there may be disagreements with administration over clinical issues. These may include restricted formulary options and an inability to control the time and number of medication administrations per day. The correctional environment itself may render it difficult or impossible to maintain confidentiality, making appropriate treatment difficult to provide. This is especially true in higher-security or segregation settings.

◆ *Many corrections cases are brought* pro se *(i.e., by the inmate/ plaintiff who is not represented by counsel).* Typically, courts allow *pro se* litigants more latitude in prosecuting their complaints than they would permit an attorney filing on a litigant's behalf. Cases that might not be permitted to proceed via counsel may last much longer when filed *pro se*. Trial judges are very liberal in allowing amended complaints to which defendants and their attorneys must respond, often several times.

Some factors inherent to correctional practice affect the risk of liability exposure. In general, inmates are more litigious than people in the community, for reasons that may include legitimate grievances regarding the context in which care is delivered. Claims of professional negligence may include common legal theories such as wrongful death/suicide; adverse drug reactions; and failures

to obtain informed consent, diagnose, or treat appropriately. Some inmates use their unscheduled time to devise unusual legal claims. While many of these claims ultimately will be dismissed as frivolous, they still must be addressed and defended. Correctional providers may be named in these claims. Finally, inmates may file actions in both state and federal court based on more than one legal theory, including licensure complaints, professional negligence claims/lawsuits, ordinary negligence claims/lawsuits, and/or civil rights claims/lawsuits. These render inmate-engendered lawsuits far more complex than patient complaints in the community.

Additionally, when the plaintiff is represented in a §1983 action, the attorney may be motivated to include as many defendants as possible and to keep them in the case as long as possible, because §1983 actions allow for the recovery of attorneys' fees. These features of correctional litigation increase the cost of defending even cases that ultimately are dismissed. Section 1983 and other civil rights actions are discussed in more detail subsequently.

While the risk of having a claim filed in correctional practice may be higher than in community practice, payouts are generally smaller for correctional cases. The second author (D.V.) reviewed data from Professional Risk Management Services, Inc. (PRMS) from 2002 to 2012 and found that less than 10 percent of correctional claims filed against PRMS-covered psychiatrists were closed with an indemnity payment. More than half of these indemnity payments were for less than $50,000, though the cost of defending these claims, especially when they include §1983 complaints, may be quite high, as noted previously.

Many cases ultimately result in a finding that some of the defendants are entitled to qualified immunity from the lawsuit. In some circumstances, public officials, but not private practitioners or other correctional contractors, are found eligible for qualified immunity. However, a recent US Supreme Court case suggests that in certain scenarios, even private providers may be entitled to qualified immunity (*Filarsky v. Delia*, 2012); that said, qualified immunity would not apply to allegations of reckless or malicious acts.

The role of the correctional psychiatrist in civil rights litigation and settlement

Habeas corpus

The doctrine of *habeas corpus* stems from the Common Law and is enshrined in the US Constitution: "The Privilege of the Writ of Habeas Corpus shall not be suspended" (US Const. art. I, §9). *Habeas* petitions are primarily used to challenge the legality of continued detentions and are occasionally brought by incarcerated individuals who seek a hearing. For example, a *habeas* petition could be brought to seek medical interventions that are being denied by the detaining institution and, as such, the medical staff could be named defendants. A correctional psychiatrist who is advised that a patient has filed for a *habeas* hearing should notify institutional management and the psychiatrist's attorney and insurance company.

Class action litigation

Many class actions have involved correctional mental health care. Often clinicians working in correctional settings welcome these litigations, as they focus the attention of the courts and, at times, the media and the public on deficiencies in care related to inadequate resources. While such lawsuits can be sensitive, especially in the earlier phases when the outcome is in doubt, correctional psychiatrists and other clinicians may also serve as sources of information for each party to the case and to the court. Chapters 3 and 66 have additional information about class action litigation.

Class actions may result in remedial court orders or private settlement agreements in which the jurisdiction agrees to modify services. During these remediation phases, policies may change and resources may be added to ensure provision of the enhanced services. Additionally, there may be court monitoring or other oversight of the case during the remediation phase. This may result in changes in how clinicians practice. It is important to be aware of such cases when working in a correctional setting to ensure that the care provided is consonant with the expectations of the court and the parties to the litigation.

External review and investigation

As noted previously, an institutionalized person may file a civil rights complaint pursuant to 42 USC §1983, civil action for deprivation of rights. In a §1983 action, a person who subjects another person "to the deprivation of any rights, privileges or immunities secured by the Constitution and laws . . . under color of any statute, ordinance, regulation, custom, or usage, of any State or Territory or the District of Columbia" is liable for that deprivation. This statute is the basis for much of the significant correctional litigation over the past half-century, including *Estelle v. Gamble* (1976) and the subsequent cases related to the constitutional obligation to provide health care and mental health care that are discussed elsewhere in this text.

Public and certain private institutions where individuals may be detained are also subject to the independent oversight of the US Department of Justice, Civil Rights Division, pursuant to the Civil Rights of Institutionalized Persons Act (CRIPA). Passed in 1980, this legislation covers institutions designed for people with mental illnesses or disabilities as well as jails, prisons, and juvenile detention centers. A CRIPA action can be initiated by the attorney general based on "reasonable cause" that a state or county, or the employees of a state or county, are

> subjecting persons residing in or confined to an institution . . . to egregious or flagrant conditions that deprive such persons of any rights, privileges, or immunities secured or protected by the Constitution or laws of the United States causing such persons to suffer grievous harm, and that such deprivation is pursuant to a pattern or practice of resistance to the full enjoyment of such rights, privileges, or immunities, the Attorney General, for or in the name of the United States . . . .

These investigations are carried out by the US Department of Justice, Civil Rights Division, Special Litigation Division. At times, the state's Protection and Advocacy for Individuals with Mental Illness group or other advocacy-oriented legal groups may join in these investigations. The role of the correctional psychiatrist in such actions is parallel to the role in class action complaints, described previously.

Other forensic issues

Confidentiality

The usual rules of confidentiality often do not apply in a correctional mental health care setting. For example, the fact that

an inmate is receiving mental health treatment is not kept confidential from custody staff for many reasons (e.g., scheduling, managing heat-related risks associated with certain medications, providing mental health input into the disciplinary process) and is apparent to other inmates based on medication passes and clinic visits. A balance needs to be maintained between the privacy rights of the mental health caseload inmate and the needs of other inmates, in addition to the security needs of the correctional facility (American Psychiatric Association, 2000). Correctional staff in special mental health units (see Chapter 22) are often considered part of the treatment team and attend treatment team meetings where confidential information is shared with all team members. Other practice variations or exceptions to the usual rules of confidentiality include

* Parole board evaluators who access the inmate's health care record without requiring consent from the inmate (varies by jurisdiction),

* Duty to protect exceptions in many jurisdictions,

* Duty to reveal knowledge of escape plans, and

* In some facilities, a vague need to know exception for security purposes.

The mental health clinician should inform their clients of the limitations of confidentiality and numerous exceptions. This should be done in a manner that does not interfere with establishing a therapeutic alliance with the inmate.

Mental health input into the disciplinary process

Little has been written regarding the importance of providing mental health input into the disciplinary process. A national survey by Krelstein (2002) demonstrated that "considerable diversity exists among the states in prison policy regarding the role of mental health personnel in the inmate disciplinary process." Metzner (2002) recommends that mental health input into the disciplinary process not address issues of responsibility (i.e., "not guilty by reason of insanity") but be limited to identifying mitigating factors related to mental illness when present, dispositional recommendations when clinically appropriate, and competency-to-proceed issues in the context of the disciplinary hearing. This quasi-forensic assessment should be done by an appropriately trained clinician who is not the inmate's clinician in order to minimize dual-agency issues.

Prison rape elimination act

The Prison Rape Elimination Act, enacted in 2003, has begun to reshape correctional attitudes and responses to sexual assault in US jails and prisons. While the forensic ramifications are still unfolding, psychiatrists working in US correctional settings need to understand their screening, training, management, and evidentiary responsibilities (National PREA Resource Center, 2013).

Summary

There are many common forensic challenges in correctional psychiatric practice. Numerous defendants are found IST each year, and some places have inadequate public mental health resources to handle this burden. Thus, correctional psychiatrists may be expected to treat illness and to restore competency. This chapter reviewed these issues and made recommendations for the correctional psychiatrist managing such cases.

Additionally, correctional psychiatrists may face allegations and investigations in addition to the more usual cases alleging professional negligence or malpractice. This chapter discussed these causes of action and made recommendations for the handling of such cases. Correctional psychiatrists need to be aware of these issues and to understand how such cases are litigated. Even more important, practitioners need an awareness of the scope and limits of their malpractice insurance policy coverage.

References

42 USC §1983: Civil action for deprivation of rights. Available at http://www.gpo.gov/fdsys/pkg/USCODE-2009-title42/pdf/USCODE-2009-title42-chap21-subchapI-sec1983.pdf, accessed December 5, 2013.

American Correctional Association (2009). *Public correctional policy on correctional mental health care.* Available at https://www.aca.org/government/policyresolution/view.asp?ID=11, accessed December 9, 2013.

American Psychiatric Association (2000). *Psychiatric services in jails and prisons: A task force report of the American Psychiatric Association,* 2nd ed. Washington, DC: American Psychiatric Association.

Annotated Code of Maryland, Criminal Procedure Article, §3-101(g), 2013, available at http://www.lexisnexis.com/hottopics/mdcode/, accessed October 28, 2013.

Annotated Code of Maryland, Criminal Procedure Article, §3-106, 2013, available at http://www.lexisnexis.com/hottopics/mdcode/, accessed October 28, 2013.

Centers for Disease Control and Prevention (2013). *Suicide and self-inflicted injury,* available at http://www.cdc.gov/nchs/fastats/suicide.htm, accessed December 24, 2013.

CRIPA, 42 USC §1997, available at http://www.justice.gov/crt/about/spl/cripastat.php, accessed October 20, 2013.

Estelle v. Gamble, 429 U.S. 97, 1976.

Filarsky v. Delia, 566 U.S. ____, 2012, available at http://www.supremecourt.gov/opinions/11pdf/10-1018.pdf, accessed December 5, 2013.

GAINS Center (2007). *Quick fixes for effectively dealing with persons found incompetent to stand trial.* Available at http://gainscenter.samhsa.gov/pdfs/integrating/QuickFixes_11_07.pdf, accessed October 20, 2013.

Hogg Foundation (2013). *Issue brief: Restoration of competency to stand trial.* Available at http://www.hogg.utexas.edu/uploads/documents/Competency%20Restoration%20Brief.pdf, accessed June 26, 2013.

Jackson v. Indiana, 406 U.S. 715, 1972.

Jones v. United States, 463 U.S. 354, 1983.

Jennings, J. L., & Bell, J. D. (2012). The "ROC" model: Psychiatric evaluation, stabilization and restoration of competency in a jail setting. In L. Labate (ed.), *Mental illnesses—Evaluation, treatments and implications.* Available at http://www.intechopen.com/books/mental-illnesses-evaluation-treatments-and-implications/the-roc-modelpsychiatric-evaluation-stabilization-and-restoration-of-competency-in-a-jail-setting, accessed June 5, 2013.

Kapoor, R. (2011). Commentary: Jail-based competency restoration. *Journal of the American Academy of Psychiatry and the Law, 39,* 311–315.

Krelstein, M. S. (2002). The role of mental health in the inmate disciplinary process: A national survey. *Journal of the American Academy of Psychiatry and the Law, 30,* 488–496.

Metzner, J. L. (2002). Commentary: The role of mental health in the inmate disciplinary process. *Journal of the American Academy of Psychiatry and the Law, 30,* 497–499.

National Commission on Correctional Health Care (2008). *Standards for mental health services in correctional facilities.* Chicago: NCCHC.

National Judicial College (2012). *Mental competency: Best practices model.* Available at http://mentalcompetency.org/, accessed October 20, 2013.

National PREA Resource Center (2013). *Prison and jail standards.* Available at http://www.prearesourcecenter.org/training-technical-assistance/prea-101/prisons-and-jail-standards, accessed December 25, 2013.

New York CPL—Criminal Procedure, §730.70 (undated). *Fitness to proceed; procedure following termination of custody by commissioner,* available at http://public.leginfo.state.ny.us/LAWSSEAF.cgi?QUERYTYPE=LAWS+&QUERYDATA=$$CPL730.70$$@TXCPL0730.70+&LIST=SEA13+&BROWSER=EXPLORER+&TOKEN=01894228+&TARGET=VIEW, accessed December 24, 2013.

Noonan, M. E., & Ginder, S. (2013). *Mortality in local jails and state prisons, 2000–2011—statistical tables.* Bureau of Justice Statistics NCJ 242186, Available at http://www.bjs.gov/content/pub/pdf/mljsp0011.pdf, accessed December 24, 2013.

Professional Risk Management Services (PRMS). (Summer 2007). Correctional psychiatry: A unique patient population and professional liability risk. *Rx for Risk—The Psychiatry Edition,* 15(3).

Sell v. United States, 539 US 166, 2003.

U.S. Constitution, art. I, §9, Clause 2. Available at http://www.archives.gov/exhibits/charters/constitution_transcript.html, accessed October 20, 2013.

Washington v. Harper, 494 U.S. 210 (1990).

CHAPTER 62

Psychological testing

Ira K. Packer and Tasha R. Phillips

Introduction

Psychological testing can be a helpful adjunct to standard clinical assessments. Tests provide additional sources of data for use in comprehensive assessments; however, they are not a substitute for clinical evaluations. This chapter includes a discussion of the rationales and purposes for using psychological testing, special issues in administering and interpreting these tests in correctional settings, and caveats about their proper use. Three categories of psychological testing are discussed: tests of cognitive abilities, tests of personality and psychopathology, and tests of symptom validity and performance validity (e.g., measures of malingering or exaggeration of psychiatric symptoms or exaggeration of intellectual deficits). Following an overview of each of these categories, the most commonly used tests in correctional settings are briefly described, including their strengths and weaknesses. A brief case vignette is presented to illustrate how some tests help with assessment. The chapter concludes with recommendations for evaluating the utility of tests and a description of a standard protocol for referral for psychological testing.

We begin with a hypothetical case example that captures some of the issues typically encountered in correctional facilities. At the end of the chapter, we provide an illustration of how some of the tests discussed could help address the issues raised by this referral.

Case vignette: referral information

Mr. Smith, aged 51, was convicted of murder and sentenced to 30 years in a maximum-security state correctional facility. During the intake interview, he reported a longstanding history of major mental illness and alcohol abuse. He described his most prominent historical symptoms as paranoid ideation, auditory hallucinations, and affective lability. He had been prescribed antipsychotic and mood-stabilizing medications in the community, with variable response. Prior to his state incarceration, he was in the county jail for approximately eight months, during which he was prescribed a mood-stabilizing medication, a first-generation antipsychotic medication, and an atypical antipsychotic medication. When he arrived at the state facility, he appeared stable, other than enduring paranoid delusions. Within a few weeks, he began to display confusion, agitation, confabulation, and repetitive verbalizations. His attending psychiatrist referred him for psychological testing to determine the nature and extent of his symptoms and to rule out feigning or exaggeration of symptoms.

Rationales for using psychological tests

The advantages of using psychological tests in an assessment include standardization, increased objectivity, and comparison to established norms. When choosing to administer a test, it is important to consider whether the test has good psychometric properties and has been found appropriate for a correctional population. Psychometric qualities include reliability in scoring items and interpreting results (i.e., not varying significantly from one rater to another or from one administration to another given close in time), validity (accurately measuring what it purports to), and having well-established normative data (e.g., Weiner, 2012).

Psychological tests employ a standard set of questions or stimuli. This reduces the variability that can typify a clinical assessment. Tests also provide an objective source of information, as they include scoring rules that are applied consistently across administrations. Furthermore, psychometrically validated tests produce norms, which allow comparisons across individuals and time. For example, a test measuring psychopathology allows the psychologist to compare the inmate's profile to that of other individuals. If the test is read ministered, it allows comparison within the individual to determine whether significant change has occurred (e.g., improvement with treatment or decompensation).

Three main categories of psychological testing can be useful in correctional settings: cognitive, personality and psychopathology, and symptom or performance validity.

Cognitive testing

Cognitive testing includes measurement of intelligence and assessment of functioning that may indicate neuropsychological impairment. Correctional settings often need a test to briefly screen intellectual ability to identify inmates with significant disabilities that could interfere with functioning within the institution. Screening tests should have high sensitivity (i.e., few false negatives) to ensure that genuinely impaired individuals are not missed. For those who screen positive, more comprehensive testing will be indicated, as discussed later. When interpreting the results of these measures, it is crucial to consider both individual (e.g., educational history, racial/ethnic background, symptoms of mental illness, level of effort/motivation) and environmental factors (e.g., noise, peer influence) that may alter performance.

Thorough measures of neuropsychological functioning require specialized training and expertise to interpret the results. The information gathered from such test batteries may reveal impairment in a range of functions, including memory, speech, executive functioning (including ability to plan and ability to inhibit responses), and visuospatial functioning. Clinical neuropsychology is a specialty area within psychology, and only those with this specialized training are qualified to interpret neuropsychological batteries and make appropriate recommendations. Most correctional settings do not have clinical neuropsychologists on site. Thus, a correctional psychologist can screen for neurocognitive impairment using some of the tests described later. However, if significant impairment is suggested, further consultation in the form of neuropsychologist testing and/or neurological examination may be needed to maintain best standard of practice.

Because there are many cognitive measures with varying purpose, comprehensiveness, and utility, a full review is beyond the scope of this chapter. Rather, several measures frequently used in correctional settings are highlighted. For each instrument, a brief description, a discussion of practical strengths and weaknesses, and key references for additional review of the instruments are included.

Screening measures

Wechsler Abbreviated Scale of Intelligence, 2nd ed. (WASI-II; Wechsler, 2011): Brief screening measure of general intellectual functioning through measures of verbal comprehension and perceptual reasoning. The WASI-II can be flexibly administered using all four subtests or only two subtests. It is strongly linked to the WAIS-IV. Because it requires individual administration, it is not optimally suitable for large-scale screenings of inmates. However, this may be offset by the brief administration time.

Kaufman Brief Intelligence Scale, 2nd ed. (KBIT-2; Kaufman & Kaufman, 2004): Similar to the WASI-II in administration and practical utility (McCrimmon & Smith, 2013).

Shipley-2 (Shipley, 2010): Brief screening measure of knowledge derived from prior learning and experiences (crystallized intelligence) and abstract reasoning abilities independent of learning (fluid intelligence). The Shipley-2 is sometimes preferred over the WASI-II and the KBIT-2 because it can be administered in a group format. However, very little research has been done on the utility of this measure. It cannot be used with non-English–speaking examinees (Kaya, Delen, & Bulut, 2012).

Beta-III (Kellogg & Morton, 1999): Brief screening measure of nonverbal intelligence. The Beta-III can be used with individuals who don't speak English, who are illiterate, or who have limited reading comprehension, and it can be administered in a group format. Although developed and normed on prison populations, very little subsequent research has been done to validate its use.

General Ability Measure for Adults (GAMA; Naglieri & Bardos, 1997): Similar to the Beta-III in administration and practical utility (Megargee, 2012).

Repeatable Battery for Neuropsychological Status Update (RBANS; Randolph, 2012): Screening measure of cognitive status across five broad domains of neuropsychological functioning: language, attention, visuospatial/constructional, and immediate and delayed memory. The RBANS has been well validated as a screening tool for cognitive status of examinees with dementia, schizophrenia, and acute and postacute traumatic brain injury. A few authors have cautioned that this measure is not good at detecting milder cognitive impairments. Thus, if an examinee does not show impairment on this measure but has behavioral indications of cognitive deficits, alternative neuropsychological testing or neurological consultation is recommended (Duff, Hobson, Beglinger, & O'Bryant, 2010; McKay, Casey, Wertheimer, & Fichtenberg, 2007).

Comprehensive measures

Wechsler Adult Intelligence Scale, 4th ed. (WAIS-IV; Wechsler, 2008): Comprehensive measure of general intellectual functioning in four domains: verbal comprehension, perceptual reasoning, working memory, and processing speed. The WAIS-IV is the latest iteration of the most comprehensive and widely used measure of general intellectual functioning in correctional, forensic, and community samples. The WAIS-IV is empirically linked to learning, academic achievement, and cognitive development. However, because of its comprehensiveness, it can take 60 to 90 minutes to administer (Benson, Hulac, & Kranzler, 2010).

Wechsler Memory Scale, 4th ed. (WMS-IV; Wechsler, 2009): Comprehensive measure of auditory, visual, and working memory. The WMS-IV is the most recent iteration of the most extensively validated measure of memory impairment. In addition to its widespread utility in assessing memory impairments, the nonverbal subtests can be adapted cross-culturally to assess impairment in stroke patients. Because of its comprehensiveness, it can take 45 to 60 minutes to administer (Hoelzle, Nelson, & Smith, 2011).

Personality and psychopathology testing

Measures of psychopathology and personality are the most commonly used tests in correctional settings (e.g., Boothby & Clements, 2000). These self-report inventories can take more than 1 hour to complete and thus are not typically administered upon the inmate's admission to the facility. Rather, they are used after an initial mental health screening finds a need for additional data to clarify the clinical formulation and diagnosis. The most commonly used tests for this purpose are the Minnesota Multiphasic Personality Inventories (MMPI-2 and the MMPI-2-RF, the Millon Multiaxial Clinical Inventory–III (MCMI-III), and the Personality Assessment Inventory (PAI). These tests do not provide definitive diagnoses. Instead, their results help generate hypotheses about diagnosis and symptom presentation that can be ruled in or out by further clinical inquiry, observation, and other collateral courses. They also can serve as a source of convergent validity with clinical diagnoses. In other words, confidence in the diagnostic assessment will increase when the clinically derived diagnosis and the profile on the objectively scored test agree. These tests also include validity scales to assess overreporting and underreporting of problems as well as consistency of responses. One advantage of self-report measures in correctional facilities is that they can be administered in a group setting, with careful monitoring by qualified staff.

These tests are typically scored by a computer program, which produces a profile. In addition, testing companies offer interpretive reports, including ones specific to correctional settings. We urge caution in using such interpretive reports without review by a qualified psychologist, however. For example, the MMPI scoring reports identify "critical items" (i.e., answers that suggest psychopathology or areas of significant concern). A review of these items with the inmate can sometimes result in reinterpretation. For example, items that would suggest paranoia about being watched in the community might reflect reality-based fears about monitoring by camera in a prison cell.

In addition to these self-report inventories, projective techniques assess psychopathology and personality styles more indirectly. The best known of these is the Rorschach inkblot test. Considerable controversy exists in the psychology community about this test; some have criticized it, claiming that many of its measures have not been sufficiently validated (Wood, Lilienfeld, Garb, & Nezworski, 2000), while others dispute these contentions (e.g., Meyer & Archer, 2001). Given this controversy, there is no consensus about the utility of this instrument. However, even its detractors acknowledge that the measure of thought disorder has good empirical support (Wood et al., 2000). Thus, the Rorschach test may be useful to assess individuals who are guarded in a self-report format or who are in the early stages of a psychotic disorder (e.g., first-break schizophrenia). Other projective techniques, such as the Draw-a-Person Test or the House–Tree–Person Test are not widely accepted, as questions have been raised about the reliability and validity of interpretation (e.g., Garb, Wood, Lilienfeld, & Nezworski, 2002).

Within this domain of psychological testing, there are broadband and narrowband measures. Broadband measures assess a wide range of symptoms of psychopathology, whereas narrowband measures assess a particular construct or cluster of symptoms. A few commonly used instruments in each subdomain are highlighted here.

Broadband measures

Minnesota Multiphasic Personality Inventory-2 (MMPI-2): 567-item true–false self-report inventory that assesses personality traits, psychopathology, and response style. In 2006, Boothby and Clements reported that the MMPI-2 is the most widely used inventory of personality and psychopathology in correctional settings. It has been extensively validated in correctional populations. However, one limitation is considerable item overlap, with use of the same item on multiple scales (e.g., Graham, 2011).

Minnesota Multiphasic Personality Inventory-2-Restructured Form (MMPI-2-RF): Revised 338-item version of the MMPI-2 designed to parsimoniously assess personality traits, psychopathology, and response style. The MMPI-2-RF is the product of a multiphase restructuring project that began more than a decade ago to improve the convergent and discriminant validity of the instrument. One significant advantage of the MMPI-2-RF compared to the MMPI-2 is that there is no overlap of scales (i.e., each item on the test is associated with only one clinical scale). However, this measure has not been as extensively researched as its predecessor, including in correctional settings (Ben-Porath, 2012).

Personality Assessment Inventory (PAI): 344-item self-report inventory to assess personality traits, psychopathology, and response style. Several studies have demonstrated the widespread utility of this measure across correctional settings. In addition to tapping constructs of psychopathology, the PAI assesses normative personality traits. However, the four-point Likert response format can be particularly challenging for examinees with limited comprehension abilities (e.g., Magyar, Edens, Lilienfeld, Douglas, Poythress, & Skeem, 2012).

Millon Clinical Multiaxial Inventory, 3rd ed. (MCMI-III): 175-item self-report inventory to assess *Diagnostic and Statistical Manual of Mental Disorders*–IV categories of personality disorders and general psychopathology. The MCMI-III focuses on personality disorders, which are prevalent in correctional settings. However, it is susceptible to overpathologizing (Rogers, Salekin, & Sewell, 2000).

Narrowband measures

Beck Depression Inventory-II (BDI-II; Beck et al., 1996): 21-item self-report instrument of current symptoms of depression. It is the most commonly used narrowband measure of depression. The BDI-II is easy to administer and has been widely used in suicide prevention research. The two-factor structure distinguishes between somatic–affective and cognitive symptoms of depression. However, the BDI-II has not been extensively validated across racial/ethnic groups.

Beck Anxiety Inventory (BAI; Beck, 1993): Similarly constructed measure of current symptoms of anxiety (Joe, Woolley, Brown, Ghahramanlou-Holloway, & Beck, 2008).

Validity testing

The third category of psychological testing relates to measures of symptom and performance validity. Symptom validity refers to the accuracy of self-reported symptoms, whereas performance validity refers to test performance (Larrabee, 2011). Symptom validity tests or embedded indicators (e.g., validity scales of the MMPI-2, MMPI-2-RF, or PAI) often rely on self-report and structured interviews to gather data about the accuracy of an examinee's reported symptoms. The obtained score is compared to profiles of individuals known to have a genuine disorder or known to be exaggerating (including groups instructed to "fake bad" when taking the test).

Performance validity tests often rely on a forced-choice testing methodology, which was introduced by Pankratz, Fautsi, and Peed in 1975. This type of testing involves a series of trials in which examinees select between two alternatives: the correct response (or target) and the incorrect response (or foil). Scores that are significantly below chance provide definitive evidence of intentionally incorrect answers (i.e., even a completely impaired examinee should obtain a 50% score by random guessing). However, because few malingerers score below chance, performance validity instruments also provide cutoff scores that are above chance but below scores obtained by individuals with genuine impairments.

For a full review on the assessment of malingering in correctional settings, see Chapter 23. However, a few frequently used symptom and performance validity instruments appropriate for correctional settings are highlighted here.

Symptom validity tests

Miller Forensic Assessment of Symptoms Test (MFAST; Miller, 2001): Brief (25-question) structured interview designed to provide an estimate of the probability of malingered psychiatric illness.

Research has demonstrated that the MFAST has good clinical utility across racial/ethnic groups and literacy levels. The interview format eliminates problems with reading comprehension but is more time-consuming (Jackson, Rogers, & Sewell, 2005).

Structured Inventory of Malingered Symptomatology (SIMS; Windows & Smith, 2005): 75-item screening instrument to assess feigned psychopathology and neuropsychological impairment. The SIMS has high sensitivity, which is a desirable characteristic for screening measures. However, some research suggests that it has a high false-positive rate—that is, it misclassifies examinees with genuine psychiatric illness as malingerers (Edens, Poythress, & Watkins-Clay, 2007).

Structured Inventory of Reported Symptoms, 2nd ed. (SIRS-2; Rogers et al., 2010): Structured interview for assessing deliberate response distortion of self-report symptoms of psychopathology. The SIRS-2 is considered the most comprehensive instrument for assessment of malingering of psychiatric symptoms. Because it typically takes 30 to 40 minutes per administration, its use is recommended only after an inmate has scored above the threshold for malingering on one of the briefer screening tests described previously. In addition, it can often result in indeterminate findings, thus limiting its sensitivity (Green, Rosenfeld, Belfi, & Rohlehr, 2013).

Performance validity tests

Test of Memory Malingering (TOMM; Tombaugh, 1996): Visual recognition test for distinguishing between malingered and *bona fide* memory impairments. The TOMM is easy to administer and has been adequately validated in criminal forensic samples. However, its established cutoff scores may result in false positives for individuals with dementia and intellectual disability (e.g., Gervais, Rohling, Green, & Ford, 2004; Ray, 2012).

Validity Indicator Profile (VIP; Frederick, 1997): Assesses motivation and effort during cognitive testing and comprises verbal and nonverbal subtests, which can be used independently or as companion measures. The nonverbal subtest can be easily administered to non-English–speaking populations. The VIP is not considered appropriate for examinees with known diagnoses of intellectual disability (Frederick, 2002).

Case vignette: psychological testing

Based on the referral information from the attending psychiatrist described previously, the psychologist selected two tests to administer during the initial assessment: the MMPI-2-RF and the RBANS. The MMPI-2-RF was selected to parsimoniously assess a wide range of clinical symptoms, personality characteristics, behavioral tendencies, and interpersonal functioning that can inform diagnosis and treatment recommendations. In addition, the MMPI-2-RF can provide information about Mr. Smith's response style. The RBANS was selected to broadly screen for potential neurocognitive impairment and to determine the need for further neuropsychological testing. The following is an example of potential findings from the psychologist's report:

Based on his responses to the validity scales (assessing overreporting and underreporting of symptoms and consistency of responses), Mr. Smith answered MMPI-2-RF items in a seemingly honest and forthright manner. Thus, his scores on the substantive scales likely present an accurate portrayal of his psychological functioning. Mr. Smith's responses indicate serious thought dysfunction. He reports prominent persecutory ideation and is likely to feel alienated, suspicious of others, and to have delusional thinking. He also reports unusual perceptions such as auditory hallucinations.

In addition, Mr. Smith has cognitive difficulties, including memory problems, poor concentration, and confusion. His cognitive complaints may be associated with his thought disturbance. He is likely to have low frustration tolerance and difficulty coping with stress. Finally, Mr. Smith reports a pattern of externalizing behavior, including antisocial conduct and substance abuse. He likely has a history of violent behavior and poor impulse control as well.

Mr. Smith scored 64 on the RBANS. Compared to other individuals his age, his score is in the severely impaired range of neuropsychological functioning. His most prominent deficits are in immediate and delayed memory as indexed by auditory and visual recall and auditory recognition tasks. Mr. Smith also has impairment in oral language and auditory and visual attention. He showed no deficits in visuospatial/constructional functioning.

Mr. Smith's test results indicate several concerns and possible diagnoses for follow-up evaluation. Specifically, he has symptoms consistent with a thought disorder, most likely schizophrenia. In addition, Mr. Smith has neurocognitive difficulties. Although his symptoms of psychosis could partially account for these deficits, further specialized neuropsychological testing is recommended to explore other etiologies. Such considerations include side effects of his psychotropic medication, Korsakoff syndrome, and early-onset dementia.

Assessing the utility of new tests for correctional settings

Although this chapter focuses on description and assessment of the most commonly used psychological tests in correctional settings, the field is constantly evolving and new tests are likely to become available. The following guidelines can help determine the usefulness of newly developed tests:

◆ Does the test have high reliability?

◆ Has the test been validated on the relevant demographic population (factors include gender, race, ethnicity, language, and age)? Particular care should be taken when choosing tests for non-English speakers, as tests cannot simply be translated into another language but require rigorous procedures to ensure preservation of the psychometric properties.

◆ Is the test valid for a correctional population? Megargee (2012) noted that the research on psychological tests in correctional setting lags behind the more extensive work in community settings. As new tests are developed and considered for correctional settings, it will be important to verify that they have demonstrated validity for that population.

Summary

This chapter reviewed the general categories of psychological testing that are appropriate for correctional settings and discussed the most widely used instruments. Well-validated psychological tests can be an important adjunct to a comprehensive mental health assessment and can help to identify psychiatric symptoms and cognitive deficits that may impair functioning in correctional institutions. In addition, testing can assist in determining the validity of symptoms reported by inmates.

Given the range of tests, with varying suitability to a correctional population, a qualified doctoral-level psychologist should make the decision about which tests to administer (International Association of Correctional and Forensic Psychology, 2010). The referral should identify the issues and questions to address, instead of requesting specific tests, to allow the psychologist to choose the best instruments. Although technicians may administer many tests, only a qualified psychologist can interpret the results. The psychologist should produce a report that explains the results, their applicability to the referral issues, and any caveats about their validity. The results can then be integrated into the diagnostic assessment and treatment plan for the inmate.

References

Ben-Porath, Y. S. (2012). *Interpreting the MMPI-2-RF.* Minneapolis: University of Minnesota Press.

Benson, N., Hulac, D., & Kranzler, J. (2010). Independent examination of the Wechsler Adult Intelligence Scale—Fourth Edition (WAIS-IV): What does the WAIS-IV measure? *Psychological Assessment, 22*(1), 121–130.

Boothby, J. L., & Clements, C. B. (2006). A national survey of correctional psychologists. In C. R. Bartol & A. M. Bartol (Eds.), *Current perspectives in forensic psychology and criminal justice* (pp. 215–222). Thousand Oaks, CA: Sage Publications.

Duff, K., Hobson, V., Beglinger, L., & O'Bryant, S. (2010). Diagnostic accuracy of the RBANS in mild cognitive impairment: limitations on assessing milder impairments. *Archives of Clinical Neuropsychology, 25*(5), 429–441.

Edens, J., Poythress, N., & Watkins-Clay, M. (2007). Detection of malingering in psychiatric unit and general population prison inmates: a comparison of the PAI, SIMS, and SIRS. *Journal of Personality Assessment, 88*(1), 33–42.

Frederick, R. (2002). Review of the Validity Indicator Profile. *Journal of Forensic Neuropsychology, 2*, 125–145.

Garb, H., Wood, J., Lilienfeld, S., & Nezworski, M. (2002). Effective use of projective techniques in clinical practice: Let the data help with selection and interpretation. *Professional Psychology: Research and Practice, 33*(5), 454–463.

Gervais, R., Rohling, M. L., Green, P., & Ford, W. (2004). A comparison of WMT, CARB, and TOMM failure rates in non-head-injury disability claimants. *Archives of Clinical Neuropsychology, 19*, 475–487.

Graham, J. R. (2011). *MMPI-2: Assessing personality and psychopathology* (5th ed.). New York: Oxford University Press.

Green, D., Rosenfeld, B., Belfi, B., & Rohlehr, L. (2013). *New and improved: A comparison of the SIRS and SIRS-2.* Paper presented at the annual meeting of the American Psychology–Law Society.

Hoelzle, J., Nelson, N., & Smith, C. (2011). Comparison of Wechsler Memory Scale-Fourth Edition (WMS-IV) and Third Edition (WMS-III) dimensional structures: Improved ability to evaluate auditory and visual constructs. *Journal of Clinical and Experimental Neuropsychology, 33*(3), 283–291.

International Association of Correctional and Forensic Psychology (2010). Standards for psychology services in jails, prisons, correctional facilities, and agencies, third edition. *Criminal Justice and Behavior, 37*, 749–808.

Jackson, R., Rogers, R., & Sewell, K. (2005). Forensic applications of the Miller Forensic Assessment of Symptoms Test (MFAST): screening for feigned disorders in competency to stand trial evaluations. *Law and Human Behavior, 29*(2), 199–210.

Joe, S., Woolley, M., Brown, G., Ghahramanlou-Holloway, M., & Beck, A. (2008). Psychometric properties of the Beck Depression Inventory-II in low-income, African American suicide attempters. *Journal of Personality Assessment, 90*(5), 521–523.

Kaya, F., Delen, E., & Bulut, O. (2012). Test review: Shipley-2 manual. *Journal of Psychoeducational Assessment, 30*(6), 593–597.

Larrabee, G. J. (2011). *Forensic neuropsychology: A scientific approach.* New York: Oxford University Press.

Magyar, M., Edens, J., Lilienfeld, S., Douglas, K., Poythress, N., & Skeem, J. (2012). Using the Personality Assessment Inventory to predict male offenders' conduct during and progression through substance abuse treatment. *Psychological Assessment, 24*(1), 216–225.

McCrimmon, A. W., & Smith, A. D. (2013). Review of Wechsler Abbreviated Scale of Intelligence, Second Edition (WASI-II). *Journal of Psychoeducational Assessment, 31*(3), 337–341.

McKay, C., Casey, J., Wertheimer, J., Fichtenberg, N. (2007). Reliability and validity of the RBANS in a traumatic brain injured sample. *Archives of Clinical Neuropsychology, 22*(1), 91–98.

Megargee, E. I. (2012). Psychological assessment in correctional settings. In I. B. Weiner, J. R. Graham & J. A. Naglieri (Eds.), *Handbook of psychology: Volume 10, Assessment Psychology* (pp. 394–424). New York: Wiley and Sons.

Meyer, G. J., & Archer, R. P. (2001). The hard science of Rorschach research: What do we know and where do we go? *Psychological Assessment, 13*(4), 486–502.

Pankratz, L., Fautsi, A., & Peed, S. (1975). A forced-choice technique to evaluate deafness in the hysterical or malingering patient. *Journal of Consulting and Clinical Psychology, 43*, 421–422.

Ray, C. (2012). Assessment of feigned cognitive impairment: A cautious approach to the use of the Test of Memory Malingering for individuals with intellectual disability. *Open Access Journal of Forensic Psychology, 4*, 24–50.

Rogers, R., Salekin, R., & Sewell, K. (2000). The MCMI-III and the Daubert standard: separating rhetoric from reality. *Law and Human Behavior, 24*(4), 501–506.

Wood, J. M., Lilienfeld, S. O., Garb, H. N., & Nezworski, M. T. (2000). The Rorschach test in clinical diagnosis: A critical review, with a backward look at Garfield (1947). *Journal of Clinical Psychology, 56*, 395–430.

CHAPTER 63

Standards and accreditation for jails, prisons, and juvenile facilities

Joseph V. Penn

Introduction

The history of medical and mental health care in America's prisons and jails is replete with examples of gross neglect and indifference. Until the early 1970s, the availability and quality of correctional health care were left to the discretion of correctional officials, with both the courts and society assuming a hands-off policy (Anno, 2001). The result was woefully inadequate health care. This chapter details the background, evolution, and current status of standards and accreditation for correctional facilities in the US.

Background

A survey of local jails conducted by the American Medical Association (AMA) in 1972 (Steinwald, Alevizos, & Aherne, 1973) revealed that first aid was the only medical care available in two thirds of the jails; not even this service was available in about 17% of the jails. Only 7% of the jails had an infirmary. On-site access to physicians, nurses, and other medical personnel was extremely limited. Although most state prisons had some medical facilities, they were typically poorly equipped and staffed primarily by unlicensed physicians and medical assistants (Anno, 2001; US General Accounting Office [GAO], 1978). In some cases, inmates with no formal medical training dispensed medications, extracted teeth, and even performed minor surgery (McDonald, 1999).

Mental health services in correctional institutions fared no better. With passage of the Mental Retardation Facilities and Community Mental Health Centers Construction Act of 1963, state mental hospitals began releasing thousands of patients with chronic and severe psychiatric disorders into communities that often lacked the resources to provide adequate and accessible alternatives to hospitalization (Lamb & Bachrach, 2001; US GAO, 2000). Unable to access mental health services, large numbers of formerly institutionalized persons with serious mental illness were left homeless, impoverished, and highly symptomatic—a combination of factors that put them at high risk for arrest and criminal prosecution (Lamb & Bachrach, 2001; Stelovich, 1979; Whitmer, 1980). As a result of deinstitutionalization and new restrictions on civil commitment, the nation's prisons and jails became the de facto psychiatric hospitals (Torrey, Kennard, Eslinger, Lamb, & Pavle, 2010). Studies of prison populations in the United States have consistently found elevated rates of serious mental illness relative to the general population (Baillargeon, Hoge, & Penn, 2010). Based on a systematic review of psychiatric surveys, Fazel and Danesh (2002) estimated that the rates of psychotic disorders and major depression among US prisoners are two- to four-fold higher than among the general population. Very few correctional institutions had the resources to provide adequate care for this large influx of inmates with debilitating mental disorders.

Over the past four decades, remarkable improvements in correctional health care have occurred thanks, in large part, to the role of several health care organizations along with the judicial actions of the federal courts. Out of increasing concern about deficiencies in health care for the imprisoned, several organizations, including the AMA and the American Public Health Association (APHA), became involved in developing standards and accreditation programs for health care delivery in prisons and jails in the 1970s (Anno, 2001). Regrettably, these early attempts at health care reform lacked enforcement power, and many correctional administrators elected to reject them. Fortunately, at roughly the same time, the federal courts began a reversal of a long-held "hands-off" doctrine regarding the rights of inmates to medical care. In a seminal case heard in 1972, a US district court found the state prison system of Alabama to be in violation of the Eighth and Fourteenth Amendments in failing to provide its inmates with adequate medical and mental care (*Newman v. Alabama*, 1972). The correctional system was placed under injunction and ordered to immediately rectify all deficiencies. Although the Alabama case was closely followed by lower-court cases that upheld specific health care rights of inmates, these decisions were largely binding only on the litigants who were specifically involved. All of this changed with the landmark case of *Estelle v. Gamble* (1976), in which the US Supreme Court affirmed that deliberate indifference to the serious medical needs of prisoners was a violation of the Eighth Amendment and ruled that the federal courts could intervene to ensure sufficient medical care (Rold, 2008). By 1995, 139 state correctional facilities were under court order or consent decree because of inadequate medical care (Stephan, 1997).

There is no question that litigation has provided much of the impetus for improved medical and mental health services in jails and prisons. In several of the class action lawsuits that involved allegations of deficient health care that have gone to trial, state governments have expended considerable resources in resisting health care reforms at enormous cost to taxpayers. As an example, the civil case against the Texas Department of Corrections (*Ruiz v. Estelle*, 1980), originally filed in 1972, dragged on for decades and cost the state millions of dollars in attorney fees and payments for the services of the court-appointed master and monitors. Faced with the prospect of such costly litigation, correctional officials have increasingly opted for compliance with national health standards and achieving accreditation (Anno, 2001; Rold, 2008).

Correctional health care standards

According to the International Organization for Standardization (n.d.), a standard is a document that provides requirements, specifications, guidelines, or characteristics that can be used consistently to ensure that materials, products, processes, and services are fit for their purpose. In correctional health care, standards serve that same purpose but also "provide a national process to keep the evolution of correctional health care practices following community-based standards" (Wallenstein, 2004, p. 3). Although standards are often established to support accreditation programs, correctional facilities need not pursue accreditation to benefit from following nationally accepted standards. Standards are offered by several organizations, including the American Correctional Association (ACA), the National Commission on Correctional Health Care (NCCHC), the Joint Commission, APHA, and regional organizations such as the Medical Association of Georgia (MAG).

The AMA jail project evolved into NCCHC, which issues separate standards manuals for jails, prisons, and juvenile confinement facilities. Updated periodically to remain responsive to contemporary concerns and practices, the NCCHC standards take a holistic approach to health care, integrating mental health services. However, since 2008, NCCHC has published standards specifically for mental health services (NCCHC, 2008). These parallel those for jail and prison health services in format and substance. However, they make more explicit what the standards require for adequate delivery of mental health services in nine areas: governance and administration, safety, personnel and training, health care services and support, inmate care and treatment, health promotion, special mental health needs and services, clinical records, and medicolegal issues.

Examples of NCCHC mental health standards under the governance and administration section are Access to Care, Responsible Mental Health Authority, Clinical Autonomy, Administrative Meetings and Reports, Policies and Procedures, Continuous Quality Improvement Program, Emergency Response Plan, Communication on Patients' Mental Health Needs, Privacy of Care, Procedure in the Event of an Inmate Death, and Grievance Mechanism for Mental Health Complaints. To illustrate the nature of these standards, the second standard, Responsible Mental Health Authority, specifies that the facility have a designated mental health authority responsible for mental health services. This standard is supported by five compliance indicators that outline the mental health authority's scope of responsibility, minimum qualifications, and other requirements. Terms are defined, and a discussion elaborates the standard's intent.

The ACA accreditation standards address all aspects of facility operations, including health care. Specifically, they encompass services, programs, and operations essential to good correctional management. These include administrative, staff and fiscal controls, staff training and development, physical plant, safety and emergency procedures, sanitation, food service, rules and discipline, and other subjects that represent good correctional practice.

Accreditation

Accreditation, as defined by the NCCHC, is a process of external peer review in which the NCCHC, a private, nongovernmental association, grants public recognition to detention and correctional institutions that meet nationally established and accepted standards for the provision of health services. The accreditation program renders a professional judgment on the quality of health services provided and assists correctional facilities in their continued improvement (NCCHC, n.d.). Among the benefits of accreditation cited by the ACA are improved staff training and development, assessment of program strengths and weaknesses, defense against lawsuits, establishment of measurable criteria for upgrading operations, improved staff morale and professionalism, a safer environment for staff and offenders, reduced liability insurance costs, and performance-based benefits (ACA, n.d., a).

There are several types of accreditation available to county, state, and federal correctional facilities and systems, regardless of the size, scope, custody level, and function of a specific facility or system. These include accreditation by the ACA, NCCHC, Joint Commission, a combination of the above, and state agencies. Accreditation is largely a voluntary process, but there appears to be a national trend toward accreditation due to several factors. One common factor leading to "voluntary" accreditation, illustrated previously and described in Chapters 3 and 66, is litigation and oversight by judges, special masters, or receivers, where a correctional facility or system may achieve removal from such oversight only by receiving national accreditation. Another recent trend is the contracting, outsourcing, or "privatization" of correctional health care services to universities, local health centers/systems, or for-profit vendors. Achieving and maintaining accreditation are often contractual obligations or expectations.

Similar to achieving and maintaining Joint Commission accreditation for hospitals and other "free world" health care centers, it is important for custody and correctional health care leadership, other involved public policy makers, budget staff, and correctional/forensic psychiatric consultants to be aware that achieving "voluntary" initial accreditation and maintaining accreditation, regardless of the type, take a great deal of planning, preparation, staff time, and resources. Similarly, achieving and maintaining correctional accreditation have significant fiscal, staffing, risk management, and budgetary implications.

Accreditation types differ depending on the facility's health care mission and its patient population. For example, some correctional systems and leaders may seek to obtain accreditation solely from either the ACA or NCCHC. Some may seek to have their infirmary, acute or tertiary medical units, dialysis centers, or psychiatric facility/unit receive Joint Commission accreditation. Some systems may seek for their psychiatric/mental health facilities to be NCCHC accredited without seeking NCCHC accreditation for their medical units. Some facilities/systems seek dual accreditation or have all three (ACA, NCCHC, and Joint Commission). The following descriptions of the primary accrediting bodies are summaries of information provided by the organizations.

National commission on correctional health care

The NCCHC originated as the AMA jail project and was incorporated as an independent nonprofit organization in 1983. Its mission is to improve the quality of health care provided in jails, prisons, and juvenile confinement facilities. Today it is the only national organization dedicated solely to improving correctional health care through standards, accreditation, certification, education, and technical assistance. The NCCHC board of directors comprises liaisons from 37 national organizations, including the American Academy of Child and Adolescent Psychiatry (AACAP), the American Academy of Psychiatry and the Law (AAPL), the American Psychiatric Association (APA), and other organizations from the fields of medicine, public health, law, and corrections, as well as state and county associations.

NCCHC's evidence-based standards represent the organization's requirements for health services (e.g., nursing, medical, dental, and mental health and psychiatric) in state and federal prisons, jails, short-term detention, juvenile detention and other confinement settings, and US Immigration and Customs Enforcement facilities. They are intended for use in evaluating the health services in correctional facilities, including those that are part of larger systems.

Mental health care has been integral to the NCCHC standards and accreditation program from the start. When the first NCCHC standards were developed in the 1970s—with the input of mental health professionals—it was decided to integrate medical and mental health standards to encourage a unified and holistic approach to inmate care. However, as the number of incarcerated persons with mental illness soared, some systems opted to manage mental health services separately from medical services. NCCHC's mental health standards and accreditation program were designed for correctional facilities in which the legal authority for mental health services is separate from their other health services and both parties are not already accredited under the standards for jails or prisons. This option enables a mental health services program to seek accreditation even if the health services counterpart does not.

More narrowly, NCCHC also offers accreditation for opioid treatment programs (OTPs) in correctional facilities. Opioid treatment is fairly rare in correctional facilities due, in part, to regulatory obstacles and institutional resistance. However, this is a lost opportunity to help addicted inmates, especially those who participate in community-based OTPs but must discontinue this treatment when they become incarcerated. To assist facilities that wish to provide such treatment, NCCHC established an accreditation program in 2004 that enables corrections-based OTPs to obtain legally required certification from the Substance Abuse and Mental Health Services Administration (SAMHSA) of the US Department of Health and Human Services. NCCHC, the only SAMHSA-authorized accrediting body that focuses on corrections, has developed standards that are based on federal regulations but tailored for this field.

Accreditation process

Approximately 500 correctional facilities participate in NCCHC's accreditation program. These facilities are diverse in terms of jurisdiction, management structure, size, and inmate population, ranging from a juvenile facility with an average daily population of 10 to a large metropolitan jail complex housing 9,000 inmates. The average size of an accredited prison is more than 1,300 inmates. NCCHC is not a membership organization, and there are no requirements to becoming accredited other than meeting the standards and adhering to NCCHC accreditation policies.

A correctional facility seeking accreditation first reviews the standards manual relevant to the setting to assess current compliance with the standards. The next step is to complete an application, followed by a self-survey questionnaire. NCCHC staff review the information on the questionnaire and work closely with the facility to help it prepare for an on-site survey. Once the facility feels ready, a survey is scheduled. The survey duration depends on the facility's size and the complexity of health services provided, but it usually lasts two or three days.

Survey teams consist of qualified, trained physicians, nurses, health administrators, and other credentialed health professionals certified in correctional health care who understand corrections and combine that knowledge with their professional expertise. They conduct a review of health records, policies, and procedures; interview health staff, correctional officers, and inmates; and tour the facility to gather information. Surveyors use the same compliance indicators listed in each NCCHC standard to measure compliance. At the end of the survey, an exit conference is conducted to discuss their preliminary findings. These reviews are collegial and educational, with the survey team offering suggestions for improvement.

An NCCHC accreditation committee then reviews the survey team's report to evaluate compliance with the standards and make an accreditation decision. The facility receives a comprehensive written report that includes recommendations to assist with standards compliance. Once accredited, the facility submits an annual report with updates on key information. Subsequent on-site visits occur about every three years.

American correctional association

Originally founded as the National Prison Association in 1870, the ACA is the oldest and largest international correctional membership association in the world. The private, nonprofit organization changed its name in 1950 to more accurately reflect its philosophy on corrections. The ACA's mission is to provide "a professional organization for all individuals and groups, both public and private that share a common goal of improving the justice system" (ACA, n.d., b). Approximately 80% of all state departments of corrections and youth services are active ACA members. Also included are programs and facilities operated by the Federal Bureau of Prisons, the US Parole Commission, the District of Columbia, and the private sector.

The ACA's Standards and Accreditation Department serves a dual mission of providing services for ACA and the Commission on Accreditation for Corrections (CAC). These services include the development and promulgation of new standards, revision of existing standards, coordination of the accreditation process for all correctional components of the criminal justice system, semi-annual accreditation hearings, technical assistance, and training for consultants involved in the accreditation process. The ACA publishes many standards manuals, primarily administration and standards manuals for the safe, effective, and professional operation of correctional agencies, including local detention facilities and county jails, state and federal prisons, juvenile facilities and/or training schools, private halfway houses or group homes, and probation and parole agencies.

Since 1989, the ACA has developed health care standards for corrections. Beginning in 1999, it began providing what it described as state-of-the-art performance-based standards, an initiative that focuses accreditation on outcome measures that are critical to the consequences of programs. Prior ACA efforts measured only the presence or absence of an operation, condition, or situation. In 2001, ACA began evaluating compliance of health care against these benchmarks. The standards manuals most relevant to correctional health and mental health staff are the *Performance-Based Standards for Correctional Health Care for Adult Correctional Institutions* (ACA, 2002) and the *Standards for Adult Correctional Institutions*, Part 4: Institutional Services, Section E: Health Care (ACA, 2003). The stated goal is to "provide appropriate and necessary health services and care for offenders." One notable goal of the performance-based health care expected practices is for correctional systems to gain experience in collecting data and providing outcome measures. These standards are under continual revision to reflect changing practice, current case law, new knowledge, and agency experience. These changes are published by ACA in the Standards Supplement.

Accreditation process

The ACA and the CAC administer the only national performance-based accreditation program for all components of the correctional/criminal justice system, including adult correctional institutions (prisons), adult local detention facilities (jails), adult community residential services facilities, adult probation and parole field services, juvenile facilities, and correctional training academies. The accreditation program and process offers the opportunity for correctional agencies to evaluate their operations and processes against national standards, remedy deficiencies, and improve the quality of correctional programs and services. ACA accreditation is available to all adult and juvenile agencies for which standards have been published. The requirements of the accreditation process are the same for all types of agencies: state, county, federal, and private. Correctional administrators initiate accreditation activities voluntarily. When an agency chooses to pursue accreditation, ACA staff provide the agency with information and application materials, including a contract, the applicable standards manual, a policy and procedure manual, and an organization summary.

All programs or facilities seeking ACA accreditation sign a contract, pay an accreditation fee, conduct a self-evaluation, and have a standards compliance audit conducted by trained ACA consultants prior to an accreditation decision by the CAC. Once accredited, all programs and facilities submit an annual certification statement to ACA. Also, at ACA's expense and discretion, a monitoring visit may be conducted during the initial three-year accreditation period to ensure continued compliance with the appropriate standards.

Accreditation and standards promulgated by other medical organizations

Joint commission

Founded in 1951, the Joint Commission (formerly known as the Joint Commission on Accreditation of Healthcare Organizations, or JCAHO) is an independent, not-for-profit organization whose mission is "to continuously improve health care for the public, in collaboration with other stakeholders, by evaluating health care organizations and inspiring them to excel in providing safe and effective care of the highest quality and value" (Joint Commission, n.d.). It is the nation's oldest and largest standards-setting and accrediting body in health care.

The Joint Commission evaluates and accredits more than 20,000 health care organizations and programs in the United States. Joint Commission accreditation and certification is recognized nationwide as a symbol of quality that reflects an organization's commitment to meeting certain performance standards. Accreditation can be earned by many types of health care organizations, including hospitals, doctor's offices, nursing homes, office-based surgery centers, behavioral health treatment facilities, and providers of home care services. Joint Commission–accredited organizations can also earn certification for programs devoted to chronic diseases and conditions, such as asthma, diabetes, and heart failure. Providers of health care staffing services can also earn Joint Commission certification. To earn and maintain the Joint Commission's Gold Seal of Approval™, an organization must undergo an on-site survey by a Joint Commission survey team at least every three years (laboratories must be surveyed every two years). Some examples of correctional health care facilities accredited by the Joint Commission include the Texas Department of Criminal Justice prison hospital located on the central campus of the University of Texas Medical Branch and several ambulatory care facilities operated by the Federal Bureau of Prisons.

Medical association of georgia

MAG formed a Committee on Correctional Medicine in 1975 to study and recommend ways to improve the delivery of health care in nonfederal prisons in Georgia (MAG, n.d.). With funding provided by the state legislature, the committee implemented a program to accredit health care facilities in state prisons and county jails in the early 1980s. The accreditation process is based on NCCHC standards and additional standards developed by the committee. More recently, the committee developed and published a set of standards for jails with an average daily population of 200 or less (MAG, 2012).

American psychiatric association and other organizations

Other national organizations, such as the APHA (2003), have promulgated standards for medical, mental health, and other correctional health services. The APA has also developed guidelines. First published in 1989, the APA guidelines are in their second edition (APA, 2000) and are being revised. Particularly challenging areas covered by these guidelines and position statements include the use of seclusion and restraint with inmates/offenders with mental disorders (Appelbaum, 2007; Champion, 2007; Metzner, Tardiff, Lion, et al., 2007) and the housing of offenders with mental illness in solitary confinement, administrative segregation, and other types of restrictive housing units.

Best health care practices in correctional settings: where are we today?

Psychiatrists and other health care staff who are new to the world of corrections must receive an orientation that helps them understand basic correctional systems, culture, environmental, and safety issues. Topics include security policies and procedures, contraband issues, hostage and other emergency situations, boundaries and communication between offenders and staff, and professionalism. Some relevant examples include the NCCHC standards (2008; see Standard P-C-09 Orientation for Health Staff) and the ACA standards (2003; see Standards 4-4082 and 4-4088).

Current national standards and/or guidelines for correctional mental health care programs emphasize the importance of mental health screening and evaluation performed by qualified personnel on all inmates as part of the admission process to a prison. Metzner, Miller, and Kleinsasser (1994) reported data from all 50 state departments of corrections regarding prison mental health screening and evaluation models. They found that most states appeared to have adopted some variation of the most recognized guidelines and/or standards (e.g., APA, NCCHC, APHA) for correctional health care systems.

Ncchc guidelines for disease management

An NCCHC Guideline for Disease Management is a consensus statement designed to help correctional health practitioners and their patients make decisions about appropriate health care for specific clinical disease states/conditions and clinical circumstances. The guidelines contain information and evidence-based recommendations on the best practices for the clinical management of specific health conditions (e.g., asthma, adolescent attention-deficit/hyperactivity disorder, opioid detoxification), with special consideration regarding the correctional housing and living environment.

NCCHC's guidelines aim to standardize, guide, and improve clinical practice in correctional institutional settings. They are based on nationally accepted medical science and practice and evidence-based studies and take into consideration special circumstances commonly found in correctional facilities. The guidelines are not meant to be prescriptive for evaluation and treatment of particular disease states. Instead, they provide recommendations on clinical management, laboratory testing, patient education, and clinical monitoring and include references to widely promulgated studies and best clinical practices. The guidelines are reviewed annually and, if necessary, updated to reflect the latest evidence-based practices. Guidelines have been developed for conditions common among incarcerated adults and juveniles (e.g., alcohol detoxification, chronic noncancer pain management, diabetes, hypertension, hyperlipidemia, obesity, hypertension, sickle cell disease).

In addition, several state correctional systems, university correctional health systems, the Federal Bureau of Prisons, and private for-profit correctional health care vendors have developed disease management guidelines and formularies in an attempt to standardize health care and reduce costs.

Position statements of NCCHC, the society of correctional physicians, and other organizations

In addition to promulgating standards, the NCCHC, the Society of Correctional Physicians, and other organizations such as the APA, AAPL, AMA, and AACAP periodically adopt position statements on topics of importance for the correctional health care field. The position statements are useful to correctional administrators and health professionals because they offer recommendations on a wide range of health-related issues. They can be of interest to policy makers and the public because they often frame the social, economic, and political aspects of contemporary correctional health care issues.

Education and certification of correctional health professionals

With increased recognition that health care delivery within correctional settings requires specialized training and expertise, national certifications are now available to correctional psychiatrists, physicians, nurses, dental staff, and other health care staff. Both the NCCHC and ACA have established separate certification processes for correctional health professionals (nurses, medical, dental, mental health staff). NCCHC has the multidisciplinary Certified Correctional Health Professional Program with specialty certification for nurses and mental health professionals. This program requires passing an examination created by a committee peer group of correctional health care experts. NCCHC also produces several correctional health publications, including the peer-reviewed *Journal of Correctional Health Care*.

ACA has a comprehensive certification program for corrections professionals. There are also three certification categories for nurses: certified corrections nurse manager, certified corrections nurse, and health services administrator.

Correctional health–specific continuing education opportunities for correctional and forensic psychiatrists include NCCHC national conferences and educational programs. NCCHC also provides correctional health consultations and technical assistance to correctional facilities and their leadership. Similarly, ACA sponsors national conferences that include health services seminars with continuing medical education opportunities for health care staff. Because of the increasing awareness of the problem of people with serious mental illness in correctional settings, the APA, AAPL, AACAP, and Society of Correctional Physicians are all dedicating educational sessions, panels, and conference presentations to correctional mental health themes.

Summary

Many challenges confront correctional health staff in serving the needs of incarcerated adults and juveniles. Effective screening, timely referral, and appropriate treatment are critical. Their implementation requires interagency collaboration, adherence to established national standards of care, and implementation of continuous quality improvement practices and research on the health needs of this vulnerable patient population. Effective evaluation and treatment during incarceration meets important public health objectives, helps improve health services, and facilitates effective transition into the community upon release. Better correctional health care for individuals as defined in national standards and accreditation programs serves the intended goal of treatment and rehabilitation.

References

American Correctional Association (n.d., a). Standards & accreditation: Benefits of accreditation. Available at: https://www.aca.org/standards/benefits.asp.

American Correctional Association (n.d., b). Vision statement. Available at: http://www.aca.org/pastpresentfuture/doc_visionstatement2.pdf.

American Correctional Association (2002). *Performance-based standards for correctional health care for adult correctional institutions.* Lanham, MD: Author.

American Correctional Association (2003). *Standards for adult correctional institutions* (4th ed.). Lanham, MD: Author.

American Psychiatric Association (2000). *Psychiatric services in jails and prisons: A Task Force Report of the American Psychiatric Association* (2nd ed.). Washington, DC: Author.

American Public Health Association (2003). *Standards for health services in correctional institutions* (3rd ed.). Washington, DC: Author.

Anno, B. J. (2001). *Correctional health care: guidelines for the management of an adequate delivery system.* Washington, DC: National Institute of Corrections.

Appelbaum, K. L. (2007). Commentary: The use of restraint and seclusion in correctional mental health. *Journal of the American Academy of Psychiatry and the Law, 35*, 431–435.

Baillargeon, J., Hoge, S. K., & Penn, J.V. (2010). Addressing the challenge of community re-entry among released inmates with serious mental illness. *American Journal of Community Psychology, 46*, 361–375.

Champion, M. K. (2007). Commentary: Seclusion and restraint in corrections—A time for change. *Journal of the American Academy of Psychiatry and the Law, 35*, 426–430.

Estelle v. Gamble (1976), 429 U.S. 97.

Fazel, S., & Danesh, J. (2002). Serious mental disorder in 2300 prisoners: A systematic review of 62 surveys. *Lancet, 359*, 545–550.

International Organization for Standardization (n.d.). Standards. Available at: http://www.iso.org/iso/home/standards.htm.

Joint Commission (n.d.). About the Joint Commission. http://www.joint-commission.org/about_us/about_the_joint_commission_main.aspx.

Lamb, H. R., & Bachrach, L. L. (2001). Some perspectives on deinstitutionalization. *Psychiatric Services, 52*, 1039–1045.

McDonald, D. C. (1999). Medical care in prisons. *Crime and Justice, 26*, 427–478.

Medical Association of Georgia (n.d.). MAG—which developed the standards for evaluating health care in jails and prisons in Georgia—surveys eight jails and 33 prisons. Available at: http://www.mag.org/organizations/correctional-medicine.

Medical Association of Georgia (2012). *Accreditation standards for jails.* Atlanta, GA: Author.

Mental Retardation Facilities and Community Mental Health Centers Construction Act of 1963, Pub. L. No. 88-164, 77 Stat. 282.

Metzner, J. L., Miller, R. D., & Kleinsasser, D. (1994). Mental health screening and evaluation within prisons. *Bulletin of the American Academy of Psychiatry and the Law, 22*, 451–457.

Metzner, J. L., Tardiff, K., Lion, J., Reid, W. H., Recupero, P. R., Schetky, D. H., . . . Janofsky, J. S. (2007). Resource document on the use of restraint and seclusion in correctional mental health care. *Journal of the American Academy of Psychiatry and the Law, 35*, 417–425.

National Commission on Correctional Health Care (n.d.). Accreditation programs: Health services: Overview. Available at: http://www.ncchc.org/health-service-accreditation-overview.

National Commission on Correctional Health Care (2008). *Standards for mental health services in correctional facilities.* Chicago, IL: Author.

Newman v. Alabama, 349 F. Supp. 278 (M.D. Ala. 1972).

Rold, W. J. (2008). Thirty years after *Estelle v. Gamble*: A legal retrospective. *Journal of Correctional Health Care, 14*, 11–20.

Ruiz v. Estelle, 503 F Supp 1265 (SD Tex 1980).

Steinwald, C., Alevizos, G., & Aherne, P. (1973). *Medical care in U.S. jails: A 1972 AMA survey.* Chicago, IL: American Medical Association.

Stelovich, S. (1979). From the hospital to the prison: a step forward in deinstitutionalization? *Hospital & Community Psychiatry, 30*, 618–620.

Stephan, J. J. (1997). *Census of state and federal correctional facilities, 1995.* Washington, DC: US Department of Justice, Bureau of Justice Statistics.

Torrey, E. F., Kennard A. D., Eslinger, D., Lamb, R., & Pavle, J. (2010). *More mentally ill persons are in jails and prisons than hospitals: a survey of the states.* Arlington, VA: Treatment Advocacy Center.

US General Accounting Office (1978). *A federal strategy is needed to help improve medical and dental care in prisons and jails: Report to the Congress.* Washington, DC: U.S. Government Printing Office.

US General Accounting Office (2000). *Mental health: Community-based care increases for people with serious mental illness.* Washington, DC: U.S. Government Printing Office.

Wallenstein, A. M. (2004, Fall). Understanding history vital for future success. *CorrectCare, 18*(4), 3.

Whitmer, G. E. (1980). From hospitals to jails: The fate of California's deinstitutionalized mentally ill. *American Journal of Orthopsychiatry, 50*, 65–75.

CHAPTER 64

Hunger strikes

Emily A. Keram

He has chosen death:
Refusing to eat or drink, that he may bring
Disgrace upon me; for there is a custom,
An old and foolish custom, that if a man
Be wronged, or think that he is wronged, and starve
Upon another's threshold till he die,
The Common People, for all time to come,
Will raise a heavy cry against that threshold,
Even though it be the King's.
                    W. B. Yeats, *The King's Threshold*

Introduction

The management of hunger strikers in correctional settings presents the psychiatrist with unique clinical and ethical challenges. The potential for such complex tensions between medical decision making and medical ethics rarely exists in other practice settings. A physician's primary consideration involves the health of his or her patient and respect for human life (World Medical Association [WMA], 2006a). These are advanced within an ethical framework that includes respect for patient autonomy, as well as physician beneficence and nonmaleficence (Beauchamp & Childress, 2012). The correctional psychiatrist who treats or evaluates a hunger striker may be involved in medical decisions that lead to opposite extremes, from death by starvation to force-feeding. Concepts such as respect for human life, respect for patient autonomy, beneficence, and nonmaleficence present new and difficult considerations in the context of a correctional hunger strike.

This chapter provides correctional psychiatrists with the historical, legal, and ethical background for working with detained hunger strikers. The psychiatric evaluation and treatment of hunger strikers within the management protocols of the institution are discussed. The lack of international consensus in this area is reviewed.

History

Self-starvation as an instrument of nonviolent coercion or protest has an ancient history. Hindu scriptures dating from approximately the fourth century B.C.E. contain the earliest reference to a hunger strike. In the Ramayana, Prince Bharata refuses to eat in an effort to compel his brother Rama to assume the throne (Menon, 2004; Narayan, 2006).

In pre-Christian Ireland, Brehon law, a system of oral law, enforced judgments by means of *troscud*—that is, fasting to cause another's distress (Higgins, 2011). When a person of high rank committed a wrong and failed to provide the requisite compensation, the wronged party had the right to sit and fast outside the house of the defendant. If the defendant ate during the fast, he was required to pay double the original fine. If he refused to make payment, he forfeited the right to be compensated for any wrongdoing against him. An identical system of justice, sitting *dhurna*, existed in ancient India (Vernon, 2007). Brehon law was codified in writing in the seventh century C.E. and survived until the seventeenth century when it was replaced by British common law. Sitting *dhurna* was outlawed in India during British colonial rule in 1860.

Hunger strikes in correctional settings have occurred regularly since the early 1900s. The English suffragette Marion Wallace-Dunlop began the first recorded prison hunger strike in 1909 (Sullivan & Romilly, 2000). She was released when British authorities feared she might die and become a martyr. Other incarcerated suffragettes took up the practice. They were force-fed, which they protested as a form of torture. Public outcry over this intervention led to the passage of the Prisoner's Temporary Discharge of Ill Health Act of 1913. Known as the "Cat and Mouse Act," it provided for the temporary release of prisoners on hunger strike when they became sick. Once recovered, the suffragettes were sent back to prison. American suffragettes also engaged in hunger strikes and were subject to force-feeding (Gallagher, 1974).

The difficult choice of whether to force-feed hunger strikers is illustrated in the inconsistent response on the part of authorities to Irish republican prisoners in the twentieth century. Irish republicans first adopted prison hunger strikes in 1917 (Beresford, 1997; O'Malley, 1991). Later that year, Thomas Ashe died after he was injured during a force-feeding. The practice of force-feeding hunger strikers was suspended. At least eight imprisoned Irish republicans died on hunger strike in the 1920s. In the 1940s, several Irish republican hunger strikers were allowed to die. When the tactic was revived in the 1970s, several members of the Provisional Irish Republican Army successfully used hunger strikes to force their release after they were held without charge in the Republic of Ireland. Several others died in England, including Michael Gaughan, who died after being force-fed. Irish republican hunger strikes in British prisons continued in 1980, receiving widespread attention. The authorities did not reinstate force-feeding. In 1981, 10 Irish republicans, including Bobby Sands, died during a hunger strike. Public support for the hunger strikers resulted in some being elected to both Irish and British parliaments. After the deaths, the British conceded to some of the prisoners' demands and the strike was ended.

Hunger strikes occur in prisons throughout the world. Among them are the South African hunger strikes of the 1980s (Reyes,

1998); the episodic hunger strikes by Turkish prisoners from 1996 through 2012 (Amnesty International, 2013; Reyes, 1998); and the ongoing hunger strikes at the US Naval Station at Guantanamo Bay, Cuba (Rubenstein & Thomson, 2013). Amnesty International provides frequent updates about custodial and noncustodial hunger strikes currently in effect around the world (e.g., Amnesty International, 2013).

International approaches to hunger strikes

Given the differing roles and priorities of prisoners, physicians, and institutional personnel involved in hunger strikes, the lack of consensus regarding their management is not surprising. Varying international conceptions of human rights contribute to these disparate approaches. Human rights and medical organizations throughout the world have published guidelines emphasizing the ethical responsibilities of correctional physicians while caring for prisoners on hunger strikes. In the United States, where competent custodial hunger strikers are force-fed, correctional policies and procedures attempt to balance the right of prisoners to engage in a hunger strike, their health, and the safety needs of the institution. In the early twenty-first century, US and European courts issued opinions on custodial hunger strikes that underscore the lack of consensus in balancing these competing interests.

Guidelines for psychiatrists and other physicians

The WMA sets out broad international standards for physicians who care for hunger strikers in custodial settings while acknowledging that varying strategies may have to be adopted by physicians according to the circumstances of the case. Nonetheless, physicians must be able to act independently from the detaining authorities and need to use their own moral judgment in particularly complex situations (WMA, 2006b, 2006c).

The WMA defines a hunger strike as a form of protest or demand through food refusal. Short-lived fasts that last less than 72 hours are excluded. All correctional physicians must be aware of the symptoms and clinical physiology of different stages of fasting in order to give accurate medical counseling to patients. Hunger strikers who refuse both nutrition and hydration for more than 48 hours are at risk for significant harm. Humans cannot survive more than a few days without fluid. Thus, correctional hunger strikes typically involve refusal of food but ingestion of adequate quantities of water. The fasting body first uses liver and muscle glycogen stores for energy. Ketosis, which subdues the sensation of hunger, soon occurs and is evident on the breath and in lab studies. Glycogen stores are depleted by about day 10 to 14; at this point, muscle including cardiac muscle becomes a substrate for gluconeogenesis. The WMA recommends close medical monitoring after a weight loss of 10 percent for lean healthy individuals. Major health problems arise at weight loss of about 18 percent. Hunger strikers should be informed that dehydration is a risk as hunger and thirst mechanisms are lost.

The WMA describes the duties of physicians caring for custodial hunger strikers. First, the physician, preferably a psychiatrist, must assess the prisoner's mental health. Their competence and motivation for food refusal should be established. If fasting is a psychiatric symptom, the underlying cause must be treated.

If the patient's mental illness impairs their safety and judgment regarding their need for treatment, the psychiatrist should follow the institution's guidelines for considering involuntary treatment. Such patients should not be allowed to fast to the point that their health is damaged. Religious fasts are not considered protest fasts and should be respected. Competent hunger strikers are aware of the reason for their hunger strike and have a rational understanding of the consequences of their food refusal.

Competent hunger strikers generally fall into two categories, distinguished by their motivations and intentions. The first seek to gain publicity to achieve a goal. They have no intention of damaging their health and often agree to artificial feeding and medical assistance at some stage of their fast. Their goals may seem petty or involve a larger principle. These hunger strikes may be prolonged. Custodial personnel might view strikers as blackmailers and allow the strike to continue to test their resolve. The psychiatrist should meet privately with these hunger strikers at regular intervals to establish the parameters at which the protester will accept medical intervention to prevent permanent health consequences.

The second type of competent hunger strikers is prepared to risk their health or life for a cause. Political hunger strikers fall into this category. These food refusers often mistrust correctional clinicians, whom they view as agents of the detaining authority. They pose a serious challenge to medical ethics, as their willingness to risk their lives inevitably raises difficult questions about whether and when to intervene and the thorny ethical question of whether feeding contrary to patients' expressed wishes can ever be justified.

Once the motivation and intention of the hunger striker have been ascertained, the psychiatrist's next duty is to establish the voluntariness of the food refusal. Some institutions use the term "voluntary total fasting" to describe a hunger strike. However, total fasting is rare. Most hunger strikers accept fluids and others accept some food. In assessing voluntariness, the psychiatrist should be aware of possible sources of coercion and pressure. These may include hunger-striking peers, family, media, and inappropriate treatment by staff members, for example, taunting, that may make it difficult for the hunger striker to stop a fast. Psychiatrists must be able to talk privately with a hunger striker. Interpreters should be neutral and not connected to the detaining authority or member of the hunger striker's peer group. The psychiatrist should discuss limits to confidentiality present in the custodial setting. If the psychiatrist suspects the presence of duress, they can recommend that the hunger striker be removed to a hospital on medical grounds. If duress is confirmed, feeding can be offered and accomplished in the hospital. If the psychiatrist cannot gain the trust of the hunger striker, consideration should be given to bringing in an external psychiatrist with no relationship to the detaining authorities. In evaluating voluntariness, the psychiatrist can discuss flaws or lack of logic in the detainee's decision making without causing undue pressure. If the decision to hunger strike appears voluntary, the decision should be respected.

Other duties of psychiatrists and other clinicians include providing accurate information on the health consequences of fasting, giving accurate advice and counseling in response to the patient's questions and in the context of the policies of the institution, maintaining confidentiality, and weighing the risks and benefits of communicating directly with the hunger striker's family. Psychiatrists and other clinicians may be in a position to act as mediators between hunger strikers and custodial authorities, particularly when they have the trust of both parties. The WPA advises that most hunger strikers want to find a way to stop their fasting and may do so if authorities make minor concessions. Physicians may be in a position to negotiate such compromises between the parties. If the demands of hunger strikers are obviously out of reach, correctional psychiatrists and other clinicians must not pretend otherwise or insinuate that a solution is achievable through mediation. They should make clear to both parties that their role is to assist in negotiations and that they are not a party to them. They should continue to provide accurate information to patients about their medical condition without interference from the detaining authorities.

The WMA describes several other duties of physicians caring for hunger striking prisoners. Clinicians should remain objective and independent. They should avoid pressure to advance the interests of any particular group by giving medical information or advice that is not evidence based. Physicians, including psychiatrists, employed by the detaining authorities or their vendors may find this challenging. Without external support from medical associations, it may be difficult for them to oppose administrative decisions imposed on them, even if they are fully aware of the ethical implications of a potentially terminal hunger strike. Medical associations have a duty to support their members who act consistent with one or more of the currently prevailing ethical guidelines. The WMA notes that, ideally, independent physicians should be permitted to counsel hunger strikers in the interest of all involved and in an attempt to avoid fatalities. In countries that allow this practice, the independent status of physicians supports their credibility.

Physicians, including psychiatrists, have a duty to manage medical and mental health conditions during a hunger strike. Extreme, inadequate nutrition causes a clinical syndrome that closely resembles true starvation. Long-term hunger strikers experience significant gaps in memory and inability to concentrate. As the body begins to experience medical and psychiatric consequences, the physician has a duty to resume a serious discussion with each hunger striker about his or her wishes. Privacy and confidentiality is of the utmost importance in order to avoid sources of coercion or interference.

Finally, physicians, including psychiatrists, have a duty to understand the moral and practical differences between artificial feeding (administration of nutrients parentally or via a nasogastric tube to which the patient has consented), force-feeding, and resuscitation. The WMA conceives of situations in which a physician may ethically participate in artificial feeding and resuscitation. In all circumstances, it is unethical for physicians to participate in force-feeding of competent individuals. Physicians must have a clear understanding of the hunger striker's wishes regarding medical intervention before the patient loses capacity for medical decision making. Prior to or in the early stages of a hunger strike, the physician and patient should have a frank discussion regarding the patient's attitude about whether and when they wish to receive artificial feeding and resuscitation at later stages of the hunger strike. In some countries, patient's advance instructions dictate the physician's intervention once consciousness is lost. In others, physicians face prosecution if they fail to intervene to save the life of the hunger striker. The physician and hunger striker should discuss this issue as well. If a physician cannot accept the patient's competent and legally permissible decision, a physician willing to act in accord with the informed advance decision of the hunger strikers should take their place. Artificial feeding generally should not involve coercion of competent patients. The WPA acknowledges that some circumstances may justify a decision to artificially feed or resuscitate a hunger striker who has lost competence, for example, when the situation that provoked the hunger strike has changed after the hunger striker has lost consciousness. Physicians should never participate in force-feeding or other measures that involve cruel, inhuman, or degrading treatment.

Most national medical association members of the WMA have shown support for the Malta Declaration and the WMA's position on the ethical management of prison hunger strikes. For example, both the American Medical Association and the British Medical Association have issued public statements against the force-feeding of detainees at Guantanamo (Nathanson, 2013; Rosenberg, 2013).

The International Committee of the Red Cross (ICRC) employs physicians who monitor the conditions of detained hunger strikers in certain settings (International Committee of the Red Cross, 2013). These physicians act as neutral parties who assess and follow protesters' medical and psychiatric condition and capacity and whether food refusal is voluntary. The goal of the ICRC physician is to assist the clinical staff caring for hunger strikers in delivering care that meets ethical standards. The ICRC also strives to ensure that the hunger strikers' dignity, humanity, and informed medical decisions are respected. It is the position of the ICRC that force-feeding of competent inmates constitutes a gross violation of medical ethics.

Case law

In the United States, case law has supported the force-feeding of custodial hunger strikers in contravention of international standards. Despite the 1990 Supreme Court finding that competent adults have the right to refuse force-feeding even if death will result (*Cruzan v. Director, Missouri Department of Health*, 1990), inmates have been unsuccessful in stopping this practice. Instead, case law relies on the finding, also in 1990, that prison authorities could force medicate a prisoner, even in the absence of a determination that the prisoner was incompetent (*Washington v. Harper*, 1990). In 2012 the Connecticut Supreme Court held that the Department of Correction could lawfully force-feed a prisoner on a hunger strike (*Commissioner of Correction v. Coleman*, 2012). The court found that the state's interest in the prisoner's health and the safety of the institution outweighed the prisoner's common-law right to bodily integrity; that force-feeding did not violate the prisoner's First and Fourteenth Amendment rights to free speech and privacy; and that the weight of international authority did not prohibit medically necessary force-feeding.

Beginning in 2002, detainees at Guantanamo Bay have held numerous hunger strikes to protest both the conditions of their confinement and their indefinite detention (Crosby et al., 2007). In 2014 the US District Court and Court of Appeals for the District of Columbia reversed their long-standing position and ruled that the courts have subject-matter jurisdiction over detainee challenges to conditions of confinement (*Aamer v. Obama*, 2014). Within a month, the first detainee had filed a motion to enjoin the force-feeding protocol at Guantanamo, arguing that they amount to torture (*Hassan v. Obama*, 2014).

In contrast to US courts, European courts have deferred to the WMA and ICRC recommendations on the management of prison hunger strikes. For example, in 2006, in *Prosecutor v. Seselj* (2006), the court directed the detaining authority to follow internationally accepted standards of medical ethics and international law and ordered medical professionals caring for a prisoner on hunger strike to seek professional advice on care and medical ethics in considering how to manage their patient.

Role of the psychiatrist in correctional hunger strikes

Correctional psychiatrists may be asked to serve several roles during prison hunger strikes. In addition to evaluating voluntariness of food refusal, reviewed previously, the psychiatrist may evaluate medical decision-making capacity, assist the patient in formulating advance instructions regarding artificial feeding and resuscitation, and provide treatment and deliver consultation–liaison services to the treatment team and correctional personnel. If possible, these responsibilities should be assigned to different individuals.

Mental health clinicians do not make value judgments on the cause of the patient's hunger strike. However, a psychiatrist has an ethical duty to report known or suspected torture or abuse. Correctional psychiatrists should know the procedures for such reporting as well as policies and laws that protect whistleblowers (Daines, 2007).

Medical decision-making capacity

It is essential to evaluate the ability of prisoners to understand the risks a hunger strike poses to their health and life before they are allowed to initiate a strike. The assessment of decision-making capacity is the same as the process in other settings. The prisoner must understand the medical and mental health consequences of fasting and subsequent food refusal. They must have intact reality testing regarding these issues. Prisoners who lack these capacities may require interventions that could include forced feedings.

The psychiatrist should be aware of the interaction of food refusal and mental state. Early in the hunger strike, anger and irritability may intensify, increasing motivation for continuing the strike even while health risks increase. These negative emotions can strengthen the need for instant gratification, in this instance, redress of the grievance, further intensifying pursuit of the strike. This may skew the prisoner's assessment of the risks and benefits of continued food refusal. The presence of psychiatric illness does not necessitate a finding of incapacity. However, if a psychiatric symptom contributes to the motivation for food refusal and can be treated, improvement may result in voluntary resumption of feeding. A prisoner with a known psychiatric history may decompensate with the stress of the hunger strike. The psychiatrist should be vigilant for signs of the re-emergence of previously stable symptoms that may affect capacity and offer appropriate treatment (Daines, 2007; Fessler, 2003).

Advance directives

Some jurisdictions allow consideration of a hunger striker's advance instructions or directives regarding artificial feeding and resuscitation. In this instance, it may be beneficial to have a psychiatrist present during discussions between the prisoner and treatment team. This gives the psychiatrist the opportunity to assess capacity in a context in which the prisoner's questions and concerns can be addressed. The treatment team can obtain a contemporaneous opinion of capacity to understand subtle or specific aspects of the risks of hunger striking. The psychiatrist can also assist both parties in identifying and working through uncomfortable affect generated by the discussion.

Treatment

In general, options for the treatment of psychiatric illness in a hunger striker are identical to those of the noncustodial population. Cognitive and supportive psychotherapy may reduce distress. Some hunger strikers will accept psychotropic medication. Institutional policy and local law should be followed in determining the need for involuntary administration of medication. In either instance, the psychiatrist should assess and monitor the prisoner's physiologic status and the presence of side effects in considering which agent to prescribe. For example, tricyclic antidepressants should be avoided secondary to their potential to aggravate orthostatic hypotension. Bupropion has been linked to seizures in patients with eating disorders and should not be used. If medication is administered involuntarily, the psychiatrist should be familiar with agents that can be administered parenterally. In some instances, insertion of a nasogastric tube may be necessary to administer medication (Daines, 2007).

Symptoms of depression overlap with symptoms that arise during a hunger strike. Examples include appetite loss, weight loss, impaired concentration, psychomotor retardation, and fatigue. Symptoms of depression that would not be expected solely due to starvation include suicidal ideation, anhedonia, depressed mood, decrease in self-worth, and guilt. Additionally, a prisoner with depression may have a sense of a foreshortened future, or may be actively or passively suicidal. They may be overwhelmed by the very real loss of control over their lives in the custodial setting. In such instances, participation in a hunger strike may restore a sense of self-worth, purpose, and autonomy. The psychiatrist should be attuned to the possible presence of these dynamics in order to optimally treat the prisoner's depression. Some euthymic inmates may develop depression during a hunger strike and accept medication while continuing to fast. If suicide becomes the motivation for continued food refusal, involuntary treatment may be required. Nasogastric feedings and intravenous fluids may be ordered to prevent suicide (Daines, 2007).

Prisoners with psychotic disorders may have capacity to participate in a hunger strike. In the absence of flagrant symptoms such as command hallucinations to refuse food or delusional beliefs regarding the purpose or consequences of the hunger strike, a psychotic prisoner may be allowed to hunger strike. Administration of involuntary medication should be decided upon as described previously. Risk of orthostasis and cardiac arrhythmias must be considered when selecting a medication and dose. The psychiatrist should be aware that dehydration can increase the risk of neuroleptic malignant syndrome (Daines, 2007).

Consultation–liaison

Psychiatric consultation–liaison services can be useful in correctional hunger strikes by providing education and improving communication. The psychiatrist can help the treatment team and custodial staff to clarify and modulate negative feelings toward the hunger striker. Helping them to understand the mental health consequences of starvation, such as anger and irritability, may decrease their perception of being personally attacked. Additionally, education regarding psychiatric symptoms may assist the treatment team and custodial staff in their interactions with the patient regarding the timing of events such as physical examinations, exercise, and cell moves. Hunger strikers in military custodial settings may be incorrectly perceived to be participating in "asymmetric warfare." The psychiatrist can provide a historical context on hunger strikes in detention and help to reframe the hunger strike by emphasizing the goals of the participants.

Regarding consultation to the treatment team, in addition to assisting in capacity evaluations and advance instructions, the psychiatrist can help clarify and maintain the professional roles and boundaries of clinicians caring for custodial hunger strikers. Some treating clinicians may find it difficult to reconcile their personal beliefs and understanding of their ethical responsibilities to the desires of their patient or the policies of the institution. The psychiatrist should be attuned to the presence of this concern and recommend that a clinician seek consultation to resolve their dilemma.

Summary

Participating in the management of a hunger-striking prisoner can pose clinical and ethical dilemmas for the correctional psychiatrist. The psychiatrist should have a clear understanding of the international guidelines for physicians on the ethical management of hunger strikes, their institution's policies and procedures on hunger strikes and force-feeding, and their willingness or ability to provide care in a setting in which their patient's wishes or the demands of their employer conflict with their beliefs regarding their professional and ethical obligations. Consultation with experts in the field may assist in balancing potentially conflicting roles and responsibilities.

References

Aamer v. Obama, No. 13-5223 (2014).

Amnesty International (2013). *Amnesty International report 2013: The state of the world's human rights* (pp. 274–275). London: Amnesty International. Available at: http://www.amnesty.org/en/library/asset/POL10/001/2013/en/b093912e-8d30-4480-9ad1-acbb82be7f29/pol100012013en.pdf. Accessed on April 30, 2014.

Beauchamp, T. L., & Childress, J. F. (2012). *Principles of biomedical ethics*. New York: Oxford University Press.

Beresford, D. (1997). *Ten men dead: The story of the 1981 Irish hunger strike*. New York: Atlantic Monthly Press.

Commissioner of Correction v. Coleman, 303 Conn. 800 (2012).

Crosby, S. S., Apovian, C. M., & Grodin, M. A. (2007). Hunger strikes, force-feeding, and physicians' responsibilities. *JAMA*, *298*(5), 563–566.

Cruzan v. Director, Missouri Department of Health, 497 U.S. 261 (1990).

Daines, M. K. (2007). Hunger strikes in correctional facilities. In O. J. Thienhaus & M. Piasecki (Eds.), *Correctional psychiatry: Practice guidelines and strategies* (pp. 8-1–8-13). Kingston, NJ: Civic Research Institute, Inc.

Fessler, D. M. T. (2003). The implications of starvation induced changes for the ethical treatment of hunger strikers. *Journal of Medical Ethics*, *29*, 243–247.

Gallagher, R. S. (1974). "I was arrested of course . . ." *American Heritage Magazine*, *25*(2), 17–24, 92–94.

Hassan v. Obama Civ. No. 04-1194 (2014).

Higgins, N. (2011). The lost legal system: pre-common law Ireland and Brehon law. In D. Frenkel (Ed.), *Legal theory, practice and education* (pp. 193–205). Athens, Greece: ATINER.

International Committee of the Red Cross (2013). *Hunger strikes in Prison: the ICRC's position*. Available at: http://www.icrc.org/eng/resources/documents/faq/hunger-strike-icrc-position.htm. Accessed on April 30, 2014.

Menon, R. (2004) *The Ramayana: A modern retelling of the great Indian epic*. New York: North Point Press.

Narayan, R. K. (2006). *The Ramayana*. London: Penguin Group.

Nathanson, V. (2013). Stop Guantanamo force-feedings. *The Guardian*, Sunday, June 16, 2013. Available at: http://www.theguardian.com/world/2013/jun/16/stop-guantanamo-force-feeding. Accessed on April 30, 2014.

O'Malley, P. (1991). *Biting at the grave: The Irish hunger strikes and the politics of despair*. Boston: Beacon Press.

Prosecutor v. Seselj, International Tribunal for the Former Yugoslavia, Urgent Order to the Dutch Authorities Regarding Health and Welfare of the Accused, December 6, 2006.

Reyes, H. Website of the International Committee of the Red Cross. *Medical and ethical aspects of hunger strikes in custody and the issue of torture*. Available at http://www.icrc.org/eng/resources/documents/article/other/health-article-010198.htm. Published January 1, 1998. Accessed on April 30, 2014.

Rosenberg, C. AMA opposes forced feedings at Guantanamo. Available at http://www.miamiherald.com/2013/04/30/3372407/guantanamo-hunger-strike-holds.html. Accessed on April 30, 2014.

Rubenstein, L., & Thomson, G. (2013). *Ethics abandoned: Medical professionalism and detainee abuse in the "War on Terror."* New York: Institute on Medicine as a Profession.

Sullivan, D., & Romilly, C. (2000). Hunger strike and food refusal. In S. Wilson & I. Cumming (Eds.), *Psychiatry in prisons: A comprehensive handbook* (pp. 156–172). London: Jessica Kingsley.

Vernon, J. (2007). *Hunger: A modern history*. Cambridge: Belknap Press.

Washington v. Harper, 494 U.S. 210 (1990).

World Medical Association (2006a). *International Code of Medical Ethics*. Available at: http://www.wma.net/en/30publications/10policies/c8/ Amended October 2006. Accessed on April 30, 2014.

World Medical Association (2006b). *World Medical Association Declaration on Hunger Strikers (Declaration of Malta)*. Available at http://www.wma.net/en/30publications/10policies/h31/ Revised 2006. Accessed on April 30, 2014.

World Medical Association (2006c). WMA Declaration of Malta—A background paper on the ethical management of hunger strikes. *World Medical Journal*, *52*(2), 36–43.

Yeats, W. B., & Kiely, D. (2005). *The King's Threshold: Manuscript materials*. Ithaca, NY: Cornell University Press.

CHAPTER 65

Responding to prisoner sexual assaults
Successes, promising practices, and challenges

Robert W. Dumond and Doris A. Dumond

Introduction

Sexual abuse in detention has been called "the most serious and devastating of non-lethal offenses which occur in corrections" (Cotton & Groth, 1982, p. 47) because of its profound impact on survivors and, ultimately society. This chapter explores the status of sexual violence in US correctional settings in the twenty-first century; examines what is known about sexual victimization in America's jails, prisons, and juvenile facilities; discusses the successes and promising practices facilitated by the Prison Rape Elimination Act (PREA) of 2003; considers the challenges that continue to exist; and makes recommendations for addressing the issues.

Sexual abuse in US jails and prisons has long been known but ignored

At the dawn of the US penitentiary movement, the Reverend Louis Dwight, president of the Boston Discipline Society (1824–1854), decried that "nature and humanity cry aloud for redemption from this dreadful degradation" of sexual abuse (Katz, 1976, p. 27). One hundred years later, Joseph F. Fishman, a federal inspector of prisons who visited 1,500 jails and prisons in the United States before 1920 (Freidman, 1993), found the problem unabated as many boys and young men were "made homosexual, either temporarily or permanently" (Fishman, 1934, p. 5). Unfortunately, it would take nearly two centuries for there to be a substantive response to "America's most open secret" (Bell, Cover, Cronan, Garza, Guggemos, & Storto, 1999, p. 196), the "plague that persists" (Dumond, 2000, p. 407), and "America's most ignored crime problem" (Lehrer, 2001, p. 24).

March to the prison rape elimination act of 2003

Following the 1990s, a decade of court cases involving staff sexual misconduct (*Cason v. Seckinger*, 2000; *Women Prisoners vs. District of Columbia Department of Corrections*, 1994); a case before the US Supreme Court of a transgender inmate sexually abused by other inmates (*Farmer v. Brennan*, 1994); groundbreaking surveys of sexual abuse in several correctional agencies (Struckman-Johnson & Struckman-Johnson, 2000; Struckman-Johnson, Struckman-Johnson, Rucker, Bumby, & Donaldson, 1996); and a series of scathing national reports about staff sexual misconduct (Amnesty International, 1999; Coomarasswamy, 1999; Human Rights Watch, 1996, 1998; Smith, 1998), this human rights violation was addressed at the national level. An innovative, bipartisan coalition of political, religious, human rights, social service, and professional organizations joined together to pursue national legislation to address all sexual violence in prisons and jails in the United States. In the summer of 2003, both houses of Congress unanimously passed PREA (117 Stat. 972-989). PREA was enacted as Public Law 108-79 in September 2003 (Dumond, 2003).

As noted by Dr. Cindy Struckman-Johnson, who served as one of the National Prison Rape Elimination Commission (NPREC) commissioners, "The passage of PREA was an unexpected victory for those who were familiar with the long-standing social and political indifference toward prison rape" (Struckman-Johnson & Struckman-Johnson, 2013, p. 340). PREA demanded a "zero tolerance" standard, focused on prevention as a top priority, and established important priorities for correctional agencies nationwide, including preventing, deterring, and detecting incidents of prisoner sexual violence; identifying and treating victims; identifying, investigating, and prosecuting perpetrators, whether inmate or staff; collecting and reporting data about prisoner sexual violence to the Bureau of Justice Statistics (BJS); establishing comprehensive training for correctional staff; developing national standards and ensuring compliance once the standards are promulgated; and creating safety for staff, inmates, and society (Fig. 65.1).

Most importantly, Public Law 108-79 assembled the resources of federal agencies within the US Department of Justice to study, address, and manage this problem, including the NPREC, the National Institute of Corrections (NIC), the Bureau of Justice Assistance (BJA), the BJS, the National Institute of Justice (NIJ), the US Attorney General's Review Panel on Prison Rape, and, most recently, the PREA Resource Center (PRC). Each of these agencies has been instrumental in crafting a blueprint for substantive

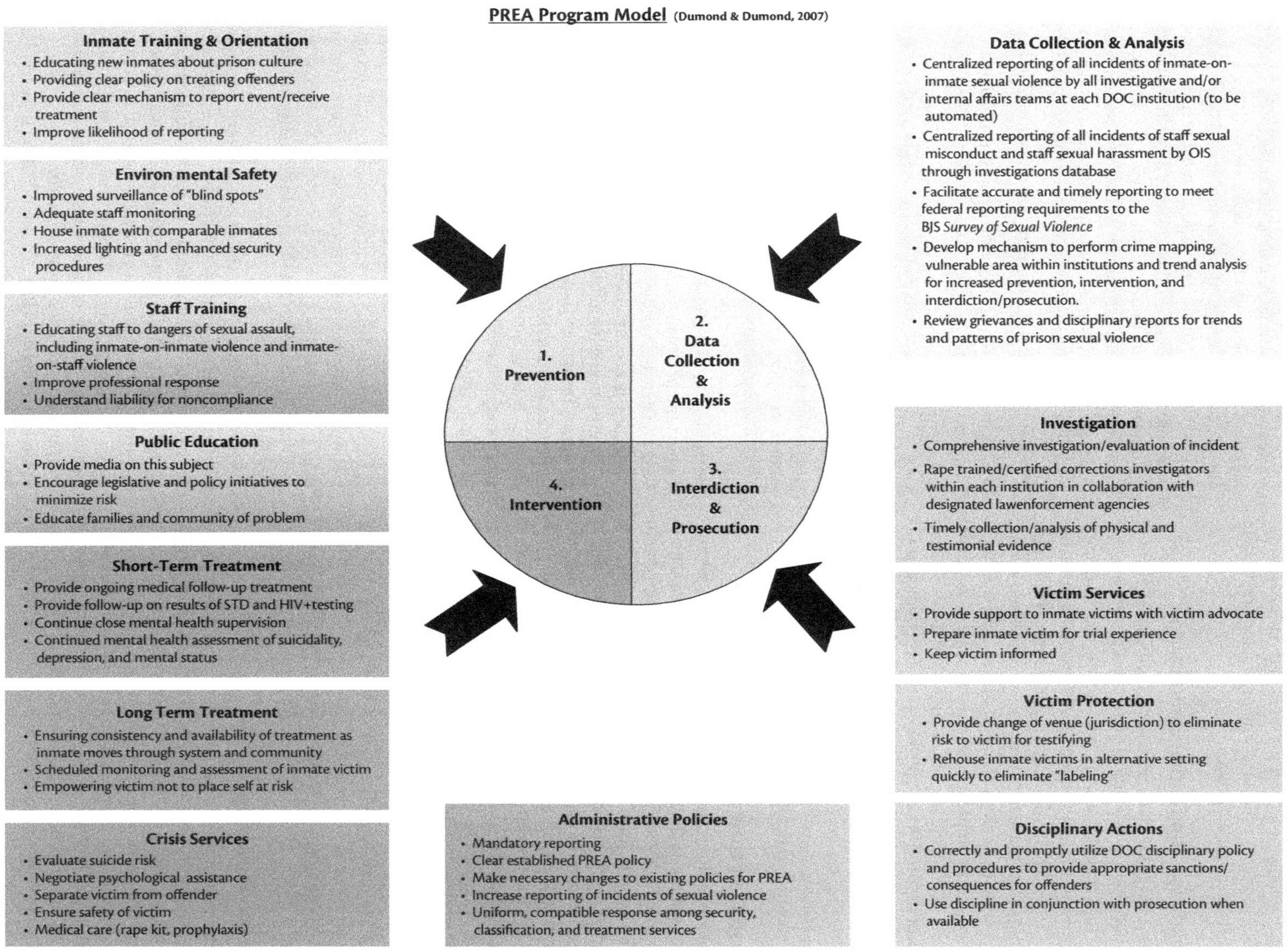

PREA Program Model (Dumond & Dumond, 2007)

Data Collection & Analysis
- Centralized reporting of all incidents of inmate-on-inmate sexual violence by all investigative and/or internal affairs teams at each DOC institution (to be automated)
- Centralized reporting of all incidents of staff sexual misconduct and staff sexual harassment by OIS through investigations database
- Facilitate accurate and timely reporting to meet federal reporting requirements to the BJS *Survey of Sexual Violence*
- Develop mechanism to perform crime mapping, vulnerable area within institutions and trend analysis for increased prevention, intervention, and interdiction/prosecution.
- Review grievances and disciplinary reports for trends and patterns of prison sexual violence

Investigation
- Comprehensive investigation/evaluation of incident
- Rape trained/certified corrections investigators within each institution in collaboration with designated lawenforcement agencies
- Timely collection/analysis of physical and testimonial evidence

Victim Services
- Provide support to inmate victims with victim advocate
- Prepare inmate victim for trial experience
- Keep victim informed

Victim Protection
- Provide change of venue (jurisdiction) to eliminate risk to victim for testifying
- Rehouse inmate victims in alternative setting quickly to eliminate "labeling"

Disciplinary Actions
- Correctly and promptly utilize DOC disciplinary policy and procedures to provide appropriate sanctions/consequences for offenders
- Use discipline in conjunction with prosecution when available

Inmate Training & Orientation
- Educating new inmates about prison culture
- Providing clear policy on treating offenders
- Provide clear mechanism to report event/receive treatment
- Improve likelihood of reporting

Environmental Safety
- Improved surveillance of "blind spots"
- Adequate staff monitoring
- House inmate with comparable inmates
- Increased lighting and enhanced security procedures

Staff Training
- Educating staff to dangers of sexual assault, including inmate-on-inmate violence and inmate-on-staff violence
- Improve professional response
- Understand liability for noncompliance

Public Education
- Provide media on this subject
- Encourage legislative and policy initiatives to minimize risk
- Educate families and community of problem

Short-Term Treatment
- Provide ongoing medical follow-up treatment
- Provide follow-up on results of STD and HIV+testing
- Continue close mental health supervision
- Continued mental health assessment of suicidality, depression, and mental status

Long Term Treatment
- Ensuring consistency and availability of treatment as inmate moves through system and community
- Scheduled monitoring and assessment of inmate victim
- Empowering victim not to place self at risk

Crisis Services
- Evaluate suicide risk
- Negotiate psychological assistance
- Separate victim from offender
- Ensure safety of victim
- Medical care (rape kit, prophylaxis)

Administrative Policies
- Mandatory reporting
- Clear established PREA policy
- Make necessary changes to existing policies for PREA
- Increase reporting of incidents of sexual violence
- Uniform, compatible response among security, classification, and treatment services

Circle diagram quadrants:
1. Prevention
2. Data Collection & Analysis
3. Interdiction & Prosecution
4. Intervention

Fig. 69.1 Prison Rape Elimination Act Program Model. BJS, Bureau of Justice Statistics; DOC, Department of Corrections; OIS, Office of Investigative Services; PREA, Prison Rape Elimination Act; STD, sexually transmitted disease. (*Source:* Dumond & Dumond, 2007.)

systemic, policy, and programmatic changes in American correctional agencies.

Successes and promising practices to date

This impressive assembly of federal partners and national initiatives has spawned important successes and promising practices in responding to prisoner sexual abuse.

National prison rape elimination commission

The NPREC was charged with conducting a thorough analysis of prisoner sexual violence in the United States, studying the causes and consequences of sexual abuse in confinement, and developing national standards to eliminate prison rape. Conducting hearings throughout the United States and hearing testimony from hundreds of correctional authorities, researchers, medical and mental health experts, community advocates, and prison rape survivors, the NPREC produced a comprehensive report on prisoner sexual violence (NPREC, 2009a) and accompanying standards for use in adult prisons and jails (NPREC, 2009b), community corrections (NPREC, 2009c), juvenile facilities (NPREC, 2009d), and lockups (NPREC, 2009e). These documents represent the collective work of the NPREC during the years of its existence (2003–2009) and provide a comprehensive roadmap and template for substantial change in US correctional practice.

National institute of corrections

The NIC became the initial clearinghouse of information for correctional agencies and established two cooperative agreements to advance training and knowledge about PREA. The first agreement involved the Moss Group, Inc., founded by Andie Moss, who was the assistant deputy commissioner in the Georgia Department of Corrections and oversaw the department's response to the *Cason v. Seckinger* class action lawsuit and was a program specialist with the NIC (1996–2002; see http://www.mossgroup.us/). The other agreement was with the American University–Washington College of Law. This resulted in End Silence: The Project on Addressing Prison Rape, established by law professor and former NPREC commissioner Brenda Smith (see http://www.wcl.american.edu/endsilence/) to provide consultation, training, and assistance. The agencies involved with each of these agreements are outstanding resources for correctional practitioners to consult; they have a plethora of print, video, and online research and training resources.

Bureau of justice assistance

The BJA implemented multiple initiatives to assist correctional agencies nationwide in responding to prisoner sexual violence, including rounds of funding of the Protecting Inmates and Safeguarding Communities initiative, which provided more than $32 million to correctional agencies. Funding was also provided for demonstration projects to establish "zero tolerance" cultures for sexual assault in correctional facilities, designed to assist correctional agencies to respond to and implement PREA standards.

Bureau of justice statistics

PREA mandated the establishment of the National Prison Rape Statistics Program under the auspices of the BJS to provide a comprehensive national data collection strategy. BJS data confirmed that sexual violence continues to be a major problem that affects thousands of prisoners and juvenile residents nationwide (Beck, Rantala, & Rexroat, 2014). Whereas previous studies of prisoner sexual violence relied on relatively small samples, the BJS data collection methodologies use a large sample pool and include a large, representative sample of correctional facilities. BJS also uses four standardized, behaviorally specific definitions: two inmate-on-inmate definitions ("nonconsensual sexual acts"—essentially acts of penetration, considered rape in most jurisdictions, and "abusive sexual contacts"—other sexually assaultive behaviors without penetration) and two staff-on-inmate definitions ("staff sexual misconduct"—sexual contact between a staff and inmate—and "staff sexual harassment"). In addition, the following four possible investigation outcomes of alleged incidents must be reported:

- ♦ Substantiated: if the incident was determined to have occurred,
- ♦ Unsubstantiated: if the evidence was insufficient to make a final determination,
- ♦ Unfounded: if the incident was determined not to have occurred, and
- ♦ Investigation ongoing: if a final determination had not been made at the time of data collection.

There had been little previous consensus on what constitutes sexual violence. By creating consistency in identifying prisoner sexual violence and mandating that all correctional agencies use the same definition, BJS has begun to assemble a national portrait of sexual abuse in prisons, jails, and juvenile facilities. Important prevalence information, developed by using broad, well-constructed national samples and statistically sound methodologies, is now available.

To fully understand the implications of these studies, it is necessary to recognize that of all crime categories, rape and sexual violence are the most underreported, making an accurate assessment of community-based occurrence rates difficult. There are three major methods to report crime: administrative records of crimes reported to law enforcement agencies (e.g., Uniform Crime Reports), victimization surveys (e.g., National Crime Victimization Survey), and self-report studies (Bartol & Bartol, 2008). BJS has developed methodologies that incorporate all three strategies. Four concurrent national correctional data collection endeavors are under way: the Survey of Sexual Violence (SSV), the National Inmate Survey (NIS), the National Survey of Youth in Custody (NSYC), and the National Former Prisoner Survey (NFPS).

The SSV belongs to the first category of data collection strategies—administrative records. The outcome most often reported upon investigation was unsubstantiated; however, in the years following initial implementation of this methodology, there has been a statistically significant increase in reports of sexual abuse (Beck et al., 2014). This increase suggests that correctional agencies are taking seriously such reports, resulting in greater willingness to report by inmate victims.

The other three BJS PREA data collection initiatives (NIS, NSYC, and NFPS) have elements of both victimization and self-report surveys. They use an innovative methodology known as ACASI (audio computer-assisted self-interviewing technology) where inmates use a laptop touchscreen and an audio feed to maximize confidentiality and minimize literacy issues. These data collection initiatives included very large samples (NIS, 2011–2012: 92,449 adult jail and prison inmates; NSYC, 2012: 8,707 adjudicated youth; and NFPS, 2012: 18,500 former inmates on active parole supervision). The reported national prevalence estimates are staggering; an estimated 80,600 inmates, juveniles, and former inmates reported one or more incidents of sexual assault by another inmate or facility staff in the past 12 months or since admission to the facility. These numbers include 57,900 (4.0%) of adult prison inmates and 22,700 (3.2%) of jail inmates (Beck, Berzofsky, Caspar, & Krebs, 2013), 1,720 (9.5%) of adjudicated youth (Beck, Cantor, Hartge, & Smith, 2013), and 2,096 (9.6%) of former state prisoners under parole supervision (Beck & Johnson, 2012). In summary, these results reveal the following:

◆ Prisoner sexual violence is common.

◆ Formal reports represent a small fraction of actual sexual assaults in jails, prisons, and juvenile settings.

◆ The predominant forms of prisoner sexual abuse are staff sexual misconduct, followed by nonconsensual sexual acts (acts legally considered rape).

National institute of justice

The NIJ has funded primary research on PREA with several notable contributions (see Goldberg & Wells, 2009), including a study of the nature of prison sexual violence in Texas, the nation's third largest prison system (Austin, Fabelo, Gunter, & McGinnis, 2006); an anthropological study of inmate culture in maximum-security prisons for men and women in the United States (Fleisher & Krienert, 2006); a project to identify effective prevention programs that exist in US prisons (Zweig, Naser, Blackmore, & Schaffer, 2006); a study to investigate the context of gender violence and safety in women's correctional facilities (Owen, Wells, Pollack, Muscat, & Torres, 2008); a review of strategies to prevent prison rape by changing the correctional culture (Zweig & Blackmore, 2008); and an examination of promising practices for managing sexual abuse in jails and juvenile facilities (English, Heil, & Dumond, 2010). As noted by Kaufman (2008, p. 25), "NIJ's work under PREA has yielded important research-based evidence to improve knowledge, practice, and policy to address sexual violence in prison."

Review panel on prison rape

Under the guidance of 42 U.S.C. §15603(b), the Review Panel on Prison Rape was charged with holding annual hearings focused on the three facilities with the highest incidence of prisoner rape and the two facilities with the lowest incidence, with an emphasis on identifying the common characteristics that relate to these findings. Since 2006, the panel has promulgated information about sexual victimization in jails and prisons and the problems faced by correctional agencies nationwide (http://ojp.gov/review-panel/reviewpanel.htm).

National standards to prevent, detect, and respond to prison rape

The national PREA standards are the vehicle to ensure compliance with PREA. These mandatory standards are the national benchmark for all correctional agencies in the elimination of prisoner sexual violence. The final standards were released by the US Department of Justice on May 17, 2012, and published in the *Federal Register* at http://www.prearesourcecenter.org/sites/default/files/library/2012-12427.pdf.

The national PREA standards provide comprehensive guidelines on all aspects of custodial sexual abuse in 11 categories: prevention planning, responsive planning, training and education, screening, reporting, response to report, investigations, discipline, health care, data collection, and audits. Monitoring of specific compliance indicators is available through the national PRC at: http://www.prearesourcecenter.org/library/search?keys&cat=4.

Many noteworthy standards are expected to significantly improve response to prisoner sexual violence. These standards include requirements that correctional agencies must do the following:

◆ Provide a coordinated response upon learning of an incident of sexual abuse (§115.65);

◆ Stipulate specific first-responder duties once an incident has been revealed (§115.64);

◆ Offer survivors forensic exams and emergency and ongoing care (§115.21; §115.82; §115.83);

◆ Attempt to make a victim advocate from a rape crisis center available (§115.21; §115.53);

◆ Improve screening/classification (§115.41; §115.42);

◆ Provide training for custody staff and specialized training for investigative, medical, and mental health staff (§115.31; §115.34; §115.35);

◆ Provide inmate education (§115.33); and

◆ Provide multiple reporting avenues (§115.51).

The national PREA standards help ensure that prisoners and detainees receive evidence-based, trauma-informed, and gender-responsive care and treatment consistent with community standards to ameliorate the devastating impact of sexual assault.

Participation of additional partners in improving the response to prisoner sexual violence

In addition to federal partners, the Moss Group, Inc., and American University–Washington College of Law, there are additional partners in the fight to more effectively manage sexual assault in prisons and jails, including Just Detention International (JDI; formerly Stop Prisoner Rape) and the national PRC.

JDI began its work in the 1970s with former prisoners who had been victims of prisoner sexual abuse. JDI has since become an international nonprofit health and human rights organizations working to end sexual violence against men, women, and youth in all forms of detention. JDI played a key role in the passage of PREA and in the deliberations of the NPREC. It continues to be involved in data collection efforts of BJS and in promulgating national standards to eliminate sexual abuse. JDI continues to advance concerns about safety in correctional settings, including groundbreaking work on violence in US detention facilities (Stop Prisoner Rape, 2006); an innovative guide to help survivors cope (JDI, 2009a); a call to protect the rights of lesbian, gay, bisexual, and transgendered individuals (JDI, 2009b); and timely, well-researched action updates. Their website (http://www.justdetention.org) has useful resources for correctional practitioners and those interested in eliminating sexual violence.

The national PRC (http://www.prearesourcecenter.org/) has become the central repository for research on trends, prevention, response strategies, and best practices in corrections. Funded through a cooperative agreement between the National Council on Crime and Delinquency (NCCD) and the BJA, the PRC provides technical assistance and resources, collaborates with federal partners, and is taking the lead in helping to implement the national PREA standards.

Future challenges and issues of concern

The recent National Inmate Survey, 2011–2012 (Beck et al., 2013) identifies high rates of sexual abuse of inmates with mental illness and inmates with a history of being sexually abused, with lesbian, gay, bisexual, and transgendered inmates being at the highest risk of victimization. US correctional facilities must make substantive changes to abate sexual abuse and improve management of inmates. The following recommendations should be considered:

There must be a sufficient number of properly trained and carefully vetted corrections security staff in all facilities. Increased numbers of staff alone will not end sexual abuse in detention. As recent BJS reports demonstrate, staff are reported as the perpetrators in more than half of alleged instances of sexual abuse. Facilities must educate their staff about the dynamics of sexual abuse and the methods for eliminating it. Struckman-Johnson and Struckman-Johnson (2000), in their study of seven Midwestern prisons, opined that "the presence of a sufficient number of motivated security staff and tight security measures appeared to limit sexual coercion among inmates" (p. 389). Correctional officers are key to intervening and responding appropriately with mentally ill or distressed inmates (Appelbaum, 2010).

All corrections staff must have adequate and appropriate medical and mental health training. Such training will enable staff to recognize prisoners with mental illness (see Chapter 9), adequately manage them, and respond appropriately to threats or incidents of sexual abuse. Ideally, facilities should put in place cross-training (Fagan & Augustin, 2011) with custody staff and mental health professionals.

Corrections mental health treatment and services for female prisoners should be trauma-informed and gender-responsive. Because of the unique pathways to incarceration and the special needs of female inmates, their treatment should be trauma-informed and gender-responsive (see Chapter 51; Bloom, Owen, & Covington, 2005; Elliott, Bjelajac, Fallot, Markoff, & Reed, 2005; Harris & Fallot, 2001). Such approaches recognize and address the ubiquitous nature of previous trauma, high rates of mental illness and addiction, and impact of gender bias within the female inmate population (Dumond & Dumond, 2010).

Corrections agencies must provide suicide training for all staff and develop strong policies and practices for managing suicide. Medical and mental health staff must recognize that the traditional responses of isolation and observation, while effective for ensuring immediate safety, are often experienced as revictimizing by survivors of sexual abuse (see Chapter 43).

Corrections agencies must ensure that inmates have access to adequate community re-entry and reintegration services. As the vast majority of inmates ultimately return to the community, it is especially important that prisoners, especially those with serious, persistent mental illness and those who have experienced sexual abuse, are provided with referrals to community mental health programs (see Chapter 15). Survivors of trauma, in particular, may be more amenable to reaching out for help in the community immediately after being released, reducing the likelihood that they will be arrested again.

Corrections departments should consider developing specialized response teams similar to the crisis intervention teams currently in operation in many jurisdictions. The NIC has developed a noteworthy model for crisis intervention teams (National Institute of Corrections, 2010a, 2010b).

Agencies must create corrections environments that focus on dignity and respect for all prisoners and ensure that those who are incarcerated are afforded legal, safe, and constitutional care and custody. Staff noncompliance with standards of professional behavior can never be tolerated and must be immediately identified and corrected by agency or facility management and supervisory staff. Corrections environments must have zero tolerance for sexual abuse and for language or behavior that demeans inmates or staff because of their race, ethnicity, religion, sexual orientation, gender, gender identity, or disability. Staff members must also be given tools for effective communication with inmates who are culturally different from them through training, mentoring, and supervision.

Continued efforts must be made to help agencies understand how the PREA standards work together. The PREA regulations are a set of groundbreaking standards that, once fully implemented, have the potential to dramatically improve safety in US corrections facilities. However, the standards for adult jails and prisons and juvenile facilities each have more than 50 provisions and run dozens of pages. All agencies must ensure that their staff understand how the standards work together.

Summary

Given the proper tools, training, and resources, corrections can and will eliminate prisoner sexual violence. However, corrections is a subset of the body politic itself and hence is subject to budget shortfalls, political pressure, and the broader attitudes of the public. Adequate financial and programmatic resources must be mobilized to ensure appropriate staff skill levels to keep jails and prisons safe. Safe, well-run jails and prisons can, if properly used, help keep communities safe. The general public will have to be convinced to join this dialogue if we are ever to have safe, constitutionally adequate correctional settings. Corrections can, and must, together with its community partners, respond with vision and leadership to make corrections facilities safe places where human rights and dignity are protected and the most vulnerable among us can emerge stronger and healthier than they went in.

References

Amnesty International (1999). *Not part of my sentence: violations of the human rights of women in custody.* New York: Author.

Appelbaum, K. L. (2010). The mental health professional in a correctional culture. In C. Scott (Ed.), *Handbook of correctional mental health* (2nd ed., pp. 91–117). Washington, DC: American Psychiatric Press.

Austin, J., Fabelo, T., Gunter, A., & McGinnis, K. (2006). Sexual violence in the Texas prison system, final report submitted to the National Institute of Justice, NCJ 215774. Available at www.ncjrs.gov/pdffiles1/nij/grants/215774.pdf

Bartol, C. R., & Bartol, A. M. (2008). *Introduction to forensic psychology: research and application* (2nd ed.). Thousand Oaks, CA: Sage Publications, Inc.

Beck, A. J., Berzofsky, M., & Krebs., C. (2013). *Sexual victimization in prisons and jails reported by inmates.* 2011-13 National Inmate Survey, 2011-12 NCJ241399. Washington, DC: U.S. Department of Justice, Bureau of Justice Statistics.

Beck, A. J., Cantor, D., Hartge, J., & Smith, T. (2013). *Sexual victimization in juvenile facilities reported by youth, 2012.* NCJ 241708. Washington, DC: United States Department of Justice, Office of Justice Programs.

Beck, A. J., & Johnson, C. (2012). *Sexual victimization reported by former state prisoners, 2008.* National Former Prisoner Survey. NCJ237363. Washington, DC: United States Department of Justice, Office of Justice Programs.

Beck, A. J., Rantala, R. R., & Rexroat, J. (2014). *Sexual victimization reported by adult correctional authorities, 2009-11.* NCJ 243904. Washington, DC: United States Department of Justice, Office of Justice Programs.

Bell, C., Cover, M., Cronan, J. P., Garza, C.A., Guggemos, J., & Storto, L. (1999). Rape and sexual misconduct in the prison system: Analyzing America's most "open" secret. *Yale Law & Policy Review, 18*(1), 195–223.

Bloom, B., Owen, B., & Covington, S. (2005). *Gender-responsive strategies for women offenders: A summary of research, practice, and guiding principles for women offenders.* NIC Accession No. 020418. Washington, DC: National Institute of Corrections.

Cason v. Seckinger (2000). 231 F.3d 777 (11th Cir.).

Coomaraswamy, R. (1999). *Report on the mission of the United States of America on the issue of violence against women in state and federal prisons* (E/CN.4/1999/68/Add.2). Geneva, Switzerland: United Nations High Commissioner. Available at http://www.unhchr.ch/Huridocda/Huridoca.nsf/TestFrame/7560a6237c67bb1180256 74c0 04406e9?Opendocument

Cotton, D. J., & Groth, A. N. (1982). Inmate rape: prevention and intervention. *Journal of Prison and Jail Health, 2*(1), 47–57.

Dumond, R. W. (2000). Inmate sexual assault: The plague that persists. *Prison Journal, 80*(4), 407–414. Available at http://www.spr.org/en/Dumond2.pdf.

Dumond, R. W. (2003). Confronting America's most ignored crime problem: The Prison Rape Elimination Act of 2003. *Journal of the American Academy of Psychiatry and the Law, 31*(3), 354–360.

Dumond, R. W., & Dumond, D. A. (2007). Correctional health care since the passage of the Prison Rape Elimination Act of 2003: Where are we now? *Corrections Today, 69*(5), 76–79.

Dumond, R. W., & Dumond, D. A. (2010). Working with female offenders: Gender-specific and trauma-informed programming. In S. Stojkovic (Ed.), *Managing special populations in jails and prisons* (volume II, part IV, chapter 13). Kingston, NJ: Civic Research Institute.

Elliott, D., Bjelajac, P., Fallot, R. D., Markoff, L. S., & Reed, B. G. (2005). Trauma-informed or trauma-denied: Principles and implementation of trauma-informed services for women. *Journal of Community Psychology, 33*(4), 461–477.

English, K., Heil, P., & Dumond, R.W. (2010). *Sexual assault in jail and juvenile facilities: promising practices for prevention and response. Final report submitted to the National Institute of Justice.* Denver, CO: Colorado Department of Public Safety, Division of Criminal Justice, Office of Research & Statistics.

Fagan, T. J., & Augustin, D. (2011). Criminal justice and mental health systems. In T. J. Fagan & R. K. Ax (Eds.), *Correctional mental health: from theory to best practice* (pp. 7–35). Los Angeles: Sage.

Farmer v. Brennan (1994). (92-7247), 511 U.S. 825.

Fishman, J. F. (1934). *Sex in prison: Revealing sex conditions in America's prisons.* New York: National Library Press.

Fleisher, M. S., & Krienert, J. L. (2006). *The culture of prison sexual violence.* Final Report of Grant No. 2003-RP-BX-1001. Washington, DC: National Institute of Justice. Available at http://www.ncjrs.gov/pdffiles1/nij/grants/216515.pdf

Freidman, L. M. (1993). *Crime and punishment in American history.* New York: Basic Books.

Goldberg, A. L., & Wells, D. (2009). NIJ Update: NIJ's response to the Prison Rape Elimination Act. *Corrections Today, 71*(3), 91–92, 94.

Harris, M., & Fallot, R. D. (2001). Designing trauma-informed addictions services. In M. Harris & R. D. Fallot (Eds.), *Using trauma theory to design service systems* (pp. 57–74). San Francisco: Jossey-Bass.

Human Rights Watch (1996). *All too familiar: sexual abuse of women in U.S. state prisons.* New York: Author.

Human Rights Watch (1998). *Nowhere to hide: retaliation against women in Michigan state prisons.* New York: Author. Available at http://www.hrw.org/hrw/reports98/women/Mich.htm

Just Detention International (2009a). *Hope for healing: information for survivors of sexual assault in detention.* Los Angeles, CA: Author.

Just Detention International (2009b). *Call for change: protecting the rights of LGBTQ detainees.* Los Angeles, CA: Author.

Katz, J. (1976). *Gay American history.* New York: Thomas Cromwell.

Kaufman, P. (2008). Prison rape: Research explores prevalence, prevention. *NIJ Journal, 259,* 24–29.

Lehrer, E. (2001). Hell behind bars: The crime that dares not speak its name. *National Review, 53,* 24–26.

National Institute of Corrections (2010a). *Crisis intervention teams: an effective response to mental illness in corrections* [Satellite/Internet Broadcast]. Aurora, CO: Author. Available at http://nicic.gov/Library/024517

National Institute of Corrections (2010b). *Crisis intervention teams: a frontline response to mental illness in corrections* [Lesson Plans and Participant's Manual]. Washington, DC: Author. Available at http://nicic.gov/Library/024797

National Prison Rape Elimination Commission (2009a). *National Prison Rape Elimination Commission Report.* NCJ226680. Washington, DC: National Prison Rape Elimination Commission.

National Prison Rape Elimination Commission (2009b). *Standards for the prevention, detection, response, and monitoring of sexual abuse in adult prisons and jails.* NCJ22682. Washington, DC: National Prison Rape Elimination Commission.

National Prison Rape Elimination Commission (2009c). *Standards for the prevention, detection, response, and monitoring of sexual abuse in community corrections.* NCJ22683. Washington, DC: National Prison Rape Elimination Commission.

National Prison Rape Elimination Commission (2009d). *Standards for the prevention, detection, response, and monitoring of sexual abuse in juvenile facilities.* NCJ22684. Washington, D.C.: National Prison Rape Elimination Commission.

National Prison Rape Elimination Commission (2009e). *Standards for the prevention, detection, response, and monitoring of sexual abuse in lockups.* NCJ22685. Washington, DC: National Prison Rape Elimination Commission.

Owen, B. A., Wells, J., Pollack, J., Muscat, B., & Torres, S. (2008). *Gendered violence and safety: A contextual approach to improving security in women's facilities.* NCJ225368. Fresno: California State University.

Smith, B. (1998). *An end to silence: Women prisoner's handbook on identifying and addressing sexual misconduct.* Washington, DC: National Women's Law Center.

Stop Prisoner Rape (2006). *In the shadows: sexual violence in U.S. detention facilities.* Los Angeles, CA: Author.

Struckman-Johnson, C., & Struckman-Johnson, D. (2000). Sexual coercion rates in seven Midwestern prison facilities for men. *Prison Journal, 80,* 379–390.

Struckman-Johnson, C., & Struckman-Johnson, D. (2013). Stopping prison rape: The evolution of standards recommended by PREA's

National Prison Rape Elimination Commission. *Prison Journal*, 93(3), 335–354.

Struckman-Johnson, C. J., Struckman-Johnson, D. L., Rucker, L., Bumby, K., & Donaldson, S. (1996). Sexual coercion reported by men and women in prison. *Journal of Sex Research*, 33, 67–76.

Women Prisoners vs. District of Columbia Department of Corrections (1994), Women Prisoners I, 877 F.Supp. 634(D.D.C. 1994).

Zweig, J. M., & Blackmore, J. (2008). *NIJ Research for Practice: Strategies to prevent prison rape by changing the correctional culture.* NCJ222843. Washington, DC: U.S. Department of Justice, Office of Justice Programs, National Institute of Justice.

Zweig, J. M., Naser, R. L., Blackmore, J., & Schaffer, M. (2006). *Addressing sexual violence in prisons: A national snapshot of approaches and highlights of innovative strategies.* Final Report. Washington, DC: Urban Institute, Justice Policy Center.

CHAPTER 66

Systems monitoring and quality improvement

Jeffrey L. Metzner

Introduction

Class action litigation that includes a focus on constitutionally inadequate correctional mental health care systems has been a major and effective force in jail and prison reform during the past four decades. Benefits to correctional mental health systems resulting from such litigation have included increased resources needed to implement basic policies and procedures that are necessary for a constitutionally adequate system (Metzner, 2009a, 2009b). Chapter 3 provides a useful summary regarding the legal basis for requiring adequate mental health services in correctional facilities.

Following the passage of the Prison Litigation Reform Act of 1995 (PLRA; 1996), the number of newly initiated consent decrees related to class action litigation involving correctional mental health services significantly decreased. This reduction in litigation followed from limiting the discretion of judges in approving such decrees that were previously allowed. Private settlement agreements and/or memoranda of agreement or their equivalents (the "Agreement") have been substituted for the consent decree process. Although the judicial enforcement specific to implementation of these Agreements is weak, the monitoring process of such Agreements is similar to those previously used with consent decrees (Metzner, 2009b).

This chapter summarizes the monitoring process frequently involved in an Agreement resulting from a class action lawsuit specific to a correctional mental health care system. Emphasis is placed on the importance of developing a quality improvement (QI) process, which should ultimately eliminate the need for an external monitor.

Quality improvement

A QI program is an essential component of an adequate correctional mental health care system (National Commission on Correctional Health Care [NCCHC], 2008b) to ensure adequate self-monitoring by the system and improvement of the care delivered in the facility. Hughes (2008) provides a useful summary of the evolution of the QI process in the health care field, which included use of techniques developed by Deming (1986) in rebuilding the manufacturing industry in post-World War II Japan.

In a correctional health care setting, the mental health care QI process is most efficient and effective when it is part of the facility health care QI committee that oversees the QI processes for medical, dental, nursing, pharmacy, medical records, and mental health care services. Each of these services often has a separate QI subcommittee that reports to the health care QI committee on a regular basis.

The mental health care subcommittee should include both line and administrative mental health care staff, nursing staff, key custody staff (e.g., deputy warden for health care), and other staff directly or indirectly involved with the mental health care delivery system. QI activities should include both process and outcome studies. The effectiveness of a health care delivery process can be assessed by a process QI study. For example, does the sick call process work, as evidenced by timely triage and clinic appointments when indicated? An outcome QI study evaluates whether the goal of a health care intervention was achieved (e.g., decreased symptoms of depression after implementation of treatment).

In correctional mental health care, if a process is not reviewed via a QI mechanism, what is believed to occur is often different from what actually occurs. This is particularly true regarding medication management issues such as timely administration of medications that have been prescribed, especially following housing transfers. Elliott (1997) described using a QI process for an initial assessment of a correctional mental health care system. He found that administrators could not accurately describe certain relevant aspects of their services (e.g., the use of psychotropic medications) related, in part, to lack of an adequate QI process.

Many correctional mental health systems have implemented a quality assurance (QA) program, which is an important component of a QI system but is not a QI system by itself. QA audits are frequently designed to determine the presence or absence of necessary data such as completion of all the elements of an initial mental health evaluation form. This is obviously important, since the form needs to be completed for both assessment and documentation purposes. Such an audit remains effective only when used for a defined period of time and with targeted levels of compliance. A QI process would not only examine the completion rate of these various elements but also would identify barriers to completion of the form and would make recommendations for overcoming these barriers. The QI process would also result in recommendations about improving the form and/or completing it independent of the identified barriers. A designated QA staff person typically performs a QA audit; this is in contrast to QI studies, which typically use line staff directly involved with the area being assessed.

Prior to class action litigation, many correctional mental health care systems had not developed an adequate QI system, and this failure often contributed to the problems in the system that resulted in the litigation. It is frequently a reflection of an inadequate QI system when a psychiatric expert can identify significant mental health care system issues during a site visit that were not known or identified by the system itself. In a correctional mental health care system, a QI process is especially important in the context of implementing an effective medication management system. Problems that may be addressed include the frequent housing transfers of prisoners and the limited windows of opportunity for medication administration due to mandatory counts, lockdowns, and other events. The QI process needs to include nursing, mental health, pharmacy, and correctional personnel, since all these disciplines are involved in medication ordering, distribution, and administration. Other examples of mental health system indicators that are often assessed via a QI process include access to care, quality and implementation of treatment plans, treatment provided in lockdown settings, and discharge planning.

Phases of class action litigation

One conceptualization of class action litigation in correctional facilities described the following three phases: "the liability phase (legally determining whether constitutional deficiencies exist), the remedial phase (developing a remedy to identified constitutional deficiencies), and the implementation phase (implementing the remedial plan)" (Metzner, 2002, p. 22).

Occasionally, the parties will agree upon joint experts for fact-finding purposes during the liability phase, although monitoring a correctional mental health system in its strictest meaning does not occur during this phase. It is more common that the attorneys for plaintiffs and defendants each have their own psychiatric experts during the liability phase. Since passage of the PLRA, such cases are often settled before trial via a negotiated settlement Agreement or similar process. The remedial plan is generally negotiated between the parties, with each side consulting with its own psychiatric experts. Most settlement Agreements include a provision for the appointment of a monitor.

Although the elements of a remedial plan will vary based on factors specific to the litigation, such as the size and type of correctional facility (e.g., jail or prison), the basic structure of the correctional mental health system that needs to be addressed in a remedial plan is well established. *Ruiz v. Estelle* (1980) mandated six minimal essential elements for such services:

- Systematic screening and evaluation;
- Treatment that is more than mere seclusion or close supervision;
- Participation by trained mental health professionals;
- Accurate, complete, and confidential records;
- Safeguards against psychotropic medication prescribed in dangerous amounts, without adequate supervision, or otherwise inappropriately administered; and
- A suicide prevention program.

National guidelines/standards and court decisions (American Psychiatric Association, 2000, 2012; *Coleman v. Wilson*, 1995; NCCHC, 2008a) have provided useful guidelines for addressing these elements in addition to enlarging this framework for a constitutionally adequate correctional mental health system.

The expanded framework includes additional elements such as discharge planning, out-of-cell structured therapeutic time for inmates with serious mental illnesses housed in lockdown units, mental health rounds in lockdown settings, and implementation of a QI process (Metzner, 2009a).

The elements of the remedial plan (i.e., the Agreement) will be operationalized via the facility's mental health care policies and procedures. In addition to the standard topics to be covered by these policies and procedures, such as mission and goal, organizational structure, and training of health care and correctional staffs (Metzner, 1997), they should address the following topics, which are often emphasized and described in detail in the Agreement related to the history of the events leading to the litigation (Metzner, 2009b):

- The screening and evaluation processes for identifying inmates with mental illnesses (see Chapter 11);
- An adequate physical plant for mental health assessment, treatment, and programming purposes (e.g., clean office space that is safe with sound privacy and climate controls);
- Staffing credentials and allocations (e.g., adequacy of staff allocations in terms of full-time equivalents);
- Adequacy of inmate access to the mental health services;
- Treatment programs available, which should include levels of care available (see Chapter 22) and the quality of these services;
- The use of seclusion and restraints, involuntary medications, and involuntary hospitalization;
- Unique correctional mental health care issues such as treatment requirements for inmates with serious mental illness in lockdown housing units, mental health rounds in such units, and mental health care input into the correctional disciplinary process;
- Medication management practices (e.g., administration of medication, documentation of medication administration);
- Suicide prevention program (see Chapter 43);
- The QI process;
- Training of both mental health and custody staffs;
- The working relationships between custody and mental health staffs;
- The working relationships between medical (including nursing) and mental health staffs; and
- Discharge planning services.

Other issues that should be addressed include obtaining informed consent for treatment and the limits of confidentiality during clinical assessments or interventions.

How the Agreement specifically addresses the details of these areas often depends on the factors that led to the litigation. For example, if one of the alleged deficiencies involved inadequate mental health staffing allocations or the use of mental health workers without appropriate credentials (e.g., licensure), the Agreement may be specific regarding caseload ratios and the type of licensure or certification needed for mental health clinicians.

One of the earliest roles of the monitor will be to review and provide consultation to the mental health director in the context of developing these policies and procedures. This tedious task, which will require multiple drafts, is crucial because implementation of these policies and procedures will be the focus of both monitoring and the initial stages of the QI process. The more difficult policies and procedures to develop include those involving involuntary treatment (particularly the use of restraints; see Chapter 26), treatment requirements for inmates with a serious mental illness housed in lockdown units, and the details of the treatment programs available, with particular reference to the residential treatment programs (see Chapter 22). These details should include staffing requirements or periodic staffing needs assessments, minimum required hours per week of structured therapeutic programs offered to inmates requiring a residential (i.e., special needs unit, intermediate care unit) level of mental health care, and the minimum frequency of clinical contacts for inmates with their psychiatrist and/or mental health clinician.

If the correctional mental health system does not have an adequate computerized management information system (MIS), numerous logbooks and spreadsheets will need to be developed for proof-of-practice purposes to facilitate the monitoring of many elements of these policies and procedures. Staff will often initially embrace such paperwork requirements but will soon find it difficult to keep the paperwork current for many reasons; these can be significantly mitigated with a computerized MIS. Without a computerized MIS, successful implementation of an adequate QI system will be extremely difficult.

Roles of a monitor

A monitor (or monitors) is usually appointed prior to the implementation phase. Initially the monitor's role is to operationalize how the remedial plan will be monitored and interpreted when sections of the plan are vague, unclear, and/or repetitive, which invariably occurs despite everyone's best efforts.

The monitor's role in the implementation phase is critical due to the importance of his or her interpretations regarding provisions of the remedial plan and assessments relevant to compliance. The monitor helps formulate the various outcome measures to be monitored via record reviews, inmate and staff interviews, QI studies, and the like. The Agreement generally defines relevant compliance terms such as noncompliance, partial compliance, and compliance. The relationships the monitor establishes with both parties (i.e., the attorneys), in addition to the key mental health and custody administrators, will have a significant impact on the success of the remedial plan's implementation. When the monitoring process is working well, it is common for the monitor to provide helpful consultation to the correctional mental health care system regarding practices that are not required by the remedial plan. However, recommendations resulting from such a consultative process should clearly be labeled as such in contrast to being requirements related to the remedial plan (Metzner, 2009b). Thoughtful selection of a monitor and clear delineation of his or her duties will help avoid dissatisfaction with the monitoring process, which often focuses on unclear or changing outcome measures, costs of the monitoring, and/or perceived monitor bias (i.e., more oriented toward the plaintiff or the defense).

A key function of the monitor is to help the system develop an adequate QI process, with elements of the Agreement being an initial focus. This learning process will be difficult but rewarding for all involved and requires much patience and mentoring. Common pitfalls initially include inadequate samples due to flawed methodology (e.g., using a completely random sample of inmates in contrast to a random sample of targeted inmates, such as inmates on the mental health caseload) and QI reports that are produced in a nonsystematic format. QI reports should be stand-alone documents (i.e., the writer should not need be present in order for a reader to understand the study purpose, results, and analysis). These reports, which do not need to be lengthy, should have subsections that include the rationale for the issue being studied, the methodology used, results, assessment of the results, and planned actions, if any.

The monitoring process

Because many of these policies and procedures will contain general provisions, the monitor will need to decide which outcome measures to use to determine whether the facility is in compliance. For example, the policy and procedure relevant to an inmate's request for mental health services (i.e., sick call) will generally require the request to be triaged by mental health staff to determine the required response time (e.g., emergent, urgent, or routine). The monitor will need to make clear the time frames required for responses to such referrals. Emergent (response as soon as possible; generally within 4 hours) and urgent (response within 24 hours) referral time frames are usually not controversial, in contrast to the time frame for routine referrals (generally 5 to 10 business days). To establish appropriate outcome measures for time frames, the monitor should obtain feedback from both parties; review national standards of correctional mental health care, such as the APA task force guidelines (APA, 2000) and NCCHC standards (2008); and consider other systems' practices as well as the specific system being monitored.

The Agreement invariably addresses the minimum frequency of on-site monitoring, which is usually every four to six months. The duration of a site visit will depend on the size and mission of the prison and the number of mental health caseload inmates. Obtaining presite information relevant to the Agreement in a timely manner (e.g., within one to two weeks) will enable the monitor to significantly reduce the number of on-site days required.

Presite information

Presite information should include data relevant to monitoring compliance with the Agreement that does not require the monitor to be on site to review. This will allow the monitor to use the limited and valuable on-site time to interview inmates and staff, observe processes such as the reception center intake assessments, and attend treatment planning team meetings and similar processes. Presite information includes staffing allocations and vacancies, new or revised policies and procedures, recent inmate population counts, mental health caseload statistics, and pertinent QI studies. Metzner (2009b) has provided a detailed list of recommended presite information to obtain.

Probably the most important presite information to obtain is a status update (i.e., a written summary that describes the steps taken toward compliance since the last site assessment) on all elements of the Agreement that are still being monitored (i.e., have not met the Agreement criteria for no longer being monitored) with proof of practices. Depending on the nature of the proof of practice (e.g., bulky logbooks), it may only be available during the site visit. Reviewing the presite information will raise many questions for the monitor to assess during the site visit and will help provide a focus for the on-site evaluation.

Review of QI reports prior to the site visit should provide information needed in determining compliance with key elements of the Agreement. The timeliness of receiving the presite information and the quality and relevance of the content are frequently predictive of the state of compliance with the Agreement. Problems with either the timeliness or content may reflect management issues. The absence of sound QI reports generally predicts significant compliance issues with the Agreement.

The on-site assessment

Site assessments often cause significant anxiety for the mental health and correctional staffs, in addition to requiring many hours of preparation. Sensitivity to their anxiety and acknowledgment of their presite preparation work will help to establish a collaborative working relationship with the staffs.

A joint opening meeting with correctional and mental health leadership provides an opportunity to receive an overview regarding significant changes in the mental health care system since the initiation of the Agreement or since the last site assessment. It is generally helpful during this meeting to review with key custody and clinical staff the issues that were identified when reviewing the presite information that involve both staffs. This meeting is also useful for scheduling various activities during the site visit, such as interviews with staff and inmates.

Following the opening meeting, it is useful to meet with key mental health staff to review in detail the status updates provided in the presite information packet. This review will often guide the monitor to request additional information or help structure questions to be asked of staff and inmates. Proof of practice is essential in determining the accuracy of the status updates provided by the correctional mental health staff. It is common to learn that the staff's perceptions and descriptions of what is occurring are very different from what is actually happening. Such a discrepancy does not usually reflect dishonesty but is related to not having reviewed the issue via adequate management audits or QI processes.

In addition to the presite data packet and information obtained from key custody and health care staff, other essential sources of information include the following:

- Interviews with line mental health staff, which includes clerical support staff;
- Interviews with mental health caseload inmates;
- Review of health care and custody records of mental health caseload inmates;
- Interviews with other health care workers whose job responsibilities involve the mental health system, such as nurses, pharmacists, and medical records staffs; and
- Interviews with correctional administrators, supervisors, and line correctional officers.

In general, the interviews with inmates and line mental health staff are most efficiently and effectively done in a group setting. It has been this author's experience that it is often challenging to obtain accurate information from both inmates and staff. When many inmates provide similar responses to clear and specific questions, it is more likely that their answers are credible; however, the answers still need to be verified via a variety of different ways, such as health care record review and asking similar questions to staff. Line staff responses may be characterized by significant omissions or inaccuracies due to different staff agendas or lack of knowledge. The monitor is more likely to obtain relevant and accurate information via group interviews if he or she provides a clear explanation regarding the purpose of the interview process and can structure and place limits on the interviewees' responses when necessary.

In general, correctional staff should not be present during group interviews with inmates, and the same usually applies with the mental health staff because the inmates' responses may be limited in the presence of either staff. For somewhat similar reasons, it is often not helpful to have supervisors present during group interviews with either custody or mental health care staffs.

The monitor should directly observe clinical activities relevant to the Agreement. For example, attending mental health treatment team meetings, custody meetings that involve mental health staff (e.g., certain classification review meetings or disciplinary hearings), and group therapy sessions will provide information that often would not otherwise be available to the monitor. It is often helpful to ask the participants questions at the end of the monitor's brief observation to clarify issues that are being monitored.

It is also important for the monitor to visit a representative sample of inmate housing units, any special needs units or other health care settings, the booking/intake area, and segregation units to answer the following questions:

- Are there environmental and physical plant issues that affect mental health care (e.g., is there adequate office/programming space to ensure sound privacy and safety during clinical assessment/treatment contacts)?
- Is there a mental health staff presence in these units?
- Is there a good working relationship between custody and health care staffs and between mental health and medical staffs?

The monitor should also observe the mental health rounding process in segregation units for similar reasons, in addition to performing a brief case-finding assessment (i.e., are there inmates with mental illnesses in segregation who had not previously been identified, or are there clinical contraindications for certain inmates in these housing units due to the nature of their mental illnesses?).

At the beginning of the monitoring process, very few of the Agreement provisions will be in compliance. The monitor can provide useful consultation to the director of mental health regarding prioritizing efforts to comply with the Agreement provisions, which often are closely related to staffing allocation and physical plant issues (both of which are often budget-driven), risk of harm to inmates or staff if lack of compliance persists, organizational structure of the mental health services, and essential infrastructure issues such as presence or absence of a computerized MIS.

Exit interviews

An exit interview is generally appreciated by the facility leadership because it helps clarify needed steps toward compliance and prepares them for the contents of the monitoring report. There should be few surprises in the exit interview because, throughout the site assessment, the monitor should be providing feedback to staff concerning pertinent findings, especially when the findings have significant ramifications for the mental health care of inmates. Even when the findings are negative, it is important to recognize positive aspects of the program to decrease the risk of the staff becoming demoralized and less motivated to improve the system. Disclaimers should be given during the exit interview about the preliminary nature of the findings, which will be more comprehensive and finalized in the report they will receive.

The monitoring report

The monitoring report should be produced on a timely basis and should address each element of the Agreement. The degree of compliance, which is generally defined in the Agreement, should be stated for each provision. For each provision or group of related provisions, it is often helpful to organize the report with the following subsections:

- Sources of information
- Findings
- Assessment of findings
- Recommendations

Production of a timely report will facilitate a more effective response by the facility because the report should serve as a blueprint for achieving compliance.

Summary

Correctional mental health systems have significantly benefited from class action litigation that includes a focus on the mental health care system related to increased resources and external monitoring of the implementation of basic policies and procedures needed for an adequate correctional mental health care system. Such monitoring should include facilitating the system's

development and implementation of a QI system that will ultimately replace the role of an external monitor and, ideally, will maintain and improve the correctional mental health care system.

References

American Psychiatric Association (2000). *Psychiatric services in jails and prisons* (2nd ed.). Washington, DC: Author.

American Psychiatric Association (2012). Position statement on segregation of prisoners with mental illness. Available at http://www.psychiatry.org/advocacy—newsroom/position-statements

Coleman v. Wilson, 912 F.Supp. 1282 (E.D. Cal. 1995).

Deming, W. E. (1986). *Out of crisis.* Cambridge, MA: Massachusetts Institute of Technology Center for Advanced Engineering Study.

Elliott, R. L. (1997), Evaluating the quality of correctional mental health services: An approach to surveying a correctional mental health system. *Behavioral Science Law, 15*, 427–438.

Hughes, R. G. (2008) Tools and strategies for quality improvement and patient safety. In R. G. Hughes (Ed.), *Patient safety and quality: An evidence-based handbook for nurses* (pp. 3:1–3:39). Rockville, MD: Agency for Healthcare Research and Quality. Publication No. 08-0043.

Metzner, J. L. (1997). An introduction to correctional psychiatry: Part I. *Journal of the American Academy of Psychiatry and the Law, 25*, 375–381.

Metzner, J. L. (2002). Class action litigation in correctional psychiatry. *Journal of the American Academy of Psychiatry and the Law, 30*, 19–29.

Metzner, J. L. (2009a). Monitoring a correctional mental health care system: the role of the mental health expert. *Behavioral Science Law, 27*, 727–741.

Metzner, J. L. (2009b). Monitoring a correctional mental health system. In C. L. Scott (Ed.), *Handbook of correctional mental health* (2nd ed., pp. 377–394). Washington, DC: American Psychiatric Publishing, Inc.

National Commission on Correctional Health Care (2008a). *Standards for health services in prisons.* Chicago, IL: Author.

National Commission on Correctional Health Care (2008b). *Standards for mental health services in correctional facilities.* Chicago, IL: Author.

PLRA, H.R. 3019, 104th Congress. (Also referenced as Pub. L. No. 104–134, §§801-810, 110 Stat. 1321–1366 (1996) (codified as amended in scattered sections of 11,18, 28, and 42 U.S.C.)

Ruiz v. Estelle, 503 F. Supp. 1265 (S.D. Texas 1980).

CHAPTER 67

Leadership, training, and educational opportunities

Raymond F. Patterson

Introduction

Services and programs for the screening, assessment, and treatment of mentally ill prisoners in correctional facilities in the United States have changed dramatically since the 1960s. These noteworthy changes can be attributed, in part, to several major legal decisions, including *Estelle v. Gamble* (1976) and *Ruiz v. Estelle* (1980), which addressed issues regarding the constitutional standard for adequate mental health services in correctional facilities (see Chapter 3). Many improvements in the development and administration of mental health services and treatment programs within our jails and prisons have derived from these decisions.

Prior to these changes, the absence or limited presence of mental health care providers was not uncommon in jails and prisons. The limited mental health services that were available were often provided by nonpsychiatric physicians, nurses, and/or "counselors" with minimal education, experience, or training in the assessment, diagnosis, or treatment of mental illness or mental conditions. The development of mental health programs was also hindered by the "prison culture" in which prisoners who did not adhere to the strict rules of behavior and comportment required of them were considered somehow defective or bad, but not ill or sick. This typically included prisoners who exhibited unusual or bizarre behaviors (i.e., disruptive, oppositional, dangerous, or other noncompliant behaviors) that may have been indications of mental illnesses, prisoners with gender identity issues, and prisoners who engaged in self-harming behaviors, including self-mutilation, serious injurious behaviors, and suicide attempts.

In addition, the Community Mental Health Services Act (1963) was passed and the movement to remove patients from state mental hospitals began with expectations that community-based care and treatment would be less expensive to state and municipal governments. Beyond cost savings, it was hoped that this would remedy unwarranted or unnecessary "warehousing" of people with mental illness in state facilities where they had remained for years. The release of thousands of patients from state or other mental hospitals, the increasingly strict and/or restrictive criteria for admission to and maintenance in mental hospitals, and limited access to community-based treatment facilities contributed to significant increases in the number of mentally ill persons in jails and prisons. This chapter focuses on the role of psychiatrists in the development and management of mental health services and programs in jails and prisons and, more specifically, on the leadership roles and related training and education opportunities available to psychiatrists who want to work in these facilities.

Leadership

This author's experience includes providing direct mental health services in jails and prisons and assessing and monitoring mental health programs provided in many correctional systems. From that experience, it is clear that the introduction of mental health professionals into these systems has frequently been met with distrust and cynicism by custody staff. This cynicism appears to come from the combined significant increase in the number of prisoners with diagnosable mental illnesses and conditions along with a history of inadequately trained mental health professionals.

A very informative article by Greifinger (2013), which focuses on the subject of cynicism by prison officials and health care professionals, notes that cynicism creates a needless hurdle to access to care and an increased risk of litigation. This author's experience is consistent with the view that, in some instances, correctional staff and prison health care providers regard inmate complaints about their health care with disbelief or as an attempt to "hustle" the provider for some other desired outcome or secondary gain. This may result in a failure to adequately assess an inmate's health care complaints or concerns and is also an endorsement of the frequently encountered correctional "culture" that presumes inmates are always "gaming" the system. In this case, the presumption is that inmates are attempting to use health care providers to satisfy their nonhealth care needs and wants. These perceptions may cause harm through failure to follow established policies and clinical guidelines, delay of an inmate's access to an appropriate level of care, and lapses in continuity and coordination of care. Such cynicism has resulted in foreseeable and/or preventable deaths from suicide (Patterson & Hughes, 2008). It is not accidental that in the federal prison system sick-call requests are referred to as "cop-outs" by both staff and inmates. Clinical leadership by psychiatrists can facilitate positive changes in this unhelpful and often harmful culture.

Psychiatric consultation to correctional facilities from a systems perspective is often obtained to improve the mental health care delivery system and avoid class-action litigation. Greifinger (2013) notes that correctional facilities that have demonstrated poor performance often have no stated mission or have a mission statement that is not understood by leadership and staff. Many lack enlightened leadership and/or accountability for health care services, among other deficiencies. Greifinger opines that among the first solutions to enact is to develop or recruit leadership. Enlightened and aware correctional administrators at the systems, facility, and even unit/tier levels recognize the need for active participation in inmate management by their mental health counterparts. Such participation is not as "guests in the House of Corrections" but as essential correctional health care staff providing treatment and assisting in the management of prisoners, particularly those with mental illnesses and others who may have behavioral difficulties or maladaptive behaviors. Such a system contributes to institutional stability, safety, and security and minimizes the risks of harm to individual inmates and custody, clinical, and other staff.

Several authors have provided introductions to and descriptions of correctional psychiatry relative to the growing populations and health care needs of persons incarcerated in prisons and jails within the United States (Metzner, 1997a, 1997b, 1998; Metzner, Cohen, Grossman, & Wettstein, 1998; Metzner & Dvoskin, 2006). Metzner (1997a, 1997b, 1998) described the essential components of adequate correctional mental health systems and the administrative structures of correctional mental health services. He emphasized the need for proper balance between security and treatment and the need for the director of mental health services or designee to have direct access to the facility's chief administrator regarding all administrative decisions that affect mental health care. These are particularly important components of mental health services delivery in any correctional setting. The role of psychiatrists as leaders in this process can take a number of avenues.

A primary avenue would be for the psychiatrist to provide direct input to the chief administrator, in addition to providing administrative and direct services. The psychiatrist should also participate in the education, training, and supervision of qualified mental health professionals, as well as collaborative consultations with other service providers, custody staff, other administrators, similar staff, or the department of mental health as needed.

The involvement of psychiatrists in leadership roles at the facility and central administrative levels presents important opportunities to define, develop, and support the treatment team concept. A psychiatrist in a leadership role may facilitate direct care service delivery and adherence to policies and procedures regarding transfers to higher or lower levels of care based on an individual prisoner's level of functioning. The level of mental health functioning and the level of mental health care required are determined by the clinical staff (see Chapter 22). The custody classification is a security determination and may include secure housing units, administrative or punitive segregation, protective custody, and other levels of custody, including maximum, medium, and minimum security levels and "camp" designations. Clinical leadership is needed to educate and work with custody staff in establishing adequate access to all levels of mental health care for prisoners as clinically indicated regardless of their custody classification. Ongoing education and training for both custody and mental health staffs are necessary in the context of these principles.

The correctional psychiatrist functions in leadership positions on multiple levels. The psychiatrist can be the leader for treatment teams that provide direct services to prisoners, from intake screening, assessment, and treatment through release and parole. Second would be leadership at the program level, in which the psychiatrist may hold a position as the chief of mental health services, chief of psychiatry, or other titles reflective of the responsibility for supervision and direction of multiple treatment teams within a facility. The third level of leadership would be at the systems level, in which the psychiatrist may be the director of mental health services for multiple facilities within a system. He or she would therefore have responsibilities not for direct service but for development of policies and procedures, training, implementation of practice guidelines, development of quality management systems including performance indicators, and management information systems for the measurement of data collection regarding morbidity and mortality, suicide prevention and management, medication management, treatment services, and peer review. The highest level of leadership would be the chief administrative officer, warden, administrator, jailer, or departmental secretary, which, in rare instances, may be a mental health professional, including a psychiatrist, and would be responsible for the health care delivered within the system and for the total operations of the system or correctional facility.

Other opportunities for psychiatric leadership include the quality management of correctional mental health care delivery, which identifies opportunities to improve care and methods to sustain practices that support high quality of care. Quality management integrates mental health assessment and treatment and provides performance measures to evaluate the effectiveness of the treatment and overall management of mentally ill offenders.

Leadership issues

The criminal justice system provides a full range of administrative and clinical opportunities for psychiatrists. The "front end" of arrest and pretrial determinations has been a longstanding component of forensic practice. The role of expert or opinion witnesses is to provide assistance to the "finder of fact" (i.e., the judge and/or jury) in pretrial proceedings related to competence, criminal responsibility, and probation. During incarceration, assessment of mental health needs, access to care, provision of treatment, and quality improvement partially constitute the jail and prison components of mental health services. The aftercare aspect of mental health services in correctional psychiatry involves individuals released on parole who need mental health treatment. It further includes individuals who, after serving a sentence in an institutional or community correctional setting, may be civilly committed for treatment as mentally disordered offenders or as sexually violent predators. These aftercare services may be delivered in secure institutional settings. This is particularly the case for inmates committed as sexual psychopaths under sexual psychopathy laws or statutes and for those civilly committed as mentally disordered offenders found to be gravely disabled or a continuing threat of harm to themselves or others. Individuals placed on parole require community-based services. All of these areas provide opportunities for psychiatric leadership, which is often missing. Historically, the lack of psychiatrists working in the criminal justice system on a full-time basis often narrowed their role to medication management, with little opportunity to advance to clinical or administrative leadership positions. Lack of familiarity and discomfort with the correctional environment both have also been barriers for psychiatrists who might otherwise assume leadership roles.

This author's experience in both traditional and correctional mental health systems has been enlightening with regard to both the similarities and the differences of service provision in these two environments. In the traditional community mental health service delivery system, the model might typically be based on treatment or recovery teams comprising practitioners from the disciplines of psychiatry, psychology, social work, and nursing; rehabilitation therapists; counselors; and direct-care services providers. Often, the de facto correctional mental health model consists of "physician and other." The physician may or may not be a psychiatrist and the "other" may be any individual defined by local custom, state regulation, or law as the "qualified mental health professional," which can vary remarkably by jurisdiction. Unfortunately, psychiatrists were often only marginally involved in the design, development, and implementation of mental health care delivery systems during the years that the need for such services increased exponentially. As a result, the organizational structure frequently excluded psychiatrists from both clinical and administrative leadership positions.

The leadership role for psychiatrists working in correctional environments is distinctly different from typical psychiatric venues, where the psychiatrist and other mental health professionals are in control and determine what services and practice models will be used. In a correctional environment, the dynamics are different in that the entity in control is not the psychiatrist or other mental health professionals, but rather the correctional structure/administration. Within correctional systems, the psychiatric and mental health leadership must understand the "correctional culture." With effective psychiatric leadership, mental health care delivery and its coordination with correctional management of prisoners both stand to be improved.

Educational opportunities

Notably, community-based psychiatric practice has evolved over time away from long-term hospitalization and long-term outpatient psychiatric treatment. The provision of long-term treatment for psychiatric conditions is more likely to occur in a correctional environment. Disorders treated in this way include major mental illnesses such as schizophrenia, bipolar disorder, major depressive disorder, and other mental health conditions, including posttraumatic stress disorder and personality disorders. Such exposure and experience can enhance the practitioner's training. The opportunities to assist individuals who may have co-occurring disorders, including substance abuse disorders and medical conditions (including dementias), are extensive. The opportunities for psychiatrists to provide direct service, lead treatment teams, and collaborate with mental health professionals in other disciplines to provide comprehensive assessments and therapeutic interventions are beneficial to the inmate and to the psychiatrist's educational and professional development.

Training for clinical and leadership positions

Traditionally, medical school curricula and psychiatric residency programs did not provide experiences and formal training for students and residents in correctional psychiatry, other than through electives in later years of training. Fortunately, this lack of training has been significantly remedied since the American Board of Medical Specialties, along with the American Psychiatric Association (APA), recognized forensic psychiatry as a subspecialty in 1992, which eventually resulted in a proliferation of forensic fellowship programs. The target population for these programs includes both traditional forensic patients (e.g., "not guilty by reason of insanity" patients) and inmates and detainees in correctional facilities. Many of these programs require clinical rotations in jails or prisons. In 2013, there were approximately 42 forensic psychiatry fellowship programs in the United States approved by the Accreditation Council for Graduate Medical Education (American Academy of Psychiatry and the Law, 2013). The American Board of Psychiatry and Neurology also requires continuing education as part of the maintenance of certification program between examinations for candidates to qualify for recertification. These educational requirements can be met by further training in correctional psychiatry lectures, seminars, and similar offerings.

For the psychiatrist practicing in correctional settings, the majority of training takes place inside correctional facilities. Departments of corrections and jail facilities all offer orientation and training for their custody officers and for employees and contractors such as psychiatrists. Corrections-specific training includes such topics as conditions of confinement, hostage negotiations and requirements, contraband, inmate counts, segregation, sound confidentiality, and special situations such as lockdowns. In most correctional training that is geared toward custody officers, there is limited training regarding mental health issues. Training typically includes screening of inmates entering the facility, mechanisms to access mental health staff, escort duties for inmates to mental health services, suicide watches and observation by custody officers, medication administration and observation by custody officers, contraband, and emergency procedures for first responders, including CPR and first aid. For mental health professionals, including psychiatrists, the "custody" training provided by correctional institutions and systems focuses on correctional and custody practices rather than on mental health issues and management, which are presented in very limited formats. Other mental health professionals who have been working at the particular facility usually conduct the "clinical" on-the-job training provided to psychiatrists and other mental health professionals.

One major resource that describes the role of the psychiatrist in providing services in jails and prisons is *Psychiatric Services in Jails and Prisons, A Task Force Report of the APA* (2000). This work highlights the principles governing the delivery of psychiatric services, offers guidelines for psychiatric services, and discusses special applications for the principles and guidelines. The National Commission on Correctional Health Care (NCCHC) has also published *Standards for Mental Health Services in Correctional Facilities* (2008), and the Joint Commission on Accreditation of Healthcare Organizations' *Standards for Behavioral Health Care* (2014) are relevant to behavioral health care in corrections.

The APA's task force report (2000) addresses key areas that include access to mental health care and treatment, quality of care, cultural awareness, suicide prevention, mental health treatment, ethical issues, services in court and other settings, jail diversion, alternatives to incarceration, and research. In addition, there is significant information on education and training that emphasizes the need for professional development for mental health clinicians working in a jail or prison. It references as appropriate those programs in the facility as well as continuing medical education activities.

Comprehensive education and training within a facility or system requires substantial cross-training of custody staff by clinical staff and clinical staff by custody staff. Cross-training should include orientation by custody staff regarding the jail/prison custody culture. Such training supports effective collaboration and includes requirements such as those for mental health screening and evaluation of inmates segregated from the general population (for protective custody, disciplinary sanctions, or administratively for individual or institutional safety). Psychiatrists need to become knowledgeable regarding lockdown units due to potential mental health concerns related to the prison environment. Considerable work has been done regarding the conditions of confinement, particularly in segregation environments, and its impact on the mental health functioning of inmates in those settings (Metzner et al., 1998; Patterson & Hughes, 2008). For inmates placed in segregation settings, cell-front rounds no less than once per week by a qualified mental health professional and more frequently as necessary should be conducted as an adjunct to determine the need for out-of-cell assessment of the mental health functioning of these inmates, the adequacy of their mental health treatment and management, and their adjustment to segregation status.

In addition to the in-house training, educational and networking opportunities for correctional psychiatrists are available via the NCCHC, which holds several meetings each year. While it is generally accepted that compliance with the published NCCHC accreditation standards does not guarantee adequate mental health services or compliance with APA guidelines, efforts to achieve accreditation indicate attempts to improve quality of care (APA Task Force Report, 2000). Other relevant organizations for similar purposes include the American Academy of Psychiatry and the Law, the American Correctional Association, and the Society of Correctional Physicians.

There have been major efforts in the education and training of mental health professionals to become more aware of and to incorporate consideration of cultural factors in the diagnosis and treatment of mental illness and disorders. Many cultural factors, including but not limited to race, ethnicity, gender, religion, education, socioeconomic status, and life experiences, are all considerations for clinicians to develop comprehensive assessments and treatment. Providing clinical services, training, and leadership in correctional environments should include consideration of these factors and the unique "culture of corrections." The very milieu of individuals involuntarily confined in a controlled setting as "punishment" for suspected or proven crimes includes the relationships between prisoner and custody and between prisoners. Terms such as "prison politics" (interactions between prisoners), lockdowns, "the hole" (isolation/segregation), "shot callers" (gang leaders), and "blood in blood out" (gang membership) are often used. The practices of counts, standing at attention when "rank" or "white shirts" (higher-ranking/administrative custody staff) are present, wall postings of "no warning shots," and agreement by staff that there be "no hostage trades" for inmates are realities in many systems. Special housing for inmates at risk of harm from other inmates because of their "paperwork" (commitment offense—sexual assault of child or high-notoriety crime) or status (gang dropout, shot caller, or mental illness) and outside yard activities requiring separation of inmates exist in many systems.

While one purpose of incarceration may be "as" punishment for crimes committed, in some systems the "culture" supports incarceration "for" punishment while incarcerated.

The psychiatrist must consider that prisoner requests for medical or mental health services may not be for primary gain (i.e., assessment and treatment) but rather for reasons frequently described as secondary gain (i.e., manipulation or malingering). It is extremely important to identify, acknowledge, and incorporate this possibility in assessment and treatment. The "two Ms" of manipulation and malingering in a correctional environment may include attempts to avoid or defer responsibility, obtain monetary rewards, or influence a familial, social, or criminal justice outcome. The secondary gain may also be based on threats to a prisoner's body integrity or social standing (particularly within a gang system), to effect a change in housing, to gain transfer to a mental health treatment environment, and/or to avoid interactions with other inmates or correctional officers. Knowledge of these terms and how to address these issues are usually part of the "on-the-job training" for mental health professionals in correctional environments and need to be appreciated by clinicians so they can become effective leaders.

Summary

The increase in the number of detainees and inmates who require mental health services has created numerous challenges for jail and prison administrators and staff. Another population needing mental health care includes arrestees who may have been diverted to community mental health programs in lieu of incarceration on the front end of the system, as well as prisoners who have been paroled or released with requirements for mental health services after release. The need for dedicated and qualified leadership for mental health services and the importance of providing appropriate education and training in correctional mental health practices offer remarkable opportunities for psychiatrists. Psychiatrists and other health care professionals must be educated and trained to provide the necessary leadership for these extraordinarily complex systems of care and confinement.

References

American Academy of Psychiatry and the Law (2013). Forensic psychiatry fellowships. Available at: http://aapl.org/fellow.php (accessed October 15, 2013).
American Psychiatric Association (2000). *Psychiatric services in jails and prisons, a task force report of the American Psychiatric Association* (2nd ed.). Washington DC: Author.
Community Mental Health Centers Construction Act (1963). Mental Retardation Facilities and Construction Act, Public Law 88-164.
Estelle v. Gamble (1976). 429 U.S. 97.
Greifinger, R. B. (2013). The acid bath of cynicism. *Correctional Law Reporter, 25*, 3.
Joint Commission on the Accreditation of Healthcare Organizations (2014). *Standards for behavioral health care.* Oakbrook Terrance, IL: Author.
Mental Retardation Facilities and Community Health Centers Construction Act of 1963. Public Law 88-164, 77 STAT 282.
Metzner, J. L. (1997a). An introduction to correctional psychiatry: Part I. *Journal of the American Academy of Psychiatry and the Law, 25,* 275–281.
Metzner, J. L. (1997.). An introduction to correctional psychiatry: Part II. *Journal of the American Academy of Psychiatry and the Law, 25*(4), 571–579.

Metzner, J. L. (1998). An introduction to correctional psychiatry: Part III. *Journal of the American Academy of Psychiatry and the Law, 26*(1), 108–115.

Metzner, J. L., & Dvoskin, J. (2006). An overview of correctional psychiatry. *Psychiatric Clinics of North America, 29,* 761–772.

Metzner, J. L., Cohen, F., Grossman, L. S., & Wettstein, R. M. (1998). Treatment in jails and prisons. In R. M. Wettstein (Ed.), *Treatment of offenders with mental disorders* (pp. 217–264). New York: The Guilford Press.

National Commission on Correctional Health Care (2008). *Standards for mental health services in correctional facilities.* Chicago, IL: Author.

Patterson, R. F., & Hughes, K. C. (2008). Review of completed suicides in the California Department of Corrections and Rehabilitation. *Psychiatric Services, 59,* 676–682.

Prison Litigation Reform Act (1996). 18 U.S.C. Section 3626(d)(2).

Ruiz v. Estelle (1980). 503 F. Supp. 1265 (S.D. Tex.)

CHAPTER 68

Role of clinical trainees

Charles L. Scott and Brian J. Holoyda

Introduction

Correctional settings are important and worthy training sites for medical students, general psychiatry residents, child and adolescent psychiatry residents, and forensic psychiatry fellows. Logically, educating future clinicians on how to best treat individuals with mental illness should occur in settings where they are most frequently treated—and in the United States, there are now three times more persons with serious mental illness in jails and prisons than in hospitals, making America's jails and prisons the new and largest mental hospitals (Torrey, Kennard, Eslinger, Lamb, & Pavle, 2010).

Despite a resulting increased need for correctional psychiatrists, most general psychiatry residency programs do not provide training in a correctional site. In an online survey of US general psychiatry residency program training directors, less than one third of responding programs reported that a correctional training site was mandatory for trainees (Fuehrlein, Jha, Brenner, & North, 2013). With the significant shift of individuals with mental illness to correctional settings, psychiatric training programs should consider the benefits that such sites can provide for both residents and staff.

Resident benefits of training in a correctional environment

Training in a correctional setting provides medical students, general psychiatry residents, and forensic psychiatry fellows a range of training experiences. First, patients seen in correctional settings typically demonstrate a broad array of psychopathology, which gives trainees the opportunity to hone their diagnostic acumen. Anxiety disorders are common among those who experience first arrest or incarceration (Gunter, Arndt, Wenman, Allen, Loveless, Sieleni, & Black, 2008). Correctional populations typically have a greater prevalence of personality disorders, including antisocial and borderline personality disorders, than those in the community (Trestman, Ford, Zhang, & Wiesbrock, 2007). Trainees may encounter psychopathic patients who often do not enter psychiatric care in the community. Comorbid substance use disorders are also more prevalent in correctional populations than in the community (Peters, Bartoi, & Sherman, 2008). Posttraumatic stress disorder, particularly among women inmates, is extremely common among incarcerated individuals (Sacks, 2004). Lastly, given the trend toward diversion of persons with mental illness into correctional settings, a disproportionate number of individuals with chronic psychotic disorders are incarcerated throughout the country (Prince, Akincigil, & Bromet, 2007). These disorders can present phenotypically similar with multiple mood, anxiety, and psychotic symptoms, which requires trainees to strengthen their skills in developing and modifying a differential diagnosis.

The constraints of working in a correctional setting can enhance trainees' basic time management and organizational skills. Depending on the specific treatment environment (general population follow-ups, crisis unit care, parole/probation clinics), a trainee may have to balance the parameters of an evaluation with the needs of the correctional setting and staff. Inmates frequently have other obligations, such as meeting with their legal counsel, visiting with family members, and attending court hearings. Similarly, correctional staff's primary obligation is to maintain the safety of the facility. Because of these and other concerns, psychiatric care may not be of primary importance to correctional staff or inmates. Trainees must learn to navigate the environment and use their time wisely in evaluation, treatment, and documentation. Furthermore, the logistical difficulties of traveling through a facility, which can take significant time, demand that the trainee be organized and prepared for the day's workload. A correctional setting, therefore, can bolster trainees' basic skills in time management, documentation, and organization.

Similarly, correctional training sites can teach trainees how to work in a collaborative, team-based model of care. Unique to jails and prisons is the presence of correctional staff who supervise inmates' activities. Psychiatric trainees may gain crucial information that is important to inmate assessment by developing rapport with these staff members who can report their concerns about the inmates they monitor. Because of this close supervision, correctional staff can provide insights into an inmate's hygienic activity, speech, attitude, psychomotor activity, and mood, as well as the presence of odd behaviors that become problematic. These tips, which signal nursing and mental health staff in inpatient psychiatric units in the community, can serve as red flags for trainees to follow up.

Learning the principles of psychopharmacology is an essential component of psychiatric training for medical students and residents (Accreditation Council of Graduate Medical Education [ACGME], 2007a). Correctional settings provide trainees with an opportunity to learn basic psychopharmacology, including the use of antidepressants, mood stabilizers, antipsychotics, anxiolytics, anti-adrenergics, and anticholinergic agents. Correctional settings often have modified drug formularies. Psychiatric trainees may be unaware that compounds commonly prescribed in the community, including bupropion (Burns, 2009), quetiapine (Tamburello, Lieberman, Baum, & Reeves, 2012), and trihexiphenidyl, are common substances of abuse in incarcerated populations. Furthermore, some patients may malinger illness to obtain medications, including sedating or activating medications. Lastly, correctional formularies are less likely to include typical substances of abuse, such as stimulants, benzodiazepines (except in cases of substance withdrawal), or opioids (Burns, 2009), requiring that a trainee learn creativity and flexibility in prescribing practices to an extent unparalleled in community settings.

Correctional settings also provide opportunities to learn other therapeutic modalities that may benefit patients. The potential to learn about substance use disorder treatments abounds, ranging from detoxification of newly incarcerated individuals, to motivational interviewing for drug diversion court participants, to pharmacological and psychotherapeutic interventions for individuals with a history of substance use disorders in parole/probation or general population clinics. There are opportunities to learn and use dialectical behavior therapy and other psychotherapeutic techniques to address borderline personality disorder and self-harm behaviors, which are common in correctional populations (Chaiken, Thompson, & Shoemaker, 2005). Although the typical inpatient or outpatient correctional treatment setting does not provide time or resources for the most dynamic forms of psychotherapy, such as psychoanalysis, the need for supportive psychotherapy is strong. Unfortunately, many systems do not have staffing levels that allow psychiatrists to routinely conduct psychotherapy beyond those psychotherapeutic interventions provided during appointments to evaluate medication need or treatment response.

As one might expect, there are opportunities to learn about forensic psychiatry within correctional settings. For example, malingering is a common problem among incarcerated individuals. Walters (2006) identified seven incentives to malinger in a correctional setting: compensation, avoidance, separation, relocation, entitlement, attention, and amusement. Recent research (McDermott & Sokolov, 2009) on malingering at a county jail, using the Structured Interview of Reported Symptoms, found that 66% of 161 subjects clinically suspected of malingering were confirmed to be malingering, with no psychiatric diagnosis (including antisocial personality disorder) predictive of malingering or nonmalingering. This finding indicates the utility of objective assessments to evaluate and potentially confirm suspected malingering. Training in a correctional setting, therefore, provides the trainee with an important opportunity to learn the use of both clinical interviewing skills and structured assessment tools to assess suspected malingering (see Chapter 23).

Box 68. 1 Potential benefits for trainees assigned to a correctional site

- Improve diagnostic abilities through exposure to a broad array of psychopathology
- Develop efficient time-management and organizational skills
- Learn to work in collaborative team-based model of care
- Appreciate role of custody in evaluating inmates
- Understand potential abuse of prescribed substances
- Enhance ability to use clinical skills and structured assessment tools to evaluate malingering

---

Given the levels of mental health care available in many correctional systems, psychiatric trainees have the opportunity to practice developing appropriate discharge plans and coordinating follow-up care for their patients, whether it be within the correctional facility, in a parole clinic, or in the community. In fact, correctional settings, with their classification levels and unique housing options, may offer more options than are available in community settings. Following acute hospitalization, the treatment team can work with correctional staff to determine whether an individual will be able to function in the general population, with a cellmate, or under other circumstances and to make recommendations based on the patient's mental status. Many correctional settings provide close monitoring and restriction of behaviors for suicidal or self-harming inmates. A correctional setting provides trainees with the opportunity to learn the skill of coordinating care for their patients. Box 68.1 summarizes potential benefits for trainees assigned to a correctional site.

Benefits for correctional staff from academic affiliations

Correctional staff receive many benefits from affiliations with teaching institutions. First, sites that teach medical students and residents create learning environments that help maintain current standards of treatment because supervising staff are expected to impart up-to-date knowledge to trainees. Second, trainees can assist with treatment for inmates, including pharmacotherapy (as appropriate to their training level), individual assessments, and group therapy. The additional personnel help lessen an often heavy workload for the correctional staff, and trainees can help deliver high-quality and timely mental health care. Third, academic affiliations give correctional staff a chance to have university appointments and to participate in research and publications. Fourth, correctional staff can help groom and recruit future colleagues by providing positive learning experiences for trainees.

Matching the requirements of training to correctional rotations

Accreditation organizations set guidelines for required training experiences and competencies that trainees must complete. For graduate medical education, including general adult psychiatry residency and forensic psychiatry fellowship programs, the ACGME (2007a) promulgates these guidelines. There are no specific guidelines for required psychiatric training experiences provided by the ACGME's undergraduate counterpart, the Liaison Committee on Medical Education. The Liaison Committee provides broad medical education accreditation standards and allows individual medical schools to determine their own graduate competencies and clinical rotations. The Association of Directors of Medical Student Education in Psychiatry (2007), however, has developed a list of recommended learning objectives in psychiatry for medical students to meet over the course of their training program.

The Association of Directors of Medical Student Education in Psychiatry (2007) has outlined learning objectives for medical students, broadly categorized into clinical skills; psychopathology and psychiatric disorders; disease prevention; therapeutics and management; and professionalism, ethics, and the law. Correctional settings offer medical students the opportunity to meet most of these objectives. Leamon, Fields, Cox, Scott, and Mirassou (2001) found that medical students who rotated on an inpatient psychiatric unit in a county jail had the same quality of teaching, level of clinical responsibility, patient variety, and level of clinical observation that they and their colleagues had with other psychiatric services. In addition, they performed no differently than their peers at other sites on all components of their clerkship grade, including National Board of Medical Examiners examination score, clinical skills grade, and oral examination grade. These findings suggest that jail psychiatric settings can be suitable training sites for medical students.

For correctional settings to serve as appropriate training sites for psychiatric residents, they should meet the requirements set forth by the ACGME. The ACGME identifies six core clinical competencies that must be integrated into a program's curriculum: patient care, medical knowledge, practice-based learning and improvement, interpersonal and communication skills, professionalism, and systems-based practice. Each clinical competency lists requirements that residents must meet during the course of training. Correctional environments are varied and include inpatient psychiatric units, general population medication clinics, parole or probation clinics, emergency psychiatric evaluations, and consultations with other medical specialties. Many of the ACGME core competency requirements can be met while at a correctional site. In fact, depending on the breadth and depth of services available in a system, a residency program could elect to fulfill most of its educational and didactic requirements in the correctional setting.

The ACGME core requirements for child and adolescent psychiatry training are also easily applied to juvenile correctional facilities, including detention facilities and community treatment programs. In addition, the ACGME core program requirements mandate that child and adolescent psychiatrists have "experience in legal issues relevant to child and adolescent psychiatry, which may include forensic consultation, court testimony, and/or interaction with a juvenile justice system" (ACGME, 2007b).

The ACGME program requirements for graduate medical education in forensic psychiatry, unlike the general psychiatry and child and adolescent psychiatry requirements, explicitly mandate training related to individuals involved with the criminal justice system. For example, the introduction to these program requirements notes that forensic psychiatry focuses on interrelationships between psychiatry and the law, including "the specialized psychiatric treatment required by those who have been incarcerated in jail, prison, or special forensic psychiatric hospitals" (ACGME, 2013, p. 1). Correctional curriculum and training experiences in addition to criminal and civil forensic evaluations are heavily emphasized throughout the forensic core requirements. ACGME forensic program requirements specific to incarcerated individuals include competence in the evaluation and treatment of incarcerated individuals; knowledge of the structure and function of correctional systems; knowledge of the structure and function of juvenile systems; knowledge of the theory and practice of sentencing the convicted offender; evaluating and managing acutely and chronically ill patients in correctional systems; and treating persons involved in the criminal justice system (ACGME, 2013).

In addition to these specific requirements, the forensic program guidelines require that fellows develop skills and habits to

Box 68. 2 Factors to maximize positive experience of trainees at correctional sites

- Assign supervisors trained in forensic psychiatry with correctional experience
- Provide on-site supervision with weekly meetings with assigned supervisor
- Provide basic training on correctional issues *prior* to site placement. Specific training may include:
  - Assessment of suicide risk
  - Potential abuse of prescribed medications
  - Evaluation of malingering
  - Steps to maintain personal safety
  - Guidelines to work with custody staff
  - Limits of confidentiality
  - Importance of maintaining personal boundaries
- Organize on-site didactic lectures
- Assign teaching responsibilities for general residents and/or medical school students
- Include fellow in quality improvement process

systematically analyze practice using quality improvement methods and implement changes with the goal of practice improvement. Jails and prisons provide opportunities for forensic fellows to participate in quality improvement activities. Typical measures of quality improvement include inmates' access to care, appropriateness of suicide risk evaluations, timely delivery of medication, and appropriate medication monitoring. Factors that increase the positive experience of all trainees' experience in a correctional environment are highlighted in Box 68.2.

Addressing trainees' concerns

Despite the apparent benefits that correctional settings afford psychiatric trainees, medical students and residents may have concerns about such a training experience. Fuehrlein, Jha, Brenner, and North (2012) recently examined general psychiatry residents' attitudes about correctional psychiatry in a residency program that used a county jail as one of its mandatory training sites. Attitudes were evaluated on a scale with 0 representing "most negative attitude" and 100 representing "most positive attitude." Overall, residents had a neutral attitude toward correctional psychiatry (mean score 54). The residents recognized the need for more psychiatrists to work in jails (mean score 84), but they expressed little likelihood of doing so after completing residency (mean score 22). The authors found statistically significant differences in residents' attitudes in the following areas: the professional rewards of working at a jail versus an inpatient setting (mean score 32 vs. 60), how often patients exaggerate symptoms in a jail versus an inpatient setting (mean score 65 vs. 45), the likelihood of negative feelings toward a patient in a jail versus an inpatient setting (mean score 42 vs. 28), and worries about assault in a jail versus an inpatient setting (mean score 52 vs. 43). Of note, there were no significant differences between the responses of residents who had completed the jail rotation and residents who had not.

These findings raise serious concerns about psychiatric trainees' perspectives on correctional psychiatry. These issues need to be addressed if there is going to be a psychiatric workforce to face the clinical needs of correctional facilities in the future. First and foremost among these issues is trainees' perception of their safety. Trainees must be safe in their work environment; if they aren't safe, they will not enjoy the experience or wish to work in a correctional setting in the future. Although jails can feel safer than general inpatient facilities, given the presence of correctional officers, panic buttons, and restricted movement of inmates (via handcuffs or ankle cuffs), many trainees are nevertheless anxious about this working environment. Because of potential fear of their patients and for their own personal safety, trainees' concerns should be addressed before they arrive at the training site to lessen fear and to increase comfort in the setting.

Another common concern is trainees' enjoyment of the correctional psychiatry experience. Residents and medical students may find it difficult or emotionally draining to treat individuals who have been charged with crimes (Fuehrlein et al., 2012) or those perceived as having a "secondary gain picture" (Bender, Hays, Klug, Matsuzaka, & Singleton, 1985). These problems are inherent in the correctional milieu, but didactic instruction on the deinstitutionalization movement and the resultant influx of persons with mental illness into correctional settings will help assuage trainees' discomfort and negative attitudes toward the incarcerated population. Similarly, lectures on commonly encountered clinical problems in this population (e.g., malingering, antisocial personality disorder) could increase trainees' comfort and serve as points of clinical growth instead of irritating obstacles to patient care.

Logistics of creating academic affiliations with correctional sites

Although a correctional site may be located near a university, academic affiliations can be challenging to coordinate. The first logical step when pursuing a potential academic affiliation with a correctional site is determining whether the basic components are present or could be developed at the site that meet the necessary criteria by the governing accrediting body. Important factors to consider when determining the appropriateness of the site include distance from the teaching institution, expected duty hours, availability of supervisors, willingness by the site to provide coverage for the trainee when off site, on-call requirements (if any), presence of quality improvement process, current working relationship between custody and mental health, supervisory responsibilities of forensic fellows for nonphysician mental health providers, availability of emergency psychiatric care, accreditation (or lack thereof) by national organizations, suicide trends, locations to interview inmates, office space, administrative support, current formulary, medical record-keeping process, and the laboratory monitoring system. The training director should also review current policies and procedures to determine whether there is a structure in place to appropriately address inmates' mental health needs and should conduct a thorough site visit to evaluate working and safety conditions.

Summary

Increasing numbers of individuals with mental illness receive their treatment in a correctional environment. Correctional settings can provide appropriate and meaningful training opportunities for both medical school students and psychiatry residents. Despite a need for psychiatrists trained in correctional psychiatry, such training is not currently available in the majority of programs. Educators interested in developing academic teaching affiliations should anticipate concerns by trainees and should be prepared to address those concerns. The opportunities for matching current psychiatric training requirements with correctional settings abound. Providing care to individuals with mental illness where they live increasingly means providing care to those persons who are in incarcerated in jails and prisons.

References

Accreditation Council of Graduate Medical Education (2007a). ACGME program requirements for graduate medical education in psychiatry. Available at www.acgme.org

Accreditation Council of Graduate Medical Education (2007b). ACGME program requirements for graduate medical education in child and adolescent psychiatry. Available at www.acgme.org

Accreditation Council of Graduate Medical Education (2013). ACGME program requirements for graduate medical education in forensic psychiatry. Available at www.acgme.org

Association of Directors of Medical Student Education in Psychiatry (2007). *Clinical learning objectives guide for psychiatry education of medical students.* Available at www.admsep.org

Bender, S. L, Hays, D. S., Klug, R., Matsuzaka, H., & Singleton, P. A. (1985). The teaching of psychiatry in the correctional setting: a new dimension in the medical school curriculum. *Psychiatric Journal of the University of Ottawa, 10,* 139–145.

Burns, K. A. (2009). Commentary: Top ten reasons to limit prescription of controlled substances in prisons. *Journal of the American Academy of Psychiatry and Law, 37,* 50–52.

Chaiken, S. B., Thompson, C. R., & Shoemaker, W. (2005). Mental health interventions in correctional settings. In C. Scott & J. Gerbasi (Ed.), *Handbook of correctional mental health* (pp. 122–127). Washington, DC: American Psychiatric Publishing.

Gunter, T., Arndt, S., Wenman, G., Allen, J., Loveless, P., Sieleni, B., & Black, D. W. (2008). Frequency of mental and addictive disorders among 320 men and women entering the Iowa prison system: use of the MINI-Plus. *Journal of the American Academy of Psychiatry and the Law, 36,* 27–34.

Fuehrlein, B. S., Jha, M. K., Brenner, A. M., & North, C. S. (2012). Can we address the shortage of psychiatrists in the correctional setting with exposure during residency training? *Community Mental Health, 48,* 756–760.

Fuehrlein, B. S., Jha, M. K., Brenner, A. M., & North, C. S. (2013). Availability and attitudes toward correctional psychiatry training: results of a national survey of training directors. *Journal of Behavioral Health Services & Research* [Epub before print].

Leamon, M. H, Fields, L., Cox, P. D., Scott, C., & Mirassou, M. (2001). Medical students in jail: the psychiatric clerkship in an outpatient correctional setting. *Academic Psychiatry, 25,* 167–172.

McDermott, B. E., & Sokolov, G. (2009). Malingering in a correctional setting: the use of the Structured Interview of Reported Symptoms in a jail sample. *Behavioral Sciences and the Law, 27,* 753–765.

Peters, R. H., Bartoi, M. G., & Sherman, P. B. (2008). *Screening and assessment of co-occurring disorders in the justice system.* Center for Mental Health Services National GAINS Center.

Prince, J., Akincigil, A., & Bromet, E. (2007). Incarceration rates of persons with first-admission psychosis. *Psychiatric Services, 58,* 1173–1180.

Sacks, J. Y. (2004). Women with co-occurring substance use and mental disorders (COD) in the criminal justice system: a research review. *Behavioral Science and the Law, 22,* 449–466.

Tamburello, A. C., Lieberman, J. A., Baum, R. M., & Reeves, R. (2012). Successful removal of quetiapine from a correctional formulary. *Journal of the American Academy of Psychiatry and Law, 40,* 502–508.

Torrey, E. F., Kennard, A. D., Eslinger, D., Lamb, R., & Pavle, J. (2010). More mentally ill persons are in jails and prisons than in hospitals: A survey of the states. Available at http://www.treatmentadvocacycenter.org/storage/documents/final_jails_v_hospitals_study.pdf

Trestman, R., Ford, J., Zhang, W., & Wiesbrock, V. (2007). Current and lifetime psychiatric illness among inmates not identified as acutely mentally ill at intake in Connecticut's jails. *Journal of the American Academy of Psychiatry and the Law, 35,* 490–500.

Walters, G. D. (2006). Coping with malingering and exaggeration of psychiatric symptomatology in offender populations. *American Journal of Forensic Psychology, 24,* 21–40.

CHAPTER 69

International perspectives and practice differences

Lindsay D. G. Thomson

Introduction

In our practice of correctional psychiatry, what unites us is much greater than what divides us. This chapter examines correctional psychiatry in an international context and explores similarities and differences in our practices and the cultural, political, and economic background to these practices. Whatever our geographical location, we must learn from other jurisdictions and other systems. Rates of imprisonment, the organization of psychiatric services, and the location of the treatment of mentally disordered offenders all vary, and it is easy to fall into the trap of assuming that your system is the "right" one. Even the use of the term "correctional psychiatry," while recognizable, is not routine in many countries, where the term "forensic psychiatry," although wider in meaning, is more commonly used. This type of psychiatry has been defined as

> a specialty of medicine based on detailed knowledge of relevant legal issues, criminal and civil justice systems, mental health systems and the relationship between mental disorder, antisocial behavior and offending. Its purpose is the assessment, care and treatment of mentally disordered offenders and others requiring similar services; risk assessment and management and the prevention of further victimization are core elements of this (Nedopil, Gunn, & Thomson, 2012).

Correctional psychiatry is, to a degree, dependent on the wider health facilities available and the existence of legislation to move individuals from correctional to health care settings and back where appropriate. Even the term "prison" has different meanings in different countries. In most of the United States, it refers specifically to correctional facilities in which the population has been convicted of major crimes and given a sentence of more than one year, whereas jails house people on remand or serving sentences of less than one year. In Europe no such distinction is made. For the purposes of this chapter, the term "prison" is used generically.

International context

Across the world, 14% of the global burden of disease is attributable to mental, neurological, and substance use disorders (World Health Organization [WHO], 2013a). Individuals with major mental disorders suffer stigma and discrimination, and their rates of employment are low. This stigma is compounded for those who have mental disorders and have also been incarcerated.

This chapter deals primarily with wealthier nations with developed systems of correctional psychiatry. In taking an international perspective on our systems of correctional psychiatry, it is important to note the differences in their demographic, political, and economic makeup. Such comparisons, while useful, are complex and limited by many legal, social, and operational differences. Table 69.1 summarizes some of these differences, along with prison population rates of countries drawn from North America, Europe, Australasia, and Asia.

Mental health

To consider the context in which we practice correctional psychiatry, Table 69.2 sets out data on mental health and demonstrates that there are significant variations in spending on mental health. The actual amount spent on forensic mental health is difficult to determine for most jurisdictions. The Schizophrenia Commission (Andrews, Knapp, McCrone, Parsonage, & Trachtenberg, 2012) estimated that schizophrenia costs £11.8 billion ($18.9 billion) per year in England and that secure and high-dependency services accounted for 19%, or £1 billion ($1.6 billion), of the mental health budget in 2010–2011. The commission recommended a realignment of resources away from prisons and institutional care to community options. It argued that community sentences and community mental health treatment are considerably more cost-effective than imprisonment. Further, given the high rates of recidivism in those currently imprisoned on short-term sentences, community-based alternatives to incarceration are potentially more effective in reducing reoffending behaviors. This view is supported by the findings of the Connecticut study (Swanson, Frisman, Robertson, et al., 2013), which reported that costs of care during 2006–2007 approximately doubled for justice-involved individuals with serious mental illness.

The last 30 years has seen a major reduction in psychiatric beds in developed nations and moves toward community care (e.g., Furedi, Mohr, Swingler, et al., 2006). There is some evidence, however, that other forms of institutional care have taken over, such as residential homes, forensic hospitals, and, of particular relevance here, prisons (Priebe, Badesconyi, Fioritti, et al., 2005).

Correctional psychiatry

There are ethical codes that apply to all who work in correctional psychiatry. The United Nations Principles of Medical Ethics states that the medical professional's role in relation to those deprived of their liberty is to assess, protect, and improve their health.

Table 69.1 An international overview of psychiatric care for prison populations

Country	Population	Political System	Health Care System	Wealth: Gross Domestic Product per Capita* Total Health Expenditure per Capita[†] (US$ and GDP%) Life Expectancy at Birth[†] Infant Mortality Rate[§] (deaths/1,000 live births)	Prison Population Rate/100,000 National Population (Walmsley, 2013)
Australia	21,507,717 (2011 census)	Federal parliamentary democracy Constitutional monarchy	Universal publicly funded system (Medicare) with a private health system	10th $41,954 $3,685/9.0% 81.98 years 4.49	130
Canada	35,000,000	Parliamentary democracy Constitutional monarchy Federal structure, 10 provinces	Publicly funded health care organized by provinces	9th $42,317 $4,443/11.4% 81.57 years 4.78	118
China	1,370,536,875 (2010 census)	Communist state President Elections to local People's Congress, with hierarchy of congresses voted by the lower congress up to National People's Congress 22 provinces, 5 autonomous regions, 4 municipalities, 2 special administrative regions	Basic health insurance covers 95% of population	93rd $9,095 $373/5.0% 74.99 years 15.20	121 Sentenced prisoners only
Denmark	5,580,516 (2012)	Parliamentary democracy Constitutional monarchy	Universal health care system	20th $37,324 $4,467/11.1% 78.94 years 4.14	73
Germany	80,600,000	Federal parliamentary democracy with 16 states President Chancellor, head of government	Comprehensive health insurance plan: 77% government funding and 23% private	17th $38,666 $4,342/11.5% 80.32 years 3.48	79
Republic of Ireland	4,600,000	Parliamentary democracy, *Taoiseach* (prime minister) Elected president, ceremonial	Public health care system with subsidized fees depending on income, age, illness, and need for continuous care	13th $40,716 $3,720/9.2% 80.44 years 3.78	88

(continued)

Table 69.1 (Continued)

Country	Population	Political System	Health Care System	Wealth: Gross Domestic Product per Capita* Total Health Expenditure per Capita† (US$ and GDP%) Life Expectancy at Birth‡ Infant Mortality Rate§ (deaths/1,000 live births)	Prison Population Rate/100,000 National Population (Walmsley, 2013)
Japan	127,300,000 (2011)	Parliamentary democracy Constitutional monarchy	Based on European civil law/statutory law Universal health insurance system	22nd $35,855 $3,120/9.2% 84.19 years 2.17	51
Netherlands	16,818,084	Parliamentary democracy Constitutional monarchy Unitary state	Dual system with state-controlled mandatory insurance for long-term treatments (27%) and obligatory private health insurance for short-term treatments (41%)	12th $41,527 $5,112/12.1% 81.01 years 3.69	82
New Zealand	4,500,000	Parliamentary democracy Constitutional monarchy	Mixed public–private system	31st $29,481 $2,992/10.1% 80.82 years 4.65	192
South Africa	52,000,000 (2011)	Parliamentary republic President, head of state, and head of government 9 provinces	Based on English law, civil and statutory Medical schemes cover 16% population, 20% private health care, remainder pay if able	83rd $11,281 $915/8.7% 49.48 years 42.15	294
United Kingdom	63,181,775 (2011 census)	Parliamentary democracy Constitutional monarchy Devolved administrations - Northern Ireland executive and assembly - Scottish government and parliament - Welsh government and assembly	England, Wales, and Northern Ireland - Common law Scotland - Common law and civil law principles National Health Service	21st $36,569 $3,433/9.6% 80.29 years 4.50	England and Wales, 148 Northern Ireland, 101 Scotland, 147
United States	317,660,000 (US POPClock Projection March 9, 2014)	Federal republic - 50 state governments and 1 federal district	Health, public and private Life expectancy 78.4 years	6th $51,704 $8,233/17.6% 78.62 years 5.90	716

(continued)

Table 69.1 (Continued)

Country	Population	Political System	Health Care System	Wealth: Gross Domestic Product per Capita* Total Health Expenditure per Capita[†] (US$ and GDP%) Life Expectancy at Birth[‡] Infant Mortality Rate[§] (deaths/1,000 live births)	Prison Population Rate/100,000 National Population (Walmsley, 2013)
European Union	500,000,000	28 member states and powers agreed by treaties Structures include European Parliament, European Council, European Commission	Court of Justice of European Union All the member states have either publicly sponsored and regulated universal health care or publicly provided universal health care	27th $31,571 –/– 79.86 years 4.43	Western Europe, 98

*Wealth gross domestic product per capita (International Monetary Fund, 2012).

[†]Total health expenditure per capita (World Health Organization, 2010): US dollars and percent gross domestic product.

[‡]Life expectancy at birth (Central Intelligence Agency, 2013).

[§]Infant mortality rate (Central Intelligence Agency, 2013): deaths/1,000 live births.

Table 69.2 International perspective on mental health

Country	Mental Health Expenditure/Total HealthBudget, %	Contribution of Psychiatric Disorder to Global Disease Burden, %	Suicide Rate/100,000 Population, male/female	Psychiatric Beds, per 100,000 Population
Australia	7.64	29.4	16.7/4.4	38.92
Canada	7.2	33.9	16.8/5.5	31.38
China	n/a	17.6	13.8/12.29	14.72
Denmark	n/a	28.8	17.5/6.4	53.91
Germany	11	30.9	17.9/6	88.68
Ireland	n/a	29.6	17.4/3.8	74.09
Japan	4.94	24.6	35.8/13.7	277.56
Netherlands	10.65	30.8	11.6/5	137.81
New Zealand	10	24.8	18.9/6.3	21.35
South Africa	n/a	5.9	n/a	23.2
United Kingdom	10.82	31.4	10.1/2.8	58.62
England	n/a			106.7
Scotland				
United States	6.2	30.9	17.7/4.5	33.8

n/a, not available.

Data from World Health Organization's *Mental Health Atlas* (2011).

The Hawaii and Madrid Declarations set out a code of ethics for psychiatrists (World Psychiatric Association, 1978, 1996). There are two areas relevant to doctors who practice correctional psychiatry. The first is the dual responsibility to the patient and to legal proceedings inherent in assessing detainees, for example, for fitness to stand trial. At the time of assessment, the psychiatrist must disclose and discuss this with the patient. Second, "under no circumstances should psychiatrists participate in legally authorized executions nor participate in assessments of competency to be executed (World Psychiatric Association, 1996)." Not all professional organizations agree, however: The American Psychiatric Association and the American Medical Association do not consider assessments of competency to be executed unethical.

WHO's Health in Prisons program aims to improve public health by improving health care in prisons. A recent report concentrating on Europe sets out standards for the governance of prison mental health. This recommendation follows from concerns that in most countries, the justice ministry, rather than the health ministry, was responsible for health in prisons and that the right to health of prisoners was often disregarded (WHO, 2013b). There has been a move in some countries, such as Italy and the United Kingdom, to separate responsibility for health in prisons from the justice ministries.

The quality of mental health care in European prisons was questioned following the identification of poor health reporting standards, screening, and assessment procedures by inadequately trained staff (Dressing & Salize, 2004). Pathways to care for those acutely psychotic in prison varied significantly according to national law and available services. Of the 24 countries studied, health care was the responsibility of the ministry of justice or prison administration in 15 countries, it was the responsibility of the ministry of health in 5 countries, and it was a joint responsibility in 4 countries. Four organizational models for the delivery of health care were identified: exclusively internal prison health care (N = 2); exclusively external health care provision (N = 4); predominantly internal prison service with some external (N = 8); and predominantly external services of the national health system but some internal prison health care services (N = 10). In this context, the terms "external" and "internal" refer to the provider of the service and not to its location (which is largely in prisons). Treatment of those with psychosis was entirely in a prison hospital in 2 countries, in a prison hospital or a psychiatric hospital in 13 countries, and in a psychiatric hospital in 9 countries.

Most comparisons found in the literature are generally limited to one continent. An exception to this is the SWANZDJSACS (Sweden, Wales, Australia, New Zealand, Denmark, Japan, South Africa, Canada, and Scotland) collaboration across five continents and nine countries (Lindqvist, Taylor, Dunn, et al., 2009). This collaboration has explored common forensic scenarios and described the likelihood in each country that an individual would be placed in prison or hospital.

Problems that arise in correctional psychiatry

Prisons are designed for containment, public safety, and rehabilitation; they are not designed to provide a therapeutic environment. The rules and environment of a prison can present challenges to a therapist, such as access to patients, provision of medication, sudden transfer of prisoners to another establishment, and poor data collection systems. Services tend to reflect historical arrangements rather than the result of careful design following a systematic assessment of need or a mirroring of those developed in the community. In addition, patients may spend many months in prison acutely psychotic while awaiting transfer to a hospital.

Often the mental health services in prisons are not truly multidisciplinary, do not reflect the working methods found in community health settings, and are not set up to meet the level of need found in the custodial population. In European countries, the need to develop such services follows from the principle of equivalence of provision of prison mental health services with those established in the community (Levy, 2011). Some argue that we should go beyond this (Exworthy, Wilson, & Forrester, 2011). In the United States, the aim in terms of quality of care is again to provide the same level that should be available in the community (American Psychiatric Association, 2000). Principle 9 of the United Nations Basic Principles for the Treatment of Prisoners states that "prisoners shall have access to the health services available in the country without discrimination on the grounds of their legal situation" (see Chapter 4).

Suicide is a particular concern in the prison population and was found in a metaanalysis to be 5 times greater in male prisoners and 20 times greater in female prisoners than in equivalent community populations (Fazel, Bains, & Doll, 2006). Completed suicide was associated with a history of past attempts, mental disorder, and alcohol misuse; current suicidal thoughts; being remanded to prison; and being placed in a single cell (see Chapter 43).

The needs of special groups such as women, young offenders, the elderly, and those with intellectual disability or comorbid diagnoses present a myriad of challenges in correctional settings and are discussed in other chapters. Co-occurring mental illness and substance misuse is very common in prisoners and increases the risk of suicide, homelessness, violence, recidivism, victimization, and physical ill health. The problem in many jurisdictions is that in prisons, mental illness and substance misuse are treated by different teams; this can lead to inconsistencies and conflict. There needs to be an integrated care model for those with dual diagnosis (see Chapter 45).

Prevalence of psychiatric morbidity in prisoners

The prevalence of mental disorders in prisoners presents a major problem. There were some 11 million prisoners detained around the world in 2013—half of them were in China, Russia, and the United States. In most of the world, rates of imprisonment have been rising more than the population rate, with a 6% increase over the past 15 years (Walmsley, 2013). The rates of incarceration in the United States have been falling since 2009 (Glaze & Herberman, 2012), but the United States still has the highest rates of incarceration in the world (Walmsley, 2013). Studies of mental disorder in prisoners across many countries show increased rates of mental disorder in comparison to those in the community. These are summarized in Table 69.3. With the exception of depression in the United States, there is no evidence that the prevalence of most disorders among inmates is increasing over time (Fazel & Seewald, 2012).

Table 69.3 Systematic reviews of psychiatric morbidity in prison

Mental Disorder	Results	Authors
Psychosis	3.6% men	Fazel and Seewald (2012)
Major depression	3.9% women	35,588 prisoners, systematic review
	10.2% men	
	14.2% women	24 countries including eight low- to middle-income countries
Alcohol abuse and dependence	18–30% men	Fazel, Bains, and Doll (2006)
	10–24% women	7,600 prisoners, systematic review
Drug abuse and dependence	10–48% men	
	30–60% women	13 studies
Personality disorder	65% men	Fazel and Danesh (2002)
Antisocial personality disorder	42% women	23,000 prisoners, systematic review
	47% men	
	21% women	62 studies in 12 countries

As well as increased morbidity, increased standardized mortality ratios have been found in white, female, and younger prisoners in a metaanalysis of studies reporting 26,163 deaths. Drug misuse was the reported cause of 18% of deaths, 8% of suicides, and 9% of homicides (Zlodre & Fazel, 2012). The immediate post-release period was the time of highest risk.

Models of care in correctional psychiatry

Prison mental health services look after different tiers of need from primary to specialist care (see Chapter 22). The mental health team in many jurisdictions will encompass all roles, from screening to specialist care, and there will seldom be a primary care service involving general practitioners or family doctors that will meet the primary mental health needs of prisoners. Most prison mental health services offer a screening service at intake and an initial assessment by psychiatric nurses or social workers with assessment by psychiatrists if required. Follow-up of prisoners is by outpatient appointment but in the prison setting. There are debates about this model. It provides ease of access to psychiatric services by individuals known to have a high level of need. It also creates considerable routine work and does not allow staff time for detailed psychotherapeutic engagement. Some prisons may operate an "in-reach" model in which local psychiatric services provide care to patients from their catchment area. This approach clearly depends on the geographical location of the prison and the home address of the prisoner.

There are three basic models of care for the acutely unwell in correctional psychiatry: prison as the psychiatric hospital, transfer to a psychiatric hospital, and a mixed model. Most countries send those found not guilty by reason of insanity to a psychiatric hospital. Many, however, have no provision for disposal to the psychiatric system for those found to be guilty but whose mental disorder was a major component of the reason for offending (Daigle, Daniel, Dear, et al., 2007). Some jurisdictions have no legal mechanisms to transfer acutely unwell psychiatric patients out of prison; instead, psychiatric units exist in the prison to care for these individuals.

In other countries (e.g., the United Kingdom), acutely unwell prisoners are transferred to a hospital. Medication for a mental disorder cannot be given in prison against an individual's wishes. Legislation exists to permit such transfers. There is considerable variation in the length of time it takes to transfer an inmate to a hospital. In England and Wales transfer may take many months, whereas in Scotland most transfers take place within one week (Fraser & Thomson, 2007). There are several potential reasons for such a significant difference within one nation: the slightly lower prison population rate in Scotland coupled with greater psychiatric bed availability and the cohesion of the forensic service, with integration of psychiatrists working in local forensic units and local prisons and those working in national prisons with the national high-security hospital.

Other states and countries operate a mixed model, having the ability to transfer patients to a psychiatric hospital and inpatient facilities in the prison setting. For example, the State of Victoria in Australia operates inpatient units in prisons and maintains the ability to transfer an inmate to a secure hospital. In reality, these models are seldom pure and depend on available facilities.

Components of a correctional psychiatry model

Successful prison mental health care requires recognition of the range and complexity of mental disorders in the prison population. Such demands include the need for services for prisoners with mental illness, learning disability, drug and alcohol problems, comorbidity, and personality disorder or problem behaviors. There are many components required for a successful correctional psychiatry model. These include screening on intake, for example using the Correctional Mental Health Screen for Men or Women (Ford, Trestman, Osher, Scott, Steadman, & Clark Robbins, 2007; see Chapter 11), and a referral system and access to hospital beds or prison inpatient facilities. There should be joint coordination with social care services and solid arrangements for through-care. Where geographically possible, there should be in-reach work by community mental health teams for existing patients or those likely to require ongoing care on release (see Chapter 15). The prison mental health team should optimally include nursing staff, psychiatrists, occupational therapists, social workers, and clinical psychologists and should have access to primary care medical and nursing staff. There should be support for self-help approaches through the chaplaincy service, listener programs in which prisoners trained by organizations such as the Samaritans listen to other prisoners who need support (Samaritans, n.d.), or access to tele-mental health programs. A range of tele-mental health services can be used in correctional settings. Videoconferencing can improve access to specialist services, supervision, and training and can be used for clinical assessments and preparation of reports. Secure telephone services, online computer technology, and a digital television platform can provide guided self-help and cognitive-behavioral programs to prisoners. These services do not replace the need for an established mental health team, but they do offer wider access to therapies, a mode of delivery that will be available on return to the community, and potential resource savings. In addition, in a prison setting, input from prison administrators and operational staff is required (see Chapter 9). There should be joint coordination between custody and health staff to consider issues of risk assessment, offending behavior, and mental health interventions.

Finally, the issue of personality disorder is central to many problem behaviors found in prisons, from failure to take part in therapeutic programs to an excessive drain on health service resources in prison by continual demands for assessment and medication. In these contexts, assessment of individuals for the presence of personality disorder would assist in their subsequent management (see Chapter 36). Mental health professionals need to engage more widely with the therapeutic work of the prison service, including offender-based programs.

Summary

Across the developed world, services for those with mental disorders in prison have been established but are seldom equivalent to those found in the community. Prisoners are largely socio-economically deprived and have high rates of mental disorders. They have often been victimized. Prisons are our new asylums: In the United States, three times as many mentally ill people are in prison than in psychiatric hospitals.

There are major differences throughout the world in terms of rates of imprisonment, place of treatment of acutely ill prisoners, and structure of mental health services in prisons. Those requiring hospital care should be transferred out of prison for treatment. Independence of health services from correctional services would promote the development of the former. One challenging issue for correctional psychiatry in some jurisdictions is capital punishment. Ethically, psychiatrists should have no role in executions and should be aware of the ethical stance of the World Psychiatric Association.

References

American Psychiatric Association (2000). *Psychiatric services in jails and prisons* (2nd ed.). Washington, DC: Author.

Andrews, A., Knapp, M., McCrone, P., Parsonage, M., & Trachtenberg, M. (2012). *Effective interventions in schizophrenia the economic case: A report prepared for the Schizophrenia Commission.* London: Rethink Mental Illness (London School of Economics).

Central Intelligence Agency (2013). *The World Factbook.* Accessed October 30, 2014 at: https://www.cia.gov/library/publications/download/download-2013/index.html.

Daigle, M. S., Daniel, A. E., Dear, G. E., Frottier, P., Hayes, L. M., Kerkhof, A., . . . Sarchiapone, M. (2007). Preventing suicide in prison, Part II. International comparisons of suicide prevention services in correctional facilities. *Crisis, 28*(3), 122–130.

Dressing, H., & Salize, H. J. (2004). Compulsory admission of mentally ill patients in European Union member states. *Social Psychiatry and Psychiatric Epidemiology, 39*, 797–803.

Exworthy, T., Wilson, S., & Forrester, A. (2011). Beyond equivalence: Prisoners' right to health. *The Psychiatrist, 35*, 201–202.

Fazel, S., Bains, P., & Doll, H. (2006). Substance abuse and dependence in prisoners: A systematic review. *Addiction, 101*(2), 181–191.

Fazel, S., & Danesh, J. (2002). Serious mental disorder in 23 000 prisoners: a systematic review of 62 surveys. *The Lancet, 359*, 545–550.

Fazel, S., & Seewald, K. (2012). Severe mental illness in 33,588 prisoners worldwide: Systematic review and meta-regression analysis. *British Journal of Psychiatry, 200*, 364–373.

Ford, J., Trestman, R. L., Osher, F., Scott, J. E., Steadman, H. J., & Clark Robbins, P. (2007). *Mental health screens for corrections.* U.S. Department of Justice, Office of Justice Programs, National Institute of Justice. NCJ 216152.

Fraser, A., & Thomson, L. D. G. (2007). Mentally disordered offenders: Experience elsewhere in the UK. *British Medical Journal* [electronic letter].

Furedi, J., Mohr, P., Swingler, D., Bitter, I., Gheorghe, M. D., Hotujac, L., . . . Sartorius, N. (2006). Psychiatry in selected countries of Central and Eastern Europe: an overview of the current situation. *Acta Psychiatrica Scandinavica, 114*(4), 223–231.

Glaze, L. E., & Herberman, E. J. (2012). *Correctional populations in the United States.* Office of Justice Programs, Bureau of Justice Statistics.

International Monetary Fund (2012). *World Economic Outlook Database.* Available at: http://www.imf.org/external/pubs/ft/weo/2012/02/weodata/index.aspx.

Levy, M. (2011). Health services for prisoners. *British Medical Journal, 342*, 351.

Lindqvist, P., Taylor, P. J., Dunn, E., Ogloff, J. R. P., Skipworth, J., Kramp, P., . . . Thomson, L. (2009). Offenders with mental disorder on five continents: A comparison of approaches to treatment and demographic factors relevant to measurement of outcome. *International Journal of Forensic Mental Health, 8*, 81–96.

Nedopil, N., Gunn, J., & Thomson, L. D. G. (2012). Teaching forensic psychiatry in Europe. *Criminal Behaviour and Mental Health, 22*(4), 238–246.

Priebe, S., Badesconyi, A., Fioritti, A., Hansson, L., Kilian, R., Torres-Gonzales, F., . . . Wiersma, D. (2005). Reinstitutionalisation in mental health care: comparison of data on service provision from six European countries. *British Medical Journal, 330*, 123.

Samaritans (n.d.). The development of Samaritans' prison listener scheme. Surrey, England: Samaritans, p. 12. Available at file:///P:/Documents/books/OUP%20Textbook/Section%2013%20Special%20Topics/The%20development%20of%20Samaritans%20listener%20scheme.pdf (accessed April 2, 2014).

Swanson, J. W., Frisman, L. K., Robertson, A. G., Lin, H. J., Trestman, R. L., Shelton, D. A., . . . Swartz, M. S. (2013). Costs of criminal justice involvement among persons with serious mental illness in Connecticut. *Psychiatric Services, 64*(7), 630–637.

Walmsey, R. (2013). *World prison population list* (10th ed.). International Centre for Prison Studies. London: University of Essex. Available http://www.prisonstudies.org/sites/prisonstudies.org/files/resources/downloads/wppl_10.pdf (accessed March 25, 2014).

World Health Organisation (2010). *Per capita total expenditure on health at average exchange rate.* Available at: http://www.who.int/gho/health_financing/per_capita_expenditure/en/.

World Health Organisation (2011). *Mental health atlas.* Geneva: WHO.

World Health Organisation (2013a). The burden of mental disorders. In J. Alonso, S. Chatterji, & Y. He (Eds.), *WHO world mental health surveys.* Cambridge: Cambridge University Press.

World Health Organisation (2013b). *Good governance for prison health in the 21st century. A policy brief on the organization of prison health.* Copenhagen: WHO Regional Office for Europe.

World Psychiatric Association (1978). Declaration of Hawaii. *Journal of Medical Ethics, 4*, 71–73.

World Psychiatric Association (1996). Declaration of Madrid. Approved at the General Assembly on August 25, 1996. Accessed October 30, 2014 at: http://wpanet.org/detail.php?section_id=5&content_id=48

Zlodre, J., & Fazel, S. (2012). All-cause and external mortality in released prisoners: Systematic review and meta-analysis. *American Journal of Public Health, 102*(12), 67–75.

CHAPTER 70

Correctional Mental Health Research and Program Evaluation

Nancy Wolff

Introduction

Mental illness, ranging from acute anxiety to schizophrenia, is endemic in prisons and jails (Gostlin, Vanchieri, & Pope, 2007). Unlike their free-world counterparts, incarcerated people have a constitutional right to mental health treatment (Metzner, 2002). Yet, despite the need for and right to mental health treatment, remarkably little reliable and valid evidence is available on the nature and level of mental illness in incarcerated people; the effects of incarceration on symptomatology; the availability and quality of medication, cognitive, and psychosocial treatment for disorders; and how context alters the effectiveness of the treatment that is available. Evidence is absent because corrections-based research is constrained by regulation, financing, and inexperience.

This chapter reviews the history of prisoner research and the evolution of federal regulations to protect prisoners as human subjects. We discuss how regulation has affected correctional mental health research (CMHR), after first defining what is meant by research and why research is needed to inform policy and practice decisions. This is followed by recommendations for building the CMHR evidence base. The intent is to help researchers, in collaboration with stakeholders, develop, design, and implement research studies and disseminate evidence to advance science and the quality of care available to incarcerated people with mental illnesses in the current regulatory environment.

Value, nature, and requirements of scientific inquiry

Every year billions of dollars are spent on research. The purpose of scientific inquiry is to generate knowledge that will advance our understanding of biological, behavioral, organizational, and social phenomena. Ultimately, the social value of empirical evidence rests on its potential to accurately inform policy and practice. Indeed, valid and reliable evidence is the hallmark of informed decision making. Without such evidence, influential decisions tend to be guided by custom, habit, and idiosyncratic preferences. Such decisions are likely to misallocate resources toward practices and policies that work against collective as well as individual interests.

Empirical evidence is derived from two primary sources: program evaluation and research. By intention but not always in application, both sources use scientific designs and qualitative and quantitative methodologies. These methods are rigorously and systematically applied to collect and analyze data toward the goal of answering questions. Their differences are primarily focus and generalizability. Program evaluation investigates the merit of a particular program from the perspective of key stakeholders with the intent of providing them with information unique to the organization, implementation, or performance of that program as it exists within a dynamic social context. By contrast, research advances scientific inquiry by pursuing theory-driven questions by using controlled designs that produce more generalizable knowledge.

CMHR is a field of scientific inquiry that centers on the etiology, epidemiology, prevention, diagnosis, and treatment of mental disorders in people who reside in a facility under the control of the criminal justice system (e.g., prison, jail, juvenile detention center). Table 70.1 summarizes the types of scientific inquiry that fall under the umbrella of CMHR, using posttraumatic stress disorder (PTSD) as an illustration. Overall, scientific inquiry of this type is person-oriented and seeks to improve the performance of the correctional mental health system in ways that yield better mental health as well as other ancillary outcomes. It also requires human experimentation. Studying people biologically, diagnostically, behaviorally, cognitively, or socially runs the risk of harming them in known and unknown ways. As such, participants in research must understand the risks as well as benefits associated with human experiments and, once fully informed, must choose freely. Informed and volitional choice is paramount in the context of human experimentation. What makes CMHR controversial is its use of incarcerated people in research as human subjects (Gostlin et al., 2007).

Evolution of prisoners as a vulnerable population

Whether incarcerated people can make an informed and voluntary choice is sharply debated (Christopher, Candilis, Rich, & Lidz, 2011; Lazzarini & Attice, 2000). The coercive nature of correctional environments is expected to chill volitional action by incarcerated people. By design, these environments are controlling, manipulative, and disempowering. Cumulatively, they pressure individuals into the mold of "prisoner," making them pliable and acquiescent to those with power. Further, because treatment services and human decency are scarce in correctional settings, prisoners may be overly responsive to research opportunities that offer relief from deprivation. That is, they may disregard

Table 70.1 Types of correctional mental health research: Example of posttraumatic stress disorder

PTSD

This disorder results from direct or indirect exposure to a traumatic event that is life threatening and produces intense and persistent feelings of fear, helplessness, or horror.

Etiology of PTSD

What are the risk factors for PTSD among incarcerated persons? How does the environment of prison (jail, juvenile detention) affect the onset and manifestation of PTSD symptoms among incarcerated men and women?

Epidemiology of Trauma and PTSD

What proportion of incarcerated people have been exposed to trauma? What is the prevalence of sexual and physical trauma? How do these rates vary by age of onset, setting, gender, race, ethnicity, mental disorder? What is the prevalence of PTSD among incarcerated men and women and how do these rates vary by mental disorder?

Prevention of Trauma and PTSD

How can the environment of correctional settings be changed to reduce the exposure to trauma and the conditions likely to trigger PTSD symptoms?

Measurement of Trauma and Diagnosis of PTSD

Are the standard measures of trauma exposure and instruments to measure PTSD symptoms and diagnose PTSD reliable and valid for a correctional population?

Treatment of PTSD

Are PTSD interventions that are effective for a community-based population effective in correctional settings? Are group-based PTSD interventions feasible in a correctional setting? Do medications enhance the effectiveness of therapy-based interventions? Are medication regimens feasible in correctional settings?

Service Delivery and Organization

Is it feasible to provide trauma-informed care to incarcerated persons? Can the culture and climate of correctional settings change to reflect a trauma-informed approach? How can the correctional system efficiently and effectively screen for PTSD?

or discount the long-term medical risks associated with human experimentation and inflate near-term, especially humanitarian, benefits (Chwang, 2010). As such, prisoners are vulnerable to being manipulated into research, becoming a population of unsuspecting "lab rats" (Sherrer, 1999).

Since the early 1940s, research involving prisoners has vacillated between two extremes: fully unrestrained to highly constrained. In recent years, it has become highly constrained, in part because of the extreme abuses of prisoners in research prior to the 1980s, a period of research history freighted with exploitation (Beecher, 1966; Hornblum, 1997). The custom of using prisoners as human subjects has roots in the patriotic fervor of World War II, when there was a growing need to conduct clinical trials dealing with malaria, influenza, dysentery, and gonorrhea and on the potential value of specific vaccines—health concerns affecting the troops (Hornblum, 1997; Lazzarini & Attice, 2000). The medical risks for which prisoners "volunteered" raised their social status among the public while also advertising their apparent willingness to be the subject of human experimentation (Cislo & Trestman, 2013).

The federal government's permissive use of prisoners in clinical studies during World War II, further sanctioned by a report published by the *Journal of the American Medical Association* (Ivy, 1949), signaled a legitimate opportunity for human experimentation to the burgeoning pharmaceutical industry in the postwar era. Prisoners were an ideal population for conducting drug trials because they were captives with few advocates; they were easily and inexpensively recruited into research; they were available in large numbers; and their movements and behavior were limited and highly controlled. Without ethical regulation on research, prisons became the clinical trial center for the pharmaceutical industry (Lazzarini & Attice, 2000; Mitford, 1973). Indeed, by the end of the 1960s, 42 US prisons supplied prisoners for clinical trials testing 85% of new drugs (Kalmbach & Lyons, 2003).

The pharmaceutical industry was not the only one exploiting prisoners. Prison-based medical staff, often in collaboration with academic researchers and with government funding, operated institutes or centers for behavioral change (Mitford, 1973). These residential settings were used to coerce prisoners into participating in "individualized treatment" designed to "rehabilitate" them. Rehabilitation was achieved through a catalogue of "positive and negative reinforcers" intended to "break the person" (Mitford, 1973). The arsenal of punishments included, among others, social isolation, beatings, electronic or insulin shock, hydrotherapy, and other abusive means of inducing privation or severe pain.

These institutes/centers provided behavioral scientists with a venue to "try out new theories" (Mitford, 1973, p. 131). One theory in particular, brainwashing, was advanced by Edward Schein, a psychology professor at the Massachusetts Institute of Technology in the 1960s. Schein, an expert in brainwashing methods, argued that brainwashing, sanitized of its political, ethical, and moral appurtenances, held promise in "the deliberate changing of human behavior and attitudes by a group of men who have relatively complete control over the environment in which the captive population lives" (Schein, Schneier, & Barker, 1961, p. 18). As part of these behavioral experiments, prisoners were used as test subjects for psychosurgery, psychoactive drugs, surgical and chemical castration, brainwashing techniques (e.g., social isolation, sensory deprivation, psychological disorientation), and other putative therapeutic practices incorporating harsh punitive or disciplinary methods. Many of these behavioral experiments were later deemed cruel and unusual punishment by the courts (Mitford, 1973).

The unmitigated and exploitive use of prisoners as "raw material for medical experiments" (Hornblum, 1997, p. 1439) and the characterization of prisons as "supermarket[s] of investigatory opportunity" (Hornblum, 1998, p. 37) were found to be unacceptable by a nation that, unlike in World War II, was now fighting an internal enemy—its own citizens who were committing civil rights violations. During the 1960s, prisoners were recharacterized as a vulnerable population that was susceptible to ethical violations through their involvement in research. Henry Beecher, in an article published in the *New England Journal of Medicine*, highlighted 22 studies that exemplified "unethical or questionably ethical" conduct in research involving prisoners. Beecher noted, quoting Pope Pius XII, that "science is not the highest value of which all other orders of values . . . should be subordinated" (Beecher, 1966, p. 367). With evidence of exploitation mounting, the 1938 Food, Drug, and Cosmetic Act was amended in 1962 to empower the federal government to regulate drug research.

Subsequent amendments of this act established the requirement that clinical investigators obtain informed consent as a condition of participation in research (1963) and articulated the requirements for informed consent (1966).

Not until 1974, with the passage of the National Research Act, were conditions for ethical research given eminent stature by the federal government. This act established the National Commission on the Protection of Human Subjects of Biomedical and Behavioral Research, which was charged with the responsibility of comprehensively investigating the basic ethical principles of biomedical and behavioral research that involved human subjects. Concurrent with the passage of the National Research Act, the US Department of Health, Education, and Welfare published in the *Federal Register* a set of regulations guiding the use of human subjects in research. These regulations, codified as Title 45 of the Code of Federal Regulations (CFR) 46 (Table 70.2), required agencies funded by the Department of Health, Education, and Welfare to establish an institutional review board (IRB) that would independently review studies involving human subjects and set criteria for informed consent. Special regulatory provisions protecting prisoners as human subjects were codified under 45 CFR 46 Subpart C (see Table 70.2). Between 1974 and 1978, the US Department of Health and Human Services (DHHS), the successor to the Department of Health, Education, and Welfare, revised

Table 70.2 Summary of regulations to protect prisoners as human subjects

---

Code of Federal Regulations Title 45, Subpart A (pertains to all adult human subjects)

♦ Establishes the requirement that research involving human subjects shall be reviewed and approved by an IRB

♦ Establishes criteria for IRB approval

♦ Establishes requirements for informed consent

Code of Federal Regulations Title 45, Subpart C (pertains only to prisoners)

♦ Establishes the requirement that the IRB must include a prisoner or a prisoner representative

♦ Limits research to four categories that involve no more than minimal risk

♦ Extends the IRB review to include whether and to what extent:

Benefits of participation are disproportionate to risks

Risks are comparable to those acceptable to nonprisoner volunteers

Subject selection is fair and independent of correctional influence

Information is presented in an accessible manner

Subjects understand that participation will have no impact on parole decisions

Additional Review Requirement for Federally Funded Prisoner Research

♦ Decisions of local IRBs must be approved by the sponsoring agency's office responsible for the protection of prisoners as research subjects

Recommended Additional Protection for Prisoner Research Funded by the National Institutes of Health

♦ Obtain a certificate of confidentiality to protect the privacy of research subjects; these certificates protect investigators and institutions from being compelled to release information that could be used to identify research subjects

---

the 45 CFR 46 regulations in accordance with recommendations advanced by the National Commission in its Belmont Report. The DHHS regulations, which became law in 1981, applied only to research funded by the DHHS. By 1991, the National Institutes of Health (NIH), along with 14 other federal agencies, adopted the Federal Policy for the Protection of Human Subjects (45 CFR 46), referred to as the Common Rule.

According to Subpart C, prisoners, defined as people confined in a penal institution (not those under probation or parole supervision), require additional protections because incarceration "could affect their ability to make a truly voluntary and uncoerced decision whether or not to participate as subjects in research." These protections require that local IRBs include a prisoner or prisoner representative on the board and limit research to four categories, all of which must pose no more than minimal risk: effects of incarceration and criminal behavior; prisons as institutional settings; health-related conditions affecting prisoners as "a class"; or research that is likely to produce positive changes in the health or welfare of the prisoner subject (45 CFR § 46.306). In addition, the approval decisions of local IRBs regarding prisoner research funded by some federal agencies (e.g., DHHS, NIH) must be certified as fully compliant with the Common Rule by the sponsoring agency's office that oversees protections of human subjects. For example, the US Office of Human Research Protections must certify prisoner research funded by the NIH. In addition, investigators conducting prisoner research funded by NIH should obtain a certificate of confidentiality—a tool that allows researchers to protect subject data from forced disclosure.

In 2004, the DHHS commissioned the Institute of Medicine to evaluate the Common Rule on prisoner research. Two years later, in a report titled "Ethical Considerations for Research Involving Prisoners," the Institute of Medicine advanced five recommended changes to Subpart C: expand the definition of "prisoner" to include those on parole or probation, ensure universally and consistently applied standards of protection, shift from a category-based to a risk–benefit approach to research review, update the ethical framework to include collaborative responsibility, and enhance systematic oversight of research involving prisoners (Gostin et al., 2007). To date, none of these recommendations has been adopted by the DHHS, but they have revitalized the debate on the feasibility of prisoner research (Christopher et al., 2011; Chwang, 2010; Cislo & Trestman, 2013; Obasogie, 2010; Thomas, 2010). Views differ on whether, if adopted, these changes would curtail (Cislo & Trestman, 2013) or expand CMHR (Obasogie, 2010).

Consequences of the common rule

The effect of federal regulation on prisoner research was swift and progressive. By 1980, only 15% of all drug testing involved prisoner participants, down from 85% in the 1960s (Kalmbach & Lyons, 2003). Similarly, the number of departments of corrections permitting any medical experiments declined from 46 in 1969 to 12 in 1975 (Hornblum, 1997; Kalmbach & Lyons, 2003). By the late 1990s, a review of institutions in the United States engaged in clinical research found that only 15% involved prisoners in their research studies (Christopher et al., 2011). This decline continued into the twenty-first century. As part of the Institute of Medicine report, a systematic review was conducted on the current prisoner research environment. Several consistent findings were reported.

First, while the majority of states and departments of corrections permitted program evaluations, administrative record reviews, and social or behavioral studies of a nontherapeutic nature (involving minimal risk), far fewer allowed therapeutic biomedical and nontherapeutic social or behavioral studies involving greater than minimal risk. Second, according to a review of the published literature from 1999 to 2005, the vast majority (94%) of published studies involved minimal risk and consisted of administrative record review (21%), program evaluation (26%), and nontherapeutic social and behavioral inquiry (41%). Articles involving biomedical studies or medical clinical trials were even more scarce (6%). This reflects the fact that only a small number of states allow therapeutic biomedical research (15 of 48 states) and even fewer allow nontherapeutic social or behavioral studies involving greater than minimal risk (5 of 48; Gostin et al., 2007).

Over time, the federal policy designed to protect prisoners from exploitation changed focus and reduced the amount of CMHR. No longer are prisoner studies exploring biomedical or medical issues with funding from the federal government. Rather, scientific inquiry focuses on low-risk behavioral and epidemiological issues funded, in large measure, by small grants from academic institutions, prison systems, private foundations, and state funds (Gostin et al., 2007). These studies provide an abundance of descriptive information about the need for services and the distribution of disorders but little evidence that directly benefits the welfare of prisoners.

In an attempt to protect prisoners, federal regulations have compressed and shifted scientific inquiry into a shrinking box of low-impact prisoner research. Prisoners are now protected from exploitation and exploration in ways that sustain the distribution of disease, disorder, and dysfunction in correctional settings. We may know more about the distribution of disease there, but we have no additional ability to change it through more effective and targeted treatment interventions.

Another consequence of doing less CMHR concerns the development and maintenance of the expertise needed to conduct research in correctional settings (Appelbaum, 2008; Cislo & Trestman, 2013; Wolff & Gerardi, 2007). Correctional environments are unique, both individually and collectively. Gaining access to them requires professional connections. Functioning within them requires an understanding of how they are organized; what motivates organizational and staff behavior; how residents are engaged, moved, counted, and routinized; and why security is not convenient. Once inside, researchers need to know how to engage correctional staff in helpful and respectful ways and keep their own staff safe and productive, while minimizing the burden on correctional staff and respecting the culture of the environment. It also requires specialized training (often provided by correctional staff), security clearances, and movement protocols for research materials (e.g., books, computers, tape recorders, interview forms). Most importantly, researchers must build an identity that is separate from but respected by correctional staff and known by potential research subjects. Being an "outsider" inside a correctional setting is met with suspicion by correctional staff and residents alike; this can impede engagement and the implementation of research. The professional capital and the expert knowledge needed to efficiently conduct prisoner research diminish with disuse, misuse, or underuse.

Resetting the balance

What constrains CMHR is concern about the exploitation of prisoners as human subjects. Subpart C attempts to protect prisoners from abuse; however, in so doing, it has also barred them from research that could improve the quality or the length of their life. Prisoner rights groups, as well as prisoners, are advocating for greater inclusion in meaningful research; they are choosing inclusion over protection (Gostin et al., 2007). Further, it is been argued that as an extension of their constitutional right to health and mental health care, prisoners have a right to participate in research testing treatments that are potentially life-saving or -enhancing (Christopher et al., 2011; Thomas, 2010). Those arguing for more influential prison research also draw heavily on extant demographic and epidemiologic evidence. They note the large and growing number of incarcerated people; the nature, breadth, and density of health and mental health problems afflicting this group; and the woeful state of the health and mental health delivery systems in these settings (Christopher et al., 2011). Yet, the concern remains about the ability of incarcerated people to give informed and voluntary consent to participate in research.

The current regulatory environment challenges social and medical scientists to design studies that directly benefit prisoners without imposing greater than minimal risks. In fact, neither the process of IRB review nor the funding constraints at the federal level prevent high-quality, influential CMHR. Researchers can effectively conduct, secure funding for, and efficiently implement research that is meaningful. For example, the National Institute of Mental Health funded a large-scale prison-based study that tested the reliability of computer versus clinician-administered screening for PTSD symptoms and addiction disorders and a randomized, controlled trial of two 12-week manualized, first-stage PTSD–addiction interventions. This study received local IRB approval in seven weeks, approval from the Office for Human Research Protections five months later, and approval for a certificate of confidentiality within one month of the application's submission. This grant was awarded on September 2, 2011, and all IRB requirements were satisfied by October 22, 2011. Subject recruitment began within six months of the award date, and 24 laptop computers, a dozen research staff, and supportive research materials entered the facility two weeks later. Nearly 700 subjects were recruited, 240 were randomly assigned to treatment, and data collection was completed within 28 months of the award date (Wolff, Huening, Shi, & Frueh, 2013).

The success of this project and others like it requires collaboration, determination, and patience (attributes required to conduct international research). The following recommendations provide guidance on how to efficiently and effectively work within Subpart C and the uniqueness of correctional settings to conduct robust, influential, and minimal-risk CMHR:

Research design and orientation: Meet with local departments of corrections and county jails to identify their interest in hosting or collaborating in research, the types of research that are permissible, and the research topics that are most appealing. Discuss issues regarding access to data, facilities, and residents, as well as the process by which publications resulting from research are reviewed.

Funding sources: Review the funding opportunities available for CMHR and acceptable to the correctional partner. For each possible funder, contact the project officer to discuss any limitations (e.g., study design, recruitment strategies) associated with funding CMHR.

Human subject review: The goal here is to minimize the effort required to gain IRB approval for research involving prisoners. This involves educating yourself and, in some cases, the local IRB on Subpart C. The steps to take include carefully reviewing the regulations for prisoners as human subjects; meeting with your IRB administrator to discuss these regulations; requesting samples of approved informed consent forms for prisoners; helping your IRB identify a prisoner representative; networking with local researchers who have conducted IRB-approved prisoner research; requesting that your IRB conduct a workshop on Subpart C; and providing your IRB with citations and web links to resources on Subpart C.

Engagement and collaboration: Establishing a presence in the correctional setting where the research will be situated is paramount. The principal investigator (PI), not the research coordinator, needs to be known by the correctional executive and line staff. The PI is the face of the research study. The more the PI is known and respected, the more the correctional staff and environment will accommodate the research study.

Trust: As outsiders, researchers are reflexively distrusted by correctional staff and residents alike. Trust is earned by showing respect for the environment, the staff, the residents, and the culture. Residents are watchful. They look for signs that the researchers are authentic in their concern, independent of the correctional system, and committed to the conditions set forth in the informed consent form. Learning the names of residents and correctional staff, talking with them in respectful and "normal" ways, and consistently abiding by the rules of the facility and protocols of the research will, over time, foster trust.

Communication: Executive and liaison correctional staff must be kept informed of progress and difficulties. Surprises are unpopular in correctional settings. It is important to update supervisory staff often and succinctly about progress. As a rule, detailed letters should be written periodically to the executive who approved the research. These letters should identify, by name, the people on site who are providing assistance, describe the assistance, and document progress.

Reciprocity: Giving back in meaningful ways to the facility and its residents is central to building productive, enduring collaborations. This might include providing training, workshops, and lectures on topics of interest; facilitating reading clubs; or sponsoring intramural activities. Staying involved with staff and residents establishes a connection that signals an intent to work together, not just acquire data for individual gain.

Summary

Without doubt, the current regulatory environment biases correctional scientific inquiry toward research that carries minimal risk. There are few randomized, controlled trials, particularly medical or biomedical, and fewer yet large-scale or national studies addressing the mental health needs of inmates or the service delivery systems responding to their needs. This is in part because researchers have not maximized the possibilities for intervention and services research under Subpart C and in part because the infrastructure for productive research–corrections collaborations has not been widely or tightly established. The opportunities for CMHR exceed the current grasp of researchers. The challenge for researchers is to see what is possible and to build the collaborations necessary to design and implement rigorous CMHR that will accurately and reliably inform practice and policy in ways that benefit people residing in correctional settings. Under current regulations, high-quality, influential CMHR can be effectively conducted, appropriately financed, and efficiently implemented. With more debate and empirical exploration, the regulatory environment may change to invite more medical or biomedical research. However, until then, the field of CMHR is vast, limited more by imagination and approach than law and funding.

References

Appelbaum, K. L. (2008). Correctional mental health research: Opportunities and barriers. *Journal of Correctional Health Care, 14,* 269–277.

Beecher, H. K. (1966). Ethics and clinical research. *New England Journal of Medicine, 274,* 367–372.

Christopher, P. P., Candilis, P. J., Rich, J. D., & Lidz, C. W. (2011). An empirical ethics agenda for psychiatric research involving prisoners. *AJOB Primary Research, 2,* 18–25.

Chwang, E. (2010). Against risk-benefit review of prisoner research. *Bioethics, 24,* 14–22.

Cislo, A. M., & Trestman, R. (2013). Challenges and solutions for conducting research in correctional settings: The U.S. experience. *International Journal of Law and Psychiatry, 36,* 304–310.

Gostlin, L. O., Vanchieri, C., & Pope, A. (2007). *Ethical considerations for research involving prisoners.* Washington, DC: Institute of Medicine, National Academies Press.

Hornblum, A. M. (1997). They were cheap and available: Prisoners as research subjects in twentieth-century America. *British Medical Journal, 315,* 1437–1440.

Hornblum, A. M. (1998). *Acres of skin: Human experimentation at Holmesburg Prison.* New York: Routledge.

Ivy, A. C. (1949). Nazi war crimes of a medical nature: Some conclusions. *Journal of the American Medical Association, 139,* 131–135.

Kalmbach, K. D., & Lyons, P.M. (2003). Ethical and legal standards for research in prisons. *Behavioral Sciences and the Law, 21,* 671–686.

Lazzarini, A., & Altice, F. L. (2000). A review of the legal and ethical issues for the conduct of HIV-related research in prisons. *AIDS & Public Policy Journal, 15,* 105–135.

Metzner, J. L. (2002). Class action litigation in correctional psychiatry. *Journal of the American Academy of Psychiatry and the Law, 30,* 19–29.

Mitford, J. (1973). *Kind and usual punishment: The prison business.* New York: Vintage.

Obasogie, O. K. (2010). Prisoners as human subjects: A closer look at the Institute of Medicine's recommendations to loosen current restrictions on using prisoners in scientific research. *Stanford Journal of Civil Rights & Civil Liberties, 6,* 41–81.

Schein, E. H., Schneier, I., & Barker, C. H. (1961). *Coercive persuasion.* New York: W. W. Norton.

Sherrer, H. (1999). The mental torture of American prisoners: Cheaper than lab rats, Part II. *Prison Legal News, 10*(4), 1–3.

Thomas, D. L. (2010). Prisoner research—Looking back or looking forward. *Bioethics, 24*(1). 23–26.

Title 45, Part 46 of the Code of Federal Regulations. Available at http://www.hhs.gov/ohrp/humansubjects/guidance/45cfr46.html (accessed October 29, 2013).

Wolff, N., & Gerardi, D. (2007). Building evidence on best practice through corrections-academic partnerships: Getting to successful practice. *Crime and Justice International, 23,* 13–22.

Wolff, N., Huening, J., Shi, J., & Frueh, B. C. (2013). *Screening for and treating PTSD and substance use disorders among incarcerated men.* New Brunswick, NJ: Center for Behavioral Health and Criminal Justice Research. Available at www.cbhs-cjr.rutgers.edu/pdfs/Policy_Brief_Oct_2013.pdf (accessed October 29, 2013).

CHAPTER 71

The Future of Correctional Psychiatry
Evolving and Recommended Standards

Kenneth L. Appelbaum, Robert L. Trestman, and Jeffrey L. Metzner

Introduction

Although recent decades have seen many advances in the knowledge base and practice standards for correctional psychiatry, in many ways the field remains in the early stages of development. As it continues to mature in the coming years, we hope and expect to see further progress. Establishment of evidence-based clinical practices and a firm foundation for ethical standards has begun, and the momentum will continue to build. In this chapter we discuss opportunities to expand the evidence base of correctional psychiatry, the need to refine practice guidelines, and the role that psychiatry might play in influencing the use of incarceration. As part of our review, we describe what we believe the future may hold for our subspecialty.

Where things stand

The broad range of topics covered in this textbook attests to the growing complexity of the field of correctional psychiatry. As reflected in some of the chapters, correctional psychiatry has areas that lack consensus or a well-established evidence base. Existing guidelines and standards do not fully address many significant clinical and ethical dilemmas that face practitioners. Professional psychiatric associations and correctional accreditation agencies have given scant attention to some of these issues or do not adequately monitor and enforce some standards that do exist.

These deficiencies take on greater significance given the prevalence of psychiatric disorders among inmates. Many individuals with the most serious mental illnesses reside in jails and prisons. The psychiatric profession would be remiss if it did not attend to their needs. Our professional organizations must promulgate clear ethical and clinical standards that support correctional practitioners. Anything short of this evades our collective responsibilities.

Relatively little research has been done in correctional psychiatry compared to other areas of psychiatric practice (Cislo & Trestman, 2013). Some of that research has relied on community-based tools and methods that do not necessarily adapt well to jail- and prison-based studies. For example, much of the basic epidemiologic data on the prevalence of mental illnesses among inmates has used screening instruments developed for use with community populations. Symptoms and behaviors (e.g., hypervigilance, anxiety, aggression) suggestive of pathology using these instruments can represent normal and adaptive findings among individuals in jails and prisons. These and other limitations have led many correctional mental health researchers to conclude that we need to greatly expand the empirical foundation of the field (Appelbaum, 2008). Chapter 70 reviews the history, challenges, and potential for correctional research in more depth.

In addition to the need for targeted research, correctional facilities differ from community settings in the opportunities they present for assessment and intervention. Incarceration, for example, enables unusually close monitoring of patients receiving an outpatient level of psychiatric care. This allows psychiatrists to more safely take a bolder approach to therapeutic trials while patients are on or off of medications. Chapters 19 and 20 discuss these opportunities for pragmatic management and diagnostic review.

Untapped prospects for innovation in assessment and intervention abound in correctional psychiatry. We also need to better understand the things we already do. For example, different models of behavioral intervention programs exist, but we lack robust findings that allow us to differentiate which programs work best for specific populations of inmates. A consensus has emerged about specific standards for some interventions (e.g., number of hours per week for out-of-cell structured and unstructured activities for inmates with mental illness in lockdown settings). These standards, however, often lack an empirical foundation. The recommended programming levels for inmates in segregation, for example, have arisen largely from a cascade of imitative court decisions without data to support their specificity. We also need to understand whether the efficacy of standard community clinical practices differs when used with inmates.

The future of correctional psychiatric practice and standards

At the most basic level, correctional psychiatrists must grapple with several questions. First, should clinical and ethical standards differ in correctional settings compared to other practice venues? Any substantial divergence in such standards requires thoughtful and thorough consideration of the implications. Second, if disparate standards are warranted, how will we establish those standards? Our professional organizations will need to devote similar attention to developing and promulgating such standards as they have to dissemination of guidelines for practice in noncorrectional settings. Third, how will our profession support correctional practitioners who find themselves under pressure to act in ways inconsistent with clinical and ethical standards? The following discussion illustrates some of the challenges we face as we try to answer these questions.

Do standards differ?

Before considering whether psychiatric practice in correctional settings should have unique clinical and ethical standards, we should first determine whether differences already exist between community and correctional activities. In what ways, if any, does our work in jails and prisons actually vary from what we do in other settings, or at least come under pressure to diverge from community-based customs? Several examples come to mind.

Confidentiality is an essential condition for psychiatric care. It is akin to creating a sterile field in surgery. It may yield under emergency circumstances but remains a prerequisite at all other times. Frequent exceptions to privacy, however, occur in some correctional settings, especially segregation or lockdown units. Routine cell-front clinical encounters breach confidentiality in a way that would never be tolerated outside of correctional facilities.

Pharmacological practices in correctional settings also tend to stray from community standards. Significant, and understandable, concerns arise about prescription of controlled substances to inmates (Burns, 2009). Many of those concerns, however, have parallels to risks associated with controlled substances for patients in the community. Nevertheless, correctional formularies often include de facto exclusions that rarely have counterparts in community medication access.

Inmates sometimes need clinical restraints, if not seclusion (Metzner, Tardiff, Lion, et al., 2007). Jails and prisons, however, are more like community outpatient settings than inpatient units. Jails, prisons, and community outpatient settings generally lack the staffing and therapeutic environments to provide seclusion or restraint in a way consistent with prevailing standards. Outpatients who need such emergency interventions typically are admitted for hospital care; however, the same does not always occur for inmates who may have clinical restraints applied in minimally therapeutic environments and with reduced procedural protections (Appelbaum, 2007).

Stigma remains an issue for psychiatric conditions in general, but more so for some disorders than others. The nature of gender dysphoria and its treatment, for example, may be difficult for many individuals, including custody officials and some mental health professionals, to grasp and accept. Correctional psychiatrists may come under pressure to endorse denials of services for individual inmates or specific disorders in general. Such pressure can place psychiatrists in conflict with prevailing clinical standards in psychiatry and in medicine in general that explicitly support access to care (American Medical Association, 2008; American Psychiatric Association, 2012).

In relation to ethical standards and practices, correctional psychiatrists are asked to do things that have no parallel in community settings. Along with other mental health staff, they may be asked to evaluate inmates prior to or while being housed in segregation for psychiatric contraindications to such placement. A growing international consensus, however, has called for the abolition of or significant restrictions on the use of solitary confinement, sometimes describing the use of isolation for periods exceeding several weeks as akin to torture (Gibbons & Katzenbach, 2006; *Godínez-Cruz v. Honduras*, 1989; Mendez, 2012; *New York Times*, 2011). In many instances, placement in segregation has an explicitly punitive purpose. Assessing the mental stability of individuals to tolerate punishment under conditions of intentionally unpleasant and stressful deprivations, and subsequently providing clinical clearances to place them under such conditions, let alone participation in torture, has no equivalent in community practice.

Similar concerns arise with inmates on hunger strikes. Some custody-initiated standards equate hunger strikes with other "situations that threaten institutional security . . . [such as] riots . . . disturbances, and taking of hostages" and call for involvement by medical personnel in formulation of the plans to respond to these events (American Correctional Association, 2003). If those plans include forced feedings for inmates who rationally and voluntarily refuse nourishment, the psychiatrist engages in an intervention that would not be sanctioned in the community and violates internationally accepted ethical norms for interactions with inmates (World Medical Association, 1975).

As the previous discussion indicates, some fundamental differences do exist between current correctional and community-based psychiatric practice. Are they warranted?

Should clinical and ethical standards differ in correctional settings?

Jails and prisons are unique environments. For example, inmates have been charged with crimes or adjudicated guilty of those crimes, and the institutional mission includes containment and public safety. Do such differences warrant clinical and ethical standards for psychiatric practice that diverge from community standards? If the correctional mission were exclusive, or even just paramount, that might sway the answer. Medical and psychiatric care for inmates, however, plays as integral a role in correctional policy and procedure as do other considerations. The US Supreme Court has recognized a constitutional mandate for clinical services (*Estelle v. Gamble*, 1976). The right to psychiatric care is fundamental, not ancillary. This suggests that justifications, if any, for divergent standards of care must be compelling.

A need exists for correctional psychiatrists, and the psychiatric profession in general, to closely examine current disparities in practice. Convenience or resource constraints provide a poor basis for disparity. Transferring inmates from segregation cells to private interview rooms, for example, requires available space and takes time and staff. Other needs compete for those resources, but confidentiality is a core component of psychiatric care and failure to provide it falls below acceptable professional, if not constitutional, standards. Comparable considerations have relevance to an analysis of clinical procedures for seclusion, restraint, or other practices.

Public safety and security considerations may also have relevance to clinical services such as treatments for gender dysphoria or availability of medications for psychiatric disorders. Potential compromises to safety and security cannot be ignored. They must be balanced, however, with the clinical consequences of a lowered standard of care. As with the issues discussed above, resource limitations provide poor justification for clinical restrictions that result in substandard care. Reasonable adaptations other than clinical restrictions (e.g., providing settings where transgendered inmates can safely receive treatment, ensuring sufficient numbers of custody staff to transfer inmates to confidential rooms for clinical encounters) require full implementation before considering the balance between clinical and security needs.

Where and how to draw an ethical line poses especially thorny challenges. Correctional systems in the United States do not always follow the most progressive inmate management practices. Individual psychiatrists may balk at working in settings they consider draconian. It would be an extreme and unnecessary reaction, however, for the profession as a whole to withdraw from serving the inmate population. One can do good work even in faulty settings. If psychiatrists, however, are required to play a role in punitive or psychologically harmful correctional practices, a thoughtful review becomes necessary. Whether these practices ultimately advance security or other penological interests is a question for custody officials to grapple with. However, even if punishment serves legitimate correctional purposes, participation by psychiatrists may not be appropriate. Does it make a difference that segregation evaluations screen some fragile inmates out of that placement when the evaluations screen other inmates in? Does it matter that some inmates tolerate prolonged segregation without showing signs of significant distress or lasting psychological harm? If ongoing monitoring of inmates in segregation can identify and remove those who begin to show significant distress, does this lessen ethical concerns about providing mental health clearances for placement in these units?

If disparate standards are warranted, how will we establish them?

An infrastructure already exists for consideration of correctional psychiatry guidelines and practice standards, but extant resources have their limitations. The American Psychiatric Association's Task Force Report on Psychiatric Services in Jails and Prisons (2000) provides mostly general principles, but they do assume compliance with the National Commission on Correctional Health Care (NCCHC)'s Standards for Mental Health Services in Correctional Facilities (2008), which has more targeted and specific standards. Neither, however, tackles in detail the type of challenging questions identified above.

NCCHC Standard MH-A-09 states that "mental health services are conducted in private" but considers this only an "important," not an "essential," standard. Essential standards represent "the critical components of a mental health care system" (Appendix H), taken into account for NCCHC facility accreditation. Thus, the lack of privacy for clinical encounters would not necessarily impede accreditation.

The American Psychiatric Association's report states that "The fundamental policy goal for correctional mental health care is to provide the same level of mental health services to each patient in the criminal justice process that should be available in the community" and that "a full range of psychotropic medications, including involuntary medication, must be available" (Sections

II.B and III.B). The NCCHC has more general essential requirements that "inmates have access to care to meet their serious mental health needs" (MH-A-01) and that *custody* and *administrative staff* support and do not interfere with the implementation of clinical decisions" (MH-A-03). Taken collectively, these standards could be read as providing support for inmate access to controlled substances, treatment for gender dysphoria, and other interventions that correctional psychiatrists deem clinically indicated. This does not always happen in actual practice, however.

The American Psychiatric Association's report gives tacit approval to segregation clearances when it calls for "regular rounds by a qualified mental health clinician in all segregation housing areas . . . in order to identify any inmate who appears to be showing signs of mental deterioration or psychological problems." NCCHC standards do the same by stating "mental health staff reviews . . . to determine whether existing mental health needs contraindicate the placement or require accommodation" (MH-E-07). Although these positions might reflect an underlying consideration of and comfort with the ethics of this role, it may instead reflect only an acceptance of the prevailing use of segregation in prisons and jails. In contrast to these stances, the American Psychological Association adopted a resolution in 2008 setting "an absolute prohibition against the following techniques . . . isolation; sensory deprivation and over-stimulation; . . . or the threatened use of any of the above techniques" and stating that "psychologists are absolutely prohibited from knowingly planning, designing, participating in or assisting in the use of all condemned techniques at any time" (American Psychological Association, 2008).

Organizations such as the American Psychiatric Association and NCCHC that have a vested interest in correctional psychiatric standards need to clarify, refine, and expand their positions in a way that offers explicit guidance and support to practitioners and correctional programs. The development, review, and promulgation of professional guidelines take time and effort to do well. Reaching consensus is not always easy, but further maturation of the field of correctional psychiatry requires this of us.

How will our profession support correctional practitioners who act in ways consistent with clinical and ethical standards?

Many correctional psychiatrists work in settings where they have no on-site peer support. They might find allies among medical colleagues and mental health professionals from other disciplines, but they often provide the sole voice on clinical and ethical standards for their own practice. Pressure from custody staff and other clinicians to bend, if not break, those standards sometimes becomes intense. This underscores the need for explicit professional guidelines that directly address the situations that correctional psychiatrists often face, such as the use of restraint and seclusion (Metzner et al., 2007). Those guidelines provide practitioners with defensible, sound, nonidiosyncratic bases for their positions if challenged.

Professional organizations can also play a more proactive role. Many of our patients who are most in need of treatment have become incarcerated. We need to have a strong voice on their behalf. This might entail outreach and advocacy efforts by professional societies, such as supporting psychiatrists in jails and prisons in their efforts to explain professional standards to correctional administrators. It may also include more formal review and commentary on policies and practices in local and national settings.

Psychiatry's potential role in the future use of incarceration

We have considered the potential evolution of clinical and ethical standards of psychiatric practice with inmates. Might psychiatrists also have something to offer to efforts to reform the nature of incarceration itself? Thoughtful but mostly abortive attempts to do this have been made in the not-so-distant past (Menninger, 1970). More recently, burgeoning rates and costs of incarceration, at least in the United States, have created fertile ground for a new wave of reforms.

Even in the absence of psychiatric input, alternatives-to-incarceration programs will likely expand. Management of many nonviolent criminals or those with only substance abuse–related crimes may shift to community settings. Psychiatrists can play a central role in designing and implementing interventions for these populations.

If diversion to community programs becomes common for less violent criminal offenders, a greater percentage of people who become incarcerated will have aggressive behaviors. As currently occurs, some of these inmates will have underlying mental disorders that contribute to their challenging behaviors. Thus, the proportion of jail and prison inmates who need psychiatric services will increase, enhancing the central role that psychiatrists and other mental health professionals already have in these facilities.

Along with treating high rates of mental illness among incarcerated individuals, psychiatrists may have contributions to make toward mitigating violent tendencies among inmates. This might entail development and expansion of behavioral programs that help people learn skills to manage emotions and avoid violence when discharged back to the community. On a more fundamental level, psychiatric insights could help correctional administrators modify some punitive and security-based policies and practices that do not reduce the risk of future inappropriate behaviors and may even exacerbate that risk (e.g., excessive use of segregation).

Finally, in countries that have or adopt a one-payer system of health care or those that have multiple but well-integrated systems, inclusion of seamless coverage for inmates would allow for greater coordination and continuity of care across community and criminal justice settings. A well-functioning national electronic medical records system would add to efficiency in care. The time might also come when inmates have routine access to electronic intranet systems for health care purposes (e.g., for submission of sick call requests or for psychoeducational materials). Developments such as these would open expanded opportunities for psychiatrists to provide services to criminal justice populations that rival the best available community services and meet the highest standards of care.

Summary

The questions and dilemmas that we have presented do not all lend themselves to easy consensus. They do, however, require attention and resolution. Custodial and clinical practices in correctional settings continue to evolve and change. Some of those changes may occur in a rapid and dramatic way. Psychiatry should stake out a place in the forefront of the ongoing debate. By being proactive instead of reactive, we will have a greater chance of influencing the outcomes and we will fulfill our responsibilities for the inmate patients we serve. No one can predict with certainty what the future holds. We feel safe, however, in predicting that incremental and perhaps revolutionary changes will occur. We hope that this textbook contributes to a picture of where things stand and a vision of where we need to go.

References

American Correctional Association (2003). *Standards for adult correctional institutions*. Lanham, MD: Author.

American Medical Association (2008). Removing financial barriers to care for transgender patients, H-185.950. Available at: http://www.ama-assn.org/ama/pub/about-ama/our-people/member-groups-sections/glbt-advisory-committee/ama-policy-regarding-sexual-orientation.page.

American Psychiatric Association (2000). *Psychiatric services in jails and prisons*. Task Force to Revise the APA Guidelines on Psychiatric Services in Jails and Prisons, Rep. No. 2. Washington, DC: Author.

American Psychiatric Association (2012). Position statement on access to care for transgender and gender variant individuals. Available at: http://www.psychiatry.org/file%20library/advocacy%20and%20newsroom/position%20statements/ps2012_transgendercare.pdf

American Psychological Association (2008). Reaffirmation of the American Psychological Association position against torture and other cruel, inhuman, or degrading treatment or punishment and its application to individuals defined in the United States Code as "enemy combatants." Available at: http://apa.org/about/policy/torture.aspx.

Appelbaum K. L. (2007). Commentary: The use of restraint and seclusion in correctional mental health. *Journal of the American Academy of Psychiatry & the Law, 35*, 431–435.

Appelbaum, K. L. (2008). Correctional mental health research: opportunities and barriers. *Journal of Correctional Health Care, 14*, 269–277.

Burns, K. A. (2009). The top ten reasons to limit prescription of controlled substances in prisons. *Journal of the American Academy of Psychiatry & the Law, 37*, 50–52.

Cislo, A. M., & Trestman, R. (2013). Challenges and solutions for conducting research in correctional settings: the U.S. experience. *International Journal of Law and Psychiatry, 36*, 304–310.

Estelle v. Gamble (1976). 429 U.S. 97.

Gibbons, J. J., Katzenbach, N. D., & Commission on Safety and Abuse in America's Prisons (2006). *Confronting confinement: A report of the Commission on Safety and Abuse in America's Prisons.* New York: Vera Institute of Justice.

Godínez-Cruz v. Honduras (1989). Inter-American Court of Human Rights.

Mendez, J. E. (2012). Report of the Special Rapporteur on Torture and Other Cruel, Inhuman or Degrading Treatment or Punishment. United Nations. Available at: http://www.ohchr.org/Documents/Issues/SRTorture/A-HRC-19-61.pdf.

Menninger, K. (1970). The crime of punishment. *International Journal of Law and Psychiatry, 9*, 541–551.

Metzner, J. L., Tardiff, K., Lion, J., Reid, W. H., Recupero, P. R., Schetky, D. H., Edenfield, B. M., Mattson, M., & Janofsky, J. S. (2007), Resource document on the use of restraint and seclusion in correctional mental health care. *Journal of the American Academy of Psychiatry & the Law, 35*, 417–425.

National Commission on Correctional Health Care (2008). *Standards for mental health services in correctional facilities*. Chicago, IL: Author.

New York Times (2011, Aug. 1). Cruel isolation. Available at: http://www.nytimes.com/2011/08/02/opinion/cruel-isolation-of-prisoners.html?_r=0

World Medical Association (1975). WMA Declaration of Tokyo—Guidelines for physicians concerning torture and other cruel, inhuman or degrading treatment or punishment in relation to detention and imprisonment. Available at: http://www.wma.net/en/30publications/10policies/c18/.

Appendix
Resources

Stacey K. Rich and Robert L. Trestman

This appendix covers a selected range of references and resources available to support correctional healthcare, including such organizations as accrediting bodies and national bodies, professional organizations, and relevant journals.

Accrediting organizations

Organization	Website	Resources
American Correctional Association (ACA)	www.aca.org/ http://www.aca.org/certification/)	Accreditation Educational programs Certification Publications and resources Technical assistance
Joint Commission	http://www.jointcommission.org/	Accreditation Educational programs Certification Publications and resources Technical assistance
National Commission on Correctional Health Care (NCCHC)	http://www.ncchc.org/	Accreditation Educational programs Certification Publications and resources Technical assistance

Selected national and professional bodies

Organization	Website	Resources
American Civil Liberties Union	https://www.aclu.org/	Publications and resources
American Civil Liberties Union National Prison Project	https://www.aclu.org/prisoners-rights/aclu-national-prison-project	Publications and resources
Bureau of Justice Statistics	http://www.bjs.gov/	Educational programs Publications and resources
Centers for Disease Control and Prevention	http://www.cdc.gov/	Educational programs Publications and resources Technical assistance
Correctional Peace Officers Foundation	http://www.cpof.org	Publications and resources
Federal Bureau of Investigation	http://www.csg.org/	Publications and resources
Federal Bureau of Prisons	http://www.bop.gov/	Publications and resources
Justice Center of the Council of State Governments	http://csgjusticecenter.org/corrections	Publications and resources
JustNet	www.nlectc.org	Publications and resources
National Archive of Criminal Justice Data	http://www.icpsr.umich.edu/icpsrweb/NACJD/	Publications and resources
National Center for Missing and Exploited Children	http://www.missingkids.com/home	Publications and resources
National Center for Victims of Crime	http://www.victimsofcrime.org/	Publications and resources
National Correctional Industries Association	http://www.nationalcia.org/	Publications and resources
National Criminal Justice Association	http://ncja.org	Publications and resources
The National Domestic Violence Hotline	http://thehotline.org	Publications and resources
National Institute of Corrections	http://www.nicic.gov/	Educational programs Publications and resources Technical assistance
National Institute of Justice (NIJ)	http://www.nij.gov/	Research and evaluation Publications
Prison Reform Trust	http://www.prisonreformtrust.org.uk/?dm_i=47L,1PZN1,1KH8TB,64FJ6,1	Publications and resources
US Department of Justice, Civil Rights Division, Special Litigation Section	http://www.justice.gov/crt/about/spl/	Publications and resources
Vera Institute for Justice	http://www.vera.org/	Publications

Professional organizations

Organization	Website	Resources
Academic Consortium on Criminal Justice Health	http://www.accjh.org/	Educational programs Publications and resources
Academy of Correctional Health Professionals	http://correctionalhealth.org/	Educational programs Publications and resources
American Academy of Child and Adolescent Psychiatry	http://www.aacap.org/web/aacap/	Educational programs Publications and resources Board certification
American Academy of Psychiatry and the Law	http://www.aapl.org/	Educational programs Publications and resources Board certification
American Bar Association	http://www.americanbar.org/aba.html	Educational programs Publications and resources
American Correctional Health Services Association	http://www.achsa.org/	Educational programs Publications
American Jail Association	http://www.americanjail.org/	Educational programs Publications and resources
American Probation and Parole Association	http://www.appa-net.org/eweb/	Publications and resources
American Psychiatric Association	http://www.psych.org/	Educational programs Publications and resources Position papers Board certification
American Psychology-Law Society	http://www.ap-ls.org/	Educational programs Publications and resources Position papers
Association of State Correctional Administrators	http://www.aca.org	Educational programs Publications and resources
Corrections Connection	http://www.corrections.com/	Publications and resources
Corrections Corporation of America	http://cca.com/	Publications and resources
Corrections Technology Association	http://www.correctionstech.org/	Publications and resources
International Association for Correctional and Forensic Psychology	http://www.aa4cfp.org/	Publications and resources
International Association of Forensic Mental Health Services	http://www.iafmhs.org/	Publications and resources
Office for Victims of Crime	http://www.ojp.usdoj.gov/ovc	Publications and resources
Society of Correctional Physicians	http://societyofcorrectionalphysicians.org/	Publications and resources
Victim Law	https://www.victimlaw.org/	Publications and resources

Selected relevant journals

American Journal of Bioethics http://www.bioethics.net/

American Journal of Public Health http://ajph.aphapublications.org/

Behavior Analysis in Offender Treatment and Prevention http://www.baojournal.com/JOBA-OVTP/index.html

Behavioral Sciences and the Law http://onlinelibrary.wiley.com/journal/10.1002/(ISSN)1099-0798

Corrections Today Magazine http://www.aca.org/publications/ctmagazine.asp

Criminal Justice and Behavior http://cjb.sagepub.com/

European Journal of Psychotherapy & Counseling http://www.tandfonline.com/toc/rejp20/current

International Journal of Law and Psychiatry http://www.ialmh.org/template.cgi?content=General/journal.htm

International Journal of Offender Therapy and Comparative Criminology http://ijo.sagepub.com/

Journal of Clinical Psychiatry http://www.psychiatrist.com/default2.asp

Journal of Correctional Health Care http://jcx.sagepub.com/

Journal of Medical Systems http://www.springer.com/statistics/life+sciences,+medicine+%26+health/journal/10916

Journal of Offender Rehabilitation http://www.psypress.com/journals/details/1050-9674/

Journal of Psychiatric Research http://www.journalofpsychiatricresearch.com/

Journal of the American Academy of Psychiatry and the Law http://www.jaapl.org/

Law and Human Behavior http://www.apadivisions.org/division-41/publications/journals/index.aspx

Mental Health Services Research http://www.springer.com/public+health/journal/11020

Prison Journal http://tpj.sagepub.com/

Psychiatric Services http://ps.psychiatryonline.org/journal.aspx?journalid=18

Violence and Gender http://www.liebertpub.com/vio#utm_source%3DTR_3rdP&utm_medium%3Demail&utm_campaign%3Dvio

Index

Note: Figures, tables, and boxes are indicated by f, t, and B.